Radiology of Infectious Diseases: Volume 2

Hongjun Li
Editor

Radiology of Infectious Diseases: Volume 2

PEOPLE'S MEDICAL PUBLISHING HOUSE

Springer

Editor
Hongjun Li
Beijing You An Hospital
Capital Medical University
Diagnostic Radiology Department
Beijing
China

ISBN 978-94-017-9875-4 ISBN 978-94-017-9876-1 (eBook)
DOI 10.1007/978-94-017-9876-1

Library of Congress Control Number: 2015943785

Springer Dordrecht Heidelberg New York London

Printed on acid-free paper

Springer Science+Business Media B.V. Dordrecht is part of Springer Science+Business Media (www.springer.com)

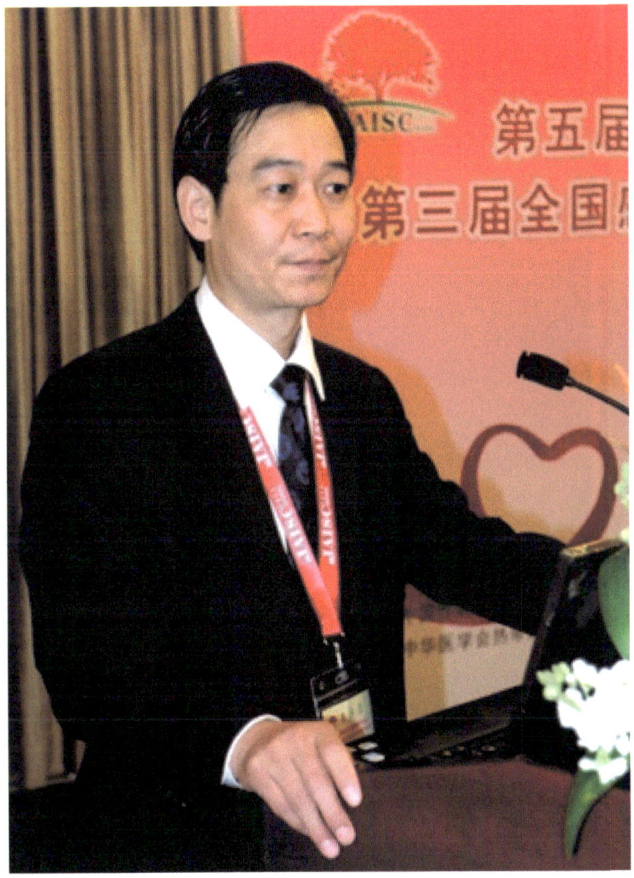

I am unwilling to alienate my wife, daughter, seniors, friends, and students. However, in order to publish this book, I had to give up my chances of enjoying family gatherings, and I had to give up chances of having good times with the seniors and my friends to write.

To my wife, Dongying Bao, I dedicate this treatise, for her support, encouragements, and trust to my persistence in academic career development.

To my daughter, Zhen Li, I dedicate this treatise, for giving me strength.

To my leaders and my team, I dedicate this treatise, to appreciate their powerful support to my work.

Hongjun Li

Foreword I

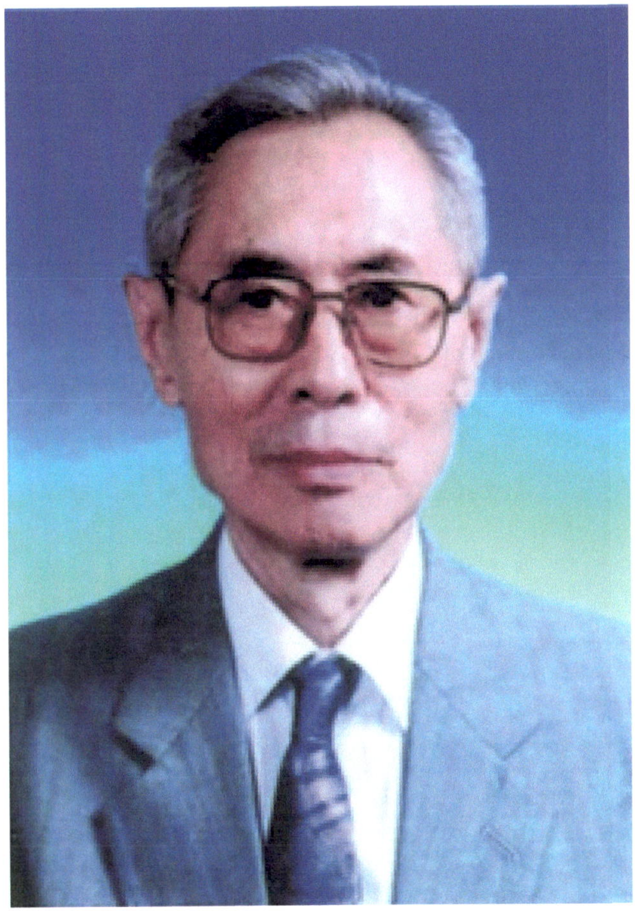

In recent years, remarkable progress has been achieved in the prevention and control of infectious diseases in China. However, along with social development, environmental and human behaviors change. As a consequence, new infectious diseases have been identified, with recurrence of traditional infectious diseases, both of which impose great challenges to the healthcare system in China. Complications of infectious diseases and their proper management are of great importance to the therapeutic outcomes of the diseases and the quality of patients' life, which deserve focused scholarly and clinical attention. Radiology, as an essential method for the diagnosis and differential diagnosis of these complications, constitutes an important procedure in the whole course of preventing and controlling infectious diseases.

Although recent years witness an increasing number of publications in radiology, those concerning infectious diseases are rare. Committed to clinical application and basic research of radiology of infectious diseases for years, Prof. Li has gained much experience and abundant data in this field. Based on his previous gains and contributions, he, as the chief editor, led his team composed mainly by professionals from the Department of Radiology at Beijing You'an Hospital to finish compiling this treatise, *Radiology of Infectious Diseases,* within 4 years.

This book falls into 3 parts, with 59 chapters in about 2 million bytes and over 3,000 figures. The comprehensive and original content makes it a treatise with newness and importance in the field of radiology. I believe and expect that the publication of this book plays a positive role in preventing and controlling the infectious diseases as well as in promoting the development of radiology.

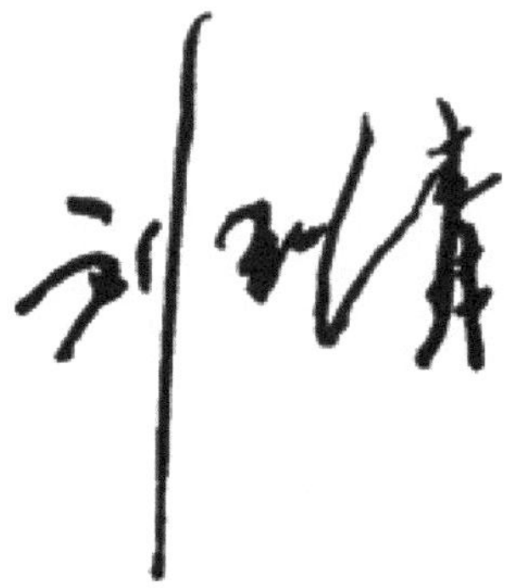

Academician of Chinese Engineering Academy
Fuwai Hospital of Chinese Academy of Medical Sciences
Beijing, China

Foreword II

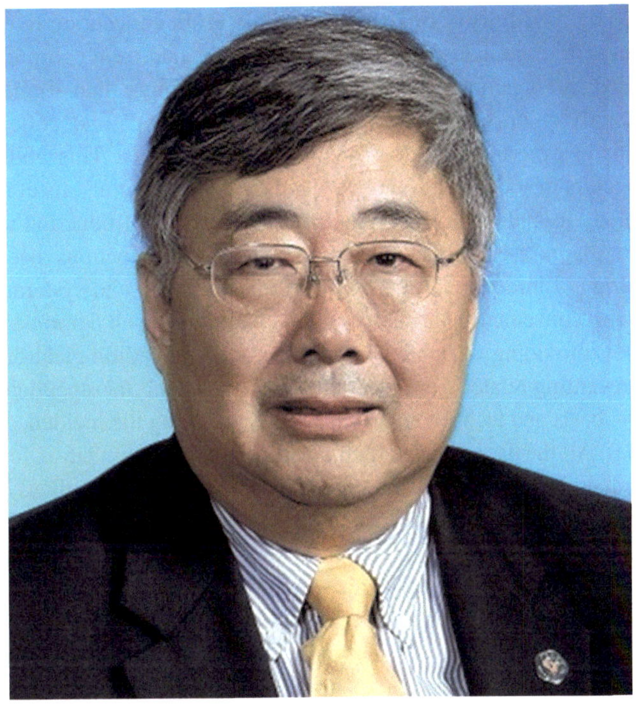

The profound changes of environment and human behaviors have produced tremendous impacts on the occurrence and prevalence of infectious diseases, such as SARS in 2004, influenza caused by H1N1 in 2009, and influenza caused by H7N9 in 2013. The current occurrence and prevalence of infectious diseases are characterized by continual emergence of new infectious diseases and recurrence of traditional infectious diseases, which impose threats to the health of human beings.

Since the common cause of death in patients with infectious diseases is the occurrence of complications, the early diagnosis and differential diagnosis of these complications turn out to be critical for the survival and quality of life of the patients. While diagnostic imaging, such as CT, X-ray, and MRI, plays an important role in the early diagnosis and differential diagnosis of complications, radiology thus constitutes an important procedure for the favorable outcomes of infectious diseases. The insufficient systematic knowledge about radiology of infectious diseases and the urgent need for its clinical application underline the compilation and publication of this book.

Currently, scientific literature on systematic theories about the clinical radiology of the 39 national legitimated and over 10 infectious diseases is still rarely found. The classical original treatise, *Radiology of Infectious Diseases*, has not been published. Previous radiological data on infectious diseases is either lost or scattered, which necessitates their collection, summarization, and systematic studies for compilation of a treatise. It is urgent to incorporate relevant resources worldwide for multiple-centered research and systematic knowledge in the field. Such a book definitely helps to avoid the embarrassment of no referential data in protecting against traditional infectious diseases.

On these accounts, Prof. Li proceeded from his 15-year observations and studies on clinical applications of radiology of infectious diseases to compile texts and data, with key points and generalizations. Based on his previous publications of ten treatises in either Chinese or English, including *Atlas of Differential Diagnosis in HIV/AIDS* (PMPH Press, Beijing), *Radiology of Influenza A (H1N1)* (Springer), and *Radiology of HIV/AIDS* (Springer), Prof. Li completed this book, *Radiology of Infectious Diseases*. He has consecutively received supports from the National Science and Technology Publishing Fund. Three of his books have been chosen as the planning project book in the program of internationally publishing referential books in Western medicine initiated by the Ministry of Health in China. From conception to completion of the manuscript, lasting for more than 2 years, the contributors had been comprehensively trained three times. Guided and organized by several professionals, more than 40 medical institutions and 50 professionals contributed to compiling the manuscript and collecting cases. The resources nationwide were incorporated for the final manuscript. This book encompasses 3 parts, with 59 chapters in about 2 million bytes and over 3,000 figures. Its contents range from imaging morphology to molecular imaging, including general introduction to medical radiology, procedures of diagnostic imaging, general introduction to infectious diseases, and specific sections of radiology of infectious diseases. The well-structured and systematic knowledge is reader friendly, with convenience for searching and reading. It well demonstrates radiology of infectious diseases, providing valuable guidance for accurate radiological diagnosis of infectious diseases, preventing related complications, and improving therapeutic outcomes. It also provides scientific basis and technological support for reducing the incidence and mortality of infectious diseases. All the firsthand data in the book lay a solid foundation for further research in radiology of infectious diseases. *Radiology of Infectious Diseases*, edited by Prof. Hongjun Li, will jointly be published by Elsevier and People's Medical Publishing House and present to domestic and international professionals a new area of medical radiology. The book will serve as an important reference for prevention, treatment, and research of infectious diseases in both fields of clinical medicine and medical radiology.

It is my great honor and pleasure to compose the foreword for this book, because it has taken the editor and contributors 4 years to complete the manuscript, with comprehensive and systematic contents as well as a highly readable style. I believe the book will improve the public cognition to infectious diseases, promote related academic communication, and advance the development in preventing and controlling infectious diseases.

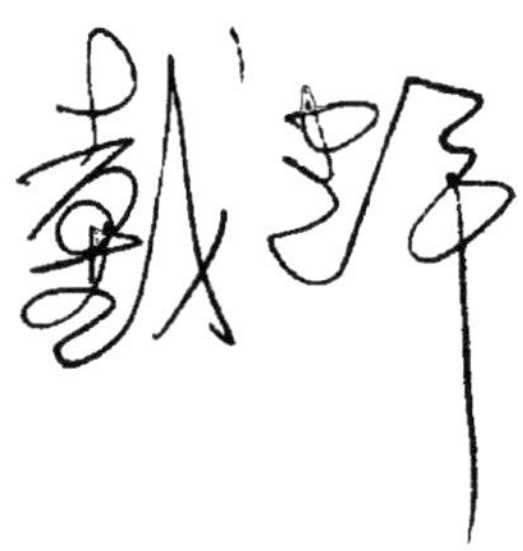

Jianping Dai
Board Chair at International Medical Communication Foundation, China
Vice President of Chinese Medical Association
Foreign Academician, Academy of American Medical Sciences

Foreword III

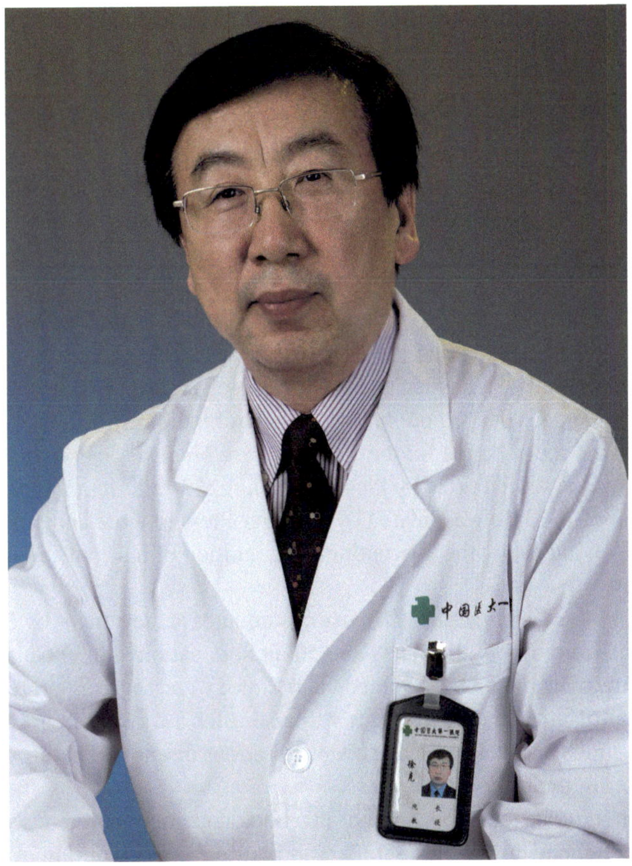

As a special group of diseases in the disease spectrum, infectious diseases, especially those highly contagious, are isolated from common health-care institutions. Within institutions specialized in preventing and controlling infectious diseases, those acute infectious conditions bear insufficient data in diagnostic imaging due to their pernicious and short courses of illness. Therefore, medical radiology contributes little to diagnosis and treatment of such diseases. Regarding those infectious diseases with a long course, due to the limitations of radiological equipments within institutions and the defects in the system for preventing and controlling infectious diseases, the radiological data may be insufficient or confined within the institution. Therefore, systematic and intensive studies in radiology of infectious diseases have been rarely conducted and reported. Meanwhile, patients with infectious diseases are excluded from those eligible to services by common health-care institutions. Scholarly and clinical attentions are rarely paid to them. Generally speaking, not only patients with infectious disease but also radiological data about infectious diseases are quarantined, which is common both domestically and internationally. In various book fairs accompanying international conferences, a treatise entitled with radiology of infectious disease is rarely found.

The past 10 years (actually even a longer period) saw dramatic changes of infectious disease spectrum that we have to pay close attention to. More infectious diseases have great crossovers with noninfectious diseases in the course of illness. The devastating SARS in 2003 perplexed the medical professionals in common health-care hospitals, leaving them no option but to establish a fever clinic for the first-line screening of SARS. And the earliest radiological data on SARS were collected and studied by first-line professionals who were not specialized in infectious diseases. This event denoted a significant turning point that the common health-care institutions may need to serve patients with infectious diseases that have not been definitely diagnosed. The field of medical radiology with traditional spectrum between infectious and noninfectious diseases should be integrated into a whole system. The radiologists from common health-care institutions and institutions specialized in infectious diseases should make joint efforts to study radiological data on traditional and newly emerging infectious diseases. The consequent scholarly achievements should be applied for prevention and control of infectious diseases. Especially, the radiologists from common health-care institutions should have knowledge about radiological data on infectious diseases to ensure its early accurate diagnosis and differential diagnosis.

As one of the pioneering radiologists dedicated to the prevention and treatment of AIDS in China, Prof. Hongjun Li has directed his team to conduct basic scientific research in the field of AIDS radiology and pathology. Their accomplishments have been widely recognized as outstanding by both domestic and international scholars. After joining Beijing You'an Hospital, Prof. Li, along with his increasing achievements, has continued his scholarly focus on radiology of HIV/AIDS and has extended his research interests into radiology of most infectious diseases. More importantly, he has led a team of radiologists nationwide specialized in infectious diseases to widen and deepen our knowledge about radiology of infectious diseases. The work was granted the second prize for the 2011 *Chinese Medical Scientific and Technological Progress Award* and the second prize for the 2012 *Beijing Scientific and Technological Progress Award*. In the year of 2013, he was invited by Springer Press to write and publish *Radiology of Influenza A (H1N1)*, indicating the international recognition of his contributions to the field of medical radiology.

This book, *Radiology of Infectious Diseases*, is another achievement by Prof. Hongjun Li, with contributions from over 40 hospitals and 50 authors nationwide in China. The book will undoubtedly fill the blank in the field of medical radiology and serve as a reference for prevention and treatment of infectious diseases. It will also offer a way for radiologists in common health-care institutions to gain knowledge about infectious diseases. Therefore, they can define infectious diseases in their daily work.

I sincerely congratulate the publication of this book and am honored to write the foreword. Meanwhile, I recommend this book to scholars and professionals working in the field of medical radiology.

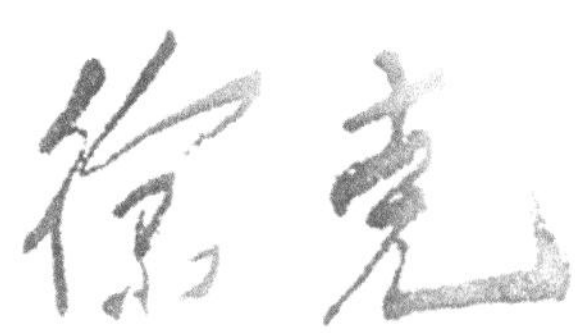

Ke Xu
Chairman, Radiology Branch of Chinese Medical Association

Preface

Definition for Radiology of infectious diseases: Radiology of infectious diseases is a discipline to primarily study the imaging features of infectious diseases caused by different pathogens, and to explore their evolution law.

Changes of the environment and human behaviors greatly impact on the occurrence and prevalence of infectious diseases, with manifestations of continual emerging of new infectious diseases and resurgence of traditional infectious diseases. All these pose threats to human health.

Since the common cause of deaths induced by infectious diseases is closely pertinent to the development of complications, early diagnosis of these complications proves key to prolonging the survival and improving the survival quality of patients with infectious diseases as well as intervention assessment. Moreover, radiology constitutes an important way for the diagnosis and differential diagnosis of the complications, which remains as a key procedure in the prevention and control of infectious diseases. Therefore, the lack of systematic theories about radiology of infectious diseases and the urgency for its clinical application underpin the compilation of this book.

Currently, studies for systematic theories on clinical radiology of the 39 legitimated and over 10 infectious diseases are still rare. No classical blue-cover treatise, *Radiology of Infectious Diseases*, has been published to guide the clinical practice. Due to the characteristic transient prevalence or outbreak of infectious diseases, the previous sporadic data on radiology of infectious diseases has been either lost or scattered, which further necessitates their collection, summarization, and systematic studies for compilation of a comprehensive treatise. It is therefore urgent to incorporate relevant resources across the whole nation and even across the world for multiple-centered studies for the compilation of a landmark book on radiology of infectious diseases. Such a book will definitely help to avoid the embarrassing shortage of referential data in the cases of resurgence of traditional infectious diseases.

Since 1998, the authors have been dedicated to radiology of infectious diseases. Till now, they have accumulated and analyzed large quantities of firsthand data and abundant clinical and research experience, which bear consecutive publications from 2006 to 2013. His published treatises, *Atlas of Differential Diagnosis In HIV/AIDS* (PMPH Press, Beijing), *Radiology of Influenza A (H1N1)* (Springer Press), *and Radiology of HIV/AIDS* (Springer Press), have been supported by the national publishing foundation for scientific and technological treatises. The books have been officially listed into the program for the international publication planning in biomedicine by the Ministry of Health in China. The nondegree curriculum for diagnostic imaging of infections and infectious diseases has been approved as a national continuing education program by the Chinese Medical Association for 5 years since 2008. *Radiology of Infectious Diseases* encapsulates clinical application and basic research in the field of radiology of infectious diseases, which fills the blank in systematic theories about radiology of infectious diseases and further develops the theoretical system of medical radiology. The publication of this book is therefore significant in preventing and controlling human infectious diseases.

The book is about relevant theoretic researches of the complication spectrum of infectious diseases regarding their radiological findings, clinical managements, pathogens, pathology, and anatomy. The book is composed of 3 parts, including 59 chapters in about 2 million bytes. The detailed case descriptions, data, and 3,000 high-quality figures demonstrate the recent development of the field to readers. Several chapters and sections incorporate registrations of morphological and molecular imaging, which include extended data for the imaging diagnosis. The book will definitely facilitate the early diagnosis of infectious diseases, especially their early noninvasive diagnosis with standardized technological guidelines and practical clinical routes. In addition, the book incorporates format styles of both Chinese and Western books, which highlights key points with brief arguments, citations from classics, as well as text along with abundant pictures. The book also includes large quantities of classical cases, which is highly practical and consultative for medical professionals of advanced, intermediate, and junior level. Many rare and precious images from clinical cases are seldom encountered in clinical practice or might be omitted due to misdiagnosis. Some imaging data are rarely found in China which are therefore cited from relevant foreign literature. These data enriches the content of this book. As most of the imaging data are presented for the first time, we hope this book provides readers a refreshing perspective for expertise.

To complete this book, we have set up an advisory committee and an experts committee for scientific design and penetrating argumentation. The composition of this book has spanned over 4 years from its outline design and writing training to the finished manuscript, which ultimately passed the peer-reviewing procedures by People's Medical Publishing House and has been published as a practical blue-cover treatise. Meanwhile, the author received invitation for its international publication by Germany Springer Press. After the signing of the transfer of copyright, its English version is to be published. Therefore, the editorial board has committed tremendous endeavors to the book, with 3 trainings on composition standards. In addition, a total of 63 medical institutions and 213 professionals contributed to the manuscript compilation, data collection, and case elaboration. Several professionals were pointed to specifically organize auditing, modification, and supplementation. As designers, advocators, and participants, I would like to express my heartfelt thanks to all the scholars and professionals who significantly contributed to the compilation of this book. I would also like to extend my sincere thanks to the senior radiologists such as academician Yuqing Liu, academician Jianping Dai (American Academy of Medical Sciences), Prof. Ji Qi, Prof. Qiyong Guo, Prof. Xiaoyuan Feng, Prof. Ke Xu, Prof. Guozhen Zhang, Prof. Xiangsheng Xiao, Prof. Jiaxing Xu, Prof. Jingxia Xie, and Prof. Daqing Ma for their persistent devotion to the field of radiology of infectious diseases. I would also like to thank the nationwide team and the team at the Department of Radiology, Beijing You'an Hospital, Capital Medical University, for their efforts and persistent contributions. Especially, I bestow my thanks to Ning Li, president of Beijing You'an Hospital of Capital Medical University, and other hospital leaders for their substantial supports. My thanks also go to those contributors for the publication and compilation of this book.

Academician Yuqing Liu, a forerunner in the field of radiology in China, is really excited at witnessing the serial publications of the treatise in both Chinese and English, such as *Radiology of HIV/AIDS* and *Radiology of Influenza A (H1N1)* as well as the manuscript of *Radiology of Infectious Diseases*, which record and signify the recent advance in medical radiology in China. He praised that our works marked a new area of medical radiology in China and enriched the theoretical system of medical radiology. When visiting China in 2011, the president of the British Science Academy acclaimed that Prof. Hongjun Li and his team at Beijing You'an Hospital had achieved significant contributions to both the Chinese people and the whole human race.

This book also covers extremely rare and even eliminated infectious diseases, with citations of pictures from domestic and foreign precious literature. The original authors of these citations have been identified, and we have requested for citations by written letters or e-mails. Hereby, I would like to express my sincere thanks to these authors for their approval and support. In light of the spread and sporadic prevalence of H7N9, this treatise will provide another powerful weapon for the battle against infectious diseases and will play a mighty role in eradicating infectious diseases that endanger human health.

There definitely exist some errors in this book. Your kindly comments are highly appreciated for the improvement of this book.

Beijing, China Hongjun Li

Acknowledgment to Contributing Institutions

Affiliated Beijing You'an Hospital, Capital Medical University, Beijing, China
University College Cork (UCC), Cork, Ireland
Department of Pathology, Capital Medical University, Beijing, China
Affiliated Beijing Ditan Hospital, Capital Medical University, Beijing, China
Affiliated Beijing Chest Hospital, Capital Medical University, Beijing, China
Affiliated Beijing Shijitan Hospital, Capital Medical University, Beijing, China
Affiliated Beijing Tiantan Hospital, Capital Medical University, Beijing, China
Affiliated Luhe Hospital, Capital Medical University, Beijing, China
The Third Affiliated Hospital, Suzhou University, Suzhou, Jiangsu, China
The Second Affiliated Hospital, Harbin Medical University, Harbin, Heilongjiang, China
Public Health and Clinical Center, Chengdu, Sichuan, China
Affiliated Huashan Hospital, Fudan University, Shanghai, China
The Eighth People's Hospital, Guangzhou, Guangdong, China
The Third People's Hospital, Shenzhen, Guangdong, China
Longtan Hospital, Liuzhou, Guangxi Zhuang Autonomous Region, China
Department of Biochemistry, Harbin Medical University, Harbin, Heilongjiang, China
The First Affiliated Hospital, Qiqihar Medical College, Qiqihar, Heilongjiang, China
Hainan Provincial Nong Ken Hospital, Haikou, Hainan, China
The City Children's Hospital, Hangzhou, Zhejiang, China
Cangzhou Heping Hospital, Cangzhou, Hebei, China
Cangzhou Central Hospital, Cangzhou, Hebei, China
The First Affiliated Hospital, Nanyang Medical College, Nanyang, Henan, China
Provincial Institution for Infectious Diseases Prevention and Control, Harbin, Heilongjiang, China
Taiping People's Hospital, Daowai District, Harbin, Heilongjiang, China
The Third People's Hospital, Harbin, Heilongjiang, China
Yantai Yuhuangding Hospital, Shangdong, China
City Kangan Hospital (former City Hospital for Infectious Diseases), Mudanjiang, Heilongjiang, China
Jingzhou Central Hospital, Jingzhou, Hubei, China
Affiliated Tumor Hospital, Chinese Academy of Medical Sciences, Beijing, China
Provincial Children's Hospital, Changsha, Hunan, China
The Third People's Hospital, Changzhou, Jiangsu, China
City Tumor Hospital, Nantong, Jiangsu, China
The First Affiliated Hospital (Xinan Hospital), the Third Military Medical University, Chongqing, China
Affiliated Tumor Hospital, Nantong University, Nantong, Jiangsu, China
City Development District Hospital, Yantai, Shandong, China
Affiliated Fifth Hospital, Sun Yat-Sen University, Guangzhou, Guangdong, China
City Public Health Medical Rescuing Center, Chongqiong, China
Peking Union Medical College Hospital, Beijing, China
The First Hospital, Shanxi Medical University, Taiyuan, Shanxi, China

City Public Health and Clinical Center, Fudan University, Shanghai, China
The Pulmonary Hospital, Shanghai, China
Ruijin Hospital affiliated to School of Medicine, Shanghai Jiao Tong University, Shanghai, China
Provincial Infectious Diseases Hospital (Provincial AIDS Care Center), Kunming, Yunnan, China
Beijing Fengtai Hospital of Integrated Traditional and Western Medicine, Beijing, China
Provincial People's Hospital, Zhengzhou, Henan, China
Provincial Tumor Hospital, Zhengzhou, Henan, China
City TCM Hospital, Nanyang, Henan, China
Baihe Town Hospital, Nanyang, Henan, China
Family Planning Guiding Center, Wolong District, Nanyang, Henan, China
Dengzhou People's Hospital, Dengzhou, Henan, China
No. 302 Hospital of PLA, Beijing, China
City Center for Disease Control, Shenzhen, Guangdong, China
The Third People's Hospital, Shenzhen, Guangdong, China
The Children's Hospital, Shenzhen, Guangdong, China
The People's Hospital of Longhua New District, Shenzhen, Guangdong, China
City People's Hospital, Shenzhen, Guangdong, China
City Hospital for Infectious Diseases, Tianjin, China
The First People's Hospital, Tianjin, China
The First Central Hospital, Tianjin, China
Zhongnan Hospital, Wuhan University, Wuhan, Hubei, China
City Central Hospital, Karamay, Xinjiang Uygur Autonomous Region, China
The Second Affiliated Hospital, Xinjiang Medical University, Urumqi, Xinjiang Uygur Autonomous Region, China
The Sixth People's Hospital, Urumqi, Xinjiang Uygur Autonomous Region, China
Maternal and Children Health Hospital of Linxiang District, Lincang, Yunnan, China
City Central Hospital, Jinhua, Zhejiang, China
The First Affiliated Hospital, Zhengzhou University, Zhengzhou, Henan, China
City Sixth People's Hospital, Zhengzhou, Henan, China
Department of Pathogenic Molecular Biology, Institute of Microbiological Epidemiology, Academy of Military Medical Sciences, Beijing, China
Lahey Clinic Medical Center
Brigham and Women's Hospital Boston
SevenHills Hospital, Mumbai
Dalin Tzu Chi General Hospital
Kaohsiung Chang Gung Memorial Hospital
Boston Children's Hospital
Yan Chai Hospital
University Hospital Southampton NHS Foundation Trust
School of Foreign Studies, Southern Medical

Contents

Contributors

Honorary Editor

Ning Li

Editor

Hongjun Li

Associate Editors

Jingliang Cheng, Puxuan Lu, Wenxiao Jia, Bailu Liu, Yuzhong Zhang, Lianchun Liang, Weimin An, Jinsheng Xu, Qingxia Zhao, Liyi Wang

Members of the Standing Editorial Committee

Feng Chen, Yanqing Gao, Chungang Guo, Yinglin Guo, Hong Wang, Xicheng Wang, Junhong Li, Li Li, Ruili Li, Xueqin Li, Zhiyan Lu, Qinghua Meng, Jiangfeng Pan, Shi Qi, Haifeng Mi, Qi Zhang, Ning He, Yanyan Zhang, Xing Wang, Cuiyu Jia, Ruichi Zhang, Yuxin Shi, Dongli Shi, Wenyan Song, Yuxin Yang, Fuchun Zhang, Xiaochun Zhang, Chengxin Yang, Dawei Zhao

Members of the Editorial Committee

Xinchun Chen, Guilin Yang, BoPing Zhou, Guoliang Zhang, Jian Lu, Xiaohua Yue, Yuejie Zheng, Jikui Deng, Chengrong Li, Yanxia He, Yingying Deng, Yungen Gan, Hongwu Zeng, Wenxian Huang, Feiqiu Wen, Jianliang Yang, Wei Zhang, Keying Zhou, Wenke Zhu, Weiye Yu, Hanwu Ma, Shujiang Mei, Xuejun Cheng, Cheng Peng, Gendong Yang, Jing Yuan, Yusen Zhou, Guangyu Zhao, ShipinWu, Guangping Zheng, Yi Cao, Zhaoqin Wang, Guoan Yang, Ping Li, Deli Zhao, Lili Liu, Xue Yin, Jinling Zhang, Lili Tang, Dong Han, Mingxiao Sun, Yang Zhao, Xuhua Yang, Han Huang, Lili Kong, Meng Huo, Guiying Li, Yungui Zhang, Huiqin Li, Lin Mao, Pengfei Tao, Mei Liu, Jun Yang, Min Yuan, Feng Feng, Su Zhou, Shuihua Lu, Heping Xiao, Xinhua Zhou, Weiren Zhang, Huixia Zhang, Jie Bai, Mengtian Sun, Jinhuan Wang, Jinxin Liu, Wenxin Hong, Xinsheng Lv, Xiaodan Wang, Chao Chen, Jingwei Wu, Guangyuan Cheng, Yuejie Yang, Bo Gao,Chunli Liu, Liucun Song, Yan Sun, Xuan Yang, Na Zhang, Dehua Yang, Xianmin Wen, Lichong Hu, Lingbin Meng, Jinsong Shen, Jinping Wu, Jia Yun, Liqing Kang, Jihuai Cao, Hanqiu Liu, Wenze Wu, Longhua Chen, Yu Lu, Jie Dai, Kui Huang, Shengxiu Lv, Heping Xu, Zhi Cao, Ganlin Xia, Danlei Mou, Xiaoxi Mao, Yunfang Li, Da Yuan, Shaohua Xu, Jinli Ding, Zhenying Xia, Shuangjun Zhao, Haiyan Zhao, Aidong

Academic Advisors

Editorial Secretaries

Author Biography

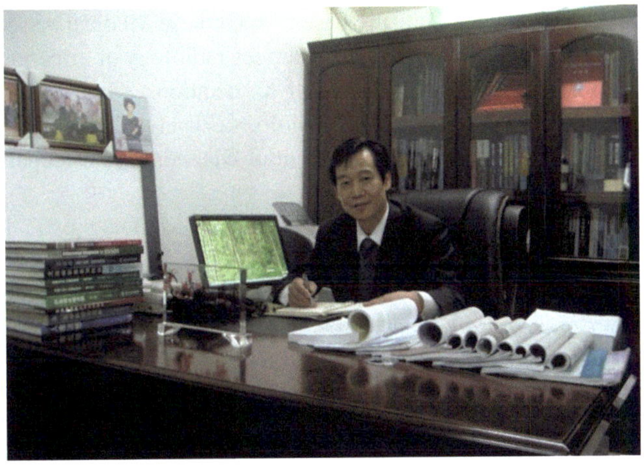

Introduction of the Chief Editor, Hongjun Li

Hongjun Li (M.D., Prof.) is a 48-year-old radiologist with an educational background in the UK. Currently, he is also a supervisor for the master's degree program in radiology. Professor Li is now offered the special government allowance from the State Council in China in recognition of his outstanding contributions to the field of medicine. He is also recognized membership in the Ten-Hundred-Thousand talent program in China at the "hundredth" level in the field of medicine. Meanwhile, he has achieved membership as one of the 215 high-level academic leaders in Beijing.

Research Direction: Radiology of Infectious Diseases

Prof. Li pioneers the first systematic disease spectra of legitimated 39 infectious diseases and other 12 infectious diseases from the perspective of radiology of infectious diseases. His contributions shed light on and improve the fundamental theories about the radiology of infectious diseases and the clinical application. In addition, his academic achievements further enrich and advance the theoretical development of medical radiology, which paves the way for future development of radiology of infectious diseases.

Current Positions

Director, Department of Radiology, Beijing You'an Hospital, Capital Medical University, Beijing, China

Deputy Dean, Department of Medical Imaging and Nuclear Medicine, Capital Medical University, Beijing, China

Chief editor, Radiology of Infectious Diseases (Elsevier platform).

Social Affiliations

Chairman member, Specialized committee on infection affiliated to Chinese Society of Radiology

Chinese Medical Science and Technology Award of the 3rd expert review committee member

National Study Abroad Foundation-funded project expert review committee member

Beijing Natural Science Foundation project expert review committee member

Chairman, Chinese Association of STD/AIDS Prevention and Control

Chairman, Society of Clinical Diagnostic Imaging for AIDS

Team director, preparatory team for radiology of infectious and contagious diseases affiliated to the section of Tropical and Parasitic Diseases, Chinese Medical Association

Academic leader, specialized collaborative group for radiology of infectious diseases, affiliated to the section of Radiology, Chinese Medical Association

Committee membership, Beijing Medical Radiology Society, Chinese Medical Association

Expert membership, experts' pool for Differential Diagnosis of Occupational Diseases in Beijing

Director, Center for Quality Control and Supervision of Diagnostic Imaging, Fengtai District, Beijing

Editorial board membership, *Chinese Medical Journal* (CMJ)

Associate editor, *Practical Radiology*

Editorial board membership, *Journal of Clinical Hepatobiliary Diseases*, *Journal of Magnetic Resonance Imaging*, *Chinese Journal of AIDS & STD*, *Beijing Medical Journal* (Infections and Research), and *Journal of Hepatic Cancer*

Academic Accomplishments

For 6 years, Prof. Li has directed or participated in 6 national and provincial scientific research projects and 3 international collaborative research projects. While conducting the research projects, he has directed or contributed to 101 research papers, including 24 published in Science Citation-Indexed journals. He also has received 17 publication fundings by the Springer and National Natural Science and Technology Publication Foundation or the Ministry of Health, editing and publishing 12 treatises including 4 in English (5 by Springer and 1 by People's Medical Publishing House) and 11 in Chinese (7 by People's Medical Publishing House, 1 by Tsinghua University Press, 1 by Chinese Medical Science and Technology Press, and 2 by Science and Technology Press). Of all the published treatises, 2 were published as national outstanding works after peer-reviewing; 3 were international publications funded by China Book International (CBI) program. Therein, within 6 months after *Radiology of HIV/AIDS* has been published, the global downloads break through more than 20,000 chapters, which achieves Springer PG praise for the work. The famous Professor Masahiro Narita from the University of Washington (American standards for infectious disease diagnosis expert of NIH) wrote a laudatory book review published in the journal *Clinical Infectious Diseases* (IF: 9.416, 2014;59(12):1811), which helps Prof. Li earn the academic status in the field of diagnostic radiology in China. In 2006, Prof. Li won the second prize for Science and Technology Progress Award issued by the national ministry or provincial government as the director of the research projects. In 2007, he won a prize for Science and Technology Progress issued by the national ministry or provincial government as the leading contributor of the research project. In 2011, he won the second prize for the Chinese Medical Science and Technology Award as the leading contributor. In 2012, he won the second prize for Beijing Science and Technology Progress as the leading contributor. In 2013, he won the first prize for Science and Technology Progress issued by the national ministry or provincial government as the leading contributor. In 2013, he won the third prize for the Chinese Medical Science and Technology Award as the leading contributor. In 2014, he won the third prize for Guangdong Province Science and Technology Progress as the leading contributor.

Part I

Radiology of Bacterial Infections

1 Anthrax

Dongli Shi and Hongjun Li

Anthrax, induced by *Bacillus anthracis*, is an acute infectious zoonotic disease. It occurs primarily due to contact of the bacterial spores in soil by herbivores, which causes skin ulceration, eschar, extensive surrounding tissue edema, and toxemia. And in some cases, even gastrointestinal anthrax, pulmonary anthrax, or meningeal anthrax occur, all of which can be complicated by septicemia.

1.1 Etiology

Bacillus anthracis is the pathogenic bacterium of anthrax in both humans and animals. It is the largest Gram-positive bacillus, with a length of 1–3 μm and a width of 5–10 μm with flat ends. The bacillus is characterized by its bamboo-like appearance arrayed in short chains, with no flagella and no motion. In environmental conditions of sufficient oxygen and appropriate temperature, spores can be formed that are about 1 μm in size and ovoid in shape, with extremely strong vitality. *Bacillus anthracis* can develop into capsules in bodies of both human and animals, which is characteristic of the *Bacillus anthracis* strain. The antigen of *Bacillus anthracis* can be divided into two parts, one as structural antigen and the other as anthrax toxin complex. There are at least four types of antigens in *Bacillus anthracis* including (1) capsular polypeptide antigens (CPA), which, in combination with capsule, are anti-phagocytic and are related to the bacterial toxicity; (2) somatic polysaccharide antigens (SPA), which are not related to the bacterial toxicity but are heat and decay tolerated and produce precipitation with corresponding antibodies, known as Ascoli reaction; (3) spore antigen (SA), which is a specific antigen and has value for serological diagnosis; and (4) protective antigens (PA), which are formed during the growth of the bacillus and are anti-phagocytic with favorable immunogenicity. Anthrax toxin is a complex comprised of three different proteins, namely, PA, lethal factor (LF), and edema factor (EF). LF or EF, when existing alone, is not bioactive. However, its combination with PA produces tissue edema and death of laboratory animals. Anthrax toxin is anti-phagocytic with immunogenicity. *Bacillus anthracis*, as an aerobic or facultative anaerobic bacillus, multiplies in common culture media, and the optimal temperature for its reproduction is 37 °C. On common agar plates, rough colonies in size of 2–4 mm can be found. But on blood agar plates, there is no hemolysis but mucous fluid in colonies. On broth culture media, thread-like sedimentation occurs.

1.2 Epidemiology

1.2.1 Source of Infection

The main source of infection is the infected herbivores such as cows, horses, sheep, and camels. Sometimes, pigs and dogs are also the source of infection. They might develop anthrax after eating foods contaminated by the bacteria. Direct or indirect contacts to their secretions and excretions by human can cause the infection. However, its transmission from person to person rarely occurs.

1.2.2 Routes of Transmission

1.2.2.1 Contact

Contact is the most common route of transmission. The direct contact of the wound to the bacteria can cause the disease. The contact to contaminated animal by-products, soil, and utensils can also cause the disease.

1.2.2.2 Inhalation

Inhalation of dusts and droplets carrying *Bacillus anthracis* can also cause the disease.

D. Shi • H. Li (✉)
Department of Radiology, Beijing You'an Hospital, Capital Medical University, Beijing, China
e-mail: lihongjun00113@126.com

H. Li (ed.), *Radiology of Infectious Diseases: Volume 2*, DOI 10.1007/978-94-017-9876-1_1

1.2.2.3 Foods and Drinks

Intake of contaminated foods and drinks can also cause anthrax.

1.2.2.4 Insects Bites and Stings

It is possible but rare for blood-feeding insects such as gadfly to transmit anthrax after biting or stinging infected animals followed by biting and stinging humans.

1.2.3 Population Susceptibility

Populations are generally susceptible to anthrax, and the high-risk populations include animal slaughters, workers processing animal by-products, animal attendants, and veterinarians. The immunity against anthrax commonly lasts for 3–6 months after the infection.

1.2.4 Epidemiological Features

Anthrax has a worldwide distribution, with more common occurrence in temperate zones and regions with poor hygienic conditions such as South America, East Europe, Asia, and Africa. In China, anthrax occurs all the year round, with a peak occurrence from July to September. Patients are commonly reported from pastoral areas, with an endemic and sporadic occurrence.

1.3 Pathogenesis and Pathological Changes

1.3.1 Pathogenesis

Experiments have demonstrated that the pathogenicity and lethality of *Bacillus anthracis* are mainly caused by its capsule and anthrax toxin. Exotoxin complex consists of three proteins, PA, EF, and LF. EF plays a complexing role in the toxic complex, inhibiting the phagocytosis of leucocytes. PA is anti-phagocytic with immunogenicity, while LF has no immunogenicity. The three components alone have no toxic effects on animals, while the combination of EF and PA can cause skin edema and the combination of PA and LF leads to pulmonary edema and death of laboratory animals. The combination of the three components produces typical toxic symptoms of anthrax, including tissue edema and bleeding following increased permeability of blood microvessels. The capsule of *Bacillus anthracis*, an invasive factor, is anti-phagocytic and facilitates the growth and spreading of the bacteria.

1.3.2 Pathological Changes

Anthrax is pathologically characterized by hemorrhage, necrosis, and edema of the involved tissues and organs. Cutaneous anthrax is characterized by anthracoid edema, eschar, ulceration, and surrounding coagulative necrosis. Pulmonary anthrax is manifested as pathological changes of hemorrhagic bronchitis and lobular pneumonia. Severe gelatinous edema of the mediastinum and lymphadenectasis surrounding the bronchi may also be found. In the cases of gastrointestinal anthrax, the pathological changes mainly occur in ileocecus, with diffusive and hemorrhagic inflammations. And there are also severe edema of surrounding intestinal walls, lymphadenectasis of mesentery, as well as bloody and serous effusion in the abdominal cavity with large quantity of *Bacillus anthracis*. In the cases of anthrax meningitis, pathological changes of obvious congestion, edema and necrosis of meninges, and cerebral parenchyma can be found. And there might be inflammatory cell infiltration and large quantity of *Bacillus anthracis* in the subarachnoid cavity when anthrax meningitis occurs.

1.4 Clinical Symptoms and Signs

The incubation of anthrax has great variance; cutaneous anthrax commonly lasting for 1–7 days, pulmonary anthrax ranging from 12 h to 12 months, and gastrointestinal anthrax lasting for 24 h. Cutaneous anthrax is the main type of naturally occurring anthrax, while bioterrorism-related anthrax is commonly pulmonary anthrax.

1.4.1 Cutaneous Anthrax

Cutaneous anthrax predominantly occurs on the exposed skin, such as the skin of the face, neck, shoulder, and hands. Small boils occur on the primary onset position, followed by hemorrhagic necrosis surrounded by large quantities of vesicles and an extending area of edema. After rupture of necrotic tissues, ulceration occurs with bloody substances forming black scabs, known as anthrax. The occurrence of cutaneous anthrax is frequently accompanied by moderate fever with a body temperature of 38–39 °C, headache, and general upset. In some cases, extensive exudative lesions as well as large areas of edema with subsequent large areas of necrosis are locally present. These lesions may further spread along lymph vessels to cause local lymphadenitis. Its invasion into the blood flow causes septicemia and even death without appropriate therapies, with a death rate of 10–20 %.

1.4.2 Pulmonary Anthrax

Pulmonary anthrax rarely occurs and is challenging for its clinical diagnosis. Most cases of pulmonary anthrax are caused by primary inhalation of the pathogenic bacteria. Occasionally, its occurrence is secondary to cutaneous anthrax. Primary symptoms of pulmonary anthrax are usually similar to common cold, such as low-grade fever, dry cough, general pain, and fatigue. The symptoms deteriorate within 2–4 days, with high fever, aggravated cough with bloody sputum, and accompanying chest pain, dyspnea, cyanosis, and profuse sweating. Death usually occurs within 24 h, and the death rate may even increase due to delayed diagnosis or treatment.

1.4.3 Gastrointestinal Anthrax

Clinically, gastrointestinal anthrax is rarely found. Generally, it can be divided into two types according to its location, oropharyngeal anthrax and abdominal anthrax. Oropharyngeal anthrax is commonly characterized by fever, ulceration in laryngeal and oropharyngeal cavities, dysphagia, and cervical swelling. Cervical swelling is often caused by the enlarged lymph nodes and soft tissue edema in the neck. However, abdominal anthrax is characterized by severe abdominal pain, abdominal distention, diarrhea, vomiting, and watery stool, all of which are induced by inflammation in the lower part of the small intestine. In some serious patients, symptoms including high fever, bloody stool, peritoneal irritation, and ascites occur. The patients with complication of septicemia die in 2–4 days due to toxic shock, and the mortality rate is 25–60 %.

1.5 Anthrax-Related Complications

1.5.1 Septicemia

Septicemia commonly occurs secondary to pulmonary anthrax, gastrointestinal anthrax, and severe cutaneous anthrax. In addition to aggravated primary local inflammation, it can also cause more serious systematic toxemic symptoms, such as high fever, chill, and failure. Patients are also susceptible to septic shock, DIC, and meningitis.

1.5.2 Anthrax Meningitis

Anthrax commonly involves the nervous system via blood flow or lymph flow, with manifestations of hemorrhagic brain parenchyma and meninges as well as abnormally enhanced meninges. The disease progresses quickly, with initial manifestations of nausea, vomiting, muscle pain, chill, dizziness, and ecchymosis. However, with 2–4 days after its onset, progressive nerve dysfunction, convulsion, and coma occur. The mortality rate is extremely high.

1.6 Examinations for the Diagnosis

1.6.1 Laboratory Tests

1.6.1.1 Smear Staining

The samples from lesions of infection should be collected, such as secretions in the deep lesions of cutaneous anthrax, sputum of patients with pulmonary anthrax, stool and vomit of patients with gastrointestinal anthrax, and cerebrospinal fluid of patients with anthrax meningitis. These samples are performed smears for microscopy. Gram staining facilitates to find typical *Bacillus anthracis*. The findings in combination with clinical symptoms facilitate the initial diagnosis.

1.6.1.2 Identification by Bacteria Culture

The positive rate by blood incubation is high, while that of damaged skin tissues ranges from 60 to 80 %. Nasopharyngeal swab for culture has a lower positive rate.

1.6.1.3 Serological Test

It is commonly applied for the retrospective diagnosis and epidemiological studies of anthrax.

1.6.1.4 Molecular Biological Assay

Specific amplification by PCR for *Bacillus anthracis* or detection of specific biomarker of the spores can be applied for both diagnosis and classification. In addition, these assays facilitate tracing the source of infection.

1.6.2 Diagnostic Imaging

1.6.2.1 X-Ray

X-ray is commonly applied to understand the involvement of lungs and intestines.

1.6.2.2 CT Scanning

CT scanning can further define the conditions of the trachea, lungs, mediastinum, hilar lymph nodes, and intestines.

1.6.2.3 MR Imaging

MR imaging is appropriate for examinations of anthrax meningitis and other complications involving the nervous system.

1.7 Imaging Demonstrations

1.7.1 Pulmonary Anthrax

1.7.1.1 X-Ray

In the early stage, X-ray demonstrates thickened pulmonary markings, blurry bilateral pulmonary hila, widened mediastinum, and pleural effusion. With the progression of the conditions, X-ray demonstrates further widened mediastinum, enlarged pulmonary hila, and increased pleural effusion.

1.7.1.2 CT Scanning

CT scanning demonstrates enlarged lymph nodes in mediastinum and hilum, mediastinal edema, thickened walls of trachea, infiltrative lesions surrounding hilum, and bloody effusion surrounding the heart and within the thoracic cavity.

Case Study 1

A female patient aged 61 years has a chief complaint of progressive shortness of breath. She also complains of substernal pain for 3 days and difficulty breathing during rests. She has a history of high blood pressure.

For case detail and figures, please refer to: Krol CM, et al. *AJR Am J Roentgenol*, 2002, 178(5):1063

1.7.2 Gastrointestinal Anthrax

1.7.2.1 Oropharyngeal Anthrax

Enhanced CT scanning demonstrates multiple enlarged lymph nodes in ovoid shape, uneven density in the lymph nodes with necrosis, and slightly blurry structures surrounding the lymph nodes in inflammatory changes (Fig. 1.1a–d).

1.7.2.2 Abdominal Anthrax

Plain CT scanning demonstrates thickened and swollen intestinal mucosa. In some cases, intestinal obstruction and ascites may be found. However, enhanced CT scanning demonstrates leakage of contrast media into the intestinal cavity during the arterial phase (Fig. 1.1e, f).

Case Study 2

A male patient aged 43 years complained of abdominal pain, nausea, vomiting, and weakness for 2 weeks.

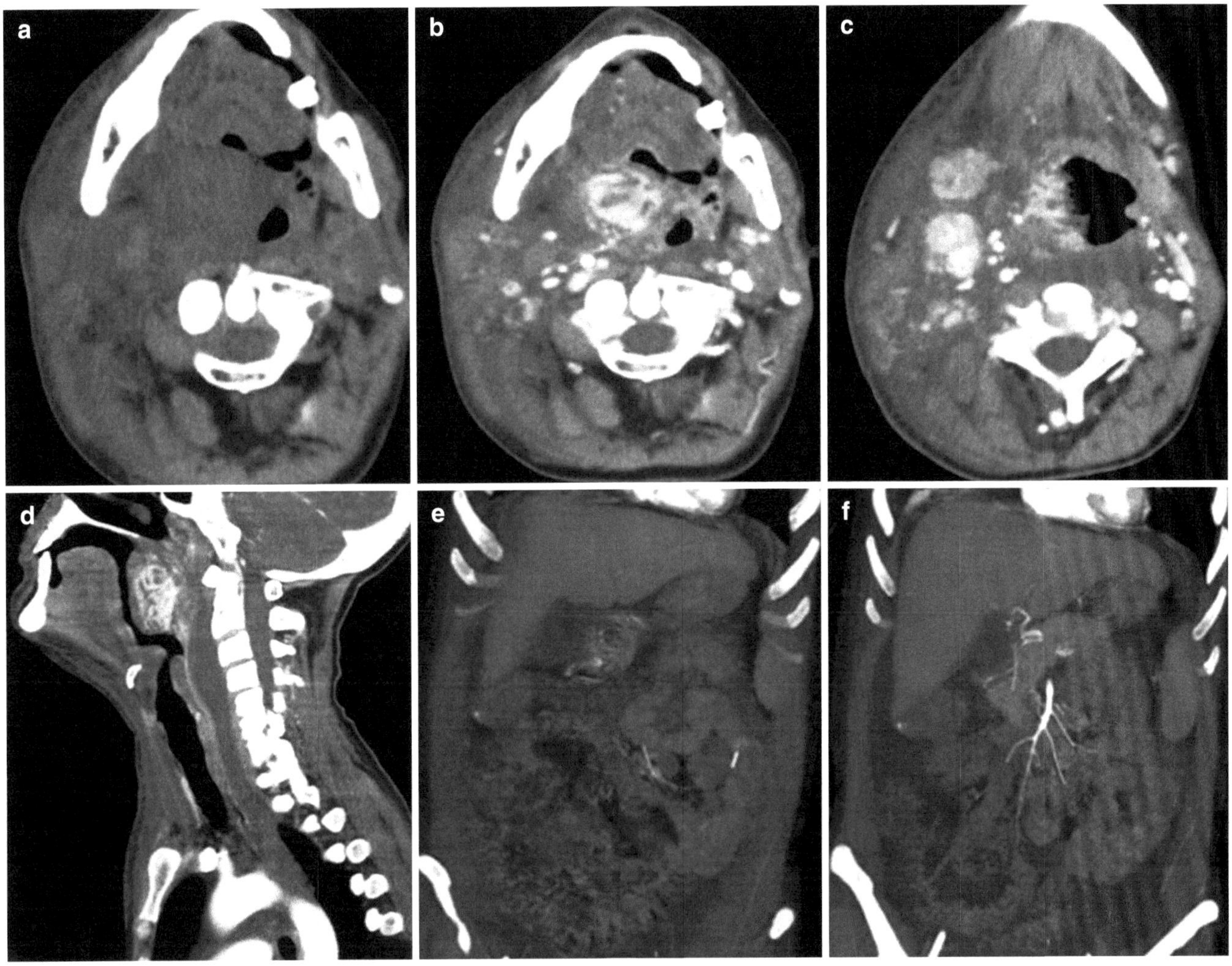

Fig. 1.1 Gastrointestinal anthrax. (**a**–**d**) Oropharyngeal anthrax. (**a**) Plain CT scanning of the neck demonstrates obvious swelling of the cervical soft tissues and narrowed cavities of nasopharynx, oropharynx, and laryngopharynx. (**b**) Enhanced scanning demonstrates multiple enlarged lymph nodes within lesions and the neck as well as uneven enhancement. In some cases, necrosis and liquefaction can be found. (**c**) Inflammatory changes can be found around the lymph nodes. (**d**) Fluid within prevertebral space can be found, which extends from oropharynx to the superior mediastinum. (**e**–**f**) Abdominal anthrax. (**e**–**f**) Coronal CT scanning demonstrates overflow of the contrast media from active stomach and jejunum, ascites, diffusive abnormal enhancement of the gastric and intestinal mucosa, and edema of small intestines (Reprint with permission from Ozdemir H, et al. *Emerg Radiol*, 2010, 17(2): 161)

1.7.3 Anthrax Meningitis

CT scanning and MR imaging commonly demonstrate hemorrhagic brain parenchyma (commonly the deep gray matter or junction of gray matter and white matter), subarachnoid space, cerebral ventricles, and meninges. Enhanced scanning or imaging demonstrates diffusive abnormal enhancement of the meninges.

Case Study 3

A boy aged 12 years was hospitalized due to sudden unconsciousness and convulsion. Physical examinations found T 37 °C and P 90/min and irregular respiration and by laboratory tests, WBC 18.7×10^9/L, ESR 3 mm/h, AST 328 U/L, ALT 93 U/L, and CRP 860 mg/L (Fig. 1.2).

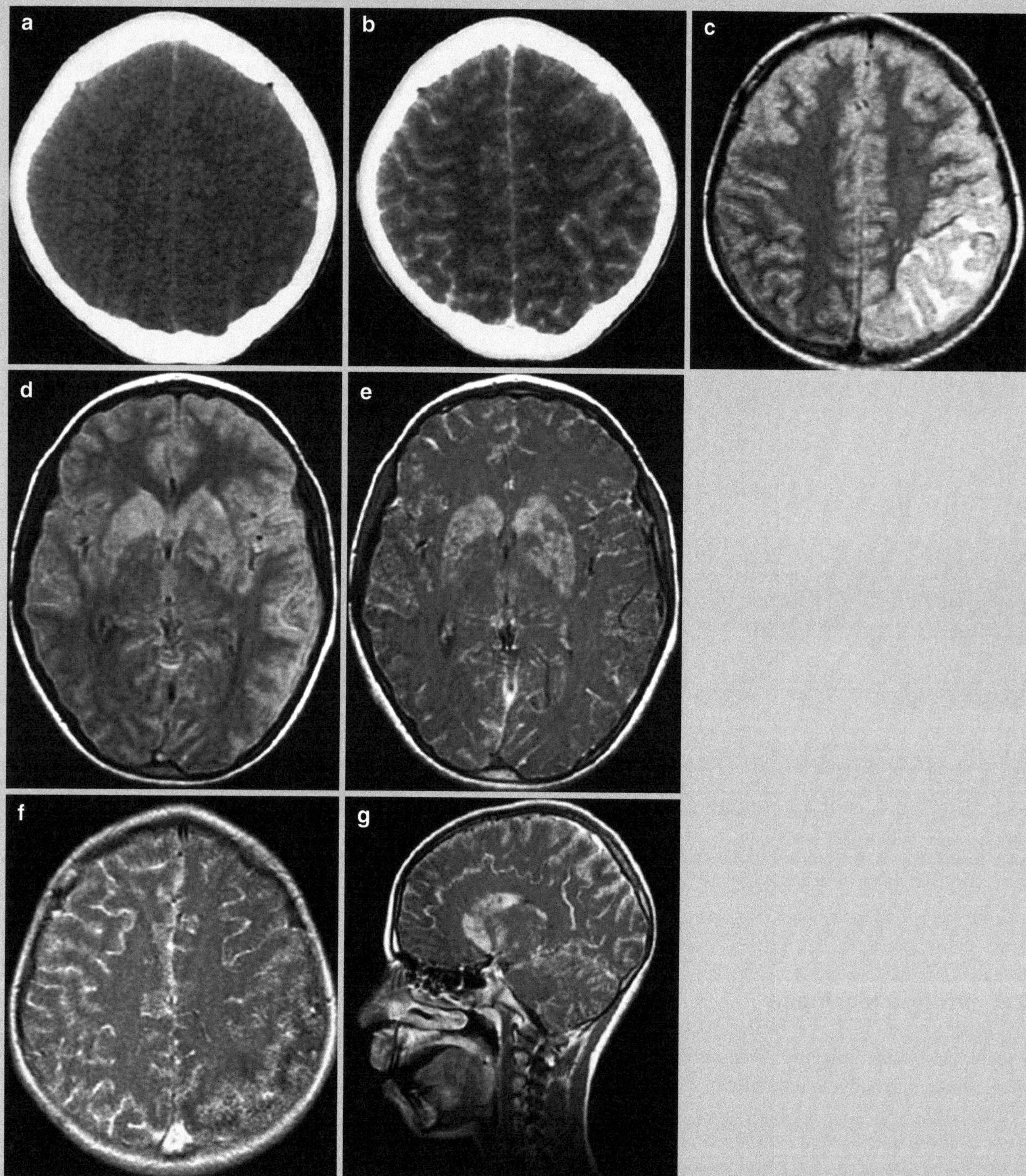

Fig. 1.2 Anthrax meningitis. (**a**, **b**) Plain CT scanning demonstrates hemorrhagic left parietal lobe and diffusive enhancement of meninges. (**c**, **d**) FLAIR imaging demonstrates high signal from the parietal lobe and basal ganglia. (**e**–**g**) Enhanced MR imaging demonstrates enhancement of the lesions in the basal ganglia and enhancement of meninges (Reprint with permission from Yildirim H, et al. *Pediatr Radiol*. 2006, 36(11): 1190)

1.8 Basis for Diagnosis

1.8.1 Epidemiological Data

The patients may have a history of visiting an epidemic area of anthrax in recent 2 weeks, with close contact to the diseased animals or their fur. Otherwise, the patients may have a history of eating meat from infected animals.

1.8.2 Clinical Manifestations and Diagnostic Imaging

1.8.2.1 Cutaneous Anthrax

The skin has typical changes of no purulent lesions, non-depressive painless edema, eschar, and ulceration. Based on these typical skin lesions, the diagnosis can be made.

1.8.2.2 Pulmonary Anthrax

Pulmonary anthrax is clinically characterized by severe dyspnea, high fever, coughing up blood, and chest pain. Chest X-ray and CT scanning demonstrate widened mediastinum, enlarged pulmonary hilum, pleural effusion, and bronchopneumonia.

1.8.2.3 Gastrointestinal Anthrax

The clinical manifestations of gastrointestinal anthrax include severe abdominal pain and diarrhea, with bloody and watery stool and bloody ascites. Imaging examinations demonstrate thickened and swollen intestinal mucosa.

1.8.2.4 Anthrax Meningitis

Clinically, anthrax meningitis is characterized by unconsciousness and convulsion. CT scanning or enhanced MR imaging demonstrates diffusive abnormal enhancement of the meninges.

1.8.3 Laboratory Tests

By routine blood test, white blood cells and neutrophils obviously increase. With assistance of positive etiological findings, the definitive diagnosis can be made, especially findings of *Bacillus anthracis* by direct smear or bacteria culture.

1.9 Differential Diagnosis

1.9.1 Cutaneous Anthrax

Cutaneous anthrax should be differentiated from special responses following smallpox vaccination. The cases of special responses following smallpox vaccination have a history of vaccination.

1.9.2 Pulmonary Anthrax

1.9.2.1 Upper Respiratory Tract Infection

Pulmonary anthrax in its early stage has similar symptoms to upper respiratory tract infection. However, by diagnostic imaging of the chest, patients with anthrax demonstrate thickened pulmonary markings, enlarged pulmonary hilum, widened mediastinum as well as bloody pericardiac and pleural effusion. These demonstrations cannot be found in cases of upper respiratory tract infection.

1.9.2.2 Lobar Pneumonia

Lobar pneumonia occurs commonly in young and middle-aged male adults. Some factors such as catching a cold, fatigue, and exposure to rain contribute to induce the occurrence of the disease. Clinically, its initial symptoms are usually high fever and chills, with following chest pain and productive cough with rust colored sputum. Chest X-ray demonstrates large flakes of parenchymal shadows with air bronchogram in the parenchymal shadows, commonly no enlarged pulmonary hilum and mediastinal lymph nodes as well as commonly no bloody mediastinal and pleural effusion.

1.9.2.3 Others

Cases of pulmonary anthrax with dyspnea should be differentiated from severe pneumonia, leptospirosis, and pulmonary plague. The corresponding differential diagnosis should be made based on the epidemiological features and etiological examinations.

1.9.3 Gastrointestinal Anthrax

Clinically, the symptoms of gastrointestinal anthrax are similar to those of dysentery, typhoid fever, and yersinia enteritis. Sometimes, gastrointestinal anthrax has acute abdominal manifestations, with obvious symptoms of toxemia. The etiological examinations of stool and/or vomit can provide evidence for the differential diagnosis.

1.9.4 Anthrax Meningitis

1.9.4.1 Subarachnoid Space Hemorrhage or Brain Parenchymal Hemorrhage

Anthrax meningitis should be differentiated from cerebrovascular diseases, such as subarachnoid space hemorrhage or brain parenchymal hemorrhage. The cases of cerebrovascular diseases can also have bloody cerebrospinal fluid and manifestations of cerebrovascular diseases. However, there are no skin lesions or primary lesions. In addition, patients with subarachnoid space hemorrhage or brain parenchymal hemorrhage generally have a history of trauma, aneurysm, or other vascular diseases. Enhanced scanning/imaging of patients with trauma demonstrates no abnormal enhancement of meninges. Cranial CTA examination of patients with aneurysm demonstrates localized thickening of blood vessels or cystic dilatation of blood vessels.

1.9.4.2 Purulent Meningitis

Plain scanning of patients with purulent meningitis demonstrates increased density of cerebral sulcus and cistern and unclearly defined boundary between cerebral gyri. Enhanced scanning/imaging demonstrates abnormal enhancement of thread-like or gyrus-like changes on the brain surface. However, brain hemorrhage rarely occurs in the cases of purulent meningitis but with obviously enlarged cerebral ventricles. There may also be hydrocephalus, cerebral infarction, and extracerebral empyema in some cases of purulent meningitis. Anthrax meningitis and the following toxemia have life-threatening conditions, with bloody cerebrospinal fluid. Therefore, immediate smear of cerebrospinal fluid can be performed to detect large bamboo-shaped *Bacillus anthracis*.

References

Krol CM, Uszynski M, Dillon EH, et al. Dynamic CT Features of Inhalational Anthrax Infection. AJR Am J Roentgenol. 2002;178(5):1063–6.

Ozdemir H, Demirdag K, Ozturk T, et al. Anthrax of the gastrointestinal tract and oropharynx: CT findings. Emerg Radiol. 2010;17(2):161–4.

Yildirim H, Kabakus N, Koc M, et al. Meningoencephalitis due to anthrax: CT and MR findings. Pediatr Radiol. 2006;36(11):1190–3.

Suggested Reading

Doganay M, Metan G, Alp E. A review of cutaneous anthrax and its outcome. J Infect Public Health. 2010;3(3):98–105.

Lv Z. Bacillus anthracis infection and its diagnosis. Chin J Clin. 2002;30(3):62–3.

Sweeney DA, Hicks CW, Cui X, et al. Anthrax infection. Am J Respir Crit Care Med. 2011;184(12):1333–41.

Xu DL. Bacillus anthracis infection. Chin J Pract Pediatr. 2002;17(11):686–7.

Xu TT, Yang YH. Diagnosis and prevention of anthrax. Chin J Pediatr. 2003;41(1):77–8.

Zheng GY. Anthrax and bacillus anthracis. Bull Biol. 2001;36(12):1–3.

Bacillary and Amebic Dysentery

2

Ruili Li, Hongjun Li, and Zheng Qi

Dysentery is an intestinal infectious disease caused by dysentery bacillus. Clinically, it is characterized by abdominal pain, tenesmus, bloody purulent stool, and frequent bowel movements. The disease commonly occurs in summers and autumns. According to its different pathogenic organisms, it can be categorized into bacillary and amebic.

2.1 Etiology

2.1.1 Bacillary Dysentery

Bacillary dysentery is a common infectious disease of the alimentary system. The pathogen, dysentery bacillus, is gram-negative pathogenic bacteria of the intestinal tract to human and primates. It is straight rod in shape and is motionless, with two types of metabolism, respiratory metabolism and fermentation metabolism. Currently, 39 serotypes (including subtype) of bacillary dysentery have been discovered. Based on the biochemical reaction and antigenic composition, bacillary dysentery can be divided into four groups: *Shigella dysenteriae* (group A), *Shigella flexneri* (group B), *Shigella boydii* (group C), and *Shigella sonnei* (group D). The bacteria have strong surviving ability in the external environment, among which *Shigella sonnei* has the strongest surviving ability. It is motionless, and 37 °C is the optimum temperature for its survival. Bacillary dysentery can be inactivated in the sunlight for 30 min, or at a temperature of 60 °C for 10 min, or at a temperature of 100 °C immediately.

R. Li • H. Li (✉) • Z. Qi
Department of Radiology Beijing You'an Hospital, Capital Medical University, Beijing, China
e-mail: lihongjun00113@126.com

2.1.2 Amebic Dysentery

Amebic dysentery, also known as intestinal amebiasis, is a gastrointestinal infectious disease caused by invasion of pathogenic *Entamoeba histolytica* into the colon wall. The patients mainly experience the symptoms of dysentery.

The trophozoite, with a diameter of 20–40 μm, moves toward one particular direction depending on pseudopodia. It can be detected in the stool or intestinal wall tissue from patients at the acute stage. Along with phagocytes and erythrocytes, it is also known as tissue trophozoite.

The cyst is commonly found in the stool of asymptomatic patients and of patients experiencing chronic conditions. It is round in shape with a diameter of 5–20 μm. The mature cyst, a serotype of *Entamoeba histolytica* containing four nucleuses, is contagious to spread the disease.

2.2 Epidemiology

2.2.1 Source of Infection

Bacillary dysentery occurs all year round, with the highest incidence rate in summers and autumns. The patients with dysentery and individuals carrying the bacteria are the sources of its infection. The cases with slight symptoms of dysentery or chronic dysentery as well as healthy individuals carrying the bacteria tend to be neglected. Patients with chronic conditions, at the convalescence stage and healthy individuals carrying cysts, are the sources of infection of amebic dysentery.

2.2.2 Route of Transmission

Bacillary dysentery commonly spreads via the route from the feces to mouth. A small quantity of bacteria can cause the infection and further its spreading from person to person. Water contaminated by amebic dysentery cysts can cause

H. Li (ed.), *Radiology of Infectious Diseases: Volume 2*, DOI 10.1007/978-94-017-9876-1_2

regional epidemic outbreak of the disease. Feces as a fertilizer as well as unthoroughly cleaned or cooked vegetables are also important factors contributing to its transmission. The disease can also spread via fingers, foods, and utensils contaminated by the bacteria cysts. Flies and cockroaches are also media for its transmission.

2.2.3 Susceptible Population

Populations are generally susceptible to bacillary dysentery, especially young children aged under 5 years. Their high incidence rate may be related to their more chance of contacting to pathogenic bacteria due to poor personal hygiene habits, poor immunity against the disease, immature neurodevelopment, and less secretion of stomach acid to kill dysentery bacillus. Populations are also generally susceptible to amebic dysentery. The patients fail to acquire immunity against amebic dysentery after its infection.

2.3 Pathogenesis and Pathological Changes

2.3.1 Pathogenesis

2.3.1.1 Bacillary Dysentery

Bacillary dysentery is pathologically characterized by purulent inflammation at the colon (including descending colon, sigmoid colon, and rectum) or at the terminal ileum. Dysentery bacillus can be pathogenic after its successful fight against the defense line of the gastrointestinal tract. It has relatively strong acid tolerance and tends to invade the small intestines via the stomach when the immunity of human body is compromised. It can rapidly reproduce in an alkaline environment with intestinal juice. Its production of both endotoxin and exotoxin stimulates the intestinal wall to increase its permeability for absorption of both toxins into the blood flow. The toxins can then be discharged from the colon mucosa to cause damages to epithelial cells, infiltration of polymorphonuclear granulocytes, colon allergy, and mucosal impairment. Based on these pathological changes, dysentery bacillus and other intestinal bacteria multiply at the mucosal surface and under the mucosa to cause further destructions, including inflammatory responses and microcirculatory disturbance of lamina propria. Local mesentery lymph nodes are subject to congestion and swelling.

2.3.1.2 Amebic Dysentery

The pathogenic effect of amoeba is from the cross-reaction between the worms and hosts, with multiple factors playing their roles. The invasiveness of *Entamoeba histolytica* is mainly manifested as resolvable destruction to host tissue. The virulence of amoeba is hereditary, but varies based on the strains. The worm strains from tropical regions with a high incidence rate have relative strong virulence due to their long-term adaptation to endobiotic parasitism. The immunity status of the host is of great importance for pathogenicity of amoeba. Both clinical data and experimental evidence have demonstrated that systemically or locally compromised immunity caused by malnutrition, infection, intestinal dysfunction, mucosal injury, as well as systemic or intestinal infection of typhoid fever, schistosomiasis, and tuberculosis facilitates the invasion of amoeba to host tissue. And the successful infection by amoeba can hardly be controlled by medications. The pathogenesis is as the following:

Mechanical Injury and Phagocytosis
The trophozoite, especially large trophozoite, can move by pseudopods in host tissue to destroy tissue and swallow and degrade damaged cells.

Contact Dissolution
Agglutinin at the surface of *Entamoeba histolytica* can absorb and dissolve host cells. Amoeba perforin is a group of small molecular protein family contained in the cytoplasmic granule of the trophozoite. When the trophozoite contacts to target cell or invades tissue, the perforin is injected to form an ion channel in the target cell, which further causes cell death due to loss of iron. Cysteine proteinase of amebic protozoa can cause cytolysis of the target cell.

Cytotoxic Effect
In 1979, Lushbaugh et al. isolated a cytotoxin from pure culture of *Entamoeba histolytica*, which was a nominated enterotoxin. The heat-intolerant protein may play an important role in occurrence of mucosal damage and diarrhea in the cases of intestinal amebiasis.

Immunosuppression and Escape
Agglutinin of amebic protozoa has anticomplementary activity, and cysteine proteinase can also degrade complement C3 into complement C3a. Therefore, the worm can escape from attacks initiated by host immunity. In addition, increased susceptibility and compromised immunity of host may complicate the disease by other intestinal bacterial infections, which, in turn, facilitate the invasion and pathogenesis of amoeba trophozoite.

2.3.2 Pathological Changes

2.3.2.1 Bacillary Dysentery

At the early stage, endotoxin secreted by dysentery bacillus and stimulated terminal nerves at the intestinal wall by inflammation cause intestinal spasm, increased enterocinesia, decreased water absorption by intestinal wall, and serous effusion from blood vessels at the intestinal wall. In addition to these pathological changes, diarrhea occurs. After that, the intestinal mucosa is subject to diffuse congestion and edema, infiltration of a large quantity of neutrophil granulocytes, and accompanying exudation of large quantities of mucus and fibrin to form grayish-white membranous structure. The membranous structure then sheds off to cause ulceration and bleeding, with further consequence of bloody mucopurulent stool. Toxic bacillary dysentery is pathologically characterized by increased permeability of systemic small artery wall, which further causes severe edema in surrounding tissue and swelling in organs such as the brain, liver, kidney, and adrenal gland.

2.3.2.2 Amebic Dysentery

Large trophozoite of *Entamoeba histolytica* invades intestinal wall to cause amebiasis, most commonly at the cecum, then the rectum, the sigmoid colon, and the appendix, but rarely at the transverse colon and the descending colon. In some cases, amebiasis may involve the entire large intestine or part of the ileum.

Amebic cyst containing four nucleuses gains its access into the gastrointestinal tract along with contaminated water or food. It can tolerate the digestion process facilitated by gastric acid and successfully passes through the stomach and the upper part of the small intestine. Then it can be digested by alkaline digestive liquid, such as parenzyme, at the lower part of the small intestine. At this time, the parasite escapes from cyst to develop into four small trophozoites, which can proliferate in binary division under appropriate conditions. They lodge in the ileocecum and run down to the colon along with stool. The small trophozoites in healthy host move downwards under the sigmoid colon along with stool, where they transform into cysts and are discharged out of host without causing any disease. Under appropriate conditions, such as gastrointestinal dysfunction, some bacteria may supply episome-like agent to strengthen the virulence of the trophozoite. The small trophozoites then release lysosomal enzyme, hyaluronidase, and proteolytic enzyme to invade the intestinal mucosa depending on the mechanical movement facilitated by their pseudopod. The cells at intestinal mucosa are subject to destructions, with erythrocytes and histiocytes swollen. And the small trophozoites develop into large trophozoites, with the following proliferation in a large quantity. The tissue at the intestinal wall is destructed to cause erosion and superficial ulceration.

Lesion at the Acute Stage

By Naked Eye Observation

At the early stage, mostly protruding grayish-yellow spots of necrosis in size of a needle tip can be observed at the mucosal surface. Otherwise, superficial ulceration is observed. The lesion is surrounded by congestion and hemorrhage. The necrotic lesion is then enlarged to appear like a round button. The trophozoites obtain their needed nutrition from dissolved and necrotic tissue fragments and erythrocytes to constantly multiply in the intestinal mucosa, destroy tissue, and penetrate the muscularis mucosae into the inferior mucosa. Due to the spongy tissue at the inferior mucosa, amoeba spreads around. After liquidation and shedding of necrotic tissue, flask-like ulcer with large base and small opening can be observed with the underneath margin, which is valuable for the diagnosis of the disease. The mucosa between ulcers is normal or has only slight catarrhal inflammation, which is different from the lesion of bacillary dysentery. In the cases with continued enlargement of the lesion, adjacent ulcerations can form tunnellike communication at the inferior mucosa with massive necrosis and shedding of its superficial mucosa. Therefore, giant ulcer forms with the underneath margin. Amebic ulcer is generally deep in location to corrode blood vessels, and massive intestinal hemorrhage may occur. In rare cases of severe ulceration, the muscular layer of the intestinal wall and even its serosal layer can be involved to cause peritonitis. Due to its gradually progressive development, adhesion of serosa to adjacent tissues is commonly observed. Therefore, acute intestinal perforation is less likely to occur.

By Microscopy

The pathological change is characterized by tissue necrolysis, with surrounding slight inflammatory responses including congestion, bleeding, as well as infiltration of small quantities of lymphocytes, plasmacytes, and macrophages. Amebic trophozoite can be observed at the interface between the ulcer margin and normal tissue as well as in the small venous lumen of the intestinal wall.

Lesion at the Chronic Stage

The pathological changes are complex, with proliferation of mucosal epithelium, granulation tissue at the ulcer base, proliferation and hypertrophy of fibrous tissue around the ulcer, coexistent tissue destruction and healing, coexistent old and new lesions, as well as repeated alternative occurrence of necrosis, ulceration, granulation tissue proliferation, and scar formation. The intestines are subject to thickened intestinal wall, narrowed intestinal lumen, and loss of normal morphology of intestinal mucosa. In some cases, due to excessive proliferation of granulation tissue, a confined lump is formed, which is known as amebic mass and is commonly found at the cecum. The trophozoites can also gain their access into the vein of the intestinal wall and invade the liver along with blood flow via the portal vein or lymphatic vessels to cause embolism of intrahepatic minor veins and their peripheral inflammation. The liver is then subject to necrosis of hepatic parenchyma and hepatic abscess that occurs more commonly at the right liver lobe. They can also move into the lung, brain, and spleen in the form of embolus to cause migratory abscess. Intestinal trophozoites can also directly spread to surrounding tissues to cause rectovaginal fistula or skin and mucosa ulcers. In some individual cases, enterorrhagia and intestinal perforation may occur, or even with complications of peritonitis and appendicitis.

2.4 Clinical Symptoms and Signs

2.4.1 Bacillary Dysentery

In recent years, due to extensive use and continual upgrade of antibiotics, the drug-resistant strain of bacillary dysentery annually increases. Due to the differences of bacteria strain, quantity, and individual difference of immunity, the clinical manifestations tend to be atypical and diversified. According to the length of the illness course, the disease can be divided into three types: acute bacillary dysentery, prolonged bacillary dysentery, and chronic bacillary dysentery. The clinical manifestations are described as the following.

2.4.1.1 Acute Bacillary Dysentery

According to the clinical manifestations, acute bacillary dysentery can be divided into four types: common type, mild type, severe type, and toxic type. The toxic type can be further categorized into three subtypes: shock subtype, brain subtype, and mixed subtype according to the severity of clinical manifestations.

Common Type

The common type has typical symptoms of bacillary dysentery, with acute onset, fever, and a body temperature of 39–40 °C. Initially, abdominal pain and diarrhea do not occur, with only symptoms of nausea, vomiting, and headache, which can be misdiagnosed as catching a heavy cold. Several hours later, paroxysmal abdominal pain and diarrhea occur. The patients experience frequent bowel movements for 10–20 times per day, which is firstly loose or watery stool and then bloody purulent stool with abdominal dragging sensation. By physical examination, the patients have abdominal tenderness at the right lower quadrant with accompanying active bowel sound and obvious tenesmus. Timely and appropriate therapy can cure the disease within several days.

Mild Type

The mild type has the most slight clinical manifestations in the cases of bacillary dysentery, with mild systemic viremia and intestinal symptoms. Generally, the patients experience slight abdominal pain and diarrhea with bowel movements of two to four times per day. The stool is watery or mushy without pus and blood. Sometimes, it is mixed with mucus. The abdominal pain can be relieved after bowel movement. Most patients do not experience fever or only low-grade fever. And the conditions tend to be misdiagnosed as common enteritis or colonitis.

Severe Type

The severe type has an acute onset and high fever with frequent bowel movements for 20–30 times per day. The stool is purulent and bloody in a small quantity. The patient experiences severe abdominal pain, serious abdominal dragging sensation, obvious tenesmus, and even reluctance to leave from the toilet. In severe cases, the patient even experiences coldness of limbs, dehydration, and sometimes even conscious disturbance due to acidosis.

Toxic Type

The toxic type occurs more commonly in children aged 3–7 years and is usually a *Shigella* infection. This type has an acute onset, firstly with only high fever and rapid increase of body temperature to 40–41 °C and accompanying headache, aversion to cold, convulsions, or circulatory disturbance. Commonly, upper respiratory infection does not occur. The gastrointestinal symptoms are also not serious, commonly occurring in 6–12 h after convulsion. The toxic type can be further categorized into the following subtypes: the shock type characterized by peripheral circulatory failure, the brain subtype characterized by brain symptoms such as brain edema and intracranial hypertension, and the mixed subtype characterized by coexistence of respiratory and circulatory failures.

Shock Subtype

In the early stage, children patients experience pale complexion, cyanosis around the mouth, coldness of limbs, pale fingernails/toenails, and rapid heartbeat and breathing. With the development of the conditions, the patient experiences grayish complexion; cyanosis of the fingernails, toenails, and lips; skin disturbance; rapid heart rate of 160 beats per minute; low dull heart sounds; weak and fine pulse; unconsciousness; oliguria or anuria; and dyspnea. In the advanced stage, the conditions may develop into heart failure, lung shock, and DIC.

Brain Subtype

The brain subtype more commonly occurs in preschoolers, with relatively rare occurrence in infants and school-aged children. Initially, the patients experience good consciousness, with sudden onset of convulsions, spasm of limbs, and uplift of eyes. These symptoms occur repeatedly in severe cases. After each convulsion, the patients have good consciousness, but the patients gradually develop weariness, irritation or drowsiness, and even coma with normal or increased blood pressure. The children patients experience pale complexion, which is more serious along with the increase of body temperature, and neurological symptoms such as headache and frequent vomiting. Occasionally, the patients experience suspended breathing, sigh-like breathing and different-sized pupils, and respiratory failure due to brain edema and encephalopathy.

Mixed Subtype

The mixed type is manifested as the coexistence of shock subtype and brain subtype, with more serious conditions.

2.4.1.2 Prolonged Bacillary Dysentery

The cases with prolonged bacillary dysentery commonly experience an illness course ranging from 2 weeks to 2 years, which is caused by prolonged incurable acute bacillary dysentery. The patients commonly experience no high fever, no abdominal pain, or no toxic symptoms, only with abdominal upset, poor appetite, and frequent bowel movements that are sometimes alternative bloody purulent stool and mucous stool. The routine stool culture shows lower positive rate than the acute stage.

2.4.1.3 Chronic Bacillary Dysentery

The patients with chronic bacillary dysentery experience an illness course of above 2 months. Its occurrence is commonly due to delayed or incomplete treatment at the acute stage or individual weakness, malnutrition, rickets, parasitism, anemia, and drug resistance.

2.4.2 Amebic Dysentery

The incubation period of intestinal amebiasis varies from 1–2 weeks to several months. Due to the earlier infection by the *Entamoeba histolytica* cyst, it is symbiotic with its host. When the host is subject to compromised immunity or intestinal infection, the clinical symptoms begin to show up. According to different clinical manifestations, it can be categorized into the following types:

2.4.2.1 Asymptomatic Type (Common in Cyst Carriers)

Although the patient is infected by *Entamoeba histolytica*, amebic protozoa are symbiotic with their host. About above 90 % of such cases show no symptoms, namely, cyst carriers, with amebic cyst detected in their stool. Under certain conditions, they can invade the tissue to cause symptoms of the disease.

2.4.2.2 Common Type

The onset is relatively chronic with mild systemic toxic symptoms. The patients commonly experience no fever but initially slight abdominal pain and diarrhea. The bowel movements are frequent, about ten times per day, and the stool is bloody with mucus. Blood and necrotic tissue are well mixed, appearing like fruit jam with a smell of decayed fish and containing amoeba trophozoites and erythrocyte aggregation, which are characteristic manifestations of the common type.

2.4.2.3 Mild Type

The mild type commonly occurs in strong healthy individuals, with slight symptoms. The patients experience bowel movements for three to five times per day, and the stool is paste-like or watery. In some other cases, the patients experience alternative occurrence of constipation and diarrhea. Otherwise, the patients experience only lower abdominal upset or dull pain and no diarrhea. The stool occasionally has mucus or a small quantity of blood, with the pathogenic cysts and trophozoites detected. The mild type has no complication and favorable prognosis.

2.4.2.4 Fulminant Type

The fulminant type is extremely rare, with a sudden and acute onset and obvious toxic symptoms such as aversion to cold, high fever, delirium, and toxic enteroparalysis. The patients experience severe abdominal pain, tenesmus, and diarrhea. The bowel movements can be as frequent as tens of times per day or even incontinence. The stools are bloody watery or watery, resembling to those in the cases of acute bacillary dysentery. However, the stools are extremely smelly and contain a large quantity of active amebic trophozoites, which is characteristically fulminant type. The patients may also experience vomiting, water loss, rapid collapse, peripheral circulatory disorder, and conscious disturbance. Even complications such as intestinal bleeding, intestinal perforation, and peritonitis occur, with poor prognosis. Delayed treatment may result in occurrence of death due to toxemia within 1–2 weeks.

2.4.2.5 Chronic Type

The chronic type occurs commonly due to inappropriate treatment at the acute stage, with alternative occurrences of abdominal pain, abdominal distension, diarrhea, and constipation. The symptoms or repeated episodes may persist for above 2 months to several years. Between episodes, the patients appear to be in good health. The repeated occurrence is commonly induced by inappropriate diet, eating and drinking too much, alcohol use, exposure to coldness, and fatigue, with diarrhea three to five times per day. The patients often experience lower abdominal distension and pain. Due to long-term intestinal dysfunction, the patients may experience emaciation, anemia, malnutrition, or neurosis. The thickened colon is palpable at the right lower quadrant with slight tenderness. The liver may be subject to enlargement with tenderness. The stool is yellowish paste-like, possibly with pus and blood. Trophozoites and sometimes cysts can be detected in the stool.

2.4.2.6 Others Type

Amebiasis may be manifested as infection of the urinary tract, reproductive system, and skin, but is extremely rare. It can also occur as a complication, which tends to be misdiagnosed.

2.5 Bacillary and Amebic Dysentery-Related Complications

2.5.1 Bacillary Dysentery-Related Complications

2.5.1.1 Dysentery Bacillus Septicemia

The disease is rare with double manifestations of bacillary dysentery and septicemia. The onset is similar to acute bacillary dysentery, but the symptoms deteriorate rapidly. It mainly occurs in infants aged under 1 year, children with malnutrition, and individuals initially with compromised immunity. The patients experience severe clinical symptoms, and the mortality rate can reach as high as 46 %. Timely medication of effective antibiotics can reduce its mortality rate.

2.5.1.2 Hemolytic Uremic Syndrome (HUS)

The disease is severe with unknown causes. It may be related to endotoxemia, cytotoxin, and immune complex deposition. And it is commonly diagnosed after sudden occurrence of hemoglobinuria (soy sauce-like color). The clinical manifestations include progressive hemolytic anemia, hypernatremia or acute renal failure, bleeding tendency, and thrombocytopenia.

2.5.1.3 Arthritis

The disease rarely occurs, which is closely related to the prevalence of *Shigella flexneri* or is secondary to *Shigella sonnei* infection. Otherwise, its occurrence is sporadic. The disease more commonly occurs at the major joints of young adult males, such as the knee, ankle, and elbow. Its occurrence is more commonly found at the major joints of lower limbs, and the lesions are asymmetrically distributed. Myotenositis and enthesitis are also characteristic manifestations of the disease. For mild type or the cases at the early stage, X-ray demonstrates no abnormalities. Following X-rays may demonstrate osteoporosis, narrowed joint cavity, and erosive changes. In severe cases, periostitis and periosteal proliferation occur. The positive rate of HLA-B27 of the disease is close to 80 %. The incidence rate of reactive arthritis is 7 % in the cases with positive *Shigella* infection, and the incidence rate of musculoskeletal symptoms (myotenositis, attachment lesion, and synovitis) is 2 % in the cases with positive *Shigella* infection. In severe cases, the disease can be complicated by ankylosing spondylitis.

2.5.1.4 Acute Infectious Toxic Encephalopathy

The disease is not directly caused by pathogens, but a series of immune responses to infection and toxin. Toxin contributes to the increase of brain vascular permeability, which further causes swelling of the nerve cells and increased water content around the vascular vessel. Therefore, acute diffuse encephaledema occurs. The toxin also contributes to cerebral vasospasm, which further causes hypoxia and ischemia of the brain tissue, with consequent occurrence of symptoms of the central nervous system.

2.5.1.5 Intussusception

In the cases of bacillary dysentery, frequent diarrhea can cause rhythm disturbance of peristalsis and more active peristalsis. The risk factors, such as structural abnormality, thin and long mesentery at the ileocecal junction in children, immature development and fixation, and large degree of ileocecal movement, cause the occurrence of intussusception. It can also be complicated by acute abdominal diseases such as intestinal perforation and appendicitis.

2.5.1.6 Other Complications

1. In the cases of severe diarrhea, dehydration, acidosis, electrolyte disturbance, hypotension, and peripheral circulatory failure may occur.
2. The senior citizens may develop myocardial infarction. Pregnant women with severe symptoms may sustain miscarriage or premature birth.
3. Prolonged chronic diarrhea may affect nutrition absorption, which further causes anemia and malnutritional edema.

2.5.2 Amebic Dysentery-Related Complications

Acute amebic dysentery-related complications can be divided into two types: enteral and parenteral.

2.5.2.1 Enteral Complications

Enteral Bleeding

Its incidence rate is less than 1 %, whose occurrence is mostly in patients with amebic dysentery or granuloma. The extensive intestinal lesions or vascular invasion at the intestinal wall by ulcers may cause bloody stool, with different quantities of blood volumes. Bloody stool with a small quantity of blood is commonly caused by superficial ulcer bleeding, while bloody stool with a large quantity of blood is caused by invasion of ulcerations to the inferior mucosa and major vascular vessels. Otherwise, massive bleeding is caused by granuloma.

Enteral Perforation
It is common in the cases of the fulminant type. Severe amoeba ulceration may deeply involve the serosa to cause perforation that is commonly found at the cecum, appendix, and ascending colon. Multiple perforations are more common, with acute perforation inducing severe diseases like diffuse peritonitis or abdominal abscess. Chronic perforation more commonly occurs, with no severe abdominal pain. The occurrence time of perforation can be hardly defined, and its diagnosis can be defined based on the finding of free-flowing gas under the abdominal diaphragm by X-ray.

Appendicitis
By autopsy of the death cases from amebic colonitis, about 6.2–40.9 % are reported to suffer from appendicitis. In China, it has been reported that only 0.9 % of the cases with amebic colonitis have appendix involved. The symptoms of amebic appendicitis resemble to common appendicitis, with acute and chronic manifestations and development into abscess. The patients experience chronic diarrhea or intestinal amebiasis. By laboratory test, the finding of amebic trophozoites or cysts in stool facilitates the diagnosis.

Ameboma
The disease is caused by formation of granuloma due to chronic inflammatory proliferative responses at the colonic wall. It more commonly occurs at the cecum as well as the transverse colon, rectum, and anus. The patients mostly experience abdominal pain and changes in bowel movements, and some patients may also experience accompanying intermittent dysentery, which may further induce intussusception and intestinal obstruction. By physical examination, the findings include palpable smooth goose egg-shaped or gut loop-like substance with mobility and tenderness at the right iliac fossa, which is demonstrated as a space-occupying lesion by X-ray. Biopsy facilitates its diagnosis.

Lumen Stenosis
It occurs in patients with chronic conditions. Fibrous tissue repair of intestinal ulcers can produce scar stenosis, with symptoms of abdominal cramp pain, vomiting, abdominal distension, and obstruction.

2.5.2.2 Parenteral Complications

Amoeba trophozoites can spread from the intestinal tract to distant organs along with blood and lymph flows to cause various parenteral complications. The involved organs include the liver, lung, pleura, pericardium, brain, peritoneum, urogenital ducts, and adjacent skin. The consequent lesions include abscess and ulceration, with hepatic abscess being more common.

Amebic Liver Abscess
Amebic liver abscess may occur at any stage of the disease or even several weeks or years after the disease is cured. The onset of amebic liver abscess is mostly long-term irregular fever, with a body temperature of above 39 °C, which is commonly the remittent type. The disease is clinically characterized by pain at the right upper quadrant or lower right chest, progressively enlarged liver, and obvious tenderness. In most cases, the lesion of abscesses is usually singular at the right liver lobe, which is related to the commonly occurring intestinal lesion at the ileocecum, whose blood flows to the right liver lobe via the superior mesenteric vein. In the cases with hepatic abscess at the left liver lobe, local symptoms and signs may be found within a short period of time. But its diagnosis is challenging.

Pulmonary and Pleural Amebiasis
The pathogens may spread from the liver or intestine, and mostly the diseases are secondary to hepatic amebiasis. Mostly via direct spread or along with lymph flow and rarely via systemic circulation, the pathogen can reach the lung, mostly at the right lung. Hepatic abscess complicated by pleural and pulmonary amebiasis accounts for 10–20 % of the cases, with common manifestations of bronchohepatic fistula, pleural effusion, pyothorax, pulmonary abscess, and pulmonary consolidation. In some cases, the disease is only manifested as chest pain, cough, and bloody sputum. Pleural and pulmonary amebiasis may be complicated by heart failure due to pneumonia, pleuritis, and myocardial toxicity.

Pericardial Amebiasis
The disease is commonly caused by penetration of amebic abscess at the left liver lobe into the pericardium, which is the most dangerous complication of the disease. Occasionally, the penetration of liver abscess may cause acute pericardial tamponade, which leads to shock and sudden death.

Brain Amebiasis
It rarely occurs and mostly is secondary to intestinal amebiasis, hepatic amebiasis, and pulmonary amebiasis. The protozoa can move from the intestine, liver, and lung to the brain along with blood flow to cause brain abscess. The symptoms resemble to purulent brain abscess. The disease has a sudden onset and rapid development. The brain parenchyma is demonstrated with multiple bleeding, malacia, and small suppurative lesion.

Amebic Peritonitis

The disease may be caused by penetration or direct spread of liver abscess and intestinal ulcers. When amebic liver abscess is complicated by peritonitis, jaundice more commonly occurs than simplex hepatic abscess. And it tends to be misdiagnosed as cholecystitis.

Urinary Tract Amebiasis

The symptoms include lower back pain and rice water-like urine. In the cases with the bladder involved, dysuria, urgent urination, and cloudy urine with blood are common. By urine test, protein, erythrocyte, leukocyte, and amoeba trophozoite can be detected.

Reproductive System Amebiasis

Amebiasis occurs at the reproductive system, such as amebic cervicitis and vaginitis with pain and bloody or bloody purulent secretions. In some cases, fistula is formed. By smear or biopsy of cervicovaginal secretions, amebic trophozoite can be detected.

Skin Amebiasis

The disease rarely occurs even in severely affected areas and tends to be clinically misdiagnosed. The lesion is commonly found at the perineal and perianal skin. It occurs secondary to chronic dysentery or penetration of amoeba in organs or local infection following surgical drainage. Occasionally, amoeba trophozoite can infect tissue around the anus along with blood flow to cause brown or dark reddish skin rashes in miliary size. The rash is flat and susceptible to bleeding that protrudes from the skin. The skin area with rash rapidly expands to cause ulcer and granuloma. Trophozoite can be detected from the lesion of the ulcer. Amebic granuloma often occurs at the perianal tissue and is secondary to dysentery with local tenderness. It tends to be misdiagnosed as condyloma, cancer, basaloma, syphilis, or tuberculosis.

2.6 Diagnostic Examination

2.6.1 Bacillary Dysentery

2.6.1.1 Laboratory Test

Routine Blood Test

In acute cases, total WBC count and the count of neutrophil granulocytes increase moderately, possibly with leftward shift of the nucleus. In chronic cases, mild anemia may be found.

Stool Examination

In typical stool from patients with dysentery, no substantial stool can be found. The stool is in small quantities, which is bright red and appears like sticky jelly, with no undesirable odor. Microscopy demonstrates large quantities of pyocytes and erythrocytes. Macrophages are also observable. In atypical cases, a small quantity of WBC is observed. The pathogenic bacteria can be detected after culture.

2.6.1.2 X-Ray

In chronic cases, barium X-ray demonstrates intestinal spasm, dynamic change, absent bag shape, luminal stenosis, and thickened intestinal mucosa or segmental intestinal mucosa.

2.6.1.3 Other Examinations

Fluorescence Antibody Staining

It is one of the rapid examinations for the diagnosis, which is more sensitive than cell culture.

Sigmoidoscopy

It demonstrates, at the acute stage, diffuse congestion of the intestinal mucosa, edema, a large quantity of effusion, superficial ulceration, and sometimes formation of pseudomembrane. At the chronic stage, the intestinal mucosa is demonstrated in grainy appearance, with formation of ulcers or polyps. Scrapings of secretion from the lesion for culture can increase the detection rate.

Staphylococcal Coagglutination Test

In recent years, it has been applied for rapid diagnosis of bacillary dysentery, which shows favorable specificity and sensitivity.

2.6.2 Amebic Dysentery

2.6.2.1 Laboratory Test

Routine Blood Test

The common type is demonstrated with normal total WBC count and cell counts. The fulminant type and the cases complicated by bacterial infection are demonstrated with increased WBC count and increased percentage of neutrophil granulocytes. The chronic cases are demonstrated with mild anemia.

Stool Examination

The stool is dark reddish with jam-like appearance and special fish odor. More substantial stool is found, with blood and mucus. Microscopy demonstrates a large quantity of erythrocyte aggregating into mass, a small quantity of leukocytes, and Charcot-Leyden crystals. The diagnosis can be defined based on the finding of mobile amebic trophozoites that can swallow erythrocytes. In chronic cases, amebic cyst can be found in the stool.

Stool Culture

By stool culture, the findings of dysentery bacillus and dysentery protozoa can define the diagnosis.

2.6.2.2 Radiological Examination

Barium enema X-ray demonstrates filling defect, stenosis, or obstruction at the lesion of ameboma. CT scanning demonstrates thickened intestinal wall and luminal stenosis.

2.6.2.3 Immunological Assay of Serum

Pure antigen of amoeba can be applied to detect specific antibody. When invasive disease occurs in the human body, the antibody is formed, and the antibody detection for cysts carriers is negative. By indirect hemagglutination test, indirect fluorescent antibody test, enzyme-linked immunosorbent assay, counter immunoelectrophoresis, agar gel precipitation test, and invasive bowel diseases including ameboma can be diagnosed, with a positive rate of 60–80 %.

2.6.2.4 Colonoscopy

Colonoscopy demonstrates scattering ulcers with different sizes, which has broad base and narrow opening as well as regular margin. Sometimes, a circle of red halo is observed. By smear of marginal ulcer or biopsy, trophozoite can be detected.

2.7 Imaging Demonstrations

2.7.1 Bacillary Dysentery

2.7.1.1 Enteric Lesions

In patients at the chronic stage, barium X-ray demonstrates intestinal spasm, dynamic change, absent bag shape, luminal stenosis, and thickened intestinal mucosa or segmental intestinal mucosa.

2.7.1.2 Arthropathy

In the early stage or for the mild type, X-ray demonstrates no abnormalities. The following X-rays demonstrate osteoporosis, narrowed joint cavity, or erosive change. In some severe cases, the patients experience periostitis and periosteal proliferation.

2.7.1.3 Toxic Encephalopathy

The white matter is mainly involved, with manifestations of diffuse symmetric swelling of the white matter in the cerebral hemisphere. The edema may be vasogenic edema or cytotoxic edema. MR imaging demonstrates extensive long T_1 and long T_2 signal shadows in the white matter under the cortex, with high DWI signal. CT scanning demonstrates low density at the corresponding sites.

2.7.1.4 Complication of Intussusception

Ultrasound

The cross section is characterized by small ring in a large ring sign, namely, concentric circle sign. The external ring is demonstrated as even low echo, which is an intestinal wall echo at the sheaths. The inner ring is demonstrated also as low echo. Between the external and inner rings, there is a high echo ring-shaped strip. However, on the longitudinal section, it is demonstrated as a pseudokidney sign.

Barium Meal Radiology

Intussusception is an acute abdominal disease, while the barium meal flows downwards slowly and hardly reaches the ileocecal junction. In addition, it poorly demonstrates the ileocecal junction. Therefore, the diagnostic rate of the disease is low. Thus the application of barium meal radiology is of no value for the diagnosis of intussusception and should be clinically avoided.

CT Scanning

At the early stage of intussusception, due to the shallow overlapping, a target-like lump with stratification surrounded by mesenteric adipose is demonstrated. As the overlapping part extends, characteristic laminar structure is present: the outer layer is featured by relative thin membrane-like structure; the middle layer is relatively thick with soft tissue density; the tissue closer to the neck of intussusceptions is thicker. This characteristic laminar structure is caused by blood circulation disturbance secondary to flip of the intestinal wall, as well as increased pressure of overlapping intestinal tube via axial peristalsis. The inner layer is commonly thinner than the middle layer. When the running course of the overlapping intestinal tube is vertical to the plane of CT scanning, the overlapping section is demonstrated with typical five concentric circles in different heights, and they are, from inner circle outwards, atrophic inner folded intestinal tube with relative high density, ring-shaped low-density mesenteric adipose with multiple small spots of shadows that are mesenteric vascular sections, high-density ring of mucosa of the middle layer, slightly low-density ring of the inferior mucosa and muscular layer of the middle layer, and high-density ring of serosa and external sheath of the middle layer. When air flows into the space between the middle layer and the outer layer, continual gas shadow can be observed in the space. In the cases with ascites or gas in the intestinal wall, blood circulation disturbance is indicated. By contrast imaging of the diseased intestinal tract and the normal intestinal tract, weaker enhancement or delayed enhancement indicates a blood circulation disorder at the intestinal wall.

2.7.2 Amebic Dysentery

2.7.2.1 Amebic Colonitis

CT scanning demonstrates extensive range with involvement of enteric lesions, including edema and diffuse thickening at the intestinal wall (Fig. 2.1). In the cases complicated by ulceration of the intestinal wall, the lesion may involve the blood vessels of the intestinal wall to cause hemafecia.

2.7.2.2 Amebic Liver Abscess

The radiological demonstrations vary at different stages of the disease. Typical liver abscess is demonstrated at the formation period of liver abscess, while atypical liver abscess is demonstrated at the suppurative inflammation period and early stage of the abscess formation. The atypical radiological demonstrations can be hardly differentiated from neoplasms. Therefore, at such stages, it tends to be misdiagnosed.

Case Study 1

A boy aged 13 years complained of diarrhea for above 2 months and bloody purulent stool for above 1 month. By stool examination, amebic cyst was demonstrated positive.

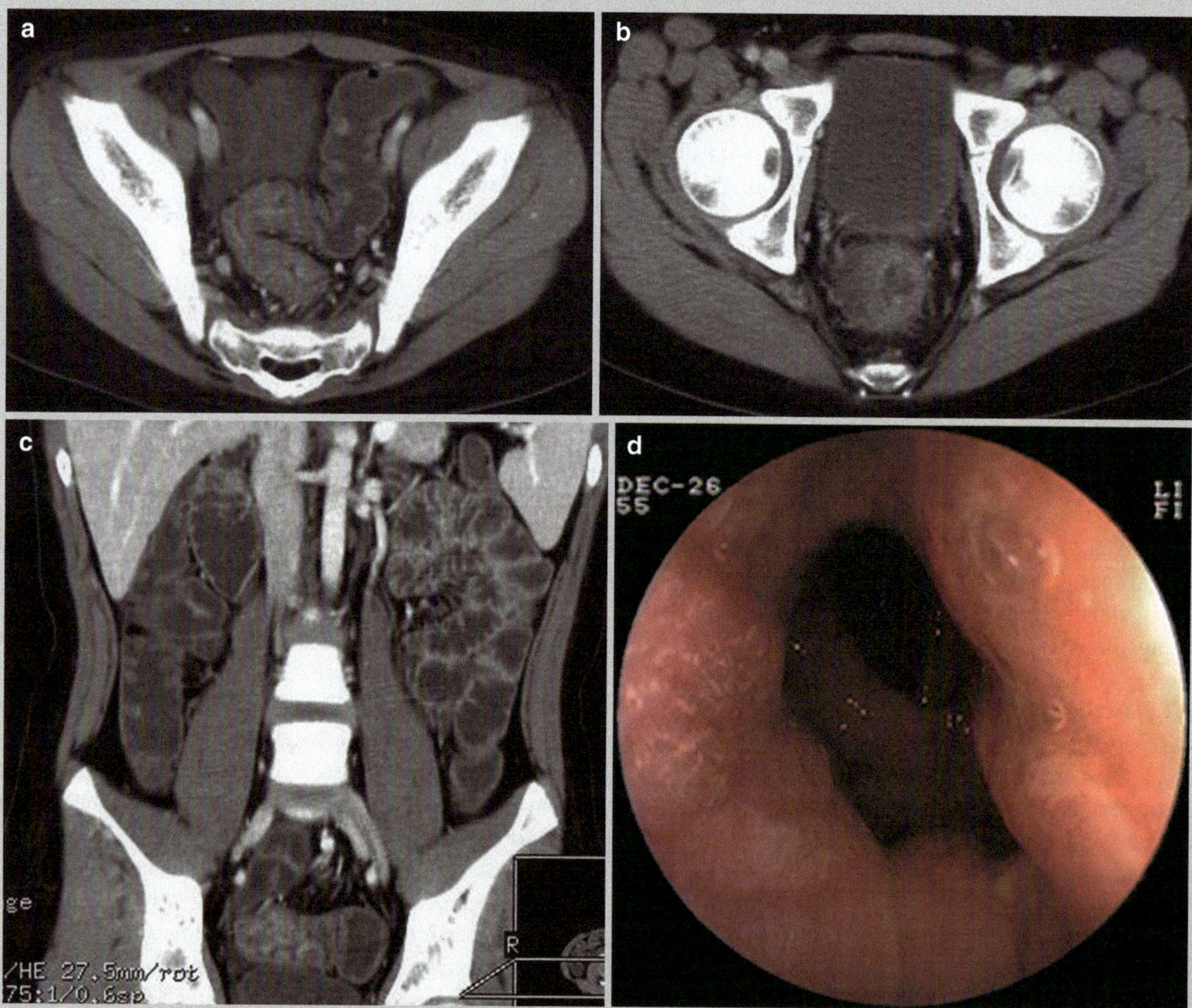

Fig. 2.1 Amoebic colonitis complicated by ulcerative colonitis. (**a–c**) Contrast CT scanning demonstrates diffuse thickening of the sigmoid colon wall and rectal wall as well as high density of abscess wall. (**d**) Colonoscopy demonstrates chronic inflammation of mucosa at the sigmoid colon and rectum

(Note: the case and the figures were provided by Tang, YH. from Ruijin Hospital, Shanghai, China)

Ultrasound

Typical Liver Abscess

Singular or multiple hypoechoic or anechoic mass is demonstrated. The abscess wall is demonstrated with strong echo and varied thickness. The outer wall is smooth, while the inner wall, irregular. Circular echo of edema is demonstrated that changes gradually from bright to dark around the abscess. The anechoic abscess cavity, strong echoic abscess wall, and hypoechoic surrounding edema form the ring-in-ring sign. In the cases with gas in the abscess, narrow and long strip of strong echo is demonstrated posterior to the lesion.

Atypical Liver Abscess

The liver is demonstrated with heterogeneous liquid dark area, which is well defined from the surrounding liver tissue. By ultrasound-guided liver puncture, typical fruit jam-colored pus with no unfavorable odor can be collected, which is of great diagnostic value.

Case Study 2

An adult male patient had a history of contact to patients with amebic dysentery in an epidemic area. By serological test, amoeba was detected positive.

(For case detail and figures, please refer to Blessmann, J, et al. *Trop Med Int Health*, 2006, 11 (4): 504.)

Case Study 3

A male patient aged 38 years experienced right upper quadrant abdominal pain, hepatosplenomegaly, and a small quantity of ascites. The bacterial culture was negative. By microscopy, amebic trophozoite was detected.

(For case detail and figures, please refer to Mandal SK, et al. *World J Gastroenterol*, 2006, 12 (25): 4109.)

CT Scanning

Typical Liver Abscess

Plain CT scanning demonstrates the abscess cavity as round or round-like low-density area. The abscess wall is demonstrated as a ring-shaped strip with slightly higher density than abscess cavity but lower density than normal liver tissue. Contrast CT scanning demonstrates obvious ring-shaped enhancement of the abscess wall and no enhancement of the abscess cavity and surrounding edema. The lesion is demonstrated as a ring-shaped target sign, which may be singular ring, double rings, and triple rings. The singular ring shows the abscess wall, without obvious surrounding edema. Double ring sign shows the abscess wall by the middle space and inner ring and surrounding edema by the outer ring (Fig. 2.2). The triple ring sign shows, from inner ring outwards, a ring with inflammatory tissue, fibrous granulation tissue, and edema as well as the other two rings of the abscess wall. The external ring is a fibrous granulation tissue, with obvious enhancement by contrast scanning. The inner ring is an inflammatory necrotic tissue, with less obvious enhancement by contrast scanning.

Atypical Liver Abscess

By plain CT scanning, the demonstrations are not characteristic, with evenly low or equal and low mixed-density shadow in the liver and poorly defined lesion boundary that is partially clear but not sharp. Contrast CT scanning demonstrates internal structure and the blood supply of the lesion, which are categorized into five typical signs:

Abscess Shrinkage Sign

It is manifested as slight to moderate enhancement of the lesion at the delayed phase. The lesion is demonstrated with equal density change like surrounding liver parenchyma. Edema strip surrounding the abscess is absent at the portal vein phase. The lesions are demonstrated to be smaller than that by plain CT scanning, or even cannot demonstrated, suggesting purulent inflammatory stage of the abscess or inflammatory response after incomplete liquefaction of abscess in liver tissue.

Peripheral Congestion Sign

By contrast scanning, the liver tissue surrounding the abscess is demonstrated with high perfusion and transient obvious enhancement at the arterial phase. The enhancement of the liver tissue is wedge shaped or in large flake, with the range confined within the liver tissue surrounding abscess or hepatic segment of the abscess. The enchantment rapidly fades away. Until the portal vein phase and early parenchyma phase, the enhancement of the surrounding liver tissue is not obvious. The detection rate of such a sign is up to 75 %. The sign is caused by decreased blood flow in the portal vein and compensatorily increased blood flow in the hepatic artery due to stenosis of the intrahepatic portal vein arising from inflammation of the portal area.

Cluster-Like Sign

Multiple tiny abscesses (<2 cm) gather into mass or fuse together, with honeycomb-like enhancement.

Petallike Sign

Petallike sign is found in the cases with multilocular abscess. Inflammatory responses can be demonstrated at the residual locular septum in the abscesses, with relatively obvious enchantment. Several adjacent septa in combination are demonstrated in a petallike sign, with mixed low-density area of less obvious enhancement.

Delayed Enhancement Sign

Long-term persistence of abscess enchantment, the lesion density being relatively higher or equal to liver parenchyma with poorly defined boundary, and shrinkage of the lesion suggest the purulent inflammation stage or proliferative reactions after destructions by purulent inflammation.

Inflammatory edema around the abscess wall and alive liver tissue with equal density enhancement are caused by capillary inflammatory congestion at the inflammatory granulation tissue of the abscess wall and its consequent increase of permeability. Therefore, slow exosmose and slow discharge of contrast agent occur.

Case Study 4

A male patient aged 31 years experienced fever and diarrhea with jam-colored stool with no known causes, tenesmus, and dull pain at the right upper quadrant. Amebic serum antibody IgM was positive.

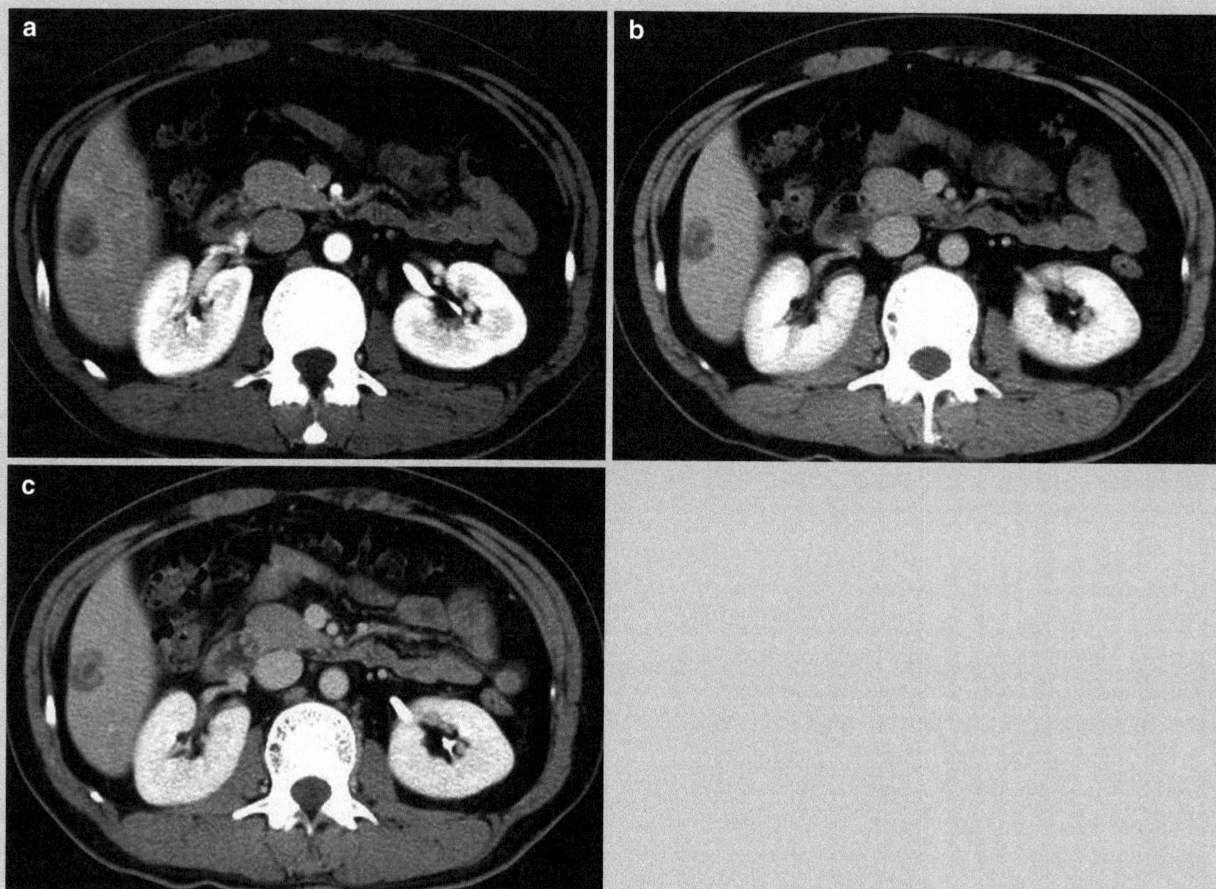

Fig. 2.2 Amoebic liver abscess. (**a–c**) CT scanning demonstrates the lesion at the right posterior inferior liver lobe with quite well-defined boundary, central low density of the abscess, and no enhancement at the artery phase, portal vein phase, and delayed phase. The abscess wall is demonstrated to be smooth with ring-shaped enhancement, which is surrounded by low-density edema strip

(Note: the case and the figures were proved by Tang, YH. from Ruijin Hospital, Shanghai, China.)

Case Study 5

An adult male experienced fever, jaundice, and abdominal pain. Amebic trophozoite was detected by microscopy.

A. Ultrasound demonstrates abscess at the right liver lobe.

B. Contrast CT scanning demonstrates abscess at the right liver lobe with inner gas density shadow during the venous phase and involved right hepatic vein.

(For case detail and figures, please refer to Singh V, et al. *Am J Trop Med Hyg*, 2008, 78 (4): 556.)

Case Study 6
A male patient aged 29 years complained of right upper quadrant pain and high fever 5 years ago. Amebic trophozoite was detected by microscopy.

Case Study 7
A female patient aged 43 years experienced fever, chills, epigastric pain, nausea, and vomiting. She was diagnosed with amebic liver abscess.

(For case detail and figures, please refer to Kim TY, et al. *Korean J Parasitol*, 2010, 48 (2): 157.)

Case Study 8
A male patient aged 37 years experienced fever and right upper quadrant pain. Enzyme-linked immunosorbent assay demonstrated positive amoeba antibody.

(For case detail and figures, please refer to Miller Q, et al. *Curr Surg*, 2000, 57 (5): 476.)

Case Study 9
A male patient aged 57 years complained of fever, poor appetite, and right abdominal pain for 15 days, which was persistent dull pain. Enzyme-linked immunosorbent assay was positive, with IgG 1:1,600.

(For case detail and figures, please refer to Sodhi KS, et al. *J EmerG Med*, 2008, 34 (2): 155.)

Case Study 10
Two patients with amebic dysentery came from an epidemic area. Their diagnosis was amebic liver abscess.

(For case detail and figures, please refer to Mortele KJ, et al. *Radiographics*, 2004, 24 (4): 937.)

MR Imaging

Typical Liver Abscess

Plain MR imaging demonstrates the abscess cavity with long T_1 and long T_2 signal. The signal of the abscess wall is slightly higher than the abscess cavity but is lower than a normal liver tissue. The edema surrounding the abscess is demonstrated with slightly low T_1WI signal and slightly high T_2WI signal, namely, the halo sign. Contrast MR imaging demonstrates ring-shaped enhancement of the abscess with even thickness, but no enhancement of the abscess cavity.

Atypical Liver Abscess

Plain MR imaging demonstrates the lesion with equal or low T_1WI signal but poorly defined contour and varied T_2WI signal that is possibly high, equal, or low, representing granulation tissue with rich blood supply, fibrous granulation tissue, and fibrous tissue, respectively. The abnormal signal at the hepatic segment is relatively low T_1WI signal, which is hardly distinguished from the lesion, but high T_2WI signal, which is even and lower than the lesion. Contrast MR imaging demonstrates obvious and delayed enhancement of the granulation tissue with rich blood supply at the artery phase, while gradually obvious enhancement of the fibrous granulation tissue along with delayed time. DWI demonstrates high signal of the abscess cavity with low ADC value.

Case Study 11
A male patient aged 24 years complained of right upper abdominal pain and fever for 5 days and tachycardia. Enzyme-linked immunosorbent assay detected positive amoeba antibody.

Case Study 12
A male patient aged 61 years complained of fever for 8 days, vomiting for 5 days, right upper abdominal pain, and both feet edema for 3 days. Enzyme-linked immunosorbent assay detected positive amoeba antibody.

The cases of 11 and 12 are published in Sarda AK, et al. *Korean J Hepatol*, 2011, 17 (1): 71.

For case detail and figures, please refer to Sarda AK, et al. *Korean J Hepatol*, 2011, 17 (1): 71.

2.7.2.3 Pulmonary and Pleural Amebiasis

Chest X-Ray and CT Scanning

The demonstrations include pleural effusion and elevated diaphragm. There are pneumonia type, round mass type, cavity type, pneumothorax type, and cardiac valve involved type. The cardiac valve involved type is demonstrated with exudative change in the medial and middle parts of both lungs and diffuse intra-alveolar exudation with hilum as the center (Fig. 2.3).

Cardiac Color Ultrasound

The chordae tendineae of the mitral valve is demonstrated with rupture and prolapsed. Moderate or severe incomplete closure of the mitral valve can be demonstrated. Pressure gradient can be detected from the right to the left venous system.

Case Study 13

A female patient aged 22 years experienced fever with a body temperature of 39.4 °C, right chest pain, fatigue, and diarrhea. She was diagnosed with pleural amebiasis.

(For case detail and figures, please refer to Uslu A, et al. *Respiration*, 2004, 71 (4): 424.)

Case Study 14

A male patient aged 52 years, an American soldier, reported a history of living in Libya for 3 months. He complained of fever, right upper abdominal pain, and bloody stool for 10 days. By enzyme-linked immunosorbent assay, amoeba antibody was detected positive in the pleural effusion. Serum IgG antibody was detected positive.

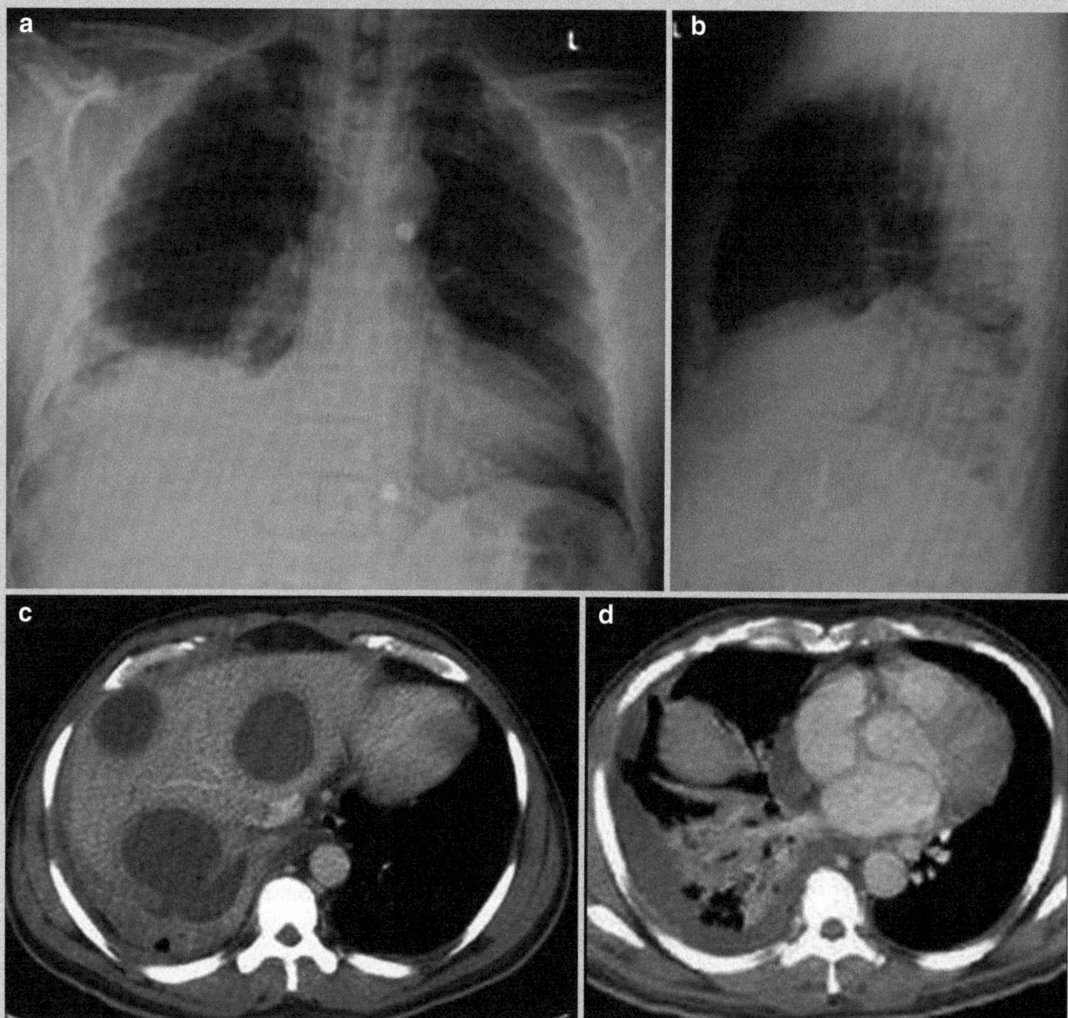

Fig. 2.3 Pulmonary and pleural amebiasis. (**a**, **b**) X-ray demonstrates elevated right diaphragm and arch line-like shadow which is laterally high and medially low, suggesting right pleural effusion. (**c**) CT scanning demonstrates multiple abscesses in the liver, the largest one in size of 7×7 cm, which involves the diaphragm, with diaphragm perforation in length of about 2.75 cm. (**d**) CT scanning demonstrates inflammation at the right lower lung lobe, right pleural effusion which skips from anterior vertebra to its contralateral counterpart, leftward shift of the mediastinum, and pericardial effusion. (**e**, **f**) Reexamination after treatment for 6 weeks demonstrates absorbed and improved inflammation at the right lung and pleural effusion and shrinkage of liver abscess (Reprint with permission from Shrestha M, et al. *Sout H Med J*, 2010, 103 (2): 165.)

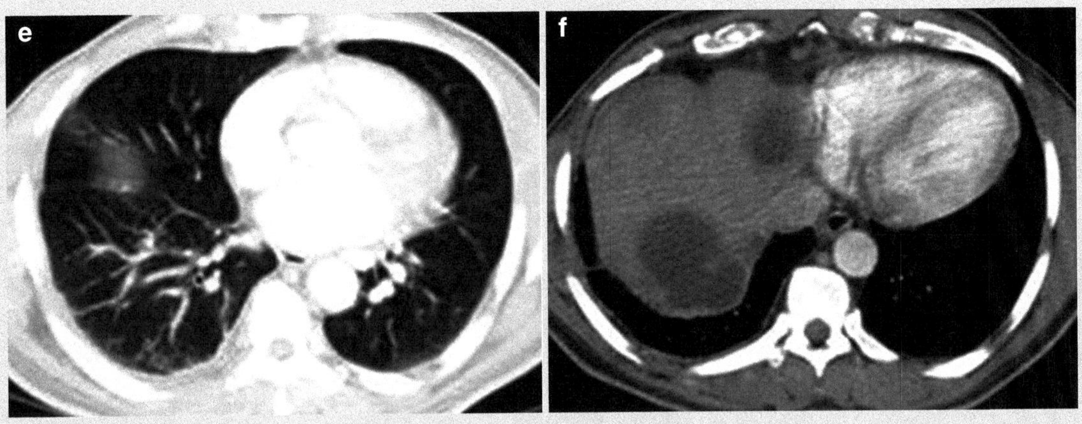

Fig. 2.3 (continued)

Case Study 15
A male patient aged 27 years, a homosexual, experienced dyspnea and right upper abdominal pain. By indirect hemagglutination test, amoeba antibody was detected positive.

(For case detail and figures, please refer to Chang HR, et al. *Intern Med*, 2010, 51 (5): 471.)

Case Study 16
A male patient aged 41 years experienced diarrhea, fever, and progressive dyspnea. He reported a medical history of amebic colonitis.

(For case detail and figures, please refer to Yokoyama T, et al. *Infect Drug Resist*, 2010, 3: 1.)

2.7.2.4 Brain Amebiasis

Brain Abscess

The cerebral parenchyma is demonstrated with multiple hemorrhage, malacia, and small suppurative foci. CT scanning and MR imaging demonstrate irregular lesion with no envelope and no surrounding ring-shaped enhancement.

Granulomatous Amebic Encephalitis

The disease is a necrotizing granulomatous encephalitis at the temporal lobe, brainstem, and cerebellum. Ventriculitis and choroiditis may also occur. It is pathologically characterized by scattering local necrotizing cystic space-occupying lesion. CT scanning and MR imaging demonstrate singular or multiple low-density or mixed-density space-occupying lesions at the basal ganglia, cerebral cortex, subcortical white matter, cerebellum, and pons, with ring-shaped enhancement by contrast scanning or imaging. The lesion may be surrounded by edema. In the cases with small lesions, solid nodular enhancement can be demonstrated, with inapparent surrounding edema (Figs. 2.4, 2.5, 2.6, and 2.7).

Case Study 17
A male patient aged 43 years complained of aphasia, generalized weakness, dizziness, and ataxia for 4 days. He reported a medication history of metronidazole to treat amebic liver abscess for 2 months, and he was diagnosed with metronidazole poisoning.

For case detail and figures, please refer to Kalia V. et al. *Indian J Radiol Imaging*, 2010, 20 (3): 195.

Case Study 18
A male patient aged 75 years experienced headache, slurred speech, and absentmindedness. He was diagnosed with granulomatous amebic encephalitis complicated by brain abscess.

For case detail and figures, please refer to Sarica FB, et al. *Turk Neurosur*, 2009, 19 (3): 256.

Case Study 19

A male patient aged 40 years experienced fever and dizziness. He was diagnosed with chronic granulomatous amebic encephalitis.

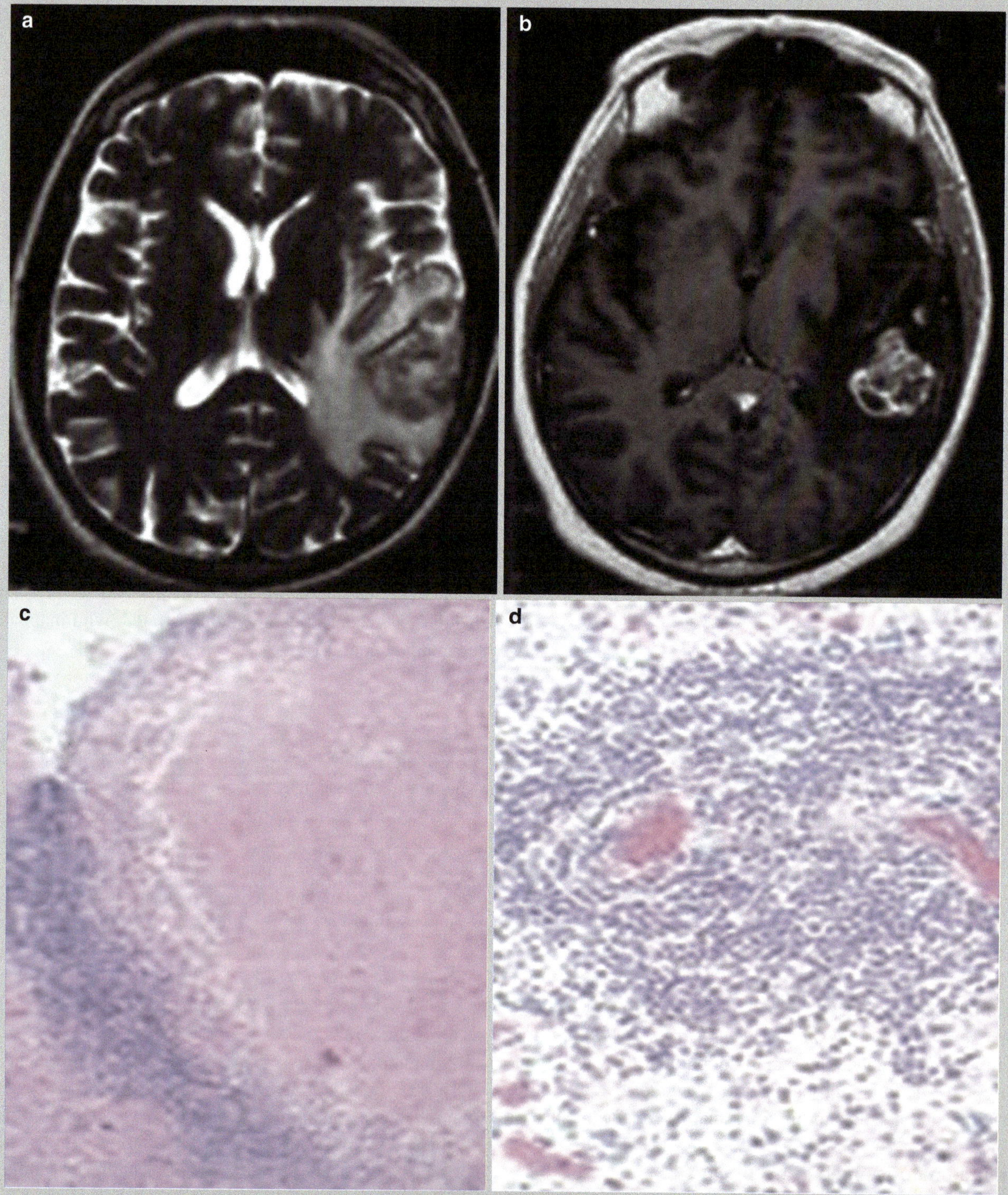

Fig. 2.4 Chronic granulomatous amebic encephalitis. (**a**) T2WI of MR imaging demonstrates mixed signal shadow at the left temporal and parietal lobes, with surrounding large flakes of edema signal. (**b**) Contrast T_1WI demonstrates floral hoop-like enchantment of the lesion at the left parietal lobe. (**c**) Microscopy demonstrates lymphocytes around cuff blood vessel (H&E staining, with original medium magnification). (**d**) Microscopy demonstrates necrotizing granulomatous inflammation (H&E staining, with original magnification) (Reprint with permission from Perez MT, et al. *Ann Diagn Pathol* 2007, 11 (6): 440.)

Case Study 20

Two cases of granulomatous amebic encephalitis. They experienced headache, fever, and behavioral abnormalities.

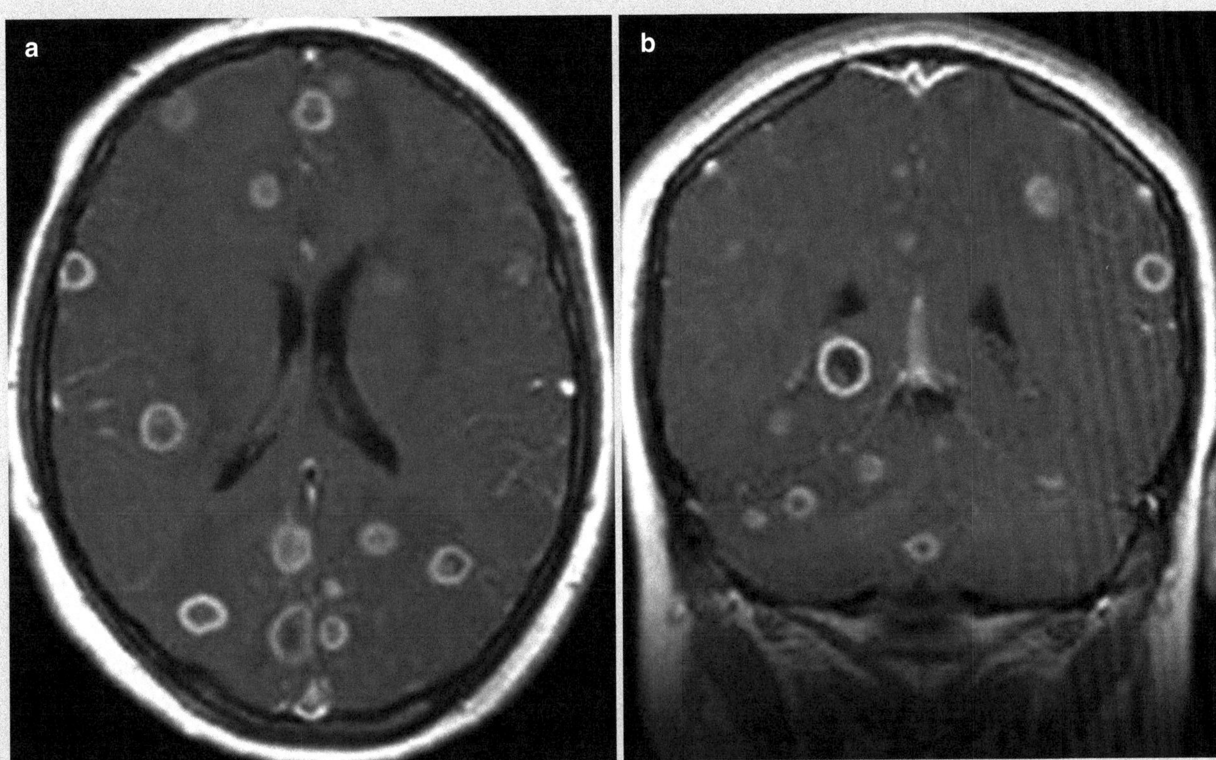

Fig. 2.5 Amoebic brain abscess. (**a**, **b**) Contrast T1WI of MRI demonstrates multiple lesions with ring-shaped enchantment in supratentorial and subtentorial brain parenchyma and involved bilateral frontal lobes, temporal lobes, and occipital lobes. Large lesions are demonstrated to be surrounded by low-density edema, with slight space-occupying effect (Reprint with permission from Schuster et al. FL, et al. *Clin Infect Dis* 2009, 48 (7): 879.)

Case Study 21

A male patient aged 55 years experienced headache, nausea, gait disturbance, paresthesia, quiver of the left arm, blurred speech, and loss of taste. He was diagnosed with amebic brain abscess.

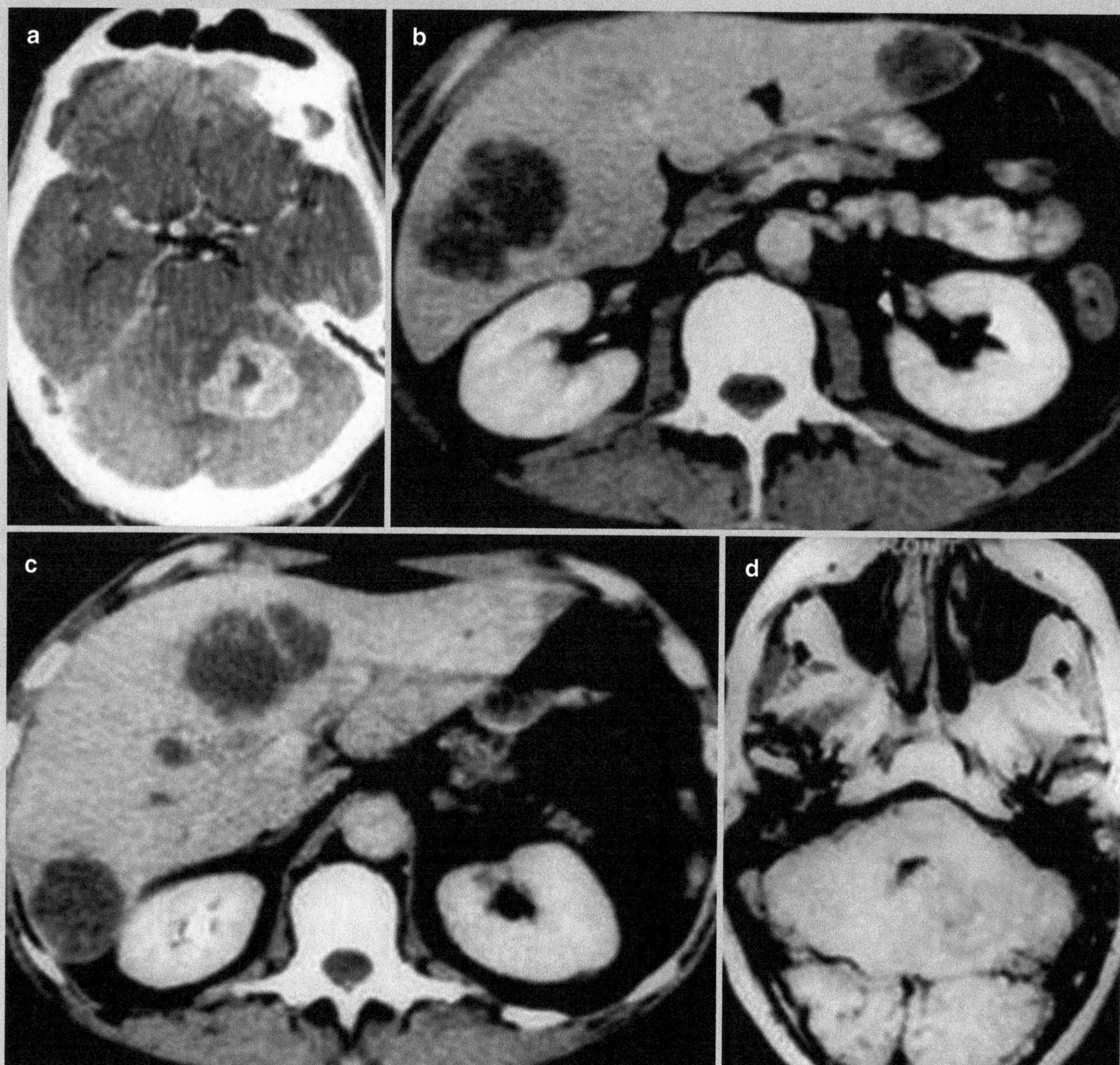

Fig. 2.6 Amoebic brain abscess. (**a**) Contrast CT scanning demonstrates ring-shaped enhancement of the lesion at the left cerebellar hemisphere, with surrounding focal edema. (**b**, **c**) CT scanning demonstrates multiple low-density lesions in the liver. (**d**) T_1WI of MR imaging demonstrates slightly low signal at the left cerebellar hemisphere. (**e**, **f**) Contrast T_1WI demonstrates obvious enchantment of the lesion. (**g**) Reexamination after treatment demonstrates obvious shrinkage of the hepatic lesion (Reprint with permission from Dietz R, et al. *J Comput Assist Tomogr* 1991, 15 (1): 168.)

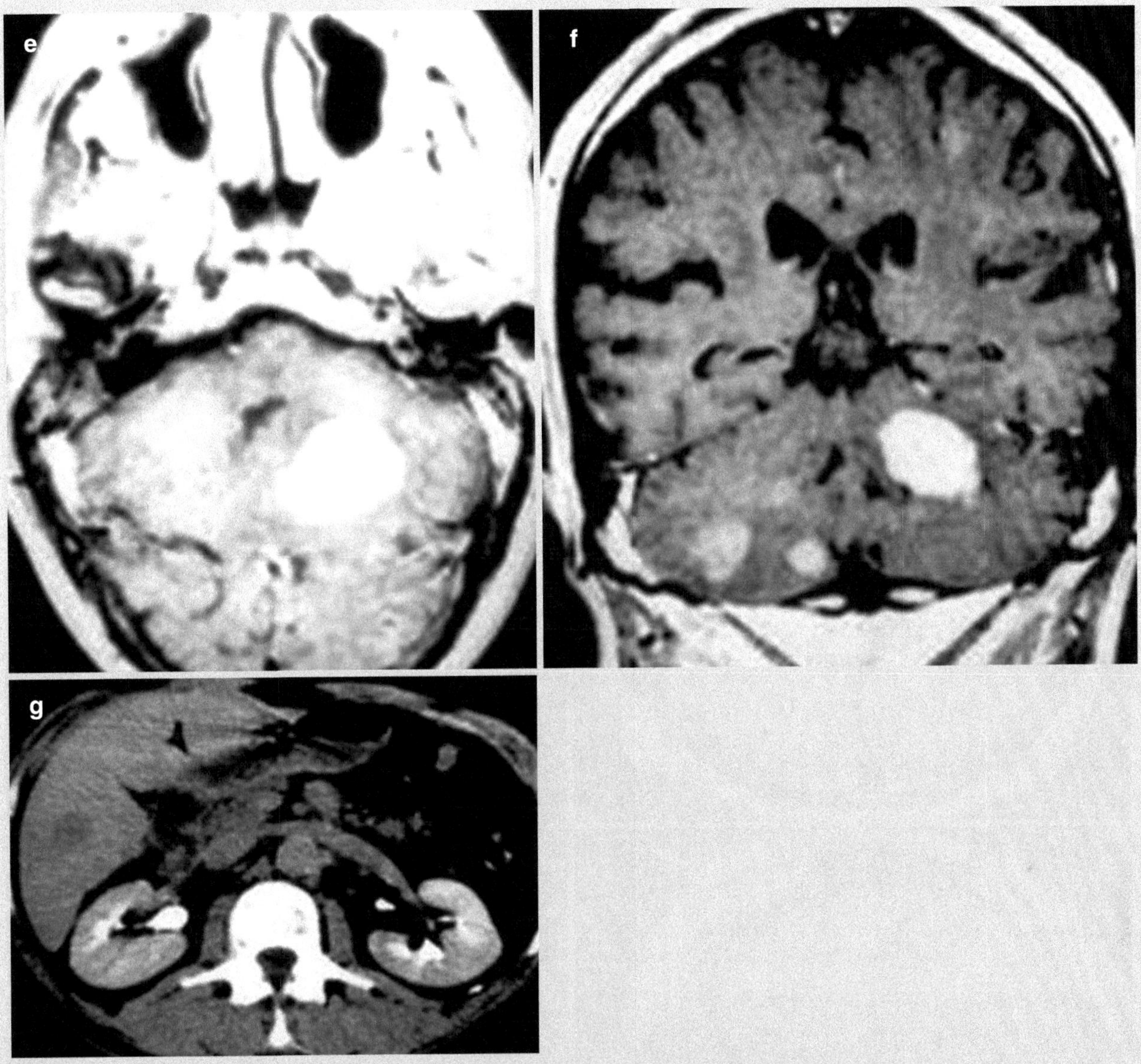

Fig. 2.6 (continued)

Case Study 22

A male patient aged 38 years, a homosexual, experienced rapid growth of a lump at the right thigh, multiple subcutaneous small nodules at the neck and face, and dizziness. By puncture and biopsy, amebic trophozoite was detected. He was diagnosed with granulomatous amebic encephalitis.

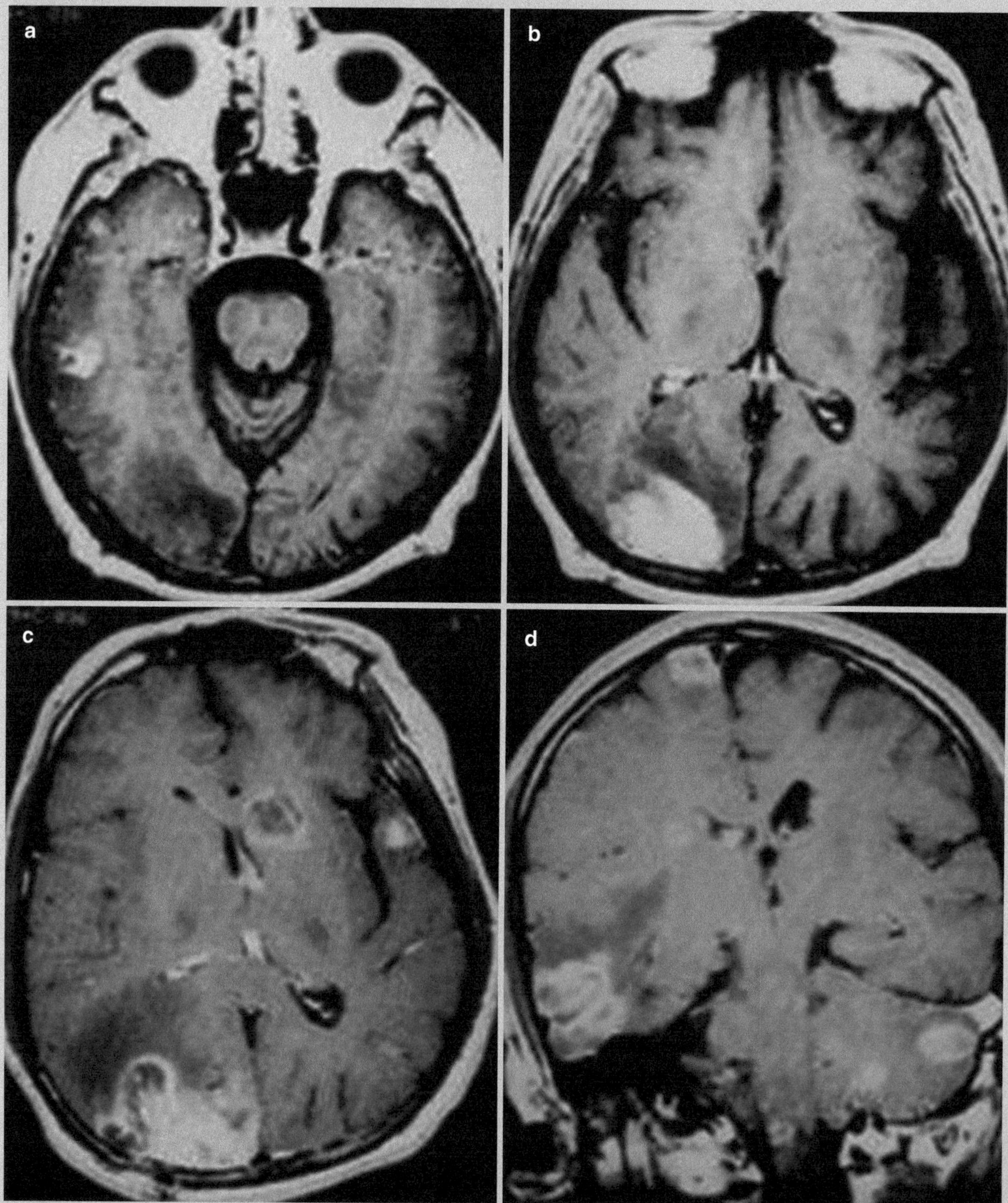

Fig. 2.7 Amoebic brain abscess. (**a**, **b**) Contrast T_1WI of MR imaging demonstrates enhancement of the lesions at the right temporal lobe and occipital lobe with surrounding edema. (**c**, **d**) Reexamination after 1 month demonstrates progress of the conditions. Contrast T_1WI demonstrates enlarged lesion at the right occipital lobe and new lesions at the left caudate nucleus and left temporal lobe. Coronary contrast T_1WI demonstrates new lesions at the right cerebral hemisphere, left cerebellar hemisphere, midbrain, and brainstem (Reprint with permission from Deol I, et al. *Surg Neurol* 2000, 53 (6): 611.)

2.8 Diagnostic Basis

2.8.1 Bacillary Dysentery

Its diagnosis is mainly based on epidemiological history, clinical manifestations, laboratory tests, and radiological demonstrations. The diagnosis can be defined based on etiological examination.

2.8.1.1 Epidemiological Data

The disease more commonly occurs in summers and autumns. The patients usually have a history of intake of contaminated food or contact to patient with bacillary dysentery.

2.8.1.2 Clinical Manifestations

Acute Atypical Bacillary Dysentery

The symptoms are mild with only diarrhea and loose stools.

Acute Typical Bacillary Dysentery

The disease has acute onset with diarrhea (with other causes excluded), abdominal pain, tenesmus, fever, bloody purulent stool or mucous stool, and tenderness at the left lower abdomen.

Acute Toxic Bacillary Dysentery

The disease has acute onset, with high fever and serious toxemic symptoms. In young children, no obvious symptoms of abdominal pain and diarrhea can be found at the early stage. By stool examination after enema or anal swab, bacillary dysentery can be found. The disease can be divided into the following types based on the clinical manifestations:

1. Shock type (peripheral circulatory failure type)
   The patients experience symptoms of infectious shock, such as pale complexion, cold limbs, fine and rapid pulse, decline of blood pressure, skin disturbances, and cyanosis.
2. Brain type (respiratory failure type)
   The patients experience symptoms of encephaledema, including irritation, convulsions, drowsiness or coma, pupil change, and even cerebral hernia and respiratory failure.
3. Mixed type
   The patients experience simultaneous symptoms of shock type and brain type, which is the most dangerous type.

Chronic Prolonged Bacillary Dysentery

The patients usually have a history of acute bacillary dysentery. The illness course usually lasts for above 2 months, and the disease is not healed.

2.8.1.3 Laboratory Tests

Routine Blood Test

At the acute stage, the WBC count slightly or moderately increases, with increased count of neutrophil granulocytes. At the chronic stage, anemia can be found.

Stool Examination

Routine Examination

By appearance, the stool has mucus, pus, and blood. By microscopy, large quantities of pyocytes or leukocytes (15 or above per high-power field) and erythrocytes are detected. The finding of phagocytes facilitates the diagnosis.

Etiological Examination

By stool culture, the positive finding of *Shigella* is the evidence to define the diagnosis.

2.8.1.4 Radiological Examination

X-ray barium demonstrates the chronic stage with intestinal spasms, dynamic change, absent bag shape, luminal narrowing, and thickening of the intestinal mucosa or segmental intestinal mucosa.

2.8.2 Amebic Dysentery

2.8.2.1 Diagnostic Principle

The chief complaints, case history, clinical manifestations, and radiological demonstrations provide references for the diagnosis. In addition, etiological examination provides important evidence to define the diagnosis. Detection of amebic pathogens in the stool provides the only reliable evidence to define the diagnosis. Generally, the patients with detectable large trophozoites are defined as present cases of amebic dysentery, while the patients with detectable small trophozoites or cysts are defined as infected cases of amebic dysentery.

2.8.2.2 Diagnostic Criteria

Symptoms and Signs

Acute Amebic Dysentery (The Common Type)

The disease is characterized by slightly chronic onset, abdominal pain, diarrhea, and moderate quantity of stool with blood and mucus. The stool is dark reddish-like fruit jam with fishy odor. The patients may also experience tenderness of the right lower abdomen.

Fulminant Amebic Dysentery

The disease has an acute onset with obvious toxic symptoms such as high fever, abdominal pain, diarrhea, dozens of bowel movements per day, and even incontinence. The stool is watery or bloody watery with extremely unpleasant odor. The patients may also experience dehydration, electrolyte disturbance, and shock.

Chronic Amebic Dysentery

The illness course lasts for above several months, with repeated occurrence of or persistent symptoms.

Etiological Examination

Stool Examination

The stool is dark reddish with mucus and special fishy odor. Microscopy demonstrates the mucus containing many erythrocytes that aggregate into mass, rare leukocytes, sometimes Charcot-Leyden crystals, and active trophozoites.

By direct smear, active trophozoites can be detected.

In clinical practice, iodine solution smear is commonly applied to detect the features and quantity of the nucleus.

Histological Examination

By sigmoidoscopy or fibro-colonoscopy, mucosal ulcers can be directly observed. Scattering prowling ulcers can be observed in different sizes, with slightly protruding margin, red halo, and mostly normal mucosa between ulcers. By biopsy or scrapings for smear, the detection rate is high.

X-Ray Barium Enema Examination

The findings include thickened intestinal wall and lumen stenosis. Focalized filling defect indicates the formation of ameboma. CT scanning demonstrates thickened intestinal wall and luminal stenosis.

Immunologic Diagnosis

For serology test, pure amebic antigen can be applied to detect the specific antibody. Indirect hemagglutination test shows relatively high sensitivity, with a positive rate for intestinal amebiasis being 98 % and for extrenteral amebiasis being 95 %. The sensitivity of indirect fluorescent antibody test is lower than IHA. Enzyme-linked immunosorbent assay has high sensitivity and specificity. Complement fixation test has important diagnostic value for extrenteral amebiasis, with a positive rate above 80 %.

Diagnostic Treatment

Clinically, the highly suspected cases whose diagnosis cannot be defined by above examinations can be administered sufficient dose of emetine by injection or oral medication of phanquinone or metronidazole for treatment. The cases with effective therapeutic efficacy can be preliminary defined as amebic dysentery.

2.8.3 Amebic Dysentery-Related Complications

2.8.3.1 Amebic Liver Abscess

Clinical Manifestations

The patients with amebic dysentery or the individuals with a past history of amebic dysentery experience clinical symptoms of upper abdominal pain or lower right chest pain, progressive hepatomegaly, and obvious tenderness.

Radiological Demonstrations

Liver or brain CT scanning demonstrates singular or multiple low-density area. MR imaging demonstrates long T_1 and long T_2 signals of the lesion. Ultrasound demonstrates low echo from the lesion. And contrast scanning or imaging demonstrates enhancement of the abscess wall and the septum, with a typical ring sign.

Puncture and Biopsy

The diagnosis can be defined after amebic trophozoites are detected in the pus.

2.8.3.2 Pulmonary and Pleural Amebiasis

Clinical Symptoms

The patients with amebic dysentery experience clinical symptoms of chest pain, cough, and bloody sputum.

Radiological Demonstrations

By radiological examinations, the patients are demonstrated with pneumonia, intrapulmonary cavity, pleural effusion, and pyopneumothorax.

Laboratory Test

By laboratory test, trophozoites of amoeba dysenteriae are detected in sputum or chest tissue.

Diagnostic Treatment

The cases with no laboratory finding of trophozoites of amoeba dysenteriae but are rapidly improved and even cured after receiving anti-amebic medication.

2.8.3.3 Brain Amebiasis

Clinical Symptoms

The patients with amebic dysentery experience symptoms of the central nervous system, such as headache and dizziness.

Radiological Demonstrations

By radiological examinations, brain abscess and granulomatous encephalitis are detected.

Etiological Examination

The definitive diagnosis should be based on the finding of amebic trophozoites and cysts at brain lesions. Otherwise, the finding of amebic trophozoites and cysts by smear, especially by early biopsy, should be the basis to define the diagnosis.

2.9 Differential Diagnosis

2.9.1 Bacillary Dysentery

In the prevailing seasons of bacillary dysentery, the cases with a history of contacting dysentery or a history of intake unhygienic food and experiencing symptoms of fever, bloody mucopurulent stool, and tenesmus should be suspected as bacillary dysentery. In summers and autumns, the patients experiencing sudden high fever, convulsions, pale complexion, coldness of terminal limbs, and rapid fine pulses should be suspected with toxic dysentery. Bacillary dysentery is clinically characterized by vomiting and diarrhea. However, the cases experiencing severe vomiting and persistent severe abdominal pain should firstly be excluded in the possibilities of other intestinal and extrenteral diseases to avoid misdiagnosis.

2.9.1.1 Acute Dysentery Should Be Differentiated from the Following Diseases

Pathogenic *E. coli* Enteritis

The disease commonly occurs in children aged under 2 years with a relatively higher incidence in those aged 5–8 months. The patients experience frequent bowel movements of mucous stool with fishy odor that is egg soup-like. Dehydration and acidosis tend to occur. By microscopy, leukocytes and pyocytes can be observed. By bacterial culture of stool, the diagnosis can be defined.

Salmonella Enteritis

Its occurrence is commonly within a family or a certain group of people, with common symptoms of vomiting and green jellylike mucus in stool. Tenesmus rarely occurs. By bacteria culture of stool, the diagnosis can be defined.

Viral Diarrhea

It is commonly acute intestinal infection caused by rotavirus or Norwalk virus, which commonly occurs in children aged under 2 years. The disease has an acute onset, with upper respiratory infection and watery or egg soup-like stool with little mucus and no fishy odor. Fecal bacterial culture is negative. Immunoelectron microscopy, enzyme-linked immunosorbent assay (ELISA), polyacrylamide gel electrophoresis, and virus isolation facilitate the diagnosis of the disease.

Amebic Dysentery

The disease is commonly found in southern area of China, and it has a chronic onset. The patients experience rarely toxemic symptoms, relatively mild tenesmus, less frequent bowel movements, and mostly right abdominal pain. The typical cases show jam-like stool with putrefactive odor. By microscopy, a small quantity of leukocytes and erythrocyte aggregation can be observed, commonly with Charcot-Leyden crystals and detectable amebic trophozoites. Sigmoidoscopy demonstrates mostly normal mucosa with scattering ulcers. It tends to be complicated by liver abscess. Ultrasound and CT scanning facilitate the diagnosis.

Vibrio parahaemolyticus Enteritis

The disease is caused by *Vibrio parahaemolyticus* (*Halobacterium salinarum*), which is a common type of bacterial food poisoning. It is clinically characterized by a history of eating seafood or salted food, rapid and simultaneous occurrence of the disease in people have dinner together, paroxysmal abdominal cramps, nausea, vomiting, and mostly no tenesmus. The stool is mucous and bloody or watery bloody with special odor. The vomits and suspected food can be collected for bacteria culture, whose result has diagnostic value.

Intussusceptions

The disease is one of the most common acute abdominal diseases during infancy and early childhood. It is also the most common cause of intestinal obstruction in children aged 3 months to 6 years, with children aged under 2 years accounting for 80 % of the cases. The typical manifestations include paroxysmal abdominal pain, vomiting, bloody stool, and abdominal mass, whose diagnosis presents no challenge. However, in the early stage, the above manifestations are atypical, and the patients experience drooping spirits, drowsiness, pale complexion, bloody stool, as well as paroxysmal crying and screaming. Such cases are susceptible to misdiagnosis or missed diagnosis. Abdominal mass is an important sign for the diagnosis of acute intussusceptions in children. Its missed diagnosis or misdiagnosis is commonly due to crying and screaming of children who show poor compliance to physical examination or insufficient expertise of the physician to palpate the abdominal mass. Anal examination is of great important value for the diagnosis of the disease. In the cases of intussusceptions, about 30 % of the patients can experience bowel movements of bloody stool by themselves. And about 60 % show bloody stool by digital rectal examination. Sometimes by digital rectal examination, a cervical-like substance can be touched, which has great diagnostic value. If necessary, enema with a small quantity of saline can be performed for early detection of bloody stool between proximal colon and rectum. By abdomen ultrasound or CT scanning, multiple concentric ring sign can be demonstrated in affected children, which facilitates to define the diagnosis.

2.9.1.2 Toxic Bacillary Dysentery Should Be Differentiated from the Following Diseases

High Fever and Convulsion

The disease often occurs in infants with a past history of repeated episodes of high fever and convulsion. Its etiological factors can be defined. After treatment for high fever, convulsion disappears along with returning of the body temperature to normal.

Toxic Pneumonia

The patients usually have a past history of exposure to coldness and experience early symptoms and signs of infective shock and pneumonia. Chest X-ray and CT scanning demonstrate pulmonary infection. No clinical manifestations of typical intestinal infection can be found. By stool examination (include anal test), no abnormalities are found.

Epidemic Encephalitis B

Toxic bacillary dysentery occurring in summers and autumns with no intestinal symptoms should be differentiated from encephalitis B. The symptoms of central nervous system in the cases of epidemic encephalitis B occur a period of time after its onset. In the extremely severe cases, their occurrence is usually 2–3 days after the onset. Such symptoms occur later than toxic bacillary dysentery. Stool examinations including anal test and enema demonstrate no abnormalities, and bacteria culture is negative. Cerebrospinal examination demonstrates changes of viral meningitis. Specific antibody IgM of encephalitis B virus positive has diagnostic value. CT scanning demonstration of encephalitis B is characterized by low-density lesion at the bilateral basal ganglia and thalamus area. The involved cerebral peduncle is the second characteristic demonstration. The cerebral cortex, brainstem, and callosum are rarely involved. MR imaging demonstrates the corresponding areas with long T1 and long T2 signal, with slightly high FLAIR signal as well as mostly high DWI signal and rarely slightly high DWI signal.

Cerebral Malaria

The disease should be differentiated from cerebral toxic dysentery. The patients usually come from epidemic area, and the seasons with high incidence rate should also be taken into account for the differential diagnosis. The manifestations are clinically characterized by intermittent sudden chills, fever, and normal body temperature following perspiration. The diagnosis can be defined based on detected *Plasmodium* in blood smear or bone marrow smear. CT scanning and MR imaging commonly demonstrate cerebral edema as well as spots of hemorrhagic focus. The sensitivity of SWI to the spots of hemorrhagic focus is higher than T_2WI and FLAIR.

2.9.1.3 Chronic Dysentery Should Be Differentiated from the Following Diseases

Chronic Amebic Dysentery

The key points for differential diagnosis are almost the same as those for acute cases.

Nonspecific Chronic Ulcerative Colonitis

The disease is an inflammatory disease commonly occurring at the colonic mucosa, mainly with lesions of ulcer and erosion. It can also involve the distal colon and spreads all over the colon as well. Its occurrence at the rectosigmoid accounts for 61.5 %. The patients experience recurrent bloody mucopurulent stool, left lower abdominal pain, fever, and tenesmus. And the disease can be misdiagnosed as chronic bacillary dysentery due to tenderness at the left lower abdomen. The patients generally experience poor conditions, with incurable prolonged disease and cannot be healed by medication of antibiotics. Multiple stool cultures fail to detect the pathogenic bacteria. Spots of bleeding can be found at the intestinal mucosa which are fragile and tend to bleeding after being touched. Barium enema X-ray or barium radiography of the entire digestive tract demonstrates thick and deranged intestinal mucosa with fine particles like change, superficial ulceration, spiculate edge of the wall, small niche, as well as absent haustra coli at the advanced stage, shortened colon, stiff intestinal wall and luminal stenosis.

Intestinal Tuberculosis

The patients may have bloody stool, which resembles to those with bacillary dysentery. It has a chronic onset, commonly secondary to pulmonary tuberculosis, with low-grade fever after noons and night sweating. By acid-fast staining of the sputum or 24-h sputum concentration, tubercle bacillus can be detected. The enteric lesions are often located at the ileocecal junction to cause tenderness at the right lower abdomen and palpable mass. Barium enema X-ray facilitates the diagnosis. Ulcerative intestinal tuberculosis is characterized by irritable sign of the affected intestinal segment by barium, Stierlin sign, thick and deranged mucosal folds, and irregular edge of the intestinal wall sometimes with jagged shape. Luminal stenosis, shortened and deformed intestinal segment, and absent ileocecal angle are also observable. Hyperplastic intestinal tuberculosis is characterized by filling defect and luminal stenosis.

Colorectal Cancer

It commonly occurs in middle aged and elderly people. In the cases complicated by local infection, the manifestations resemble to bacillary dysentery. The differential diagnosis should be based on digital rectal examination, enteroscopy, and mucosal biopsy. Barium X-ray demonstrates growth of the cancer in the intestinal lumen, commonly with lobulated or cauliflower-like filling defect, luminal stenosis, irregular contour, stiff wall, and destructed rectal mucosa. Otherwise, localized smooth regular luminal stenosis or ring-shaped stenosis is observed. CT scanning and MR imaging often demonstrate localized thickness of the intestinal wall, irregular soft tissue mass, luminal deformation and stenosis, and involved adjacent tissue with poorly defined boundary. The development of cancer can be well defined, including the severity, range, size, shape, and its invasion into the surrounding tissue, as well as lymphatic or hepatic metastasis, and microstructure of the intestinal wall. These understandings facilitate the choice of surgical approach and the post-operative examinations.

2.9.2 Bacillary Dysentery

The symptoms vary in severity and have no characteristic manifestations. Therefore, the patients with chronic diarrhea or undefined abdominal symptoms with no known causes should all be suspected as bacillary dysentery. Typical intestinal amebiasis has a relatively chronic onset with mild toxic symptoms and tends to occur repeatedly. In the cases with jam-like stool, the diagnosis presents no challenge. But its definite diagnosis is depended on the finding of pathogen in stool or tissues. And the diagnosis of atypical cases depends on serological test, colonoscopy, diagnostic treatment, and radiological examinations.

In the cases with chronic diarrhea as the dominant symptom, it should be differentiated from other invasive intestinal bacterial infection, schistosomiasis, balantidiasis, trichinosis, and nonspecific chronic ulcerative colonitis. In the cases with non-dysenteric symptom as the dominant symptom, it should be differentiated from intestinal tuberculosis, colon cancer, and Crohn's disease. Amebic liver abscess should be differentiated from subphrenic abscess, primary liver cancer, and hepatic capsulitis cholelithiasis.

2.9.2.1 Bacillary Dysentery

The disease has an acute onset with severe systemic toxic symptoms. Antibiotic is effective to treat the disease. Stool microscopy and bacterial culture facilitate the diagnosis.

2.9.2.2 Schistosomiasis

Schistosomiasis has a chronic onset and a long illness course. The patients usually have a history of contact to contaminated water, intermittent diarrhea, hepatosplenomegaly, and increased blood eosinophilia granulocytes. The diagnosis can be defined based on the finding worm eggs by intestinal mucosa biopsy, positive stool hatching, or detectable worm egg-soluble antigen in the blood.

2.9.2.3 Intestinal Tuberculosis

In most cases, primary lesion of tuberculosis can be found. The patients experience consumptive fever, night sweating, malnutrition, and yellowish congee-like stool with mucus but less pus and blood. And diarrhea and constipation occur alternatively. Gastrointestinal X-ray facilitates the diagnosis.

2.9.2.4 Rectal Cancer

The disease often occurs in elderly people. The patients with left rectal cancer experience changed habit in bowel movement, soft stool with blood, and progressive abdominal distension. The patients with right rectal cancer experience progressive anemia, emaciation, irregular fever, and unsmooth defecation with paste-like stool. Occult blood test is positive, sometimes with a small quantity of mucus and no fresh blood. In the advanced stage, abdominal mass is mostly palpable. Barium enema and fiberoenteroscopy facilitate the diagnosis.

2.9.2.5 Nonspecific Chronic Ulcerative Colonitis

Clinically, the disease can be hardly differentiated from chronic intestinal amebiasis. Multiple pathogenic detections may bear negative results, and serum amoeba antibody detection may be negative. Ineffective treatment by specific therapies supports the diagnosis of the disease.

References

Blessmann J, Khoa ND, Van An L, et al. Ultrasound patterns and frequency of focal liver lesions after successful treatment of amoebic liver abscess. Trop Med Int Health. 2006;11(4):504–8.

Choudhrie AV, Kumar S, Gopalakrishnan G. Residual amoebic liver abscess in a prospective renal transplant recipient. Saudi J Kidney Dis Transpl. 2012;23(1):99–101.

Deol I, Robledo L, Meza A, et al. Encephalitis due to a free-living amoeba (Balamuthia mandrillaris): case report with literature review. Surg Neurol. 2000;53(6):611–6.

Dietz R, Schanen G, Kramann B, et al. Intracranial amebic abscess: CT and MR findings. J Comput Assist Tomogr. 1991;15(1):168–70.

Kalia V, Vibhuti, Saggar K. Case report: MRI of the brain in metronidazole toxicity. Indian J Radiol Imaging. 2010;20(3):195–7.

Kim TY, Lee YS, Yun JH, et al. A case of probable mixed-infection with Clonorchis sinensis and Fasciola sp.: CT and parasitological findings. Korean J Parasitol. 2010;48(2):157–60.

Mandal SK, Chakraborty PP, Bhattacharjee R, et al. An unusual cause of dyspnoea complicating right upper abdominal swelling. World J Gastroenterol. 2006;12(25):4109–11.

Miller Q, Kenney JM, Cotlar AM. Amebic abscess of the liver presenting as acute cholecystitis. Curr Surg. 2000;57(5):476–9.

Mortelé KJ, Segatto E, Ros PR. The infected liver: radiologic-pathologic correlation. Radiographics. 2004;24(4):937–55.

Perez MT, Bush LM. Fatal amebic encephalitis caused by Balamuthia mandrillaris in an immunocompetent host: a clinicopathological review of pathogenic free-living amebae in human hosts. Ann Diagn Pathol. 2007;11(6):440–7.

Sarda AK, Mittal R, Basra BK, et al. Three cases of amoebic liver abscess causing inferior vena cava obstruction, with a review of the literature. Korean J Hepatol. 2011;17(1):71–5.

Sarica FB, Tufan K, Cekinmez M, et al. A rare but fatal case of granulomatous amebic encephalitis with brain abscess: the first case reported from Turkey. Turk Neurosurg. 2009;19(3):256–9.

Schuster FL, Yagi S, Gavali S, et al. Under the radar: balamuthia amebic encephalitis. Clin Infect Dis. 2009;48(7):879–87.

Shrestha M, Shah A, Lettieri C. Dyspnea and dysentery: a case report of pleuropulmonary amebiasis. South Med J. 2010;103(2):165–8.

Singh V, Bhalla A, Sharma N, et al. Pathophysiology of jaundice in amoebic liver abscess. Am J Trop Med Hyg. 2008;78(4):556–9.

Sodhi KS, Ojili V, Sakhuja V, et al. Hepatic and inferior vena caval thrombosis: vascular complication of amebic liver abscess. J Emerg Med. 2008;34(2):155–7.

Yokoyama T, Hirokawa M, Imamura Y, et al. Respiratory failure caused by intrathoracic amoebiasis. Infect Drug Resist. 2010;3:1–4.

Suggested Reading

Chang HR, Lee JJ, Lin CB. Pleural empyema secondary to rupture of amoebic liver abscess. Intern Med. 2012;51(5):471–4.

Christopher PR, David KV. Antibiotic therapy for Shigella dysentery. Cochrane Database Syst Rev. 2010;4(8):67–84.

Hannu T, Mattila L, Siitonen A, et al. Reactive arthritis attributable to Shigella infection: a clinical and epidemiological nationwide study. Ann Rheum Dis. 2005;64(4):594–8.

Kuo CY, Su LH, Perere J, et al. Antimicrobial susceptibility of Shigella isolates in eight Asian countries, 2001–2004. Microbiol Immunol Infect. 2008;41(2):107–11.

Misra SP, Misra V, Dwivedi M. Ileocecal masses in patients with amebic liver abscess: etiology and management. World J Gastroenterol. 2006;12(12):1933–6.

Yang SJ, Ren H. Studies of infectious diseases. Beijing: People's Medical Publishing House; 2008.

Brucellosis

3

Yuxin Yang, Xinsheng Lv, and Bailu Liu

Brucellosis, also known as undulant fever, is an acute or chronic bacterial infectious zoonosis caused by *Brucella* that threatens the health of humans and farming animals. The clinical symptoms include persistent fever, excessive sweating, joint pain, and hepatosplenomegaly of different degrees. The disease has a globally extensive distribution and has been legally listed as the class B infectious diseases in China.

3.1 Etiology

Brucella is Gram-negative polymorphous coccobacillus with no flagella. It does not form spore or capsule, producing only endotoxins. The Committee of Brucellosis from WHO categorized *Brucella* into 6 species with 19 biotypes, among which the species of *B. abortus*, *B. suis*, *B. melitensis*, and *B. canis* are pathogenic to humans, with variant pathogenicity. *Brucella* can produce three types of antigens: antigen A, M, and G3. The antigen A is mostly found in *B. abortus*; the antigen M is mostly found in *B. melitensis*; and the antigen G3 is a common antigen. Therefore, cross immune response occurs between different *Brucella* species, and vaccine against only one species can be developed to protect humans and animals against brucellosis.

Brucella can survive in a wide range of environmental conditions, which are especially tolerant to coldness and dryness. It can survive in the secretions and excretions of infected animals, dry soil, furs, and milk products for several weeks to several months. However, it is sensitive to antibiotics, ultraviolet rays and other various radiations, heat, and commonly used chemical disinfectants. For instance, it can be killed by 3 % bleaching powder solution within several minutes.

3.2 Epidemiology

3.2.1 Source of Infection

Infected livestock is the main source of infection, including the most commonly infected goats and sheep, followed by infected pigs and cattle, and rarely infected dogs. Other animals, such as infected deer and horses, can also be the source of infection. The disease rarely spreads from person to person.

3.2.2 Route of Transmission

3.2.2.1 Infection via Contact to the Skin or Mucosa

Direct contact to diseased farm animals or their vaginal secretions or excretions is one of its routes of transmission. Otherwise, inappropriate safety measure during feeding, slaughtering, and processing the furs and meat of diseased farm animals cannot sufficiently protect the workers from infecting the disease via skin, small wound, or eye conjunctiva. In addition, contact to contaminated environment or utensils by diseased farm animals can also indirectly transmit the disease.

3.2.2.2 Infection via Gastrointestinal Tract

Intake of contaminated food, water, uncooked dairy product, unthoroughly cooked meats, and diseased animal organs can cause the infection.

3.2.2.3 Infection via Respiratory Tract

The pathogenic bacteria can contaminate the environment by formation of bacteria containing aerosol, which can also lead

Y. Yang (✉)
Department of Radiology, The Sixth People's Hospital, Urumqi, Xinjiang Uygur Autonomous Region, China
e-mail: yangyuxin6068@163.com

X. Lv
Department of Radiology, City Central Hospital, Karamay, Xinjiang Uygur Autonomous Region, China

B. Liu
CT Department, The Second Affiliated Hospital, Harbin Medical University, Harbin, Heilongjiang, China

H. Li (ed.), *Radiology of Infectious Diseases: Volume 2*, DOI 10.1007/978-94-017-9876-1_3

to the infection after its access into the human body along with breathing.

3.2.2.4 Other Routes of Transmission

Other routes of transmission include bacteria-carrying flies and bites by bacteria-carrying ticks.

3.2.3 Susceptible Population

Populations are generally susceptible. The high-risk groups include veterinarians, farmers, butchers, workers processing furs, and persons eating contaminated food or products. The patients can acquire strong immunity after cured. The infection of different serotypes of *Brucella* has cross immune response, therefore, with rare occurrence of repeated infection. Residents living in epidemic areas can acquire the immunity after asymptomatic infection.

3.2.4 Epidemiological Feature

Brucellosis is distributed globally, with occurrence in nearly all provinces in China. However, it mainly prevails in some provinces with large farming areas. It occurs in all seasons. In late springs and early summers, after its occurrence peaks in farming animals for 1–2 months, its occurrence in humans increases to peak.

3.3 Pathogenesis and Pathological Changes

The pathogenesis of the disease is complex and still remains incompletely known. Bacteriotoxin and allergic reactions play different roles in the pathogenesis of the disease.

After *Brucella* gains its access in human body via skin or mucosa, most of them are eliminated by immune responses mediated by polymorphonuclear leukocytes (PMNL) and macrophagocytes. However, those who survived the bactericidal activities continue to invade the local lymph nodes along with lymphatic vessels to multiply themselves, where the primary lesions are formed. After its multiplication to a certain quantity in the lesions, the bacteria break through the lymphatic barrier into the blood flow to induce bacteremia. After the thallus is broken to release endotoxin and other substances, toxemia occurs. Along with the blood flow, the bacteria can be disseminated into the liver, spleen, bone marrow, or kidneys to cause new lesions, with occurrence of local or systematic infection. The pathogenic bacteria can repeatedly enter into the blood flow to cause repeated aggravation of clinical symptoms, such as undulant fever. When T lymphocytes at the lesions are sensitized by *Brucella* with following contact to the antigen, cytokines are released to activate and induce chemotaxis of macrophagocytes for repeated phagocytosis and elimination of the pathogenic bacteria. At this time, infective granuloma can be found, especially in the liver and spleen.

After the pathogenic bacteria gain their access into human body, they invade the blood flow to induce inflammatory reactions in lymph nodes or bone marrow. After that, infective lesions are formed near the joint capsular ligament or under the articular cartilage and in the bone marrow, with manifestation of epithelioid nodules. By microscopy, infiltration of epithelioid cells, lymphocytes, and plasma cells can be observed around the lesions. Spinal necrosis and suppuration may occur in some cases to form sequestrum. The intervertebral disk is also possibly subject to destruction, even with bony fusion of adjacent vertebrae.

The pathological changes of brucellosis may be systemic, mainly including inflammatory exudation, degeneration, necrosis, hyperblastosis, and granuloma. The disease may involve any organs and tissues, with occurrence of inflammations and granuloma at the liver, spleen, lymph nodes, and marrow, such as arthritis and osteomyelitis, testitis, epididymitis, endometritis, neuritis, neurodocitis, meningitis, endocarditis, myocarditis, and pneumonia. The patients at the chronic stage may experience fibrosclerosis, which further leads to body dysfunctions.

3.4 Clinical Symptoms and Signs

Brucellosis is a systemic disease with complex clinical symptoms of different severities. Its incubation period lasts for 1–3 weeks, averagely 2 weeks. In some cases, the incubation period may prolong as long as several months. Generally, the illness course is divided into acute and chronic stages.

3.4.1 Acute Stage

Most cases have a chronic onset with symptoms of fever, profuse sweating, arthralgia, and testicle swelling.

3.4.1.1 Fever and Profuse Sweating

Fever is mostly low-grade fever or irregular fever. The typical undulant fever is characterized by fever for 2–3 weeks, followed by an interval about several days or weeks and recurrence of fever, which may repeat for several rounds. During fever, the toxic symptoms are inapparent. However, after the body temperature returns to normal, the symptoms aggravate.

Profuse sweating is another characteristic symptom of the disease. The patients commonly experience profuse sweating during nights or when the body temperature drops in early mornings. In some cases with no fever, profuse sweating also occurs.

3.4.1.2 Arthralgia

Arthritis may involve one or more joints, but is more commonly found at the major joints such as the knee, waist, hip, shoulder, and elbow. The lesions are asymmetric and migrating, with stabbing pain or intractable dull pain. Its occurrence is mostly related to fever and fails to be effectively treated by common pain-relieving medications. In some cases, arthritis may be manifested as inflammation at the joint synovium, joint sheath, or tissues surrounding the joint.

3.4.1.3 Testitis

Testitis is also a characteristic symptom of the disease, which is mostly unilateral swelling of the testis with apparent pain and tenderness.

3.4.1.4 Other Symptoms

Enlarged liver, spleen, and lymph nodes are common. Some patients may experience neuralgia of the ischiadic nerve, lumbosacral nerve, and intercostal nerve due to the involved nerve root or nerve trunk. In some rare cases, meningoencephalitis or cerebrospinal meningitis occurs.

3.4.2 Chronic Stage

The illness course usually lasts for above 1 year after the acute stage. Some patients may experience only chronic stage, with no case history of acute stage. The chronic stage is nonspecific, which can be categorized into two types. One type includes systemic nonspecific symptoms resembling to neurological syndrome. The other type includes repeated sweating, local organ or tissue damages, arthralgia, neuralgia, or inflammation of organs or tissues. Some other scholars categorized the chronic stage into active type and static type.

3.5 Brucellosis-Related Complications

3.5.1 Bone and Joint Complications

The most common complication of brucellosis, occurring in more than 40 % of the cases, is bone and joint involvement. The common complications include lumbosacral arthritis, ankylosing spondylitis, osteomyelitis, and bursal synovitis, among which lumbosacral arthritis is the most common. Brucellosis is more rarely complicated by paravertebral abscess than by spinal tuberculosis. The complication of spondyloarthropathy with multiple joints involved after the infection of *Brucella* is commonly believed to be caused by immune complexes. Arthralgia is the most common symptom of brucellosis, which is the most typical and characteristic symptom of brucellosis. Arthralgia of brucellosis is characterized by occurrence at the major joint, knee, and spine. Otherwise, it is characterized by simultaneous involvements of multiple joints. At the acute stage, the patients mostly experience migrating joint pain. At the chronic stage, the patients mostly experience fixed joint pain. Occurrence of arthralgia is commonly related to climate and physical activities, and its main causes include osteoarthropathies and inflammation of tissues surrounding the joint.

3.5.2 Complications of the Digestive System

Brucellosis caused by *B. melitensis* resembles to viral hepatitis, with extremely rare occurrence of liver cirrhosis after necrosis. Some patients experience nausea, vomiting, and abdominal upset. Ileitis, colonitis, and spontaneous bacterial peritonitis rarely occur. The liver is commonly involved, with normal or slightly increased indicator levels for liver function but various histological findings of the liver. Brucellosis caused by *B. abortus* is pathologically characterized by epithelioid granuloma, which can be hardly distinguished from nodular lesions. Brucellosis caused by *B. suis* is manifested as liver abscesses. It has been reported that acute and chronic cholecystitis is related to brucellosis.

3.5.3 Complications of the Respiratory System

Inhalation of aerosols containing *Brucella* is a way of infecting brucellosis, especially when workers are slaughtering infected farm animals. It has been reported that the respiratory complications of brucellosis include hilar and paratracheal lymphadenectasis, interstitial pneumonia, bronchopneumonia, pleural effusion, and empyema. *Brucella* is rarely isolated from the sputum coughed up by patients.

3.5.4 Complications of the Urogenital System

In male patients with brucellosis, testitis and epididymitis are the most common complications. Although *Brucella* was once found in human sperm bank, the cases infected via sexual transmission have been rarely reported yet. The kidney is also rarely involved, but some clinical symptoms of brucellosis resemble to renal tuberculosis. Female patients with brucellosis have been occasionally reported to sustain pelvic abscess and salpingitis. Infection of *Brucella* during pregnancy can cause abortion or intrauterine transmission to the fetus. Therefore, during pregnancy, timely diagnosis and treatment against brucellosis can increase survival rate of the fetus. Brucellosis has been rarely reported to transmit from mother to infant via breastfeeding.

3.5.5 Complications of the Cardiovascular System

Infective endocarditis is the most common clinical manifestation of brucellosis and is also the most common cause of death in the cases of brucellosis. About 2 % of the cases with brucellosis develop endocarditis, with more common involvement of aortic valve than mitral valve. The treatment for endocarditis caused by brucellosis requires combined use of antibacterial agents and valve replacement therapy.

3.5.6 Complications of the Neurological System

Brucellosis complicated by encephalopathy refers to various neurological complications related to brucellosis. In the cases of brucellosis caused by *B. melitensis*, about 5 % have their central nervous system involved, most commonly with meningoencephalitis and meningitis. Brucellosis complicated by meningitis may be either acute or chronic, occurring mostly at the late stage of illness course. By examination of the cerebrospinal fluid, the protein can be found with an increase, with normal or slightly low level of blood sugar and predominant lymphocytes. *Brucella* is rarely isolated from the cerebrospinal fluid, but its specific antibody can be detected in the cerebrospinal fluid or serum. The other complications of the central nervous system include cerebral vasculitis, mycotic arterial aneurysm, cerebral and epidural abscess, cerebral infarction, cerebral hemorrhage, and cerebellar ataxia. The complications of the peripheral nervous system include radiculopathy, Guillain-Barré syndrome, and poliomyelitis-like syndrome (PLS).

3.5.7 Complications of the Skin

The skin diseases complicating brucellosis include skin rash, nodule, papule, erythema nodosum, and ecchymosis. The patients with brucellosis caused by *B. suis* infection are more likely to experience skin ulceration, abscess, and purulent lymphangitis.

3.5.8 Complications of the Eyes

Although eye diseases rarely occur to complicate brucellosis. Various eye diseases have been reported to complicate brucellosis, most commonly uveitis. Other eye diseases complicating brucellosis include chronic iridocyclitis, keratitis, and multifocal choroiditis. Most of these eye diseases complicate brucellosis in its advanced stage, which is possibly related to immune mediation. Therefore, steroids are usually needed to treat these eye diseases complicating brucellosis.

3.6 Diagnostic Examinations

3.6.1 Laboratory Test

3.6.1.1 Routine Blood Test

The WBC count in peripheral blood is detected normal or slightly low, with relatively increased count of lymphocytes.

3.6.1.2 Bacteriological Test

By cultures of blood, bone marrow, cerebrospinal fluid, and pus, *Brucella*, the pathogenic bacteria, can be isolated. The culture of bone marrow witnesses the highest positive rate, and its positive finding defines the diagnosis.

3.6.1.3 Serological Test

Serum Agglutination Test (SAT)

SAT can be simply operated with high specificity, which is therefore commonly applied in clinical practice. The agglutination titer of single serum sample being no less than 1:160 has diagnostic significance. At the acute stage, its positive rate can reach 80–90 %. Micro-agglutination test (MAT) and standard tube agglutination test (RBPT) can also be simply operated with high sensitivity. However, MAT and RBPT bear certain false-positive results, which are, therefore, applied for screening.

3.6.2 Diagnostic Imaging

3.6.2.1 Ultrasound

Ultrasound is simple and convenient for operation and diagnosis, which has certain diagnostic value for cardiac infection, pericardial infection, hepatosplenomegaly, superficial infection of lymph nodes, and testis involvement of brucellosis. Ultrasound is the basic examination for assessment of brucellosis.

3.6.2.2 X-Ray Radiology

X-ray radiology is simple and convenient for operation and diagnosis. It can be performed to assess pulmonary lesions of brucellosis as well as bone and joint changes at its late stage. However, due to overlapping of the images and unfavorable resolution of images, its sensitivity to lesions is insufficient. It is only appropriate for preliminary assessment of the lesions and is the examination of choice for brucellosis.

3.6.2.3 CT Scanning

CT scanning is an important examination for brucellosis, which has important diagnostic value for chest lesions, abdominal lesions, neurological lesions, joint lesions, spinal lesions, and paravertebral lesions. By CT scanning, the lesions at the chest, abdomen, and other organs can be effectively assessed. The sectional scanning and image reconstruction can well define the histological changes of diseased tissues. Therefore, clinical diagnosis can be made. However, it unfavorably demonstrates early lesions at the neurological system, joints, and spine.

3.6.2.4 MR Imaging

MR imaging has favorable resolution to soft tissues and can demonstrate from any perspective to well-defined abscesses and their surrounding tissues. MR imaging can earlier demonstrate abnormal signals at the vertebra, joint, and neurological system. Compared to CT scanning, it can earlier and more clearly demonstrate tissue involvement and its range, which is then an important supplementary radiological examination for brucellosis. DWI can demonstrate dispersion coefficient of water molecules in brain tissues and, therefore, define the range of brain tissue lesions at the early stage of the infection. Currently, MRS has been applied for radiological diagnosis of brucellosis. However, its diagnostic value for brain lesions of brucellosis has not been clarified. PWI can define the range and severity of organ lesions in the cases of brucellosis. It plays the same role as DWI in the early diagnosis of lesions.

3.6.2.5 PET and PET/CT

Until recently, their application in diagnosis of brucellosis has not been reported, which possibly is related to their nonspecificity to the lesions and its high cost.

3.7 Imaging Demonstrations

Brucellosis is most commonly involved in the spine as well as the bone and joint, with simultaneous involvements of the respiratory system, digestive system, circulatory system, and reproductive system. The patients commonly experience fever of different degrees, sweating, major joint pain including the sternoclavicular joint, sacroiliac joint, knee, hip, and elbow. Clinically, myocarditis, meningitis, and testitis may also occur.

3.7.1 Bone and Joint as Well as Spinal Brucellosis

3.7.1.1 Ultrasound

Only swelling of the soft tissues and articular effusion can be demonstrated by ultrasound.

3.7.1.2 X-Ray Radiology

At the acute stage, X-ray demonstrates only swelling of the joint and its surrounding soft tissues, while at the chronic stage, the lesions are demonstrated to involve the spine and major joints to cause bone changes. Within 2 or 3 months after the onset, confined bone destruction occurs. Extensive bone repair is one of the characteristic demonstrations of brucellosis by X-ray, with lesions of diffuse bone sclerosis under the cartilage and around the destructive lesion, narrowed interarticular space, even bony rigidity, and ossification at the attachment of tendons and ligaments.

Spine

Brucellosis may involve the spine, with manifestations of erosive osteoclasia and reactive osteosclerosis at the connective tissues between the vertebral end plate and intervertebral disk. Syndesmitis may induce ossification and calcification of the ligament. X-ray demonstrates the early lesions as multi-vertebral multifocal irregular worm-bitten-like destructions. And X-ray demonstrates the late lesions as the proliferation, sclerosis, and formation of bony spur in beak shape, known as bony bridge, that extends outward or toward vertebral margin. The vertebral center can also be involved with rapid occurrence of sclerosis but no formation of deep bone destruction. No compression to vertebra can be found. Arthritis of small vertebral joints mostly occurs at adjacent vertebra with lesions, with destructed irregular articular surface, progressive narrowing until absence of interarticular space, and bony rigidity. Calcification of ligament commonly occurs at the inferior lumbar vertebrae, with manifestations of gradual development from bottom-up of cords like calcification at the anterior and posterior ligaments. Spinal brucellar osteomyelitis is manifested as bony destruction of vertebra, narrowed intervertebral space, paravertebral abscess, and ligament ossification.

Sacroiliac Joint

The joint is commonly subject to bilateral lesions, with narrowed interarticular space, irregular bone destruction, and surrounding sclerotic response.

Shoulder

Concerning the shoulder, bones at the tendon, synovium, attachment of ligament such as the lateral tubercle of humeral head, coracoid acromial, and exterior end of clavicle are subject to focalized superficial small cystoid bone destruction, with possible occurrence of calcification of the tendon and synovium.

Other Major Joints at the Limbs

At the acute stage, the major joints at the limbs are subject to swelling of surrounding soft tissues osteoporosis, following narrowed interarticular space, cystoid destruction inferior to the articular cartilage, and small bone erosion at the articular attachment. At the advanced stage, the articular surface is subject to sclerosis, which is unsmooth with bone hyperplasia and possible occurrence of articular bony fusion (Fig. 3.1).

Case Study 1

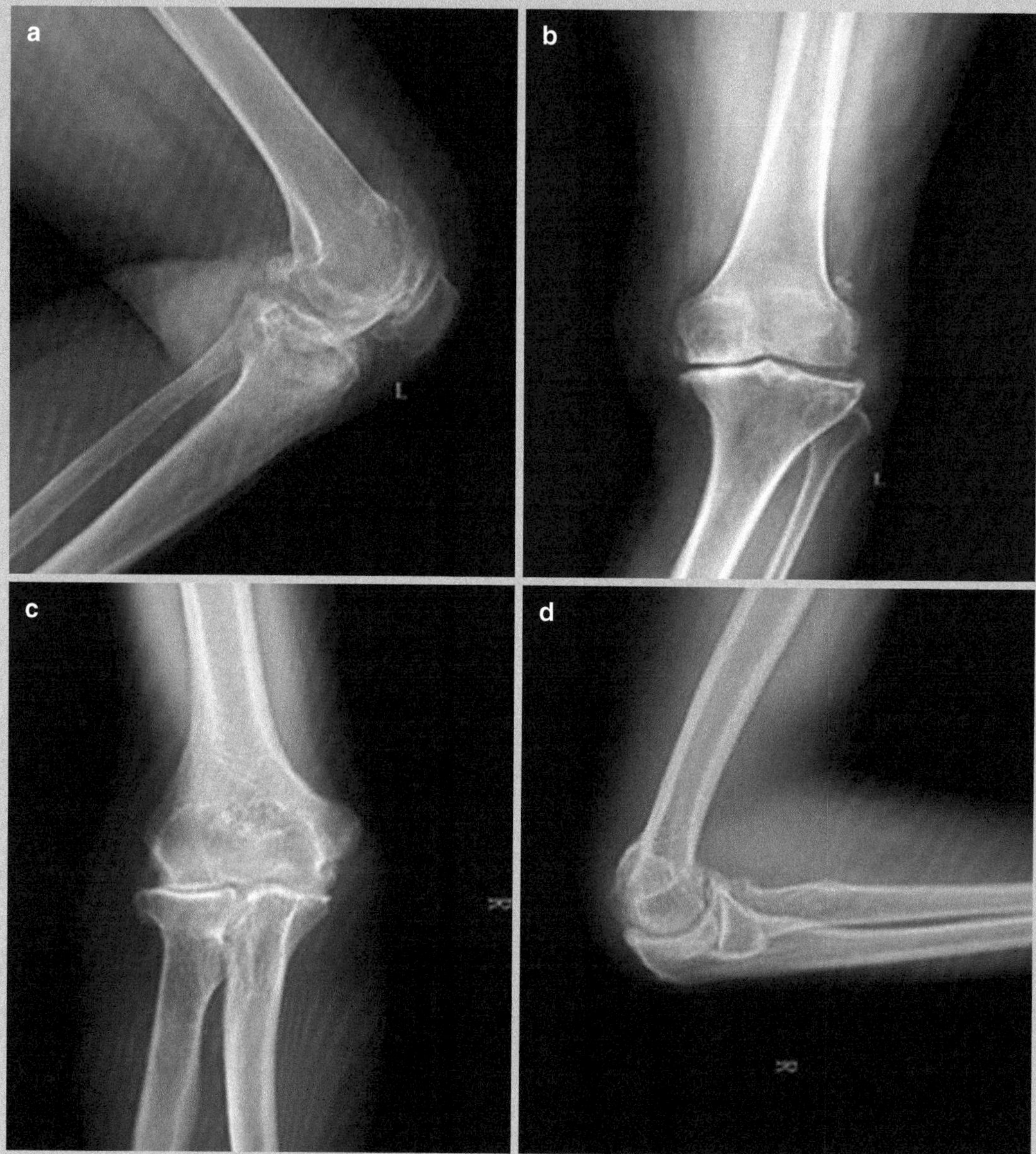

Fig. 3.1 Articular brucellosis. (**a–d**) At the late stage of the illness course, X-ray demonstrates narrowed interarticular space, sclerosis of articular surface, and bone hyperplasia at articular margin. In some cases, there are also bone destruction and articular effusion in a small quantity

3.7.1.3 CT Scanning

CT scanning demonstrates small multiple lesions of vertebral bone destruction, which are mostly confined at the vertebral margin. Around the lesions, obvious hyperplasia and sclerosis are demonstrated. In the newly formed bone tissues, new destruction lesions are mixed. The synovial cartilage or intervertebral disk is subject to destruction with equal density shadows. The joint surface is subject to hyperplasia and sclerosis, with increased density of adjacent bone and formation of paravertebral abscess in a small quantity. By contrast CT scanning, the margins of soft tissue and abscess are enhanced. At the early stage, the spine is demonstrated with small cystoid bone destruction at multiple vertebrae, with ring-shaped sclerosis at their margin. Such sclerosis mostly occurs at the superior and inferior margin of vertebra and the vertebral margin is subject to obvious osteoproliferation and osteosclerosis. At the late stage, the destruction area extends to the vertebral center, with compressed vertebra and wedge-shaped deformation of the vertebra (Figs. 3.2, 3.3, and 3.4).

Case Study 2

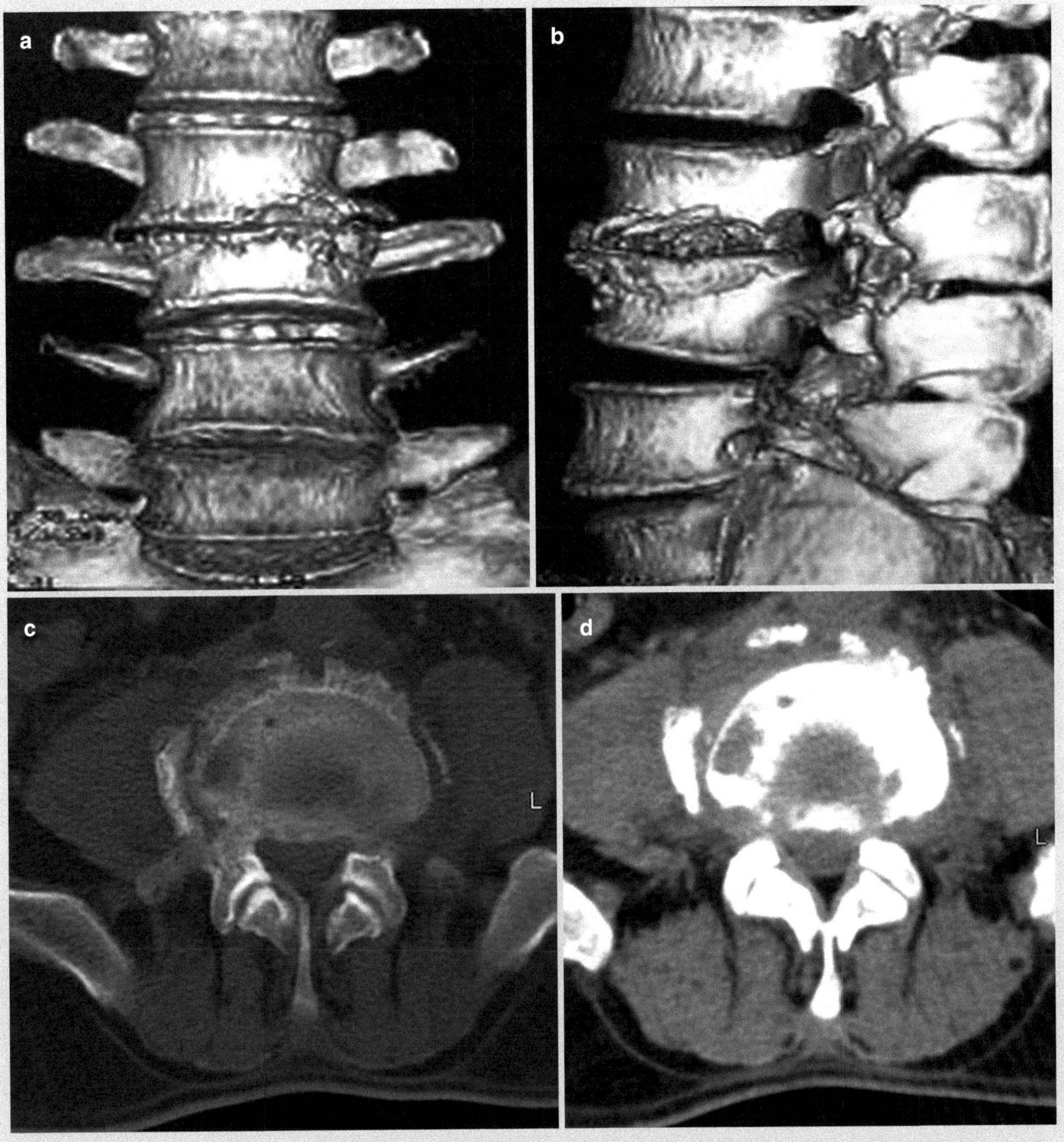

Fig. 3.2 Brucellar spondylitis. (**a–d**) CT scanning demonstrates osteoproliferation and bone destruction at the lumbar vertebrae, with narrowed intervertebral space. The vertebral margin is demonstrated with proliferation, hypertrophy, and ossification of the periosteum to form liplike or bank-like osteophytes. The newly formed osteophytes and the destructive lesions between them constitute characteristic lacelike vertebra. The osteophyte of adjacent vertebrae is demonstrated to connect with each other to form lateral-lateral vertebral fusion. Periostitis occurring at the transverse process is demonstrated as cap-like thickening at the top of the transverse process

Case Study 3

A male patient aged 24 years complained of lower back pain for 6 months that aggravated with accompanying numbness and pain at the right lower limbs for 1 month. He reported a history of working as a shepherd and lamb delivery. The serological agglutination test for *Brucella* was demonstrated positive.

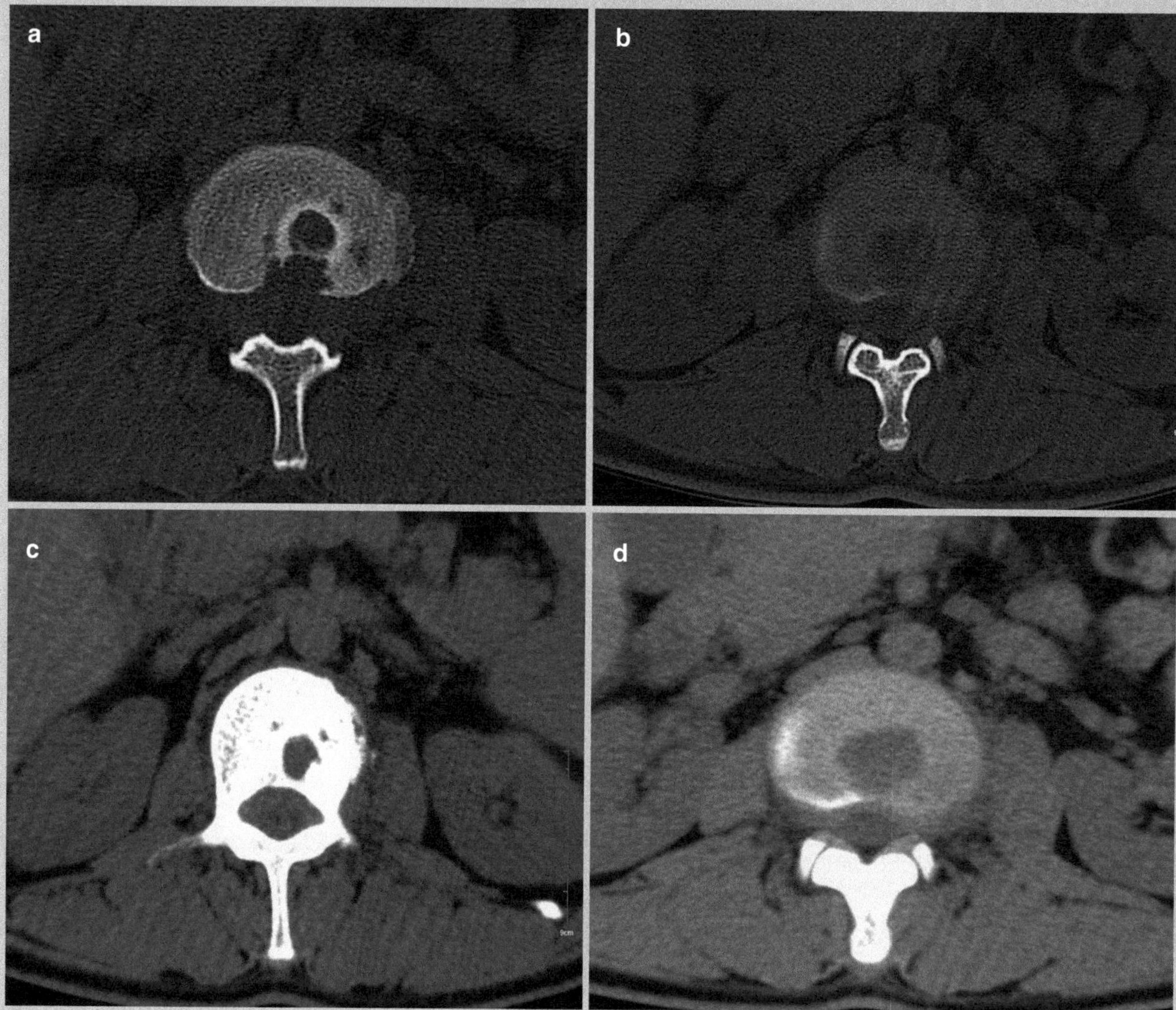

Fig. 3.3 Brucellar spondylitis. (**a**, **b**) Plain lumbar CT scanning demonstrates multiple bone destructions at the vertebra by bone window, with proliferation and sclerosis at the vertebral margin. The intervertebral disk is demonstrated with inner low-density lesions. (**c**, **d**) Soft tissue window demonstrates strips of low-density shadow around the diseased vertebra, which is actually formation of paravertebral abscess

Case Study 4
A male patient aged 47 years complained of lumbar pain, muscular pain at the lower limbs, and joint pain for 1 year. Serological agglutination test for *Brucella* demonstrated positive.

(Note: Cases 3 and 4 as well as the corresponding figures were provided by Liu BL at the Second Affiliated Hospital, Harbin Medical University, Harbin, China.)

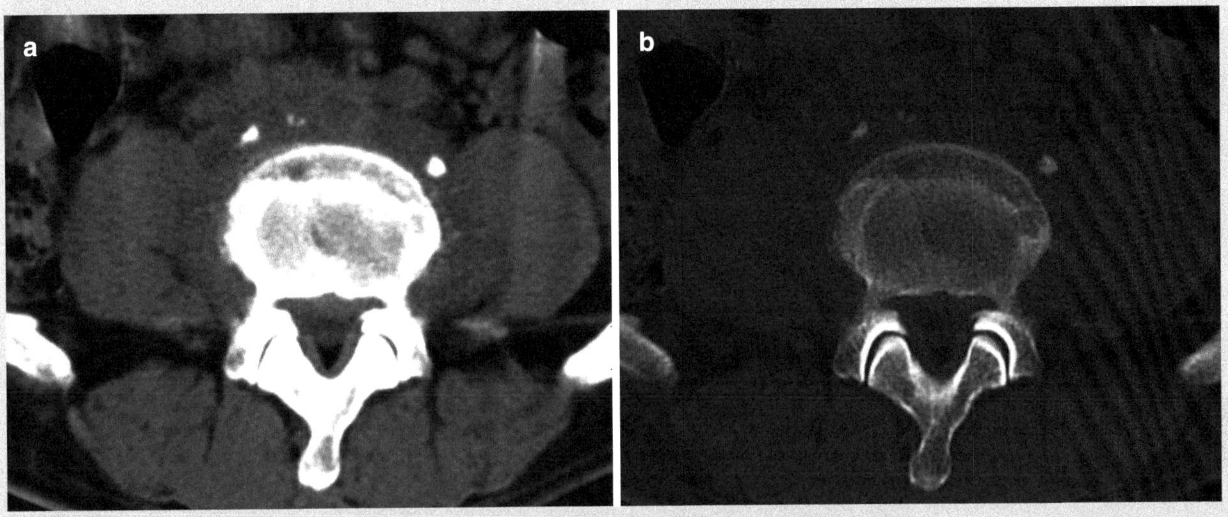

Fig. 3.4 Brucellar spondylitis. (**a**, **b**) Plain lumbar CT scanning demonstrates vertebral osteoproliferation, low uneven density shadow surrounding the vertebra with poorly defined boundaries. The vertebra is demonstrated with poorly defined interface to bilateral psoas majors. The psoas majors are demonstrated with slightly outward shift

3.7.1.4 MR Imaging

Spinal margin bone destruction is the most common in the cases of brucellosis. The lesions are mostly multiple, invading vertebral margin of 1–2 vertebrae. In some rare cases, 3 vertebrae are involved. In the early stage, T1WI demonstrates low signal of different sizes, while T2WI, equal or high signal. After several weeks, bone defect lesions can be demonstrated as lower T1WI signal shadow, with no enhancement by contrast imaging. The lesions are demonstrated with irregular worm-bitten-like or sawlike appearance, with small surrounding abscess. In the cases of central spine type of brucellosis, the central lesions are demonstrated with rapid sclerosis, with no formation of deep bone destruction, no deformed vertebra due to compression. Vertebral proliferation and sclerosis are demonstrated by MR imaging as equal, high, or low signal. Early intervertebral disk involvement is demonstrated by T2WI and fat suppression imaging as increased signal at the intervertebral disk with different degrees, which are defined as edematous change, with no destructive effect on the vertebral end plate. Development of intervertebral disk involvement is demonstrated as thinner intervertebral disk, narrowed intervertebral space, and its connection to vertebral destruction, with irregular shape and formation of abscess. Paravertebral abscess is commonly demonstrated as long T1 long T2 signals. Contrast T1WI demonstrates marginal enhancement, with thick wall, well-defined boundary, and small abscess that do not exceed the length of diseased vertebra. There is no sign indicating downward flow of abscess fluid. The surrounding fat space is well defined. The MR imaging demonstrations of brucellosis at other joints are similar, commonly joint ossification, swelling of surrounding soft tissues, and articular effusion in a small quantity (Figs. 3.5, 3.6, 3.7, 3.8, and 3.9).

Case Study 5

A male patient aged 57 years was hospitalized due to lower back pain, accompanying muscular soreness and pain at both lower limbs and joint pain for more than 6 months.

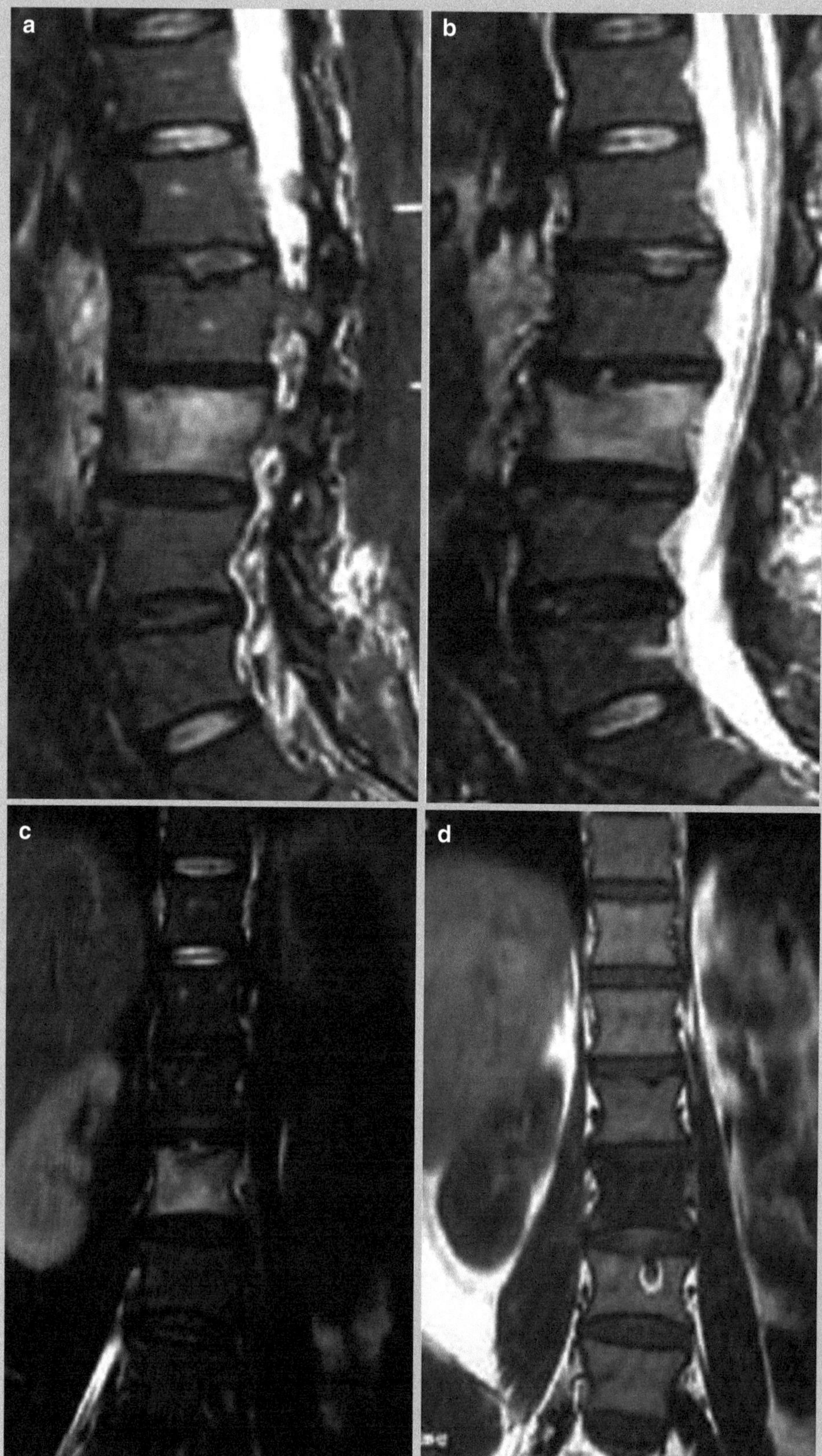

Fig. 3.5 Brucellar spondylitis. (**a–j**) MR imaging demonstrates patches of long T1 mixed slightly long T2 signals at the vertebrae of L2 and L3, with narrowed intervertebral space at the L2–L3, and strips of mixed slightly long T2 signal at the peripheral vertebra. Contrast imaging demonstrates abnormal signal with obviously uneven enhancement at the diseased vertebra and its periphery

Fig. 3.5 (continued)

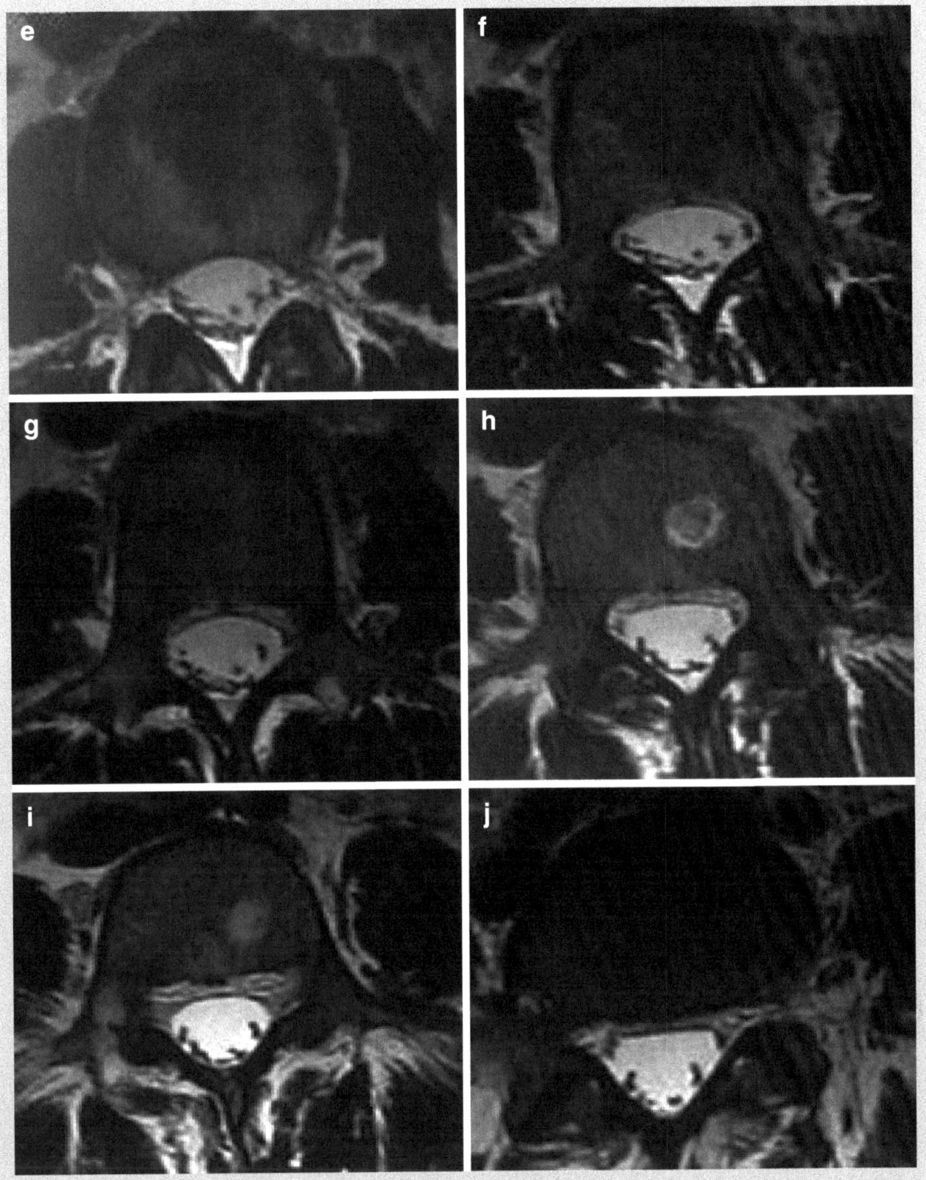

Case Study 6

A male patient aged 51 years complained of intermittent lower back pain for more than 2 months.

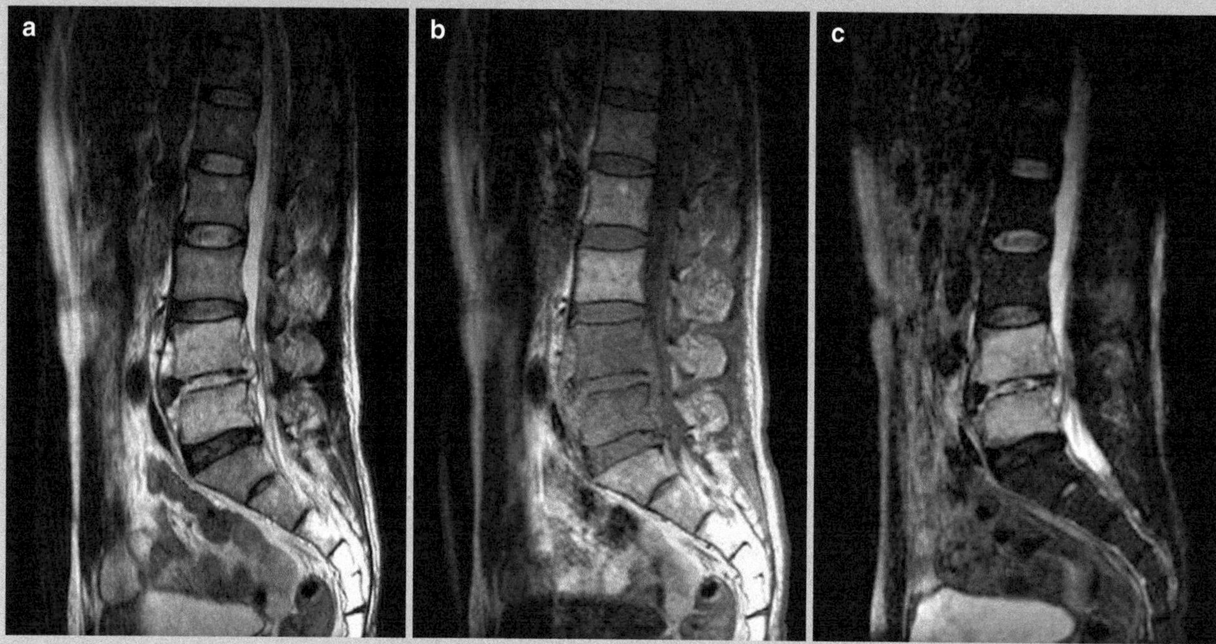

Fig. 3.6 Brucellar spondylitis. (**a–c**) MR imaging demonstrates slightly deformed L4–L5 with long T1 long T2 signals. By contrast imaging, the whole vertebra is demonstrated with homogeneous enhancement, and the intervertebral disk is demonstrated with uneven enhancement

Case Study 7

A male patient aged 64 years was hospitalized due to lower back pain, accompanying muscular soreness and pain at the lower limbs and joint pain for more than 6 months. He reported lower back pain with no known causes about half a year ago, with accompanying muscular pain at the lower limbs and major joint pain at the lower limbs. Recently, he received serological agglutination test for *Brucella* at the local CDC, with positive findings. And then he paid his clinic visit in our hospital. By laboratory tests, WBC count is 4.98×10^9/L, GR % 64.1 %, ESR 50 mm/h, and CRP 10.8 mg/L. The clinical diagnosis was brucellar spondylitis. The symptoms disappeared after he received treatment for 2 months.

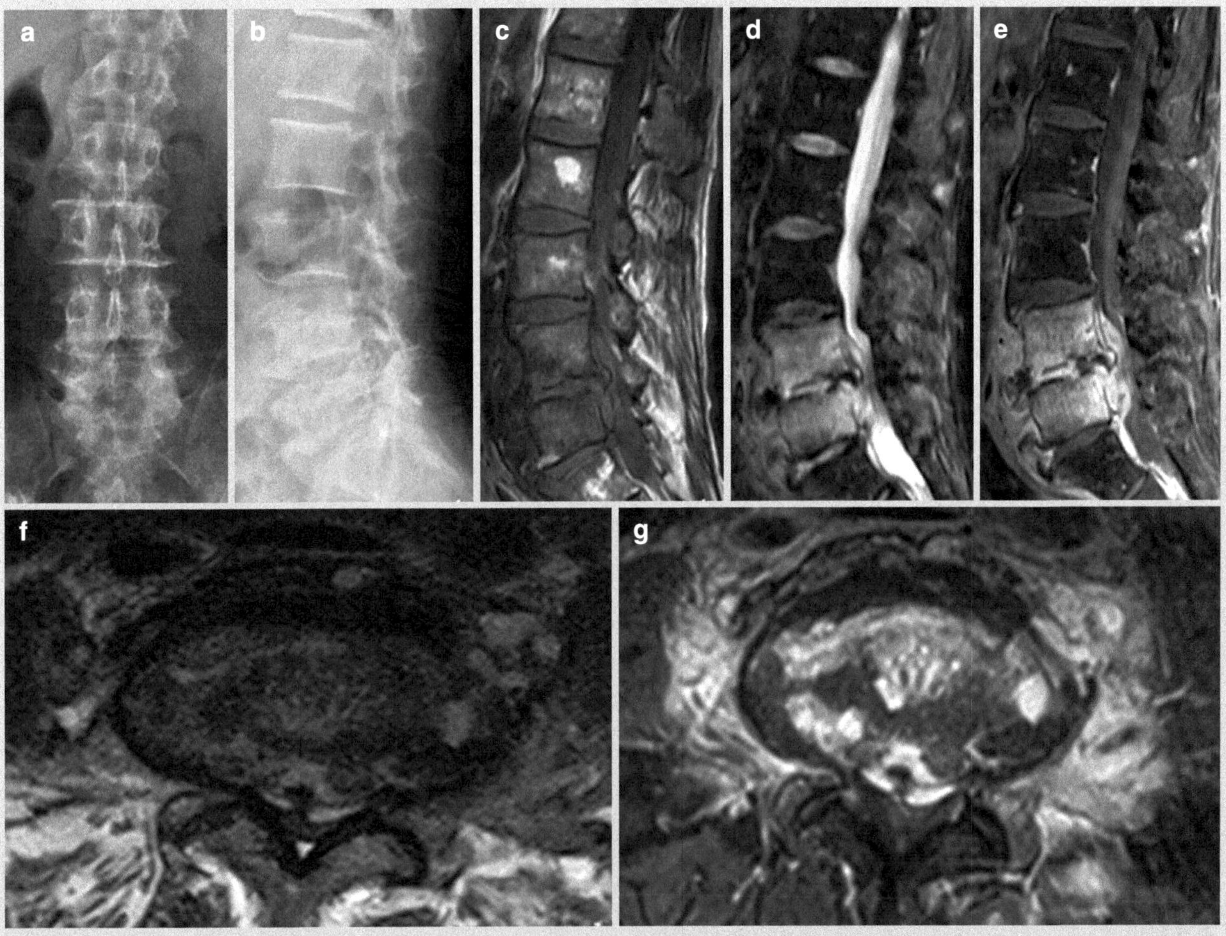

Fig. 3.7 Brucellar spondylitis. (**a**, **b**) Lateral and anterior-posterior imaging demonstrates intact sequence of lumbar vertebrae, obvious osteoproliferation at L2–L5 and bone destruction at the posterior margin of L5. (**c**, **d**, **f**) MR imaging demonstrates intact sequence of the lumbar vertebrae, diffuse slightly long T1 and long T2 signals at L4 and L5, no involvement of the appendices, obvious osteoproliferation at the L4 and L5, focalized destruction of the inferior end plate of the L4 and superior end plate of L5. The intervertebral space is demonstrated to be narrowed at L4–L5 and L5–S1, with internal long T2 signal and disk protrusion. Its posterior dural sac is demonstrated to be obviously compressed. And the paravertebral soft tissues are demonstrated with obvious swelling. The psoas major is involved. (**e**, **g**) Contrast imaging demonstrates obvious enhancement of the L4 and L5, irregular enhancement of intervertebral disk at L4–L5, obvious diffuse enhancement of the paravertebral soft tissues, enhancement of anterior and posterior longitudinal ligaments, and patches of enhancement at the left erector muscle of spine (Note: the case and figures were provided by the Department of Radiology, You'an Hospital, Beijing, China)

Case Study 8

A male patient aged 53 years was hospitalized due to intermittent fever and muscular pain for 23 days. He experienced fever 23 days ago, which was more severe after noons and during nights. He had the highest body temperature of 40 °C, with accompanying chills and aversion to cold. After clinic visit of a community-based clinic, he was diagnosed with viral infection and received medications for 4 days. His body temperature then returned to normal, but he began to experience muscular pain of the neck, with restricted cervical motions. Five days before his admission, the patient began to experience recurrence of fever with no known causes, with a body temperature of 38.7 °C and accompanying aversion to cold, chills, and lumbar paravertebral muscular pain. By physical examination after admission, the neurological system was normal, with normal brain nerves, muscle tension of limbs, and muscular strength. By bilateral finger-nose test and heel-knee-tibia test, he had favorable stability and accuracy. By bilateral needle stabbing, the sensation was symmetric. Tendon reflex of the limbs were symmetric and appropriate. No bilateral pathological signs were induced. The neck is soft; the Kernig test positive; and Patrick test positive. One week after the admission, the blood bacterial culture indicated growth of *Brucella*. Reexamination by standard tube agglutination test for *Brucella* is positive. The patient reported long-term intake of raw milk. The clinical diagnosis was brucellosis.

(For case detail and figures, please refer to Guo YJ et al. *Chinese Journal of Contemporary Neurology*, 2013, 13 (1): 49.)

Case Study 9

A female patient aged 42 years was hospitalized due to intermittent fever for 11 months, lower back pain for 7 months, and weakness of both lower limbs for 1 month. Her lower back pain is persistent. By physical examination, tenderness is near the spinous process of L3 and L4 and no reflex pain. By straight leg raising test, the right leg 70° and the left leg 90°, with muscular atrophy of both lower limbs. By laboratory test, WBC is 6.6×10^9/L, and the antibody titer of *Brucella* was 1:16.

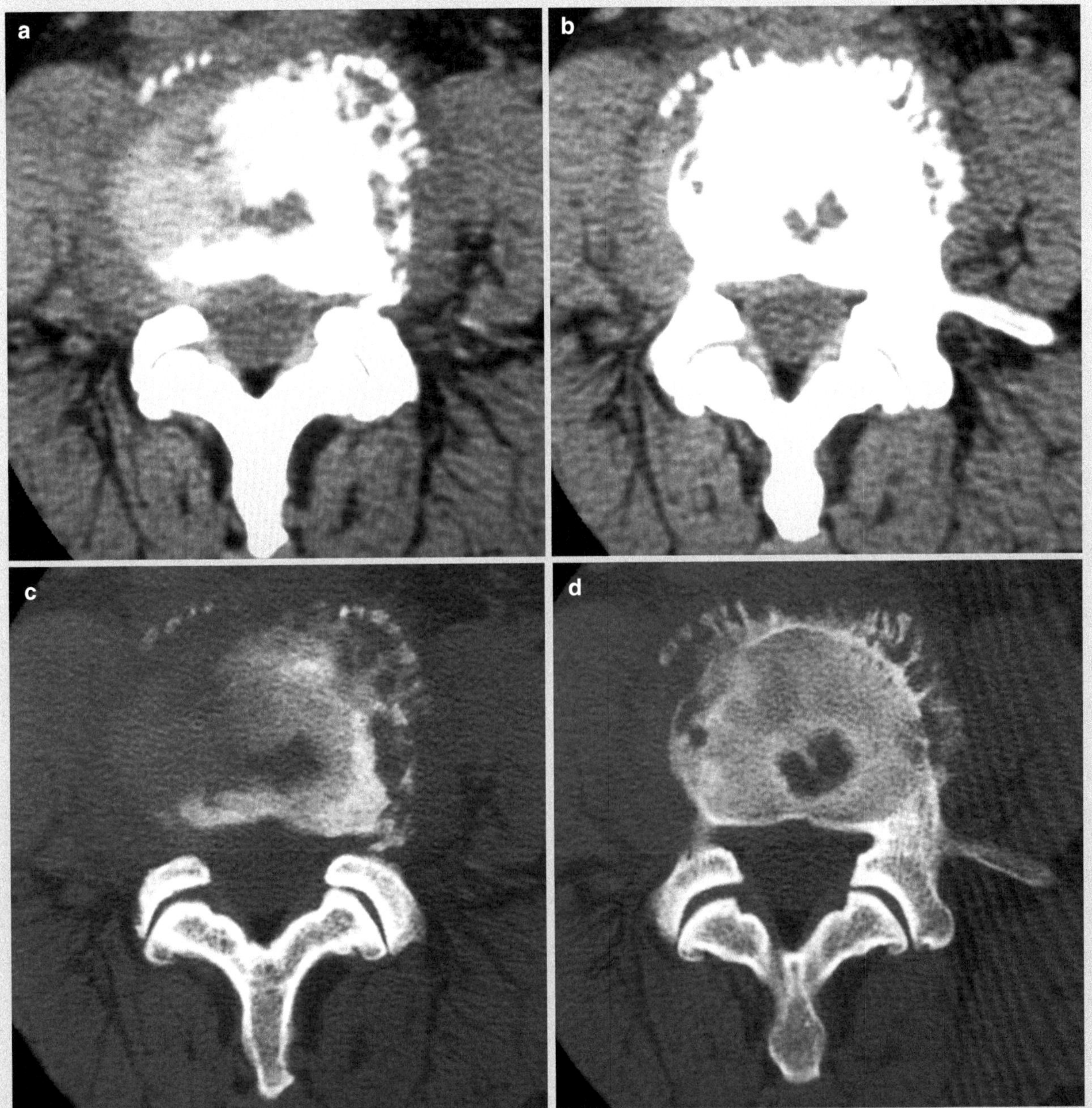

Fig. 3.8 Brucellar spondylitis. (**a–d**) CT scanning demonstrates multiple irregular bone destruction at the vertebral endplate of L4, with marginal sclerosis and no sequestrum. The bone destruction area is demonstrated to be surrounded by multiple lacelike osteophyte, with swelling of vertebral marginal soft tissue. (**e**, **f**) MR imaging demonstrates patches of long T1 and long T2 signals at the vertebrae of L3 and L4, with poorly defined boundaries. The corresponding intervertebral space is demonstrated to be narrowed, with swelling of paravertebral soft tissue and slightly compressed dural sac. (**g**, **h**) Pathology demonstrates chronic inflammation, formation of granuloma, fibrin-like exudation in a small quantity and accompanying small abscesses

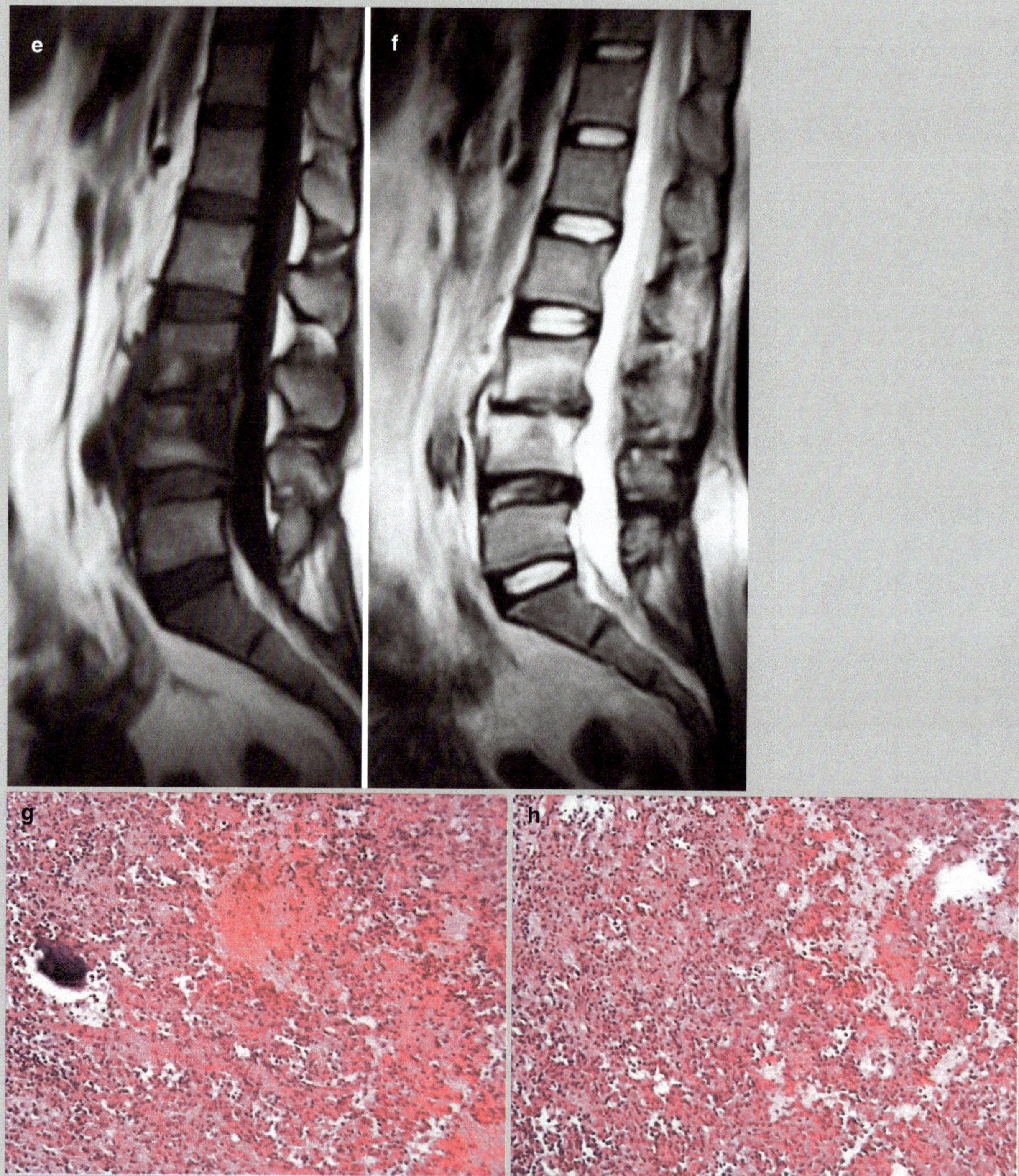

Fig. 3.8 (continued)

Case Study 10

A male patient aged 40 years worked in the industry of farming animals. He was hospitalized due to fever, lower back pain, and pain at both lower limbs for 6 months. By physical examination, reflexes of both lower limbs were normal; straight leg raising test was positive. By laboratory test, standard tube agglutination test was positive; tube agglutination test was positive.

(The Cases 9 and 10 as well as corresponding figures were provided by Kang LQ at Diagnostic Imaging Center, Central Hospital of Cangzhou, Cangzhou, Hebei, China; and Cao JH at Radiology Department, Heping Hospital, Cangzhou, Hebei, China.)

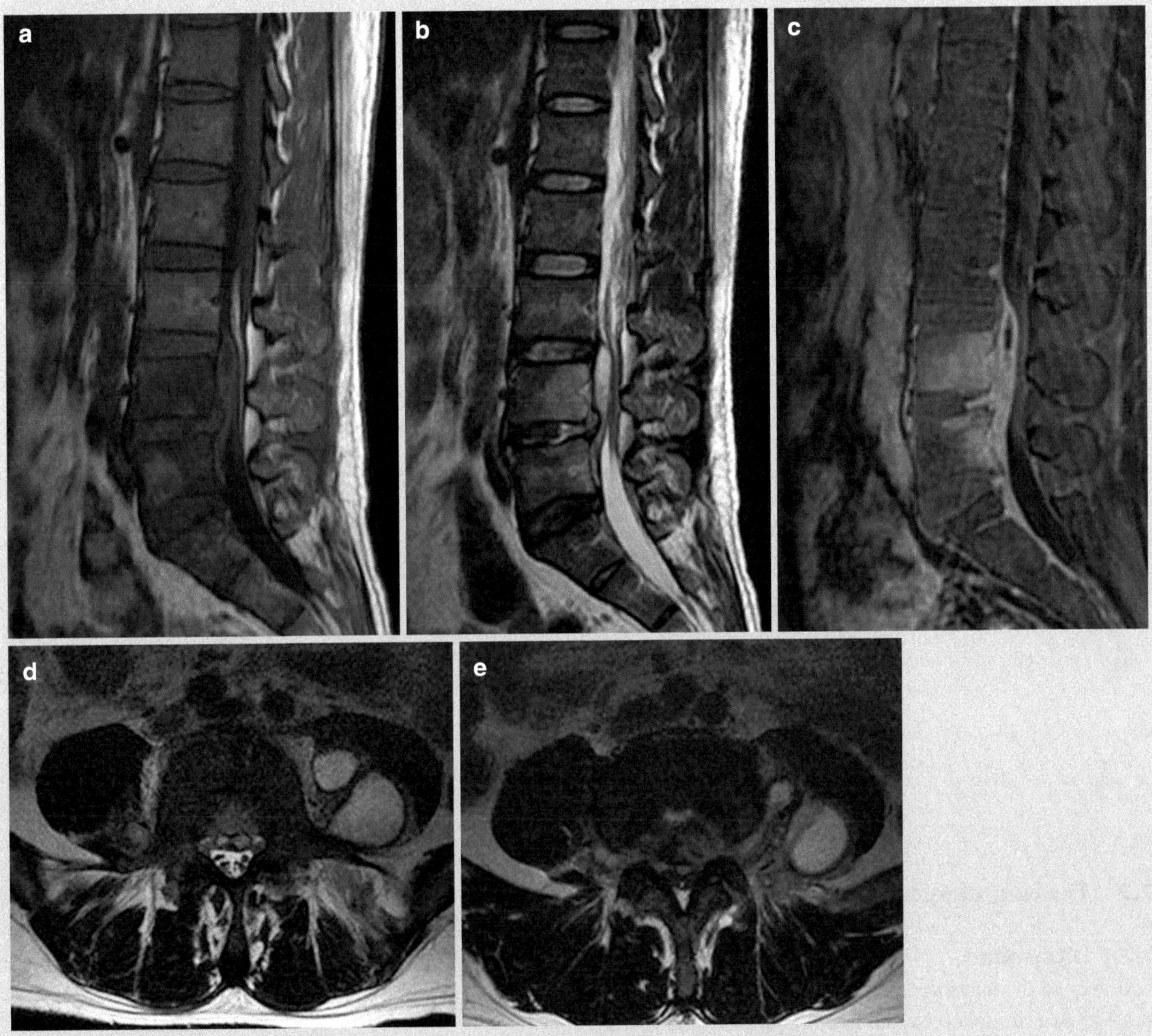

Fig. 3.9 Brucellar spondylitis and paravertebral abscess. (**a**–**e**) MR imaging demonstrates vertebrae of L1–L5 with patches of long T1 and long T2 signals, with poorly defined boundaries. Intraspinal epidural abscess is demonstrated to connect with intervertebral disk with abnormal signal. (**f**–**i**) Contrast imaging demonstrates multiple paravertebral abscesses in different sizes, which is more obvious at the left psoas major. The abscess wall is demonstrated with enhancement, and the dural sac is demonstrated to be obviously compressed

Fig. 3.9 (continued)

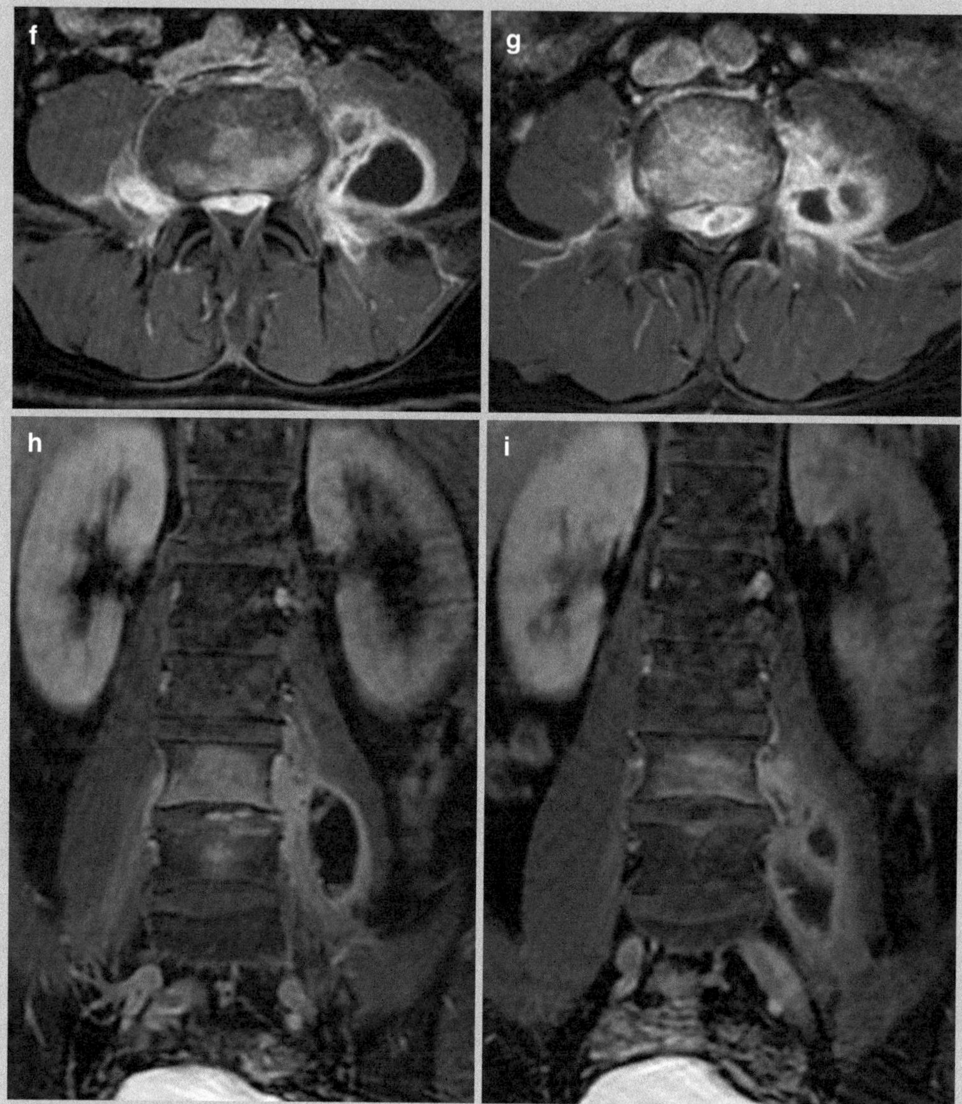

3.7.2 The Neurological System

3.7.2.1 Ultrasound

By ultrasound, no abnormalities can be demonstrated. In the cases with arteries involved, the artery is demonstrated with thickened wall, unsmooth lining, thinner artery, and even interrupted artery.

3.7.2.2 CT Scanning

CT scanning demonstrates the basal cistern to be narrowed or even absent. There are also swollen spinal cords and hydrocephalus. In the cases with the brain and spinal parenchyma involved, small flakes of low signal shadows are demonstrated. Contrast scanning demonstrates slight enhancement of the meninges. In the cases with cerebral abscess, the thickened abscess wall is demonstrated with enhancement by contrast scanning. Cranial CTA demonstrates uneven thickness of arteries. In some individual cases, interrupted arteries can be demonstrated.

3.7.2.3 MR Imaging

MR imaging demonstrates the basal cistern to be narrowed or even absent. There are also swollen spinal cords and hydrocephalus. In the cases with the brain or spinal parenchyma involved, small flakes of low signal shadows are demonstrated. By contrast imaging, the meninges are demonstrated with slight enhancement. In the cases with cerebral abscess, the thickened abscess wall can be demonstrated with enhancement by contrast imaging (Figs. 3.10 and 3.11).

Case study 11

A patient complained of headache for more than 3 months and accompanying weakness of the right limbs for almost 1 month.

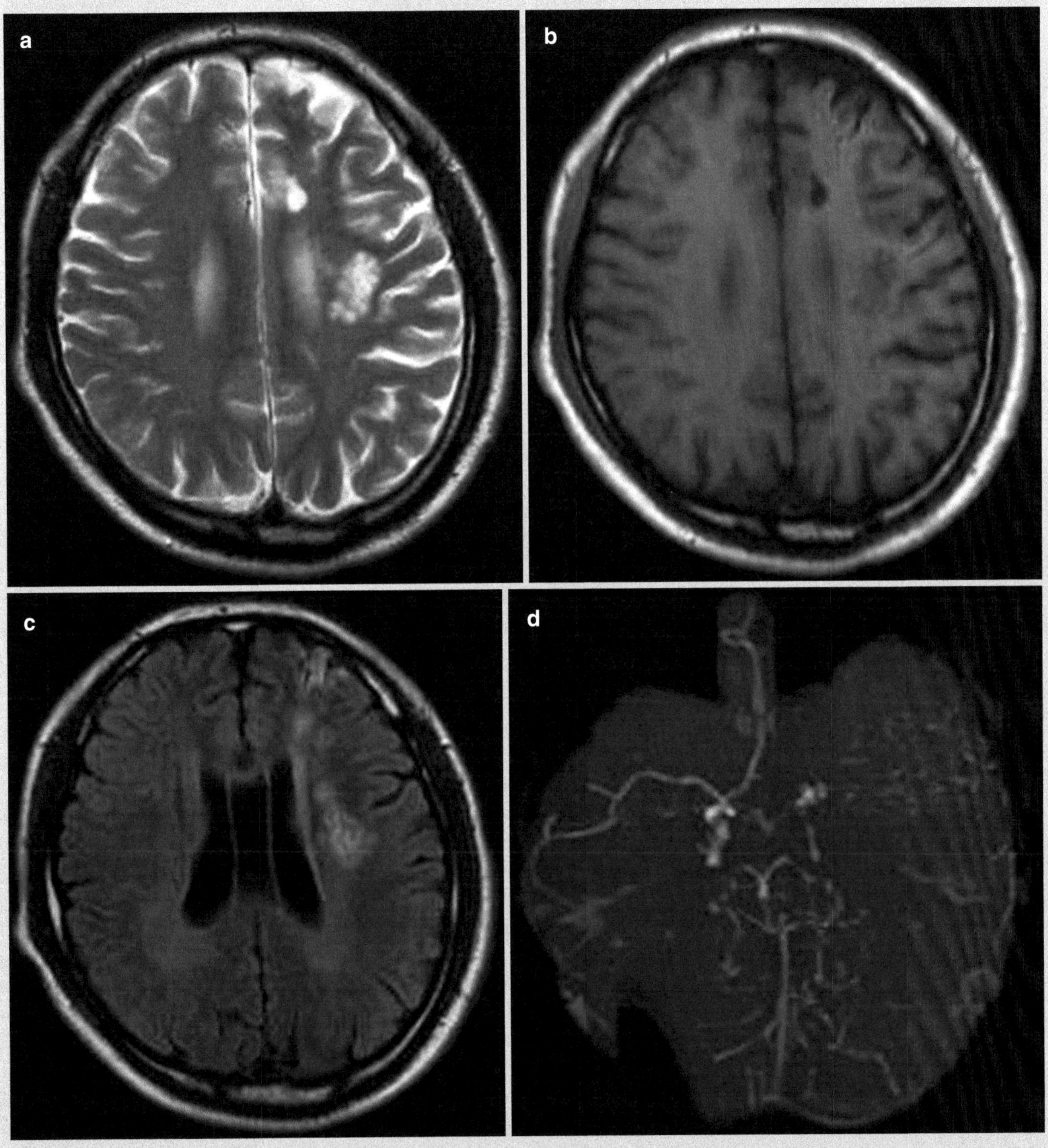

Fig. 3.10 Neurological brucellosis. (**a**–**d**) MR imaging demonstrates multiple flakes of long T1 and long T2 signals at the left basal ganglia and the frontal lobe; uneven thickness of the left cerebral middle artery. The demonstrations indicate brucellar arteritis

Case Study 12
A patient complained of headache for more than 6 months. By lumbar puncture and following examination of the cerebrospinal fluid, the findings indicated brucellar meningitis.

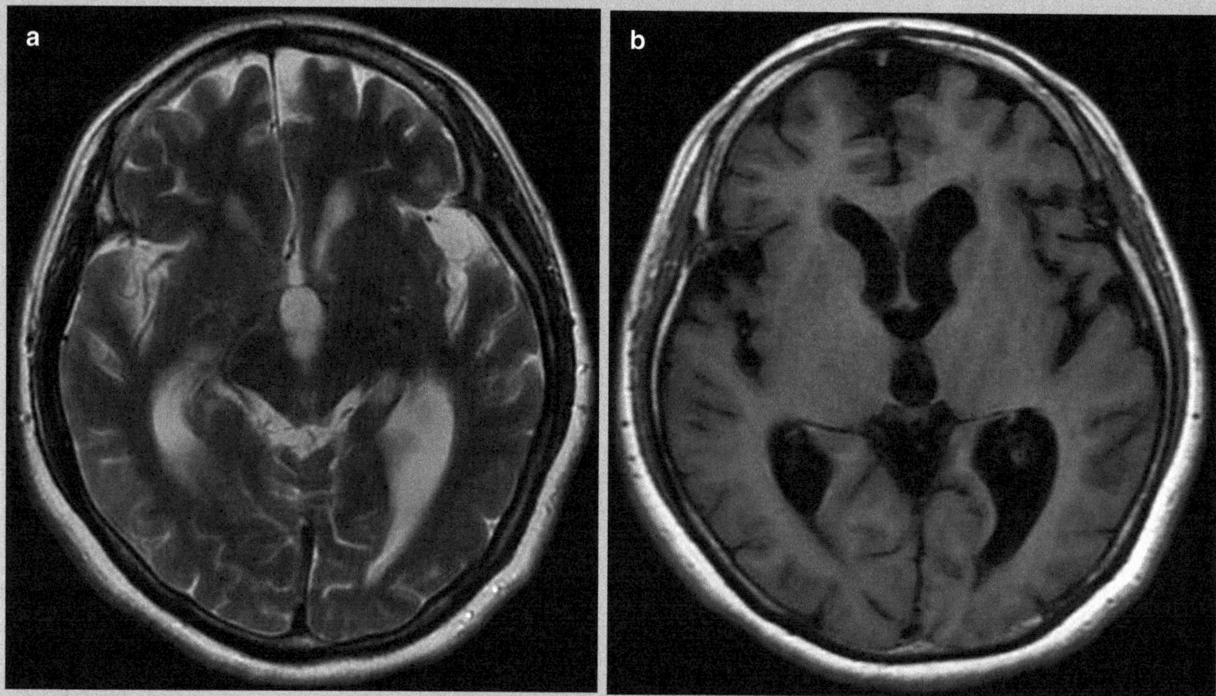

Fig. 3.11 Neurological brucellosis. (**a**, **b**) MR imaging demonstrates dilated ventricular system of the brain, suggesting hydrocephalus

3.7.3 The Respiratory and Circulatory Systems

3.7.3.1 Ultrasound

In the cases with pulmonary infection, no abnormalities are demonstrated. In the cases with pleural effusion, fluid dark area can be demonstrated. In the cases with mitral valve involved, adhesion or incomplete closure of mitral valve can be observed.

3.7.3.2 X-Ray Radiology

X-ray demonstrates the mediastinum with confined or symmetrical wideness, indicating mediastinal lymphadenectasis. X-ray also demonstrates thickened lung markings in both lungs with grid-like change, suggesting interstitial pneumonia. In other cases, X-ray demonstrates thickened lung markings at both lungs that concentrate at the middle and medial parts of the lung fields, and small flakes of shadows along the lung markings, suggesting bronchopneumonia. By X-ray, small nodules in both lungs, pleural effusion, and pyothorax can also be demonstrated. In addition, confined round-like infiltration shadows with poorly defined boundaries can also be demonstrated, with internal transparent area and thickened pleura.

3.7.3.3 CT Scanning

CT scanning demonstrates ground glass opacities, thickened bronchial vascular bundles, thickened interlobar pleura and septum. The margin is demonstrated with fine spots of nodules. The middle and lower lung fields are demonstrated with flakes and nodules of high-density shadows. There are also mediastinal or hilar lymphadenectasis, interstitial pneumonia, and bronchopneumonia. In addition, nodular shadows at the lungs, pleural effusion, pyothorax, and thickened pleura can be observed (Fig. 3.12).

Case Study 13
A patient complained of cough and fever for 3 months and above. Laboratory test indicated brucellar pneumonia.

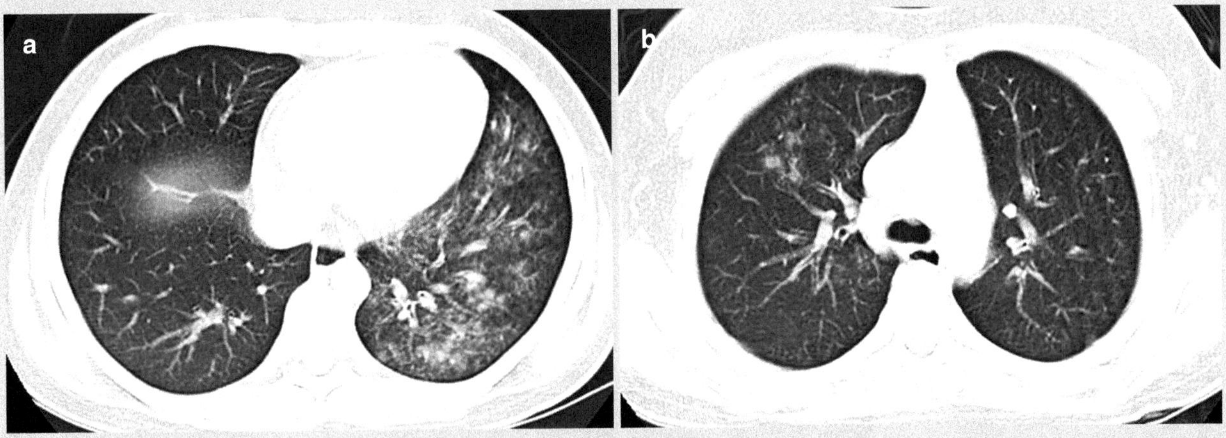

Fig. 3.12 Brucellar pneumonia. (**a**, **b**) CT scanning demonstrates multiple ground glass shadows and small nodular shadows in both lungs, suggesting bronchopneumonia

3.7.3.4 MR Imaging

MR imaging demonstrates pleural effusion or pyothorax. Regurgitation or myxoma caused by incomplete closure or stenosis of mitral valve may also be observed. In some cases, the pleura is subject to thickening, with high-signal shadow.

3.7.4 The Digestive System

3.7.4.1 Ultrasound

The demonstration is hepatosplenomegaly. In the cases with infection, abscess cavity with thick wall and poorly defined boundary can be demonstrated. Abdominal lymphadenectasis can also be observed.

3.7.4.2 X-Ray Radiology

X-ray generally fails to demonstrate the definite lesions. In some individual cases, hepatosplenomegaly can be demonstrated.

3.7.4.3 CT Scanning

CT scanning, in some rare cases, demonstrates inguinal lymphadenectasis; in most cases, it demonstrates hepatosplenomegaly or hepatic abscess. Hepatic abscess is commonly demonstrated with multilayered enhancement of abscess wall with poorly defined boundary. In some individual cases, mass-like high-density shadow can be observed.

3.7.4.4 MR Imaging

MR imaging demonstrates hepatosplenomegaly as well as plump liver and spleen. T2WI demonstrates as slightly high signal. The incidence rate of splenomegaly is higher than hepatomegaly by about 25 % (Fig. 3.13). Liver abscess is rarely observed. The lesions are demonstrated with long T1 long T2 signals. By contrast imaging, the abscess wall is demonstrated with multilayered enhancement and poorly defined boundary.

Case Study 14
A patient complained of hepatalgia and intermittent fever for above 2 months. By laboratory test, the diagnosis was defined to be brucellosis.

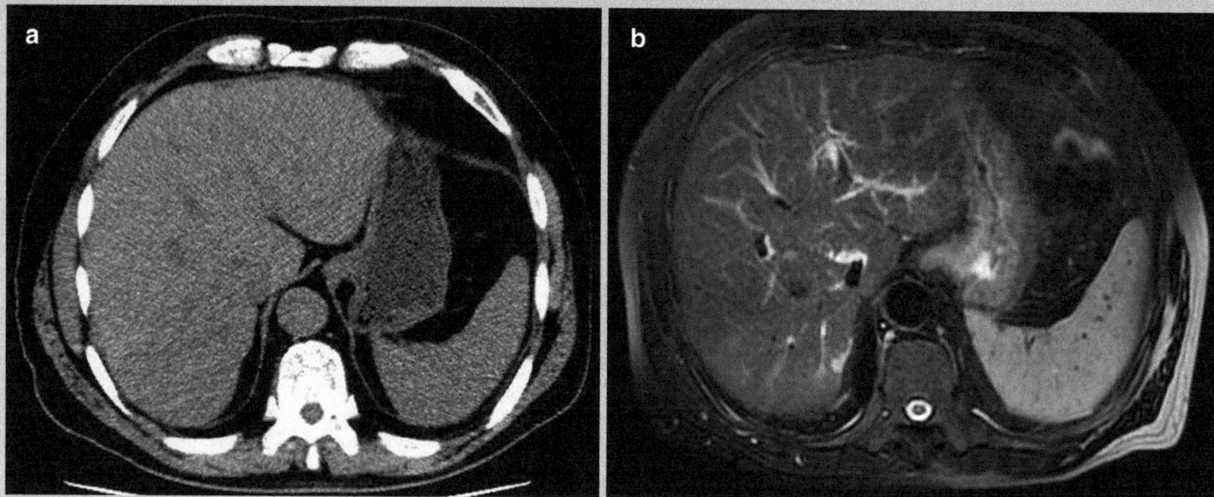

Fig. 3.13 Brucellosis complicated by liver and spleen lesions. (**a**, **b**) Both CT scanning and MR imaging demonstrate enlarged liver and spleen, with smooth margin and no abnormal densities and signals

Case Study 15
A patient complained of night fever with a body temperature of 38.5 °C for 2 months, with accompanying night sweating, joint pain, and weakness. By laboratory test, the diagnosis was defined to be brucellosis.

(For case detail and figures, please refer to Chourmouzi D, et al. *Cases Journal*, 2009, 2: 7143.)

3.7.5 The Urogenital System

3.7.5.1 Ultrasound

High echo is demonstrated from the kidney, with swollen testicles and scrotal effusion. In the cases with infection, abscess can be demonstrated with thick wall and poorly defined boundary. Abdominal lymphadenectasis can rarely be demonstrated.

3.7.5.2 X-Ray Radiology

In some individual cases, calcification in the kidney can be detected.

3.7.5.3 CT Scanning

In some rare cases, lymphadenectasis can be observed. In the cases with renal infection, irregular calcification shadow can be demonstrated. In the cases with secondary abscess, its boundary is poorly defined, which is extremely rare (Fig. 3.14).

Case Study 16
A patient complained of fever, joint pain, lower back and back pain, and night sweating for 1 month. After surgical operation, biopsy demonstrated brucellosis with renal infection.

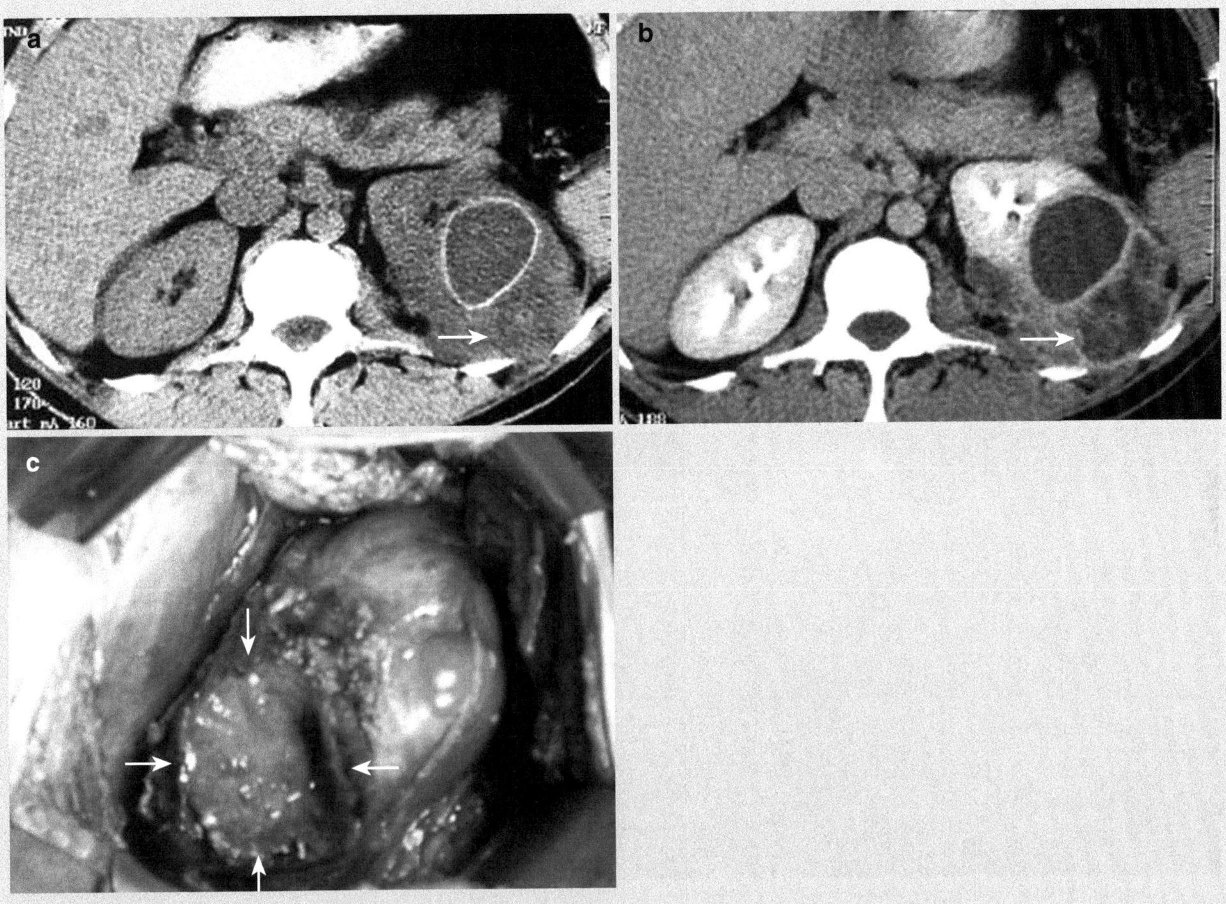

Fig. 3.14 Renal abscess and brucellosis complicated by renal infection. (**a**) CT scanning demonstrates enlarged superior pole of the left kidney due to an oval-shaped abscess that is smooth and intact with high density and thick wall. The lesion is surrounded by irregular low-density lesion, with poorly defined boundary (indicated by *arrow*). (**b**) Contrast scanning demonstrates slight enhancement of the abscess wall and ring-shaped enhancement of the surrounding low-density lesion (indicated by *arrow*). (**c**) During the operation, the abscess at the left kidney and the abscess with internal fluid discharged are observed (indicated by *arrows*) (Reprint with permission from Onaran et al. 2005, 12 (12): 1058)

3.7.5.4 MR Imaging

Brucellosis complicated by renal abscess is rarely found, with demonstrations of long T1 long T2 signals. Contrast imaging demonstrates enhancement of the abscess wall. In the cases with testicles involved, imaging demonstrates swollen testicles, increased T2WI signal, and scrotal effusion (Fig. 3.15).

Case Study 17

A patient complained of scrotal pain and swelling as well as local fever for above 3 months. Laboratory test demonstrated brucellosis.

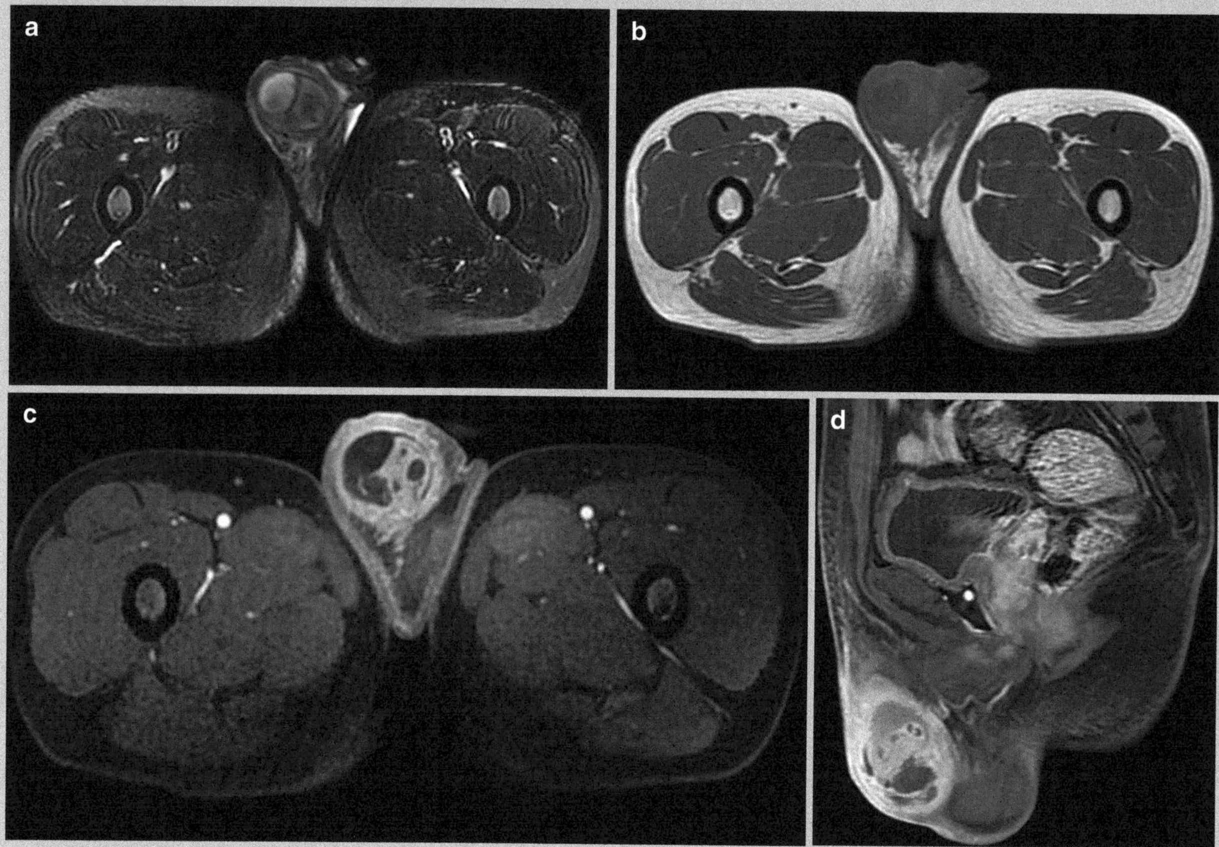

Fig. 3.15 Brucellosis complicated by testicular lesion. (**a–d**) MR imaging demonstrates swollen testicles with uneven long T1 and long T2 signals. By contrast imaging, enhanced septum is demonstrated

3.8 Diagnostic Basis

3.8.1 Brucellosis

3.8.1.1 Epidemiology

The patient usually has a history of close contacts to farming animals or farming animal products carrying *Brucella* prior to the onset. Otherwise, the patient is a resident living in an epidemic area or is closely related to the manufacture, use, and research of the bacterial strains.

3.8.1.2 Clinical Manifestations

The clinical manifestations include fever (including low-grade fever) that persists for days or weeks, profuse sweating, muscle and joint pain, and fatigue. There may be also swellings of the liver, spleen, lymph nodes, and testicle as well as other suspected symptoms.

3.8.1.3 Laboratory Test Findings

Slide test for brucellosis is positive or standard tube agglutination test is positive. Otherwise, observations at 24 h and

48 h after skin allergy test demonstrate at least one finding of the red swollen skin area being above 2×2 cm.

3.8.1.4 Bacteria Isolation

Brucella can be isolated from blood, bone marrow, other body fluids, and excretions of the patients.

3.8.1.5 Serological Test

Standard tube agglutination test shows a titer above 1:100. For individuals with a history of vaccination against brucellosis within the past 6 months and a SAT titer above 1:100, a reexamination by SAT demonstrates at least 4 times increase of the titer after 2–4 weeks. Otherwise, complement fixation test demonstrates a titer of above 1:10. Human immunoglobulin titer is demonstrated to be above 1:400.

3.8.2 Brucellosis-Related Complications

3.8.2.1 Osteoarticular and Spinal Complications

1. The patients with brucellosis have clinical symptoms of migrating pain of systemic joints whose occurrence is related to fever.
2. By radiological examinations, swellings of joint and the surrounding soft tissue are observed at the acute stage, bone changes at the chronic stage. Early and extensive bone repair is a characteristic radiological demonstration of osteoarticular and spinal complication of brucellosis. The demonstrations include diffuse bone sclerosis under the cartilage and around the destructed lesion, narrowed interarticular space, and even bone rigidity as well as ossification of tendon or ligament attachments.

3.8.2.2 Neurological Complications

1. The patients with brucellosis show clinical manifestations of neurological symptoms.
2. By radiological examinations, such as CT scanning and MR imaging, demonstrate narrowed or absent basal cistern, swollen spinal cords, and hydrocephalus. In the cases with brain parenchyma involved, small flakes of low-density shadows can be observed. Cranial CTA or MRA demonstrates uneven thickness or stenosis of arteries and even interrupted arteries.

3.8.2.3 The Respiratory System

1. The patients with brucellosis show clinical symptoms of cough, chest pain, and other respiratory symptoms.
2. By radiological examinations, interstitial pneumonia is demonstrated as thickened lung markings at both lungs in grid-like change; bronchopneumonia is demonstrated as thickened lung markings at the middle and medial parts of both lungs as well as small flakes of shadows along the lung markings.

3.8.2.4 The Digestive System

1. The patients with brucellosis show clinical symptoms of nausea, vomiting, abdominal upset, and other digestive symptoms.
2. By radiological examinations, enlarged and plump liver and spleen can be observed, with slightly increased T_2WI signal compared to the normal control. Hepatic abscess is rarely observed.

3.8.2.5 The Urogenital System

1. The patients with brucellosis show clinical symptoms of fever, lower back pain, nephric mass, swelling and pain of the testicles, regional scrotal redness and swelling, as well as other urogenital symptoms.
2. By radiological examinations, renal abscess is observed, with enlarged testicles, increased T_2WI signal, and scrotal effusion.

3.9 Differential Diagnosis

3.9.1 Spinal Tuberculosis and Pulmonary Tuberculosis

Spinal tuberculosis mainly causes bone destruction, with common involvements of the anterior vertebra in worm-bitten-like appearance. It is commonly accompanied by osteoporosis, with small masses or sand-like sequestrum, spinal angulation, and paravertebral cold natured abscess. However, paravertebral cold natured abscess is rarely found in the cases of brucellosis complicated by spondylitis. The commonalities of both diseases include destruction of involved vertebra, deformed vertebra, and narrowed or absent intervertebral space, which present challenges for their differentiation, especially at the early stage. Spinal tuberculosis is characterized by vertebral destruction, with common manifestations of abnormal morphology of the involved vertebra and formation of spinal angulated posterior process. Brucellosis complicated by spondylitis is manifested as marginal bone destruction of adjacent vertebrae, normal morphology of vertebra, or only slightly wedge-shaped deformation. The bone destruction is gradually replaced by irregular dense new bone, with more bone repair than bone destruction. At the vertebral margin, a large quantity of osteophytes is produced. Sometimes, there are also ossification of anterior ligament or posterior longitudinal ligament, vertebral fusion, sclerosis of small articular surface, and absent interarticular space.

Pulmonary tuberculosis is clinically manifested as low-grade fever after noons, emaciation, and night sweats. It may be complicated by HIV infection or immunodeficiency. By chest X-ray, specific changes can be demonstrated. Both tuberculosis and brucellosis have manifestations of enlarged lymph nodes. The lymphatic tubercles commonly adhere and fuse into mass, whose rupture with discharge of pus causes fistulas and scars. However, enlarged lymph nodes in the cases of brucellosis are rarely subject to rupture.

3.9.2 Rheumatoid Arthritis

Rheumatoid arthritis is manifested as a symmetric multiple peripheral small joint pain with swelling and joint dysfunction. At the advanced stage, the joints are subject to deformity, with rheumatoid factors positive. Hand X-ray demonstrates osteoporosis and narrowed interarticular space.

3.9.3 Osteoarthritis

Osteoarthritis commonly occurs in population aged above 50 years. The joint pain is characterized by pain after physical activities that alleviates after rests. The disease involves weight-loading joints, such as the knee and hip. By X-ray, osteoproliferation and nodules are demonstrated, with no obvious acceleration of erythrocyte sedimentation rate (ESR).

References

Chourmouzi D, Boulogianni G, Kalomenopoulou M, et al. Brucella liver abscess; imaging approach, differential diagnosis, and therapeutic management: a case report. Cases J. 2009;2:7143.

Guo YJ, Yi L, Liu L, et al. Neurobrucellosis: three case reports and literature review. Chinese Journal of Contemporary Neurology, 2013,13 (1): 49.

Onaran M, Sen I, Polat F, et al. Renal brucelloma: a rare infection of the kidney. Int J Urol. 2005;12(12):1058–60.

Xiao DL. Handbook for prevention and control of Brucellosis. Beijing: People's Medical Publishing House; 2008.

Yang XX, Du W, Du ZQ. Misdiagnosis of brucellosis as skeletal tuberculosis: report of 7 cases. Chin J Misdiagnosis. 2006;4(8):1777.

Yang XM, Shi W, Du YK, et al. Clinical radiology of Brucellar spondylitis and spinal tuberculosis: a comparative study. J Clin Radiol. 2008;27(2):234.

Zhou DH, Sun HZ, Li XX, et al. Epidemic situation of brucellosis in China and diagnosis of brucellosis complicated by osteoarthritis by CT scanning. Chin J Mod Radiol. 2008;5(7):652.

Suggested Reading

CDC, Ministry of Health, P.R.China. Handbook for prevention and control of brucellosis. Beijing: People's Medical Publishing House; 2008.

Franco MP, Mulder M, Gilman RH, et al. Human brucellosis. Lancet Infect Dis. 2007;7(12):775–86.

Guzey FK, Emel E, Sel B, et al. Cervical spinal brucellosis causing epidural and prevertebral abscesses and spinal cord compression: a case report. Spine J. 2007;7(2):240–4.

He ZH, Li X. Clinical manifestations and radiological demonstrations of spinal tuberculosis. J Pract Med Tech. 2006;13(9):1459–60.

Liu Z, Li YY, Yang DK, et al. Radiological demonstrations of chronic spinal brucellosis. Pract Radiol. 2008;23(9):1041–3.

Lv XL, Yang JY, Li SH. MR imaging demonstrations of brucellosis complicated by spondylitis. Inner Mongolia J Med. 2008;40(3): 305–7.

Ministry of Health, P.R. China. GB15988-1995 Diagnostic criteria and therapeutic principles for brucellosis. Beijing: People's Medical Publishing House; 1995.

Cat Scratch Disease

4

Qi Zhang, Hongjun Li, and Xinhua Zhang

Cat scratch disease (CSD), an infectious zoonosis, is caused by *Bartonella* and a cat scratch or bite. Though its clinical manifestations are variable, it has common manifestations of local skin lesions and enlarged lymph nodes. It is a self-limited disease, with a natural disease course ranging from several weeks to several months. During recent years, the incidence rate of CSD has been increasing due to the popularity of raising pets.

4.1 Etiology

In 1889, cat scratch disease was firstly reported by Henri Parinaud, which was described as Parinaud's oculoglandular syndrome. In 1931, Robert Debre, a French doctor, discovered that Parinaud's oculoglandular syndrome is related to cat. He announced his discovery to the public in the year of 1950, but its pathogen was still unknown. In 1983, Wear et al. successfully isolated the pathogens of CSD from the patients' diseased lymph nodes, skin tissues, and conjunctival tissues. It was not until in 1992 that *Bartonella henselae* was identified as the pathogen of CSD by using PCR technique. By serological test or molecular genetic test, most cases with obvious clinical symptoms of CSD can be demonstrated to be *Bartonella* infection.

Bartonella henselae is categorized into the genus of *Rochalimaea*, the family of *Rickettsiaceae*, and the order of *Rickettsiales*. It is a slender polymorphic Gram-negative bacillus with a size of 0.3–1.0 × 2.6–3.0 μm. Being lack of glycolytic enzymes, *Bartonella henselae* remains inactive in a series of biochemical reactions, showing negative results in oxidase test, catalase test, esculin test, hippurate hydrolysis, and nitrate reduction test.

Q. Zhang • H. Li (✉) • X. Zhang
Department of Radiology, Beijing You'an Hospital, Capital Medical University, Beijing, China
e-mail: lihongjun00113@126.com

4.2 Epidemiology

4.2.1 Source of Infection

The main source of infection is the cats carrying *Bartonella henselae*, especially kittens aged under 1 year or newly adopted cats. Other sources of infection include dogs and monkeys. Its transmission from person to person has not been reported. The onset of the disease does not occur in cats carrying the pathogens.

4.2.2 Route of Transmission

Human is commonly infected by CSD via scratch, bite, or close contact to cat or other animals. Some cases of CSD are infected via flea bite.

4.2.3 Susceptible Population

It has been reported that CSD occurs in above 40,000 persons each year worldwide, with higher incidence in young adults and adolescents. About 80 % of CSD cases are in an age group under the age of 21 years. Its occurrence is more common in autumns and winters, with male patients being significantly more than female patients. Patients with HIV infection have seriously suppressed immunity, and such patients are more vulnerable to CSD infection by a cat carrying the pathogen.

4.2.4 Epidemiological Features

CSD is a globally sporadic but acute infectious disease, which more commonly occurs in autumns and winters of the temperate zone. However, its occurrence has no seasonal changes in the tropical zone.

H. Li (ed.), *Radiology of Infectious Diseases: Volume 2*, DOI 10.1007/978-94-017-9876-1_4

4.3 Pathogenesis and Pathological Changes

4.3.1 Pathogenesis

The pathogenesis of CSD still remains elusive. It may be related to the histocompatibility antigen between some components of *Bartonella* and the vascular wall of impaired tissues and organs, which may induce the human body to produce impaired immunological recognition. Subsequently, inflammation of local vascular walls and thrombus occur. Meanwhile, hyperplasia corpuscles form in the lymph nodes to cause compromised immunity and immune dysfunction or even immune deficiency. As a result, systemic multiple system lesions occur, with involvement of the central nervous system, bone lesions, thrombocytopenia, angioma, hepatitis, and endocarditis.

4.3.2 Pathological Changes

The affected lymph nodes have different degrees of swelling, with dark red sections, on which needle tip-sized yellowish particles may be found. Under a microscope, the lymphatic structure can still be observed, with expanded germinal center. The characteristic lesion is granulomatous inflammation of lymph nodes with accompanying microabscesses, which is mainly distributed in the cortical and paracortical areas. The microabscess is composed of neutrophils and necrotic cell debris, which usually has irregular morphology, with characteristic star-shaped abscess and surrounding hyperplasia of histiocytes and lymphocytes. By Warthin-Starry (WS) silver staining, the swallowed bacteria can be found in the lymphoid sinus of diseased lymph nodes and in the macrophages surrounding the microabscess, which are black granular bacteria.

4.4 Clinical Symptoms and Signs

In the typical cases, local singular or several erythematous papules can be found in 3–14 days after scratched by a cat. The pain is slight that tends to be neglected by the patient. Within 5–50 days after scratched by a cat, about 90 % of the infected cases show swollen draining lymph nodes, which are more common in the head and neck region, armpit, elbow, and groin. The swollen lymph node is commonly unilateral, singular, or small, which can spread to the secondary lymph nodes with more obvious swelling. In about 25 % of the infected cases, suppuration of lymph nodes may occur, with occasional penetration to form sinus tracts or fistula. Some patients may experience systemic symptoms of fever and fatigue. Most patients can heal simultaneously within 2–4 months.

The rarely found types of CSD include ocular CSD, cerebral CSD, hepatic and splenic CSD, musculoskeletal CSD, mammary CSD, and systemic CSD.

4.5 Cat Scratch Disease-Related Complications

The complications of cat scratch disease rarely occur, including encephalopathy, chronic severe organ lesions (hepatic granulomas and osteomyelitis), arthropathy (arthralgia and arthritis), and erythema nodosum. Other complications include transient maculopapule, polymorphic erythema, thrombocytopenic purpura, parotid gland swelling, multiple angioma, and organs purpura (more commonly found in patients with HIV infection), all of which rarely occur in patients with CSD.

4.6 Diagnostic Examinations

4.6.1 Laboratory Tests

4.6.1.1 Smear

Warthin-Starry silver staining is the best way to detect *Bartonella* because it can amplify the pathogens for more favorable microscopic examination. By Gram staining, the stained bacteria are fine and small, with poor effects of staining.

4.6.1.2 Culture of the Pathogen

Bartonella grows slowly on the blood agar medium. Typical colonies can be found after culturing for 12–14 days and sometimes even 45 days. Therefore, the culture of the pathogen cannot provide early diagnosis of CSD.

4.6.1.3 Molecular Biological Examination

In recent years, *Bartonella* infection can be detected and defined by gene sequencing methods, including nested-PCR amplification, PCR situ hybridization, and PRC sequencing detection. However, these examinations have complex operational procedures and require more complicated equipment. Therefore, these examinations cannot be routine examination in the community hospitals.

4.6.1.4 Serological Test

Immunofluorescence antibody assay (IFA) is mainly applied to detect IgG antibody of *Bartonella*, but it is not a favorable assay for detection of IgM antibody. In addition, different individual observers may obtain different test results. IFA is also not suitable for automatic operations and large-scale sample detection.

4.6.2 Diagnostic Imaging

CT scanning and MR imaging are commonly applied to examine the nervous system and digestive organs. Ultrasound, CT scanning, and MR imaging all can detect the swollen lymph nodes. Especially, ultrasound is convenient to be performed. However, lymphadenitis of CSD demonstrated by ultrasound is nonspecific.

4.7 Imaging Demonstrations

4.7.1 Ultrasound

Ultrasound demonstrates enlarged lymph nodes that are round like with clearly defined boundaries. In these enlarged lymph nodes, low even or generally even low echo can be observed, commonly with accompanying high echo from intact hilum of lymph nodes. The posterior echo is slightly enhanced. Color Doppler ultrasonography shows cord-like blood flows stretching into the lumps, some being abundant like branches or flames. Most of these flows are artery blood flows with a relatively low RI, which has similar resistance parameters to artery blood flow of other common inflammatory lymph nodes.

4.7.2 CT Scanning

CT scanning demonstrates singular or multiple enlarged lymph nodes with accompanying central necrosis. Extensive peripheral edema occurs in the proximal lymphatic drainage channel. CT scanning reveals that many swollen lymph nodes fuse into a cluster and some have central low-density necrotic area. In the fat space surrounding the enlarged lymph nodes, there are high-density cord-like inflammatory infiltration shadows, sometimes with accompanying surrounding edema. Contrast CT scanning demonstrates slight enhancement, ring-shaped enhancement, or no enhancement. Pan SH believed that CT scanning has certain diagnostic value for CSD. He stated that for the cases with enlarged and purulent draining lymph nodes, contrast CT scanning can reveal the central necrosis and liquefaction in these enlarged lymph nodes, with no obvious enhancement. However, marginal enhancement can be obvious due to vascular hyperplasia and abundant blood supply.

4.7.3 MR Imaging

MR imaging demonstrates round-like enlarged lymph nodes, with equal to low T1 signal and low or high T2 signal. The homogeneity of signal in lymph nodes is related to its qualitative changes.

4.7.3.1 The Early Stage

In the cortex of enlarged lymph nodes, multiple granulomas form with internal scattering neutrophils in different quantities. In this stage, both T1 and T2 signals of the lymph nodes are homogeneous. By contrast imaging, moderate even enhancement can be demonstrated. The imaging demonstrations are not characteristic, which hardly provides evidence for differential diagnosis from other inflammatory granuloma.

4.7.3.2 The Middle Stage

Microabscesses form in the granulomas. When necrosis is obvious, the abscesses are commonly polygonal, which is known as starlike abscesses. In this stage, equal or low T1WI signals and high T2WI signals of necrotic areas can be demonstrated, with marginal enhancement. The imaging demonstrations are also not characteristic, which are similar to those of lymphoid tuberculosis with caseous necrosis (Fig. 4.1).

4.7.3.3 The Advanced Stage

Fibrosis occurs in the granulomas. Meanwhile, stellate fiber septum can be found in the lymph nodes. Both T1WI and T2WI signals are low. The enhancement of the fiber septum is related to its maturity. By contrast imaging, fibroblast-based fiber septum is enhanced, while fibrocyte-based fiber septum is not enhanced. The stellate fiber septum appears like flower buds at the center of flower petals, with petallike enhancement around the septum. In this stage, MR imaging demonstrations of the lymph nodes are characteristic, which can be the evidence for the diagnosis of CSD. Extensive subcutaneous edema can be found adjacent to the swollen lymph nodes, in cord-like T1WI low signals and T2WI high signals. By contrast imaging, the cord-like shadows are demonstrated with no enhancement. These changes indicate inflammatory lesions, which is the evidence for the differential diagnosis from neoplasms.

Case Study 1

A female patient aged 33 years complained of enlarged mass in the left breast with accompanying redness, swelling, fever, and pain for more than 2 months. She received a surgical incision for drainage, but with poor therapeutic effectiveness. She denied a history of contact to pets. By physical examination, a lump in size of 8×5 cm can be palpated in the upper quadrant of the left breast and the deep mammary areola. The lump is hard and nearly immobile with unclearly defined boundary and tenderness. Several hard lymph nodes in a diameter of 1.5 cm can be palpated in the left armpit. By ultrasound, disorderly and uneven echoes can be found on medial gland of the left breast nipple, with flakes of low echo covering an area of about 2.2×2.0 cm. The echoes have irregular morphology with unclearly defined boundaries and no obvious internal liquid echo. Several lymph nodes can be found in the left armpit, with the larger ones in size of 1.7×1.0 cm. The interface between cortex and medulla is well defined, with thickened cortex. By color Doppler ultrasonography, a small quantity of blood flow signals can be found in the periphery. Surgical removal of the inflammatory lesions in the left breast was performed, with removal of tough grayish white and grayish pink lump in a size of about 5×4 cm. The pathological diagnosis was pyogenic granulomatous inflammation of the left breast (mammary CSD). By special stainings, PAS staining was negative, WS staining positive, silver methenamine staining negative, and acid-fast staining with no finding of acid-fast bacillus. By immunohistochemical staining, CD68 was positive.

For case detail and figures, please refer to Lu J, et al. *Chinese Journal of Medical Ultrasound* (*Electronic Edition*), 2012, 9(6): 567.

Case Study 2

A female patient aged 36 years complained of painful lymph nodes in the right humeral epicondyle and in the armpit soft tissue for 2 weeks and persistent low-grade fever for 3 days. She had symptoms of localized pain and swelling as well as erythema lesion. She reported a history of a cat bite of her right index finger 6 weeks ago.

For case detail and figures, please refer to Wang CW, et al. *Clin Imaging*, 2009, 33 (4): 318.

Case Study 3

A girl aged 12 years complained of a painful lump in the right medial armpit and moderate fever with a body temperature of 38 °C for 2 days. She reported a history of kitten scratch 1 month ago, with no symptoms of cough, sore throat, running nose, and diarrhea. By blood culture, no growth of organism was found.

For case detail and figures, please refer to Wang CW, et al. *Clin Imaging*, 2009, 33 (4): 318.

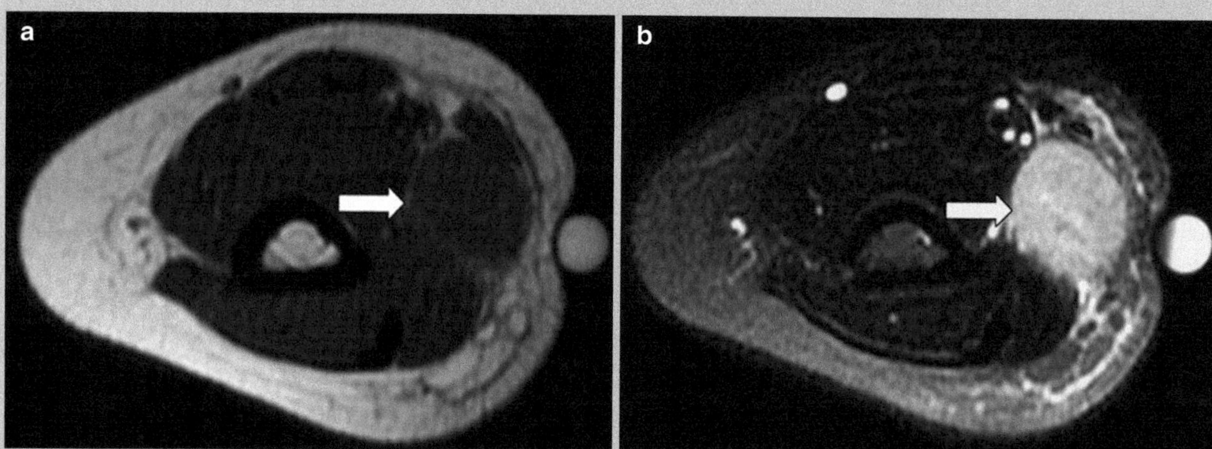

Fig. 4.1 CSD lymphadenitis in the right armpit. (**a**) MR imaging demonstrates oval nodules in the right armpit, with surrounding edema. T1WI signals are equal (indicated by *arrows*). (**b**) T2WI fat-suppression sequence demonstrates high signals. (**c**) After the injection of contrast agent, centers of the lesions are enhanced (indicated by *asterisk*) (Reproduced with permission from *Wang CW*, et al. *Clin Imaging*, 2009, 33 (4):318)

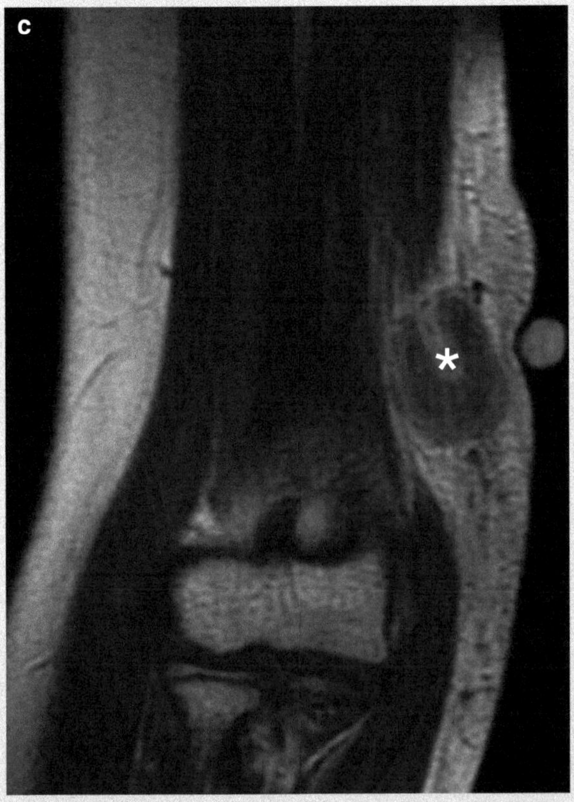

Fig. 4.1 (continued)

Case Study 4
A female patient aged 18 years was hospitalized due to a lump in her left elbow for 1 week. She denied histories of upper limb infection, trauma, as well as skin wound and bleeding at the location of the lump. By physical examination, the lump was moderately hard and mobile, with slight tenderness and a smooth surface. There was no distal radiating pain when it was pressed. Preoperatively, she was misdiagnosed with angioma. The following pathological examination defined the diagnosis of CSD lymphadenitis.

For case detail and figures, please refer to Zhang WQ, et al. *Practice of Radiology*, 2008, 23 (7): 789.

Case Study 5
A male patient aged 48 years complained of general upset, fatigue, epigastric pain, and no enlarged lymph nodes. He denied a history of contact to cat. Ultrasound indicated multiple nodules in the liver. His liver function is normal. The pathological examination after surgery defined the diagnosis of hepatic CSD.

For case detail and figures, please refer to Marsilia GM, et al. *Int J Surg Pathol*, 2006, 14 (4): 349.

Case Study 6
A girl aged 13 years was hospitalized due to systemic tonic convulsion and unconsciousness. Since day 10 after the hospitalization, she began to experience enlarged lymph nodes in the left groin and fever, with response to pain stimulations. It was reported that she raised a pet dog and cat at home. On day 1 of her hospitalization, she experienced nine episodes of convulsion, which was relieved after intravenous infusion of diazepam and was further improved after intravenous medication of midazolam and phenytoinum natricum. The patient gradually regained her consciousness. On day 2 of her hospitalization, she began to receive oral medication of carbamazepine. By cerebrospinal fluid examination, WBC count was 2 cells/μl, protein 0.22 g/L, bacterial culture negative, and herpes simplex virus negative. By immunofluorescence, IgG antibody titer was 1:512. The blood samples collected from the dog and cat at her home were detected, with *Bartonella* positive in the cat and *Bartonella* negative in the dog. The clinical diagnosis was defined to be cerebral CSD. The patient was cured after 3 months.

For case detail and figures, please refer to Ogura K, et al. *Eur Neurol*, 2004, 51 (2): 109.

4.8 Diagnostic Basis

4.8.1 Clinical Diagnosis

Item 1. The patient has a history of contact to animals, commonly dogs and cats, and has a history of animal scratch or bite.

Item 2. CSD skin antigen test is positive.

Item 3. Enlarged lymph nodes, with all laboratory tests, are negative for other etiological factors.

Item 4. Biopsy of the lymph node tissue bears findings in consistency to histopathology of CSD, including necrotic granuloma and microabscesses. By WS staining, *Bartonella henselae* is detected.

The patient having three conditions of the above four can be clinically diagnosed with CSD. The following serological tests (IFA and ELISA-IgM) can define the diagnosis. In addition, conjunctivitis with accompanying preauricular lymphadenectasis (Parinaud's oculoglandular syndrome) is one of the important indicators of CSD, which facilitates the diagnosis.

4.8.2 Radiological Diagnosis

4.8.2.1 Ultrasound

1. Multiple fused enlarged lymph nodes.
2. The swelling has well-defined boundary, with thick and coarse envelope.
3. The swelling has cortex and medulla, with target-like change.
4. Color Doppler ultrasonography demonstrates cord-like blood flows stretching into the swelling, and some have abundant blood flow like branches or flames.

4.8.2.2 CT Scanning

The enlarged lymph nodes are singular or multiple and multiple enlarged lymph nodes fuse into clusters. Low-density necrosis can be found at the center of some enlarged lymph nodes. In the fat space surrounding the enlarged lymph nodes, high-density cord-like inflammatory infiltration shadows can be found, possibly with surrounding edema. Contrast imaging demonstrates slight enhancement, ring-shaped enhancement, or no enhancement.

4.8.2.3 MR Imaging

By MR imaging, local lymphadenitis is demonstrated as uneven lumps with surrounding edema in long T1 and long T2 signals. Contrast scanning demonstrates marginal enhancement of the lesions. When granuloma is found to have fibrosis, stellate or rose sign can be demonstrated, which is a characteristic imaging demonstration.

4.9 Differential Diagnosis

4.9.1 Soft Tissue Angioma

The lesions can be singular or multiple, with nodular or diffuse growth and mostly with no envelope. T1WI demonstrates equal or slightly high signal, while T2WI demonstrates obviously increased signal intensity. There are commonly nonvascular tissue components in the neoplasm, such as fibrous tissue, hyperplastic vascular smooth muscle, thrombus, and calcification. Enhanced imaging demonstrates flakes of enhancement of the lesions with gradually increasing enhancement. The flow void phenomenon and phlebolith in the lesions facilitate to establish the diagnosis.

4.9.2 Neurogenic Neoplasm

Neurogenic neoplasms in the limbs are relatively larger, often with uneven signals. Some scholars believe that neoplasm in the flexor area or with accompanying muscular atrophy strongly indicates a diagnosis of neurogenic neoplasm.

4.9.3 Lymphatic Tuberculosis

The lesions of lymphatic tuberculosis commonly fuse into masses to form a garland-like shape with marginal enhancement. The finding of spots of calcification in the lymph nodes facilitates the diagnosis. In the cases of CSD lymphadenitis with formation of abscess and necrosis, characteristic marginal enhancement can be found. The multiple lymph nodes have well-defined boundaries with no fusion and with no internal spots of calcification.

References

Lu J, Zhong DR, Jiang YX, et al. Ultrasonic and pathological manifestations of mammary cat scratch disease: with attached 2 case reports. Chin J Med Ultrasonography (Electronic Edition). 2012;9(6):567–8.

Marsilia GM, La Mura A, Galdiero R, et al. Isolated hepatic involvement of cat scratch disease in immunocompetent adults: enhanced magnetic resonance imaging, pathological findings, and molecular analysis–two cases. Int J Surg Pathol. 2006;14(4):349–54.

Ogura K, Hara Y, Tsukahara H, et al. MR signal changes in a child with cat scratch disease encephalopathy and status epilepticus. Eur Neurol. 2004;51(2):109–10.

Wang CW, Chang WC, Chao TK, et al. Computed tomography and magnetic resonance imaging of cat-scratch disease: a report of two cases. Clin Imaging. 2009;33(4):318–21.

Zhang WQ, Yu RS, Chen Y. MR imaging for the diagnosis of elbow CSD lymphadenitis. Pract Radiol. 2008;23(7):788–90.

Suggested Reading

Ji X, Lv JG, Chen GF. CT demonstrations and pathological diagnosis of cat scratch disease. J Clin Radiol. 2004;23(7):610–2.

Pan SH. CT demonstrations cat scratch disease. J Pract Radiol. 2003;19(11):1017–8.

Ren MJ, Wang P. Ultrasonic diagnosis of cat scratch disease lymphadenitis. Chin Med Record. 2012;13(3):76–7.

Wu SM, Zhang ZY, Zhang ZQ. Newly emerging infectious diseases and re-emerging infectious diseases. Shanghai: Shanghai Science Education Press; 2010.

Zhang LX, Zhou XZ. Modern studies of infectious diseases. Beijing: People's Military Medical Press; 2010.

5 Chlamydia pneumoniae Pneumonia

Xing Wang, Hongjun Li, and Zhenying Xia

Chlamydia pneumoniae (CP) is a new species of *Chlamydia* discovered in the 1980s, which has a widespread distribution across the world. It can cause human diseases such as pneumonia and is an important pathogen of human respiratory tract infections. Currently, the occurrence of CP infection has been increasing among community-acquired pneumonia in children and adults, which has prevailed in many regions both in China and in other countries.

5.1 Etiology

Chlamydia pneumoniae (CP) is part of the *Chlamydiaceae* family and is a gram-negative pathogen.

5.1.1 Morphology and Structure

Under an electron microscope, *Chlamydia pneumoniae* is in the shape of a typical pear, with the long axis being approximately 0.44 μm, the short axis being about 0.3 μm, and an average diameter of about 0.38 μm. Its nucleus is round in shape with an average diameter of 0.24 μm, locating at the center of the cell. There is a wide protoplasm zone between the nucleus and the cell membrane (Fig. 5.1).

5.1.2 Features Found by Culture

CP can only parasitize in cells and cannot be cultured in vitro. Therefore, cell subculture is commonly used for its reproduction. The sensitive cell lines to CP include HEP-2 and H-292.

X. Wang • H. Li (✉) • Z. Xia
Department of Radiology, Beijing You'an Hospital, Capital Medical University, Beijing, China
e-mail: lihongjun00113@126.com

5.1.3 Antigenicity

CP has genus-specific antigen and species-specific antigen. So far only one serotype of CP has been found, and the DNA homogeneity of different CP strains isolated in different regions of the world is above 94 %. The restriction endonuclease maps of different CP strains are basically identical, with standard strains of TW-183 and AR-39. The standard strains have been demonstrated to be the same strain and is renominated as TWAR.

5.1.4 Resistance

Chlamydia is tolerant to cold but intolerant to heat. Only 1 % of CP can survive in the blood preserved at a room temperature of 22 °C for 24 h. About 77 % of CP can survive at a temperature of −75 °C for 3 days. CP has low virulence and the bacteria within three generations are not lethal for chicken embryos. Its antibacterial spectrum against drugs resembles to other chlamydia and it is resistant to sulfa drugs.

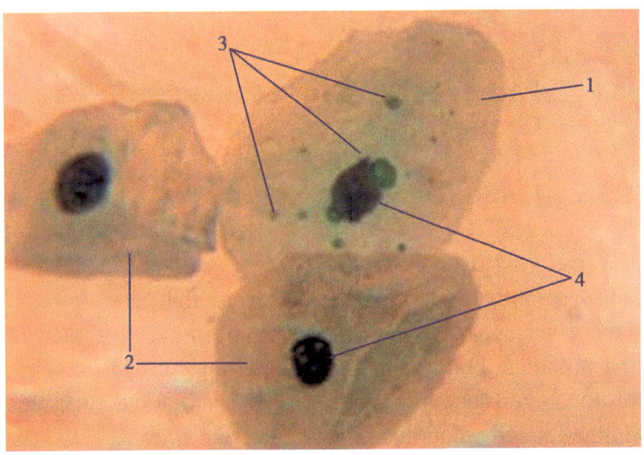

Fig. 5.1 Micrograph of Chlamydophila (Chlamydia) pneumoniae in an epithelial cell in acute bronchitis: *1* infected epitheliocyte, *2* uninfected epitheliocytes, *3* chlamydial inclusion bodies in cell, *4* cell nuclei

H. Li (ed.), *Radiology of Infectious Diseases: Volume 2*, DOI 10.1007/978-94-017-9876-1_5

5.2 Epidemiology

5.2.1 Source of Infection

CP is only parasitic in humans and it has no animal hosts as its reservoir. Therefore, the patients with CP infection, human carriers of CP, and asymptomatic patients with CP infection are the sources of its infection. Its average incubation period lasts for about 30 days.

5.2.2 Route of Transmission

CP spreads to the surrounding air via droplets by sneezing, coughing, and talking or via respiratory secretions. The inhalation of the droplets by susceptible people causes the infection. Otherwise, contaminated hands by these droplets in the environment also cause the infection.

5.2.3 Susceptible Population

People with no history of CP infection are all susceptible population.

5.2.4 Prevalence

CP infection has no significant regional and gender differences. A small-scale prevalence may occur in family, school, military troop, and other working areas with concentrated population. Its occurrence can be found all year round, which is more common in alternating period between springs and summers. Seroepidemiological studies demonstrate most people have a history of CP infection during their lifetime, which is commonly persistent and repeated. So far, no effective vaccine has been developed for its prevention.

5.3 Pathogenesis and Pathological Changes

5.3.1 Pathogenesis

5.3.1.1 Pathogenicity

CP is an obligate intracellular bacterium that reproduces by binary fission. It has a unique cycle from the protomer via the reticulate body to inclusion body and then back to the protomer and can reproduce in human alveolar macrophages, epithelial cells, endothelial cells, smooth muscle cells, and neutrophils. The pathogen can produce endotoxins resembling gram-negative bacteria, whose pathogenicity is related to lipopolysaccharide, major outer membrane proteins, heat shock proteins, and cytokines of the pathogen. Its invasion into the human body mainly triggers the reactions of mononuclear macrophages. The alveolar macrophages as the reservoir and carrier of the pathogen cause its persistent infection in the human body.

5.3.1.2 Immune Responses

The infection of CP can induce specific cellular and humoral immunity, but with weak and transient protective effect. Therefore, CP infection is commonly persistent, repeated, or asymptomatic.

5.3.2 Pathological Changes

CP firstly adheres to susceptible columnar or goblet mucosal epithelial cells and reproduces utilizing the energy from the host cell. In the early stage, CP parasitizes in the bronchial epithelial cells to cause cell toxicity and inflammatory infiltration. The involved bronchi and their surrounding pulmonary interstitium therefore have congestion, edema, and destructed epithelial cells. When the immune response is triggered, immune complexes and delayed-type hypersensitivity are produced; self repair is induced. Meanwhile, bronchiole stenosis and occlusion as well as focal emphysema of distal alveoli and lobules occur. Along with lesion development, large quantities of inflammatory exudates, destructed interstitium, bleeding, endotoxoid effects, and immune impairments further affect pulmonary parenchyma. Extrapulmonary lesions can also be found due to endotoxoid effect and the effects of immune complexes.

5.4 Clinical Symptoms and Signs

The incubation period of CP is comparatively long and the clinical manifestations of its infection lack specificity. The patients with no or slight symptoms are common.

CP infection mainly causes respiratory infections, including upper respiratory tract infections such as sinusitis, otitis media, and pharyngitis as well as lower respiratory tract infections such as bronchitis and pneumonia, which is mostly atypical pneumonia. The symptoms of community-acquired pneumonia caused by CP infection are generally mild, with a sore throat and coarse voice at the onset and occurrence of cough (commonly dry cough), fever, chest pain, headache, general upset, and fatigue several days later. In the cases with the lung lobes involved, rales can be heard. In some mild cases, the symptoms are self-limited. Since CP shares common antigens with human heart, liver, kidney, brain, and other organs, therefore, autoantibodies of the corresponding organ are produced after its infection as well as the formation of immune complexes which causes extrapulmonary organ lesions. The possibly involved organs and tissues include gastrointestinal tract, cardiovascular system, blood, skin, muscles, and joints, with corresponding clinical symptoms.

5.5 CP Pneumonia-Related Complications

CP infection may involve multiple extrapulmonary systems to complicate the primary infection. The related complications are more common in adults than in children.

5.5.1 The Cardiovascular System

In 1988, Aikku et al. reported that CP infection is possibly related to occurrence of coronary artery lesions. After that, many other scholars reported CP pneumonia is related to occurrence of arteriosclerosis-induced coronary heart disease and acute myocardial infarction. CP infection in adults may impair coronary artery to cause atherosclerosis and plaque formation. Therefore, coronary heart disease and acute coronary artery injury syndrome consequently occur. CP infection can cause acute myocarditis and endocarditis, with different severity of clinical symptoms. The common symptoms include chest distress, shortness of breath, fatigue, precardial upset, palpitation, arrhythmias and increased myocardiac enzymes. In the severe cases, the manifestation may be lethal fulminant myocarditis, especially in the cases with concurrent *Chlamydia psittaci* infection. In addition, there is also international case report about the concurrent hemorrhagic pericarditis.

5.5.2 The Nervous System

In recent years, it has been gradually recognized that the central nervous system diseases caused by CP infection are the most serious and most common complications of CP infection. In most cases, the CNS complications are encephalitis and meningitis. In addition, the cases of CP infection complicated by cerebral infarction, cerebral Reye's syndrome, Guillain-Barre syndrome, brainstem syndrome, and multiple sclerosis have also been reported.

5.5.3 Reactive Arthritis

CP infection occasionally causes reactive arthritis. After the onset of CP pneumonia symptoms for 3 weeks, asymmetric and progressively deteriorating arthritis may occur. Both serological tests and PCR detection can confirm the diagnosis of chronic CP infection.

5.5.4 Autoimmune Diseases

It has been occasionally reported that CP infection has certain correlationship with antineutrophil cytoplasmic antibody (ANCA)-associated glomerulonephritis, Still's disease, and systemic lupus erythematosus.

5.5.5 Other Complications

CP infection can also cause abdominal aortic aneurysm, hepatitis, thyroiditis, erythema nodosum, and other complications. In addition, it has been found that CP infection has certain correlationship with sarcoidosis and chronic granulomatous diseases, which needs further studies to elucidate such correlationship.

5.6 Diagnostic Examinations

5.6.1 Laboratory Tests

5.6.1.1 Routine Blood Test

Routine blood test is the most commonly applied examination for the diagnosis. The patients with CP infection commonly have normal level of WBC count. But in serious cases, the WBC count increases.

5.6.1.2 Etiological Detection

The respiratory secretions can be collected for immediate culture and isolation of the pathogen. However, such an examination has a low positive rate. HEP-2 or HL cells can also be applied for a 24-h culture, with following staining by monoclonal antibody. In such a way, the specific inclusions can be detected.

5.6.1.3 Serological Test

Micro-immuno Fluorescence (MIF)

MIF is currently the standard and the most commonly used examination for serological diagnosis of *Chlamydia* infection. The diagnostic criteria of MIF for CP infection are as follows: (1) The cases of acute infection have an increase of double sera antibody titer by above four times, or $IgM \geq 1:16$, or $IgG \geq 1:512$. (2) The cases with a past history of infection have $1:16 \leq IgG < 512$. (3) The cases with no past history of infection have $IgG < 1:16$. (4) The cases with chronic infection have $IgA > 1:8$.

ELISA

The finding of antibody titer being no less than 1:64 or double sera antibody having an increase by above 4 times has diagnostic significance. However, CP has cross reactivity with other species of *Chlamydia*.

Immunofluorescence (IF)

IF is a rapid diagnostic test for CP infection. The fluorescence-labeled species-specific monoclonal antibody (MOMP monoclonal antibody) can recognize the antibody of CP or intracytoplasmic inclusion to define its serotype. It shows no cross reaction with *Chlamydia trachomatis* and *Chlamydia psittaci* but has a low sensitivity to define the diagnosis.

5.6.1.4 Molecular Biological Examination

Using DNA probe and polymerase chain reaction (PCR), the DNA of CP can be detected in the specimen of sputum, respiratory secretion, or serum. Such an examination has both high specificity and sensitivity but requires complicated technical equipment. These genetic tests are commonly applied to confirm the findings after culture and in the epidemiologic studies.

5.6.2 Diagnostic Imaging

5.6.2.1 Chest X-ray

Chest X-ray facilitates the understanding of the pulmonary lesions, which is an important examination for the diagnosis of CP pneumonia.

5.6.2.2 CT Scanning

CT scanning is commonly applied for the examination of CP pneumonia. It can more truly demonstrate the size, morphology, quantity, and distribution of the lesions as well as changes after therapies. Such findings provide guidance for clinical treatment.

5.6.2.3 MR Imaging

MR imaging can be applied for the diagnosis of central nervous system infections caused by CP infection.

5.7 Imaging Demonstrations

5.7.1 Chest X-ray

X-ray commonly demonstrates unilateral segmental pneumonia. The serious cases can be demonstrated having wider range of lesions, which may even involve both lungs. Accompanying pleurisy or pleural effusion may occur.

Case Study 1

A female patient aged 33 years, with recurrent hemoptysis of unknown and accompanying chest pain.

For case detail and figures, please refer to Ma, QH. et al. *Journal of Practical Radiology*, 2007, 23 (4): 465.

Case Study 2

A female patient aged 40 years, with cough, fever, and chest pain.

For case detail and figures, please refer to Ma, QH. et al. *Journal of Practical Radiology*, 2007, 23 (4): 465.

5.7.2 CT Scanning

The common demonstrations include flakes or pulmonary segmental/lobular parenchymal shadow, ground glass opacity, reticulate opacity, and small nodular opacity. The lesions are commonly in lobular distribution, which are more common in both lower lungs and can be singular or multiple.

Case Study 3

CP pneumonia

For case detail and figures, please refer to Shao, F. et al. *Journal of Practical Clinical Pediatrics*, 2010, 25 (18): 1411.

Case Study 4

A patient aged 66 years

For case detail and figures, please refer to Liu, JL. et al. *Modern Medical Radiology*, 2010, 19 (3): 165.

Case Study 5

A patient aged 79 years.

For case detail and figures, please refer to Liu, JL. et al. *Modern Medical Radiology*, 2010, 19 (3): 165.

5.8 Diagnostic Basis

The clinical manifestations of CP pneumonia are nonspecific. And its definitive diagnosis is completely based on the laboratory findings. However, in clinical practice, the comprehensive understanding of the following aspects facilitates the clinical diagnosis.

5.8.1 Epidemiological Features

The patients are commonly the elderly and young people under the age of 20 years. There may be a history of contact within 1 month before the onset. And its occurrence may cause a small-scale prevalence, which is commonly sporadic all year round.

5.8.2 Clinical Manifestations

The clinical manifestations are nonspecific. The patients with pneumonia and symptoms of cough, fever, and scanty phlegm who show no therapeutic response to penicillin or cephalosporin antibiotic therapy should be suspected as having CP pneumonia.

5.8.3 Laboratory Findings

The diagnosis is mainly based on the laboratory findings, including pathogen isolation, serological test, and detection of DNA by PCR.

5.8.4 Imaging Demonstrations

X-ray commonly demonstrates infiltrative lesions in a singular lung lobe or lung segment. The lesions can be found at any part of both lungs and more commonly at the lower lung lobes and peripheries. In the serious cases, the lesions extensively involve both lungs, with occasionally accompanying pleural effusion. CT scanning mainly demonstrates flakes or segmental/lobar consolidation opacity, ground glass opacity, reticulate opacity, small nodular opacity, and signs of bronchial pneumonia.

5.8.5 Extrapulmonary Manifestations

CP pneumonia is commonly accompanied by erythema nodosum, otitis media, endocarditis, acute myocardial infarction, diarrhea, thyroiditis, encephalitis, arthritis, and Quran-Barre syndrome. These conditions should be taken into account for the diagnosis.

5.9 Differential Diagnosis

CP pneumonia should be distinguished from *Mycoplasma pneumoniae* (MP) pneumonia, viral pneumonia, and psittacosis pneumonia.

5.9.1 *Mycoplasma pneumoniae* Pneumonia

The clinical manifestations of CP pneumonia and MP pneumonia are similar, both with main symptoms of dry cough and fever. However, CP pneumonia has a chronic onset. The period from the infection to clinic visit due to its onset is usually longer than that in the cases of MP and other respiratory infections. Both conditions may be accompanied by extrapulmonary diseases such as erythema nodosum, otitis media, and encephalitis. And both conditions show no therapeutic response to penicillin or cephalosporin antibiotic therapy. Clinically, CP pneumonia is difficult to be differentiated from MP pneumonia. And the differentiation is mainly based on pathogen identification.

5.9.2 Viral Pneumonia

The clinical manifestations of both CP pneumonia and viral pneumonia can be fever and cough. X-ray demonstrates no characteristic findings. Both conditions show no therapeutic response to penicillin or cephalosporin antibiotic therapy. However, viral pneumonia commonly has an acute onset with serious systemic symptoms. Their differentiation is mainly based on pathogen identification.

5.9.3 Psittacosis Pneumonia

Human psittacosis pneumonia is caused by *Chlamydia psittaci*. Both *Chlamydia psittaci* and *Chlamydia pneumoniae* are categorized into the genus of *Chlamydia*. Being different from CP pneumonia, most patients with psittacosis pneumonia have a history of contact to poultry or have a history of inhaling bird feces.

References

Liu JL, Tuo LC. High-resolution CT scanning demonstrations of mycoplasma pneumoniae pneumonia and Chlamydia pneumoniae pneumonia. Mod Med Radiol. 2010;19(3):165–7.

Ma QH, Chen Q, Wang JG, et al. Imaging demonstrations of Chlamydia pneumoniae pneumonia during its outbreak. J Pract Radiol. 2007;23(4):465–8.

Shao F, Wang YJ, Lin Y. Clinical manifestations and imaging demonstrations of Chlamydia pneumoniae pneumonia in neonates. J Pract Clin Pediatr. 2010;25(18):1411–2.

Suggested Reading

Cai BQ. Union medical college respiratory diseases. Beijing: China Union Medical College Press; 2004.

Cheng RC, Bai XP, Cui L. Pathomechanism of atherosclerosis caused by Chlamydia pneumoniae infection. Chin J Gerontol. 2004;24(5):472–3.

Chen WQ, Liu GH, Xing ZB. Imaging demonstrations of Chlamydia pneumoniae pneumonia. Hainan Med. 2003;14(4):12–3.

Itoh I, Ishida T, Hashimoto T, et al. Chest radiograph of atypical pneumonia: comparison among Chlamydia pneumoniae, ornithosis, and mycoplasma pneumoniae pneumonia. Kansenshogaku Zasshi. 2000;74(11):954–60.

Migliorini L, Canocchi V, Zanelli G, et al. Outbreak and persistence of Chlamydia pneumonia infection in an Italian family. Infez Med. 2003;11(3):157–60.

Nong GM. Clinical manifestations of Chlamydia pneumonia and extra-pulmonary manifestations of Chlamydia infection. J Pract Clin Pediatr. 2009;24(16):1222–4.

Sessa R, Pictro MD, Santlno I, et al. Chlamydia pneumoniae infection and atherosclerotie eorolqary disease. Am Heat. 1999;137(6):1116–9.

Weng XH, Pan XZ, Wang DM. Modern studies of infectious diseases. Shanghai: Shanghai Medical University Press; 2001.

Zhang JH. Epidemiological studies of Chlamydia pneumonia. J Pract Clin Pediatr. 2009;24(16):1217–9.

6 Cholera

Junhong Li

Cholera is a fulminating infectious disease caused by *Vibrio cholerae*, with seven pandemics in human history. Cholera has an acute onset, rapid transmission, and serious damages to human health and is one of the important reasons for diarrhea in Asia and Africa. It is an internationally quarantined infectious disease and has been categorized into Class A infectious disease in China. The severity of its clinical manifestations varies, with commonly slight symptoms. The typical symptoms include acute painless diarrhea and vomiting, which may result in dehydration and muscle spasm, and even electrolyte balance disturbance, circulatory failure, and acute renal failure in serious cases. It has a high mortality rate when without timely and appropriate emergency rescuing.

6.1 Pathogen

Vibrio cholerae is categorized into the family of *Vibrionaceae* and the species of vibrio. It has heat-tolerant somatic O antigen and heat-intolerant flagellar H antigen. The H antigens of *Vibrio cholerae* mostly are the same, while the O antigens are of high specificity that can be divided into two types: group specificity and type specificity. This is the basis for the grouping and typing of *Vibrio cholerae*.

6.1.1 Classification

According to the biochemical properties of *Vibrio cholerae*, antigen specificity, and pathogenicity, the Center for Diarrhea Control of WHO classified *Vibrio cholerae* into the following three serogroups.

J. Li
Department of Emergency Medicine,
Beijing You'an Hospital, Capital Medical University,
Beijing, China
e-mail: 18901367819@163.com

6.1.1.1 *Vibrio cholerae* O_1

This group is the main pathogenic group of bacteria. Based on the biological properties, it can be divided into two biotypes: classical biotype and El Tor biotype. According to its different O antigens, *Vibrio cholerae* O_1 can also be divided into three types: Inaba, Ogawa, and Hikojima.

6.1.1.2 *Vibrio cholerae* Non-O_1

This serogroup cannot be agglutinated by polyvalent serum of *Vibrio cholerae* O_1, which is, therefore, also known as non-agglutinated vibrio. Generally, its serotypes from O_2 to O_{138} have no pathogenicity. *Vibrio cholerae* O_{139} was first identified during the cholera epidemic in India and Bangladesh in 1992, which cannot be agglutinated by the polyvalent sera of *Vibrio cholerae* O_1 and *Vibrio cholerae* non-O_1 (serotypes O_2-O_{138}). The serotype O_{139} has the same toxin genes as *Vibrio cholerae* O_1, but has stronger toxigenicity than *Vibrio cholerae* O_1. In addition, it has powerful capacities in disseminating and proliferating and can cause even more serious clinical symptoms.

6.1.1.3 Atypical *Vibrio cholerae* O_1

Atypical *Vibrio cholerae* O_1 can be agglutinated by polyvalent serum of *Vibrio cholerae* O_1, but cannot produce enterotoxins in both in vitro and vivo. Therefore, it has no pathogenicity.

6.1.2 Morphology and Culture

Vibrio cholerae is a Gram-negative, curve-shaped, or comma-shaped bacterium. It is 1.5–3.0 μm in length and 0.3–0.4 μm in width. At the end of the thallus, it has an active flagellum that is four to five times as long as the thallus. By dark-field microscopy of hanging drops, *Vibrio cholerae* shuttles back and forth like falling stars. Direct smear of patient's feces shows that *Vibrio cholerae* arranges in tandem like a shoal of fish. The morphology, staining, culture, and biochemical properties of *Vibrio cholerae* and serogroup O_1

H. Li (ed.), *Radiology of Infectious Diseases: Volume 2*, DOI 10.1007/978-94-017-9876-1_6

are almost the same. *Vibrio cholerae* O_1 has no capsule, while *Vibrio cholerae* O_{139} has a layer of thin capsule. *Vibrio cholerae* is a facultative anaerobe and grows well in ordinary culture medium. In alkaline environment, it grows and reproduces rapidly. Generally, 1 % alkaline peptone water (APW) with a pH value of 8.4–8.6 is used for its multiplying culture that can inhibit the growth of other bacteria. On alkaline plate, the bacterial colony is round in shape which is smooth and transparent with a diameter of 2 mm. *Vibrio cholerae* O_{139} can grow in APW without sodium chloride or with sodium chloride at a concentration of 30 g/L, but cannot grow in APW with sodium chloride at a concentration of 80 g/L.

6.1.3 Toxin

Vibrio cholerae produces three toxins: type I, type II, and type III. Type I is an endotoxin that is the major ingredient for preparation of bacterial vaccine to cause vaccine immunity. Type II is an exotoxin, namely, cholera enterotoxin, that is the metabolite produced by *Vibrio cholerae* during its replication in an organism. It has been proved that the serious diarrhea in cases of cholera is caused by this exotoxin which has antigenicity and can induce the body to produce neutralizing antibody. Type III toxin hardly plays a role in pathogenesis of cholera.

6.1.4 Resistance

Vibrio cholerae is sensitive to heat, dryness, sunlight, chemical disinfectants, and acid and is tolerant to low temperature and alkali. It can be killed by exposure to dryness for 2 h, by exposure to a temperature of 55 °C for 10 min and 100 °C for 1–2 min, or by exposure to water with 0.5 ppm chlorine for 15 min. It can only survive for 4 mins in normal gastric acid. *Vibrio cholerae* can survive for a long period of time under natural conditions. For instance, El Tor biotype *Vibrio cholerae* can survive in river water for 1–3 weeks and even above 1 year under appropriate conditions.

6.2 Epidemiology

6.2.1 Overview

Since 1817, seven cholera pandemics occurred, with the first six pandemics caused by classical biotype *Vibrio cholerae* and the last pandemic caused by El Tor biotype *Vibrio cholerae*. In 1992, the serotype O_{139} of *Vibrio cholerae* caused an epidemic of cholera in India and Bangladesh, which then gradually affected the surrounding countries and regions. Since the spread of cholera in China in 1820, the cases of cholera have been reported in China during each pandemic of cholera.

6.2.2 Epidemiological Feature

Cholera sporadically occurs all year around, with more common occurrence in summers and autumns from July to October. Geographically, cholera more commonly occurs along the river and the coast. However, prevalence of cholera is likely to occur in inland areas.

6.2.3 The Source of Infection

The patients with cholera and the carriers of *Vibrio cholerae* are the source of infection of cholera. The cases with slight symptoms and asymptomatic infection are difficult to be diagnosed. Therefore, their quarantine and treatment are commonly delayed, which contributes to its spreading.

6.2.4 Route of Transmission

Cholera is a gastrointestinal infectious disease. Water and food contaminated by the feces or other excrements of the patients with cholera and the carrier of the bacteria can cause transmission. In addition, contacts to patients or carriers during daily life activities and the flies also contribute to its transmission. It has been demonstrated in recent years that either El Tor biotype or *Vibrio cholerae* O_{139} can spread via contaminated aquatic products like fish or shrimps.

6.2.5 Population Susceptibility

People are generally susceptible to cholera, with more common occurrence of asymptomatic infection but rare occurrence of symptomatic infection. After its infection, certain immunity can be acquired. Antibodies against the bacteria and the enterotoxin can be produced in the human body after its infection, but with a short-term persistence. Therefore, secondary infection is likely to occur.

6.3 Pathogenesis and Pathological Changes

6.3.1 Pathogenesis

After the intake of *Vibrio cholerae* into the human body, the onset of cholera is dependent on the immunity and secretion of gastric acid of the human body as well as the quantity and virulence of *Vibrio cholerae*. In the cases of secretion of normal gastric acid that is not diluted, the gastric acid can kill the *Vibrio cholerae* to terminate its further pathogenic process. Thus, the disease fails to occur. Under unusual conditions, *Vibrio cholerae* gains its access to the intestinal tract via the stomach and then passes through the mucous layer of the intestinal mucosa under the effects of flagellar movement and the protease generated by the bacteria. It adheres to brush-like epithelial cell edge at the upper intestinal mucosa under the effects of toxin-mediated pilus and the bacterial hemagglutinin and does not invade the intestinal submucosa. After the adhesion, it multiplies in a large quantity in the alkaline environment of small intestine and generates cholera enterotoxin.

The cholera enterotoxin consists of two subunits: A and B. The subunit B can identify GM1 ganglioside receptor on the epithelial cells of intestinal mucosa to bind to it. Then enzymatically active subunit A separates itself from the cholera enterotoxin to gain its access into the cells of intestinal mucosa. Thereby, it continuously activates adenylyl cyclase (AC) and the activated AC transforms adenosine triphosphate (ATP) continuously into cyclic adenosine monophosphate (cAMP). After the concentration of intracellular cAMP increases, the crypt cells at the intestinal mucosa are stimulated to excessively secrete water, chloride, and carbonate. Meanwhile, the uptake of sodium by intestinal villus cells is inhibited, leading to aggregation of water and sodium chloride in enteric lumen that causes severe watery diarrhea. Cholera enterotoxin can also increase the mucus secretion by the goblet cells of the intestinal mucosa, which results in a large quantity of mucus in the watery feces. In addition, diarrhea tends to cause dehydration and decreased secretion of bile. Therefore, the rice-water stool may also be observed.

Due to serious diarrhea and vomiting, water and electrolytes in the body are lost in large quantities. Therefore, dehydration and electrolyte balance disturbance occur. In the cases of serious dehydration, circulatory failure may even occur. In the cases receiving delayed correction of dehydration, long-term shock occurs to further develop into acute renal failure. Although the lost fluid by patients with cholera is isotonic fluid, the potassium contained in the fluid is about two to five times as much as serum potassium, and the sodium and chlorine are slightly less than those in the serum. In the second rehydration therapy, potassium should be added timely for the cases with urination. Otherwise, severe hypokalemia may occur, leading to arrhythmia and degeneration of renal tubular epithelial cells that further aggravates renal failure.

In the cases of cholera, metabolic acidosis is common. Because diarrhea causes massive loss of bicarbonate radically and dehydration causes peripheral circulatory failure, anaerobic metabolism occurs due to a lack of oxygen in the tissue. The excessively produced lactic acid can cause and aggravate metabolic acidosis. Acute renal failure and failed discharge of metabolic acidic substances are also the reasons for occurrence of metabolic acidosis.

6.3.2 Pathological Changes

The main pathological changes are a series of changes caused by severe dehydration, with no serious organ damages. The main pathological changes include skin dryness, subcutaneous and muscular dehydration, and shrinkage of the heart, liver, and spleen due to dehydration. There may also be nephromegaly, capillary dilation in glomerulus and renal interstitium, renal tubular degeneration, and necrosis. In terms of gastrointestinal tract, there are dry and wrinkled serosa of the gastrointestinal tract, mild inflammation of the intestinal mucosa, intestines filled with rice-water fluid, and sticky turbid bile in the gallbladder.

6.4 Clinical Symptoms and Signs

The incubation period lasts for 1–3 days. In rare cases, the patients experience dizziness, fatigue, or mild diarrhea 1–2 days before the onset of the disease. Symptoms caused by classical biotype and serotype O_{139} are relatively serious. El Tor-biotype-induced symptoms are mostly mild and the infection of El Tor biotype is also commonly found in asymptomatic pathogen carriers.

6.4.1 Clinical Staging

The course of a typical case can be divided into three stages.

6.4.1.1 Vomiting and Diarrhea Stage

The stage begins with severe diarrhea, followed by vomiting. Generally, fever cannot be found, with rare cases showing low-grade fever.

Diarrhea

Diarrhea is characterized by no tenesmus and no abdominal pain. Paroxysmal abdominal colic pain may be found in rare cases. The stool is firstly yellowish loose, followed by yellowish watery. In the cases of severe diarrhea, rice-water-like stool is discharged. In the cases with intestinal bleeding, meat water-like stool is discharged that contains a large quantity of pathogenic bacteria with no fecal odor. The frequency of diarrhea ranges from several times to dozens of times even with fecal incontinence. Cholera caused by serotype O_{139} *Vibrio cholerae* is characterized by fever and abdominal pain, with possible occurrence of extraintestinal infections like bacteremia.

Vomiting

Vomiting generally occurs following diarrhea and is commonly projectile with no accompanying nausea. Vomits are firstly food in the stomach and then watery substances. In serious cases, rice-water-like substances are vomited. Twenty-four hour after the onset, vomiting tends to be relieved. In slight cases, no vomiting is observed.

6.4.1.2 Dehydration Stage

Due to severe diarrhea and vomiting, water and electrolytes in the body are massively lost to cause dehydration, electrolytes disturbance, and metabolic acidosis. In severe cases, circulatory failure occurs. The course of this stage generally ranges from several hours to 2–3 days, and its duration depends on appropriateness of the therapies and the time administering them.

Dehydration

Dehydration can be divided into three types: mild, moderate, and severe. Mild dehydration is characterized by slight dryness of skin mucosa and slight loss of skin elasticity. Generally, it refers to water loss of about 1,000 ml and the quantity of water loss is about 2–3 % of the body weight. Moderate dehydration is characterized by poor elasticity of the skin, sunken orbital socket, mild hoarseness of the voice, decreased blood pressure, and decreased volume of urination. It refers to water loss of about 2,500 ml and the quantity of water loss is about 4–6 % of the body weight. In severe cases of dehydration, the water loss is about 7–14 % of the body weight and the symptoms include dry and wrinkled skin, loss of skin elasticity, hoarseness, and choleraic complexion. In the cases with the water loss exceeding 15 % of the body weight, the patients experience hypovolemic shock, circulatory failure, acidosis, and acute renal failure, which are life-threatening.

Circulatory Failure

Circulatory failure is water-loss shock caused by severe dehydration. It can lead to peripheral coldness, misty skin, threading, and rapid pulse that even may not be felt and decreased blood pressure. Subsequently, consciousness disturbance occurs due to insufficient blood supply to the brain and cerebral hypoxia, with manifestations of irritation and upset and following sluggishness, drowsiness, and even coma.

Metabolic Acidosis

The clinical manifestations include rapid respiration. In severe cases, deep and slow respiration known as Kussmaul respiration occurs, possibly with mental and conscious disturbance such as drowsiness, delayed sensory responses, and even coma.

Muscle Spasm

Severe hyponatremia causes spasms of gastrocnemius and musculus rectus abdominis, with clinical manifestations of muscular pain and rigidity.

Hypokalemia

Clinical manifestations include decreased muscular tension, decreased or absence of knee reflex, abdominal distension, and arrhythmia. ECG demonstrates prolonged Q-T period, downward migration of ST segment, low and flat T wave, and obvious U wave.

6.4.1.3 Convalescence Stage or Response Stage

During this stage, diarrhea and vomiting terminate, with absence of symptoms and increased urine volume in most cases after correction of dehydration. The patients are physically improved. However, due to improved condition of the blood circulation in rare cases, the residual endotoxin in the intestinal lumen is absorbed into the blood flow to cause fever of different degrees. The body temperature can be up to 38–39 °C and returns to normal after 1–3 days.

6.4.2 Clinical Classification

According to the degrees of dehydration, blood pressure, and urine volume, cholera can be clinically divided into three types: mild, moderate, and severe.

6.4.2.1 Mild Cholera

It has a chronic onset, with diarrhea of ten times per day. The stool is loose or watery loose. Accompanying vomiting is not found. The whole course lasts for 3–5 days, with no obvious manifestations of dehydration.

6.4.2.2 Moderate Cholera (Typical Cholera)

Typical diarrhea and vomiting occur, with diarrhea of 10–20 times per day in a large amount of watery or rice-water-like stool. There are also obvious signs of dehydration. Blood pressure drops, with a systolic pressure of only 70–90 mmHg. Urine volume decreases, with less than 400 ml urination within 24 h.

6.4.2.3 Severe Cholera

Patients have typical diarrhea and vomiting and severe dehydration that leads to circulatory failure. Symptoms include rapid and thready pulse that may even fail to be felt, significant drop of blood pressure with a systolic pressure being lower than 70 mmHg that may even fail to be detected, and urine volume being lower than 100 ml within 24 h.

In addition to the abovementioned three clinical types, there is another type with rare occurrence, namely, explosive or toxic type that is also known as dry cholera. Such a type has acute and sudden onset. The conditions may rapidly progress into toxic shock with following occurrence of death with no occurrence of diarrhea and vomiting.

6.5 Cholera-Related Complications

6.5.1 Acute Renal Failure

In the early stage of the disease, dehydration occurs due to severe diarrhea and vomiting, with following occurrence of oliguria. At this time, oliguria is prerenal, which can be improved with increased urine volume by timely rehydration to avoid renal failure. In the cases with delayed rehydration, dehydration aggravates to cause shock. Due to insufficient blood supply in the kidneys, renal tubular ischemic necrosis may occur, with symptoms of oliguria, anuria, and azotemia.

6.5.2 Acute Pulmonary Edema

Due to severe dehydration in cases of cholera, immediate rehydration is commonly required. Therefore, acidosis should be simultaneously corrected. Otherwise, pulmonary edema is likely to occur because metabolic acidosis results in pulmonary hypertension. The common clinical manifestations include sudden occurrence of severe dyspnea, orthopnea with accompanying cough, expectoration of pink foamy sputum, irritation, cyanotic lips, excessive perspiration and overwhelming moist, and wheezing and rales in both lungs.

6.6 Diagnostic Examinations

6.6.1 Laboratory Tests

6.6.1.1 Routine Laboratory Tests

Routine feces examination shows many epithelial cells and rare erythrocytes or leukocytes. Routine urine test demonstrates proteins or cells and cellular casts and increased blood urea nitrogen. Routine blood test demonstrates increased hemoglobin, erythrocyte, and leukocyte due to concentrated blood, and continual observation of these indicators can facilitate assessing dehydration and its therapeutic efficacy. In addition, there are normal or decreased serum potassium and chlorine as well as decreased adhesive force of carbon dioxide, whose dynamic change demonstrates the conditions of dehydration and acidosis.

6.6.1.2 Etiological Examination

Smear and Staining

Feces or early culture smear can be prepared for Gram staining and microscopy. Positive finding includes Gram-negative and slightly curved vibrio, with no spore and no capsule, while the serotype O_{139} can produce capsule.

Bacterial Culture

Bacterial culture is the most important examination to define the diagnosis.

Dynamic and Immobilization Test

Fresh feces are used for hanging drop examination or dark-field microscopy. The finding of actively shuttling vibrio like falling stars demonstrates the dynamic test positive. The finding of static bacteria after addition of O_1 serogroup antiserum indicates O_1 *Vibrio cholerae* in the specimen. The finding of static bacteria after addition of O_{139} serogroup antiserum indicates O_{139} serotype in the specimen. This test can be used for rapid diagnosis of cholera during an epidemic.

Serologic Examination

Serologic examination is mainly applied for epidemiologically retrospective diagnosis of cholera. And it is commonly applied to define the suspected cases with negative feces culture. Double sera from the acute stage and convalescence stage are collected for examination. An above four times increase of antibody titer has diagnostic significance.

RCR Nucleic Acid Detection

In such a way, the gene sequence encoding enterotoxin of *Vibrio cholerae* can be detected. It is fast, with high sensitivity and specificity.

6.6.2 Diagnostic Imaging

Radiological examinations are not routinely performed for the diagnosis of cholera. Such examinations are commonly applied for the examination and diagnosis of cholera-related complications.

6.7 Diagnostic Imaging

6.7.1 Acute Renal Failure

Ultrasound demonstrates enlarged volume of kidneys, thickened cortex with enhanced echo, decreased echo of medulla, well-defined interface between cortex and medulla, as well as increased resistance index of intrarenal artery and interlobar artery.

6.7.2 Acute Pulmonary Edema

Chest X-rays demonstrate mild cases with no positive findings (Fig. 6.1). In the cases with complication of acute pulmonary edema, chest X-rays and CT scanning demonstrate the following findings.

6.7.2.1 Pulmonary Interstitial Edema

Chest X-Rays

The findings include thickened branches of the left and right superior pulmonary veins, blurry shadows of lung marking and hilar blood vessels, cuff sign of the bronchus that is more common in the anterior segment of the upper lobes, linear shadow of the septum where Kerley B line is the most common, and subpleural edema that is commonly complicated by enlarged heart shadow and small quantity of pleural effusion. Among all these findings, blurry pulmonary marking and the septal lines are the main signs of pulmonary interstitial edema.

CT Scanning

CT scanning demonstrates thickened hilar vascular shadows and thickened and blurry branches of pulmonary blood vessels. In most cases, these demonstrations are more serious in middle inner lung fields, with vascular thickening in the upper lobe being more obvious than that in the lower lobe. Sometimes, demonstrations of complicated pulmonary emphysema are found.

6.7.2.2 Pulmonary Alveolar Edema

X-Rays

The diameter of nodular opacities is 0.5–1.0 cm, with poorly defined boundaries. The nodular shadows rapidly fuse into patches or large flakes of shadow that involves multiple pulmonary segments, with visible air bronchogram. The shadows have central distribution and a typical butterfly sign can be found. In rare cases, scattering distribution is found, with intrapulmonary consolidation shadows extensively distributing in the inner, middle, and outer zone of the lung fields. Unilateral lung distribution or asymmetric distribution in both lungs is occasionally found, with atypical demonstrations. The lesions are firstly found in the inferior lung as well as medial and posterior lung that rapidly develop to superior, lateral, and anterior lung. The lesions show rapid dynamic changes, with obvious changes in 1–2 days or even within several hours. Pleural effusion is common that are mostly small quantities of bilateral pleural effusion.

CT Scanning

CT scanning demonstrates alveolar consolidation shadows in both lungs in small flakes or fused large flakes with visible air bronchogram. The lesions are relatively more obvious at the inferior lung, near the hilus, or at the lower fields of both lungs.

Case Study 1

The diagnosis was mild type of cholera infected by serogroup O_1.

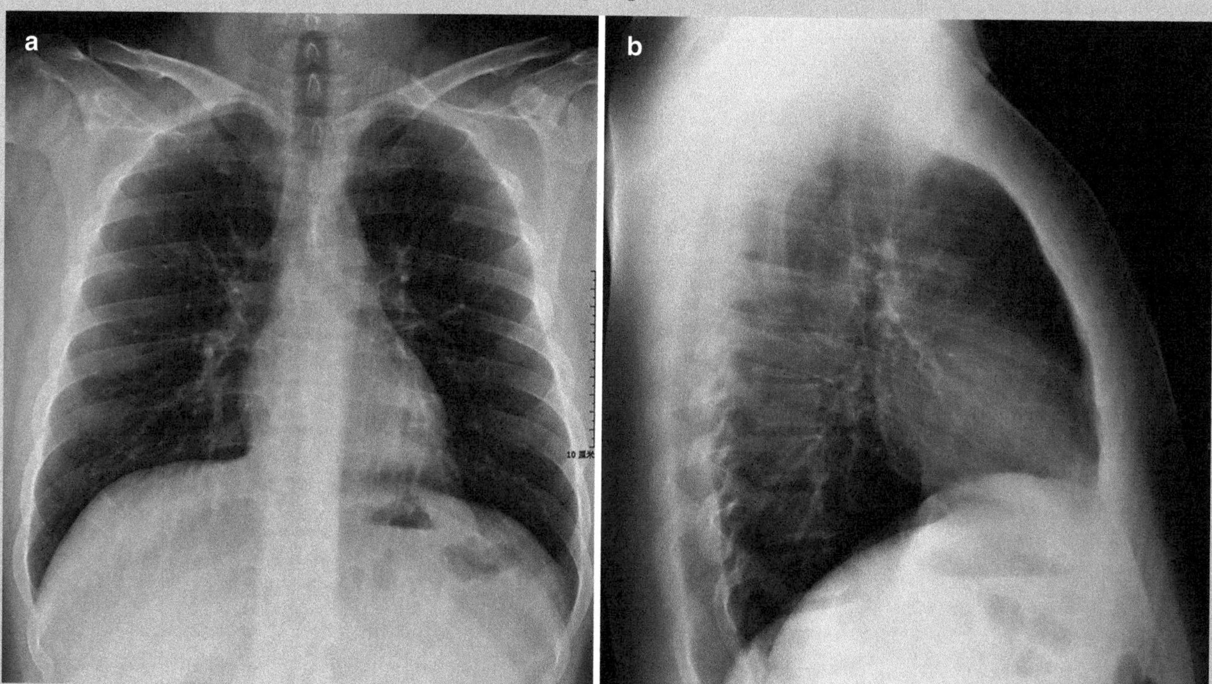

Fig. 6.1 Mild case of cholera infected by serogroup O_1. (**a**, **b**) X-rays demonstrate no obvious abnormalities

6.8 Diagnostic Basis

6.8.1 Diagnosis of Cholera

In epidemic areas of cholera during prevailing seasons, any patients with diarrhea and vomiting should be suspected with cholera. Therefore, bacteriological examination of feces should be performed for exclusive diagnosis. All patients with typical symptoms should be treated as cholera cases prior to the definitive diagnosis.

6.8.1.1 Diagnosis of the Suspected Cases

The cases with one of the following conditions should be suspected with cholera:

1. The patients with typical symptoms of cholera and no definitive results by etiological examinations.
2. During an epidemic of cholera, the patients have a definitive history of contact to patients with cholera and have symptoms of vomiting and fever, but have no other lesions for examination.

The suspected cases should be quarantined and sterilized, with a following report. Feces culture should be performed daily. In the cases with two consecutive feces cultures being negative, the cases should be excluded as cholera, with a following corrected report.

6.8.1.2 Clinical Diagnosis

The cases with one of the following conditions should be clinically diagnosed as cholera:

1. The patients have a typical symptom of diarrhea, and *Vibrio cholerae* O_1 or O_{139} serogroup is detected in their living environment.
2. During an epidemic of cholera, a typical symptom of diarrhea occurs.

6.8.1.3 Definitive Diagnosis

1. Patients have diarrhea, and *Vibrio cholerae* O_1 or O_{139} serogroup is detected from bacterial cultures of feces, vomits, or anus swab.
2. *Vibrio cholerae* O_1 or O_{139} serogroup is detected from bacterial cultures of feces, vomits, and anus swab, and the patients have diarrhea in 5 days before or after the detection.
3. During an epidemic of cholera, the patients have typical symptoms of cholera, with no finding of *Vibrio cholerae* by bacterial culture of feces. However, an above four times increase of double sera agglutination titer is detected.

6.8.2 Diagnosis of Cholera-Related Complications

6.8.2.1 Acute Renal Failure

1. Patients with cholera have sudden and obvious decrease of urine volume and accompanying rapid deterioration of renal function.
2. Laboratory tests facilitate to define the diagnosis.
3. Ultrasound demonstrates morphological changes of kidneys including enlarged volume of the kidney and thickened cortex.

6.8.2.2 Acute Pulmonary Edema

Chest X-rays demonstrate Kerley B lines and hilar butterfly signs or manifestations of pneumonia.

6.9 Differential Diagnosis

6.9.1 Differential Diagnosis of Cholera

6.9.1.1 *Vibrio parahaemolyticus* Colitis

Most cases have an acute onset and a history of intake of contaminated food. The symptoms are nausea, vomiting, abdominal pain, and diarrhea that are less severe than those in the cases of typical cholera. Differential diagnosis mainly depends on bacteriological examination of feces.

6.9.1.2 *Escherichia coli* Enteritis

The disease has a sudden and acute onset and persons who eat together have a simultaneous onset. The symptoms are characterized by vomiting and diarrhea as well as paroxysmal abdominal pain before bowel movements. Feces are commonly yellowish watery, with no pus or blood.

6.9.1.3 Viral Enteritis

It is often caused by human rotavirus and occurs more commonly in autumns. Rare patients have symptoms of the upper respiratory tract, while most patients have symptoms of fever, diarrhea, and vomiting and mostly no abdominal pain. The patients discharge yellowish watery stool, and by feces examination, human rotavirus is positive.

6.9.1.4 Acute Bacillary Dysentery

The patients experience symptoms of fever, abdominal pain, tenesmus, and bloody stool with pus, based on which it can be distinguished from cholera. The patients of mild type only experience diarrhea and loose mucous stools. It should be distinguished from the mild type of cholera based on the bacteriological examination of feces.

6.9.2 Differential Diagnosis of Cholera-Related Complications

6.9.2.1 Pulmonary Interstitial Edema

Pulmonary interstitial edema should be differentiated from pneumonia and lymphangitic carcinomatosis. Pneumonia is commonly caused by viral or mycoplasma infection. The patients with pneumonia have fever and normal heart size. The patients with lymphangitic carcinomatosis have a history of malignancy, with lymphadenectasis and normal heart size. Its lesions are not widely distributed like pulmonary edema.

6.9.2.2 Pulmonary Alveolar Edema

Pulmonary alveolar edema should be distinguished from pneumonia. The patients with pneumonia have normal size of heart shadow whose location by imaging is irrelevant to gravity. The lesions of pulmonary edema occur rapidly, with rapid dynamic changes of the shadows and with no clinical manifestation of pneumonia.

Suggested Reading

Gong ZY, Yang XP. General introduction to the prevalence and control of cholera worldwide in the year of 2010. Dis Surveill. 2011;26(12): 1009–11.

Hu RH, Ren H, Zhang P. Epidemiology and molecular epidemiology of cholera. Int J Epidemiol Infect Dis. 2006;33(4):268–70.

Li N. Oxford studies of infectious diseases (translated version). Beijing: People's Medical Publishing House; 2011.

Li JH, Zhu H. Advances in the studies of major antigens of vibrio cholerae O1 and O139 serogroups. Lett Biotechnol. 2010;21(4): 593–6.

Maiden MC, Bygraves JA, Feil E, et al. Multilocus sequence typing: a portable approach to the identification of clones within populations of pathogenic microorganisms. Proc Natl Acad Sci U S A. 1998;95(6):3140–5.

Peng WW. Studies of infectious diseases. Beijing: People's Medical Publishing House; 2003.

The Ministry of Health in P.R. China. Diagnostic criteria for cholera. Beijing: People's Medical Publishing House; 2008. WS289-2008.

Yang SJ, Ren H. Studies of infectious diseases. Beijing: People's Medical Publishing House; 2007.

Zhang J, Zheng JH, Ai L. The recent studies of cholera vaccines and their prospects. Chin J Infect Dis. 2009;27(6):381–4.

7 Diphtheria

Yinglin Guo, Xue Yin, and Bailu Liu

Diphtheria is an acute respiratory infectious disease caused by *Corynebacterium diphtheriae*. It is clinically characterized by mucosal congestion and swelling in the pharynx, larynx, and nose with a grayish pseudomembrane. The bacterial exotoxins can cause systemic poisoning symptoms and even can cause toxic myocarditis and peripheral nerve paralysis in some serious cases.

7.1 Etiology

Corynebacterium diphtheriae is classified into the genus of *Corynebacterium*. It is a group of gram-positive aerobic bacteria with a diameter of 0.3–0.8 μm and a length of 1–5 μm. The *Corynebacterium diphtheriae* are irregularly arranged, commonly in a shape of fence, V, Y, or L. The bacterium has one or two enlarged rodlike endings, therefore is known as corynebacterium. Without capsule and flagella, it produces no spores. However, it has densely stained particles in the thallus, which are commonly referred to as the metachromatic granules and facilitate the differential diagnosis. These metachromatic granules can be absent in the aged bacteria. Only those *Corynebacterium diphtheriae* infected by bacteriophage are capable of producing exotoxin, which is also known as diphtheria toxin and is the main etiological factor contributing to the occurrence of disease. Diphtheria toxin is unstable and can be developed into toxoid after treated by 0.3–0.5 % formaldehyde solution for vaccination or for preparation of antitoxic serum.

Corynebacterium diphtheriae is tolerant to external environment, for instance, it is coldness and dryness tolerant. It can survive for 12 weeks in the dry pseudomembrane and for several days in toys and clothing. Being sensitive to hotness and humidity as well as chemical disinfectants, it can be killed at the temperature of 58 °C for 10 min or in 5 % phenol solution for 1 min. In addition, it can survive for only several hours in direct rays of sunlight.

7.2 Epidemiology

7.2.1 Source of Infection

Patients with diphtheria and *Corynebacterium diphtheriae* carriers are the source of infection. Due to its infectivity during the ending period of latency, patients with asymptomatic infection, mild symptoms, nasal diphtheria, and cutaneous diphtheria play an important role in spreading diphtheria. During the convalescent period, the bacteria-carrying period commonly lasts for no more than 4 days and sometimes it may last for a maximum of 12 days. The bacteria-carrying rate in healthy population is usually 0.1–5 %, and it can reach 10–20 % during the prevailing period of the disease.

7.2.2 Route of Transmission

Corynebacterium diphtheriae commonly spreads along with droplet to invade the respiratory tract. It may also spread via direct contact to contaminated hands, toys, and utensils or indirectly along with dusts. Outbreak of diphtheria may occur due to transmission via contaminated milk and food. Occasionally, the disease can be transmitted via wounded skin or mucosa.

7.2.3 Susceptible Population

Generally, populations are vulnerable to diphtheria and children are especially susceptible to diphtheria. The neonatal can acquire immunity via placenta and breast feeding, which fails

Y. Guo (✉)
Department of Radiology, Taiping People's Hospital, Daowai District, Harbin, Heilongjiang, China
e-mail: guoyinglinhmu@126.com

X. Yin • B. Liu
CT Department, The Second Affiliated Hospital, Harbin Medical University, Harbin, Heilongjiang, China

H. Li (ed.), *Radiology of Infectious Diseases: Volume 2*, DOI 10.1007/978-94-017-9876-1_7

to persist for more than 1 year. After infection of diphtheria, persistent immunity can be acquired. However, some patients sustain diphtheria for several times during their lifetime.

7.2.4 Epidemiological Features

Diphtheria occurs worldwide and its occurrence is more common in temperate zone. Diphtheria occurs all year round and more commonly in winters and springs. Its occurrence is commonly sporadic, with occasional prevalence or outbreak.

7.3 Pathogenesis and Pathological Changes

7.3.1 Pathogenesis

The invasive capacity of *Corynebacterium diphtheriae* is weak, which invades the respiratory tract or the surface of the skin to reproduce at the surface of the mucosa. In such cases, the bacteria only cause mild inflammatory responses in local tissues, commonly with no further invasion into deep tissues and the blood flow. Diphtheria toxin is the main pathogenic substance of the bacteria, which can cause cell damage, fibrin exudation, and leukocyte infiltration. The diphtheric pseudomembrane (DPM) is present due to the coagulation of a large quantity of fibrin with diphtheric necrosis tissues, inflammatory cells, and bacteria to cover the lesion surface. Pharyngeal DPM and the tissues under DPM show a close adhesion, whose separation by force can cause bleeding, which is a characteristic lesion of diphtheria. Due to the presence of cilia on the mucosa of larynx, trachea, and bronchi, the DPM is loosely attached to the mucosa whose separation from the mucosa may cause choking. The uptake of diphtheria toxin is associated with the position and the distribution of DPM. The extensively distributed DPM can cause large quantity of uptake of diphtheria toxin, therefore leading to serious toxic symptoms. The uptake of nasal diphtheria toxin has the largest quantity, therefore causing the most serious symptoms. The uptakes of laryngeal and bronchial diphtheria toxin have the smallest quantity, therefore leading to mild general symptoms.

7.3.2 Pathological Changes

The most significant pathologic changes of diphtheria are toxic myocarditis and diphtheric neuritis. Toxic myocarditis is characterized by cardiac enlargement as well as fatty, hyaline, and granular degenerations of myocardium and myocardial fiber breakage with involvement of the conduction system. Neuritis commonly occurs in peripheral motor nerves, with common involvements of cranial nerve pairs of IX and X. The specific pathological changes include fatty degeneration of myelin as well as swollen and broken nerve axons but rare occurrence of necrosis. Other pathological changes may also occur, including cloudy and swollen kidney, shedding of renal tubular epithelial cells, and adrenal degenerations. The liver may be found with fatty degeneration and hepatocytic necrosis.

7.4 Clinical Symptoms and Signs

The incubation period of diphtheria ranges from 1 to 7 days, most commonly 2–4 days. According to the position of pseudomembrane, it can be categorized into different types: pharyngeal diphtheria, laryngeal diphtheria, nasal diphtheria, and diphtheria at other positions.

7.4.1 Pharyngeal Diphtheria

Pharyngeal diphtheria is the most commonly found diphtheria. Its lesions are confined within areas of the tonsils, pharynx, and their surrounding tissues and pharyngeal diphtheria accounts for about 80 % of diphtheric cases. According to the size of pseudomembrane and the severity of the symptoms, pharyngeal diphtheria can be divided into 4 types as the following.

7.4.1.1 Mild Pharyngeal Diphtheria

The general symptoms are mild. Patients may have fever and slightly reddish and swollen tonsils. The pseudomembrane is in a shape of spot or small flake, confined in the superior part of the tonsils. In some cases, pseudomembrane can barely be found or no pseudomembrane can be found, but there are positive findings with *Corynebacterium diphtheriae* culture.

7.4.1.2 Common Pharyngeal Diphtheria

The common type of pharyngeal diphtheria has a chronic onset, with symptoms of fatigue, poor appetite, nausea and vomiting, sore throat, and headache, as well as mild to moderate fever. By physical examination, tonsillar enlargement of I–II degree may be found, with large flaky well-defined inseparable pseudomembrane on the tonsils and accompanying enlarged submaxillary lymph nodes of tenderness.

7.4.1.3 Serious Pharyngeal Diphtheria

The general symptoms of this type are serious, with manifestations of high fever, pale complexion, extreme fatigue, nausea and vomiting, as well as decreased blood pressure in some serious cases. By physical examination, obvious tonsillar and pharyngeal congestion can be found. The pseudomembrane is thick and widely distributed, with a color of gray yellowish or even black and accompanying stink smell. The pseudomembrane may extend to palatine arches, posterior wall of the pharynx, nasopharynx, and even oral mucosa.

Patients also may have enlarged cervical lymph nodes, edema of the soft tissues surrounding lymph nodes, myocarditis, and peripheral nerve paralysis. The spreading of exotoxin into the cervical soft tissues may cause edema that is known as bullneck.

7.4.1.4 Critical Pharyngeal Diphtheria

The onset and progression of this type are acute, with serious general toxic symptoms. Patients commonly have a body temperature of above 40 °C, with accompanying irritation, shortness of breath, pale complexion, and decreased blood pressure. Symptoms as cardiac enlargement, arrhythmia, or toxic shock, as well as hemorrhage and thrombocytopenia, may also occur. The distribution of pseudomembrane is more extensive than that in the cases of serious type, with a dense black color and a rotten stink smell. The tonsils and pharynx can be found seriously enlarged, which negatively affects breathing and swallowing. In the cases of this type, serious symptom of bullneck is common, with obvious edema of soft tissues from the neck to the supraclavicular fossa. The death rate of this type of pharyngeal diphtheria is extremely high and death commonly occurs within 6–10 days after the onset.

7.4.2 Laryngeal Diphtheria

Laryngeal diphtheria is commonly caused by downward development of the serious type of pharyngeal diphtheria. Primary laryngeal diphtheria is rarely found. In the cases of laryngeal diphtheria, the uptake of exotoxin is in a small quantity causing mild toxic symptoms. It is characterized by barking-like cough, with hoarseness and even aphonia. In some cases, laryngeal obstruction induced 3 depression signs and cyanosis may even be found during inhalation. Pseudomembrane can extend to involve the trachea and bronchi whose shedding may lead to suffocation and even death.

7.4.3 Nasal Diphtheria

Nasal diphtheria is commonly secondary to laryngeal diphtheria, while primary nasal diphtheria is rarely found. Nasal diphtheria is frequently found in infants and young children, with a small range of lesions and mild systemic symptoms. The clinical manifestations commonly include nasal obstruction, mucosal bloody nasal discharge, involved red and erosive skin around the nostrils with scabs, and white pseudomembrane on the nasal vestibule or nasal septum.

7.4.4 Diphtheria of Other Positions

Diphtheria of other positions is occasionally found. Cutaneous diphtheria is common in tropical regions. And diphtheria may occasionally occur at the positions including wound, eye conjunctiva, ears, oral cavity, vulva, umbilical cord of the neonatals, and esophagus. Such cases of diphtheria commonly show local pseudomembrane with mild general symptoms.

7.5 Diphtheria-Related Complications

7.5.1 Myocarditis

Myocarditis is the most common complication of diphtheria and the leading cause of death in diphtheric cases, whose incidence is 10–25 %. It is commonly found in serious cases of diphtheria, often occurring at week 2–3 of the whole illness course. The disease usually has an acute and asymptomatic onset, with common clinical manifestations of decreased cardiac output, cardiac arrhythmia, and congestive heart failure. ECG demonstrates T wave or ST changes, possibly with conduction block and arrhythmia. The early stage of myocarditis is caused by severe toxemia, commonly with a poor prognosis and even occurrence of sudden death. And it eventually progresses into myocardiopathies due to its effects on the surrounding circulation.

7.5.2 Peripheral Nerve Paralysis

It is common in serious cases of diphtheria at week 3–4 of the whole illness course. In some cases, it lasts even for 3 months. The common clinical manifestations include motor nerve-involved flaccid paralysis, most commonly at the soft palate and the posterior wall of the pharynx. Symptoms like strong nasal sound, irritated coughing during food intake, and absent reflex of uvula palatine may be found. Paralysis at the facial muscle, ocular muscle, and limb muscle may also occur. Generally, peripheral nerve paralysis can be cured, with no sequela.

7.5.3 Bronchopneumonia

It is common in infants, frequently as a secondary infection. Patients with laryngeal diphtheria, especially cases with pseudomembrane extending down to the trachea and bronchi, are vulnerable to bronchopneumonia.

7.5.4 Other Complications

Diphtheria can be secondary to other bacterial infections, leading to cervical lymphadenitis, otitis media, sepsis, toxic nephropathies, and other complications.

7.6 Diagnostic Examinations

7.6.1 Laboratory Tests

7.6.1.1 Routine Blood Test

An increase of the peripheral WBC count is found, with an average of $10–20 \times 10^9$/L. The proportion of neutrophils is higher than normal range, with left migration of the nucleus. In some serious cases, toxic granulation and thrombocytopenia can be found.

7.6.1.2 Bacteriological Test

Tissues harvested at the interface of pseudomembrane and mucosal membrane undergo smear examination and culture. Consequently, gram-positive bacilli and *Corynebacterium diphtheriae* are commonly found. If necessary, *Corynebacterium diphtheriae* virulence test can be performed to define the diagnosis.

7.6.1.3 Serological Test

By fluorescent antibody method, *Corynebacterium diphtheriae* can be detected under a fluorescence microscope for its early diagnosis.

7.6.2 Diagnostic Imaging

For patients without complications of diphtheria, diagnostic imaging is not recommended. For diphtheric patients with myocarditis, electrocardiography (ECG) and cardiac ultrasound are recommended for diagnosis and differential diagnosis. For diphtheric patients with bronchopneumonia, chest X-ray is recommended to define the diagnosis. For the cases with no abnormal findings by chest X-ray but with obvious clinical symptoms, chest CT scanning is recommended to define the diagnosis.

7.7 Imaging Demonstrations

7.7.1 Bronchopneumonia

7.7.1.1 Chest X-Ray

Chest X-ray may demonstrate normal findings or only increased thickened pulmonary markings. For serious cases, the chest X-ray can demonstrate small flakes of blurry shadows with uneven density, which distribute along with pulmonary markings in the middle and inferior fields of the lungs. Such findings indicate inflammatory infiltration and exudation in the bronchi and alveoli.

7.7.1.2 CT Scanning

CT scanning can demonstrate thickened vascular bundles in bronchi of the middle and lower fields of both lungs. The foci are small flakes of triangle-like parenchymal shadows which may fuse into a large flake of parenchymal shadow.

7.7.2 Head and Neck

For cases with mucosal congestion and swelling in the pharynx, larynx, and nose and grayish white pseudomembrane, CT scanning can demonstrate swollen tonsils and soft tissue swelling in the uvula, the soft palate, the posterior wall of pharynx, nasopharynx, and larynx. For the cases with other secondary bacterial infection, accompanying cervical and submandibular lymphadenectasis may also be found (Fig. 7.1).

Case Study

A female patient aged 76 years has a body temperature of 37.8 °C, with a history of high blood pressure.

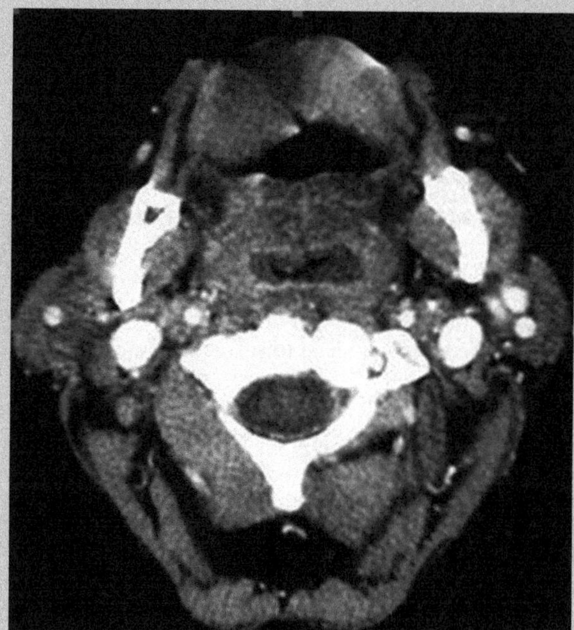

Fig. 7.1 Pharyngeal diphtheria. Enhanced CT scanning of the nasal sinus demonstrated soft tissue swelling of the uvula, the soft palate, the oropharynx, and nasopharynx (Reprint with permission from Khodaei I, et al. *J Laryngol Otol* 2008, 122(12): 1397)

7.8 Basis for Diagnosis

7.8.1 Clinical Diagnosis

In combination with the season, the region, and the history of contact within the most recent week, the clinical cases with a sore throat and inseparable grayish white pseudomembrane at the nasopharynx that is bleeding after forceful swabbing should be diagnosed as diphtheria. In smear of tissues harvested from the margin of the pseudomembrane, gram-positive corynebacteria with metachromatic granules can be microscopically found, which defines the diagnosis.

7.8.2 Laboratory Diagnosis

By bacteria culture, *Corynebacterium diphtheriae* is detected, with positive findings by virulence test.

7.8.3 Diagnostic Imaging

CT scanning demonstrates swollen tonsil as well as soft tissue swelling of the uvula, soft palate, posterior wall of the pharynx, nasopharynx, and larynx. For the cases with secondary infection of other bacteria, the accompanying cervical and submandibular lymphadenectasis can be found.

For the cases with complication of bronchopneumonia, both chest X-ray and CT scanning demonstrate enhanced and blurry pulmonary markings and spots of shadows along with pulmonary markings in the middle and lower fields of both lungs. With the condition progressing, the spots of shadows may be fused into large flakes of parenchymal shadows.

7.9 Differential Diagnosis

7.9.1 Pharyngeal Diphtheria

7.9.1.1 Acute Tonsillitis

It is characterized by an acute onset, fever, sore throat, and red and swollen pharynx. By examination, the tonsils can be found with spots or small flakes of yellowish white exudates that can be wiped away with no bleeding.

7.9.1.2 Oral Candidiasis

It is a disease commonly occurring in newborns and infants, with accompanying indigestion and malnutrition. The symptoms include fever or no fever and white and thin mucosal membrane in the oral cavity that is more common in bilateral positions of the cheeks and can be wiped away. *Candida albicans* can be found by smearing or culture.

7.9.1.3 Ulcerative Angina

Necrotic ulcers and pseudomembrane can be found in the pharynx, commonly accompanied by gingivitis that causes bleeding and oral stink smell. By the smear of throat swabs, fusobacteria and spirochetes can be found.

7.9.1.4 Infectious Mononucleosis

The tonsil is found to have white membrane that wears off slowly. By the smear and culture, no *Corynebacterium diphtheriae* can be found. And antitoxin therapy against diphtheria produces no therapeutic response. In the peripheral blood, abnormal lymphocytes can be found and heterophile agglutination test is positive.

7.9.2 Laryngeal Diphtheria

7.9.2.1 Acute Laryngitis

In the early stage, laryngeal diphtheria can be hardly distinguished from acute laryngitis that is commonly caused by viral or bacterial infections. Laryngeal diphtheria has an acute onset and serious symptoms, with similar clinical manifestations to those of diphtheria including pharyngeal congestion. By indirect laryngoscopy, the larynx and vocal cord have different degrees of congestion and edema, with no pseudomembrane. Generally, the symptoms are slight during daytime and serious during sleeping at nights. No growth of *Corynebacterium diphtheriae* can be found by laryngitis culture.

7.9.2.2 Intratracheal Foreign Body

Patients have a history of inhaling foreign body, with severe coughing. Thereafter, the coughing is paroxysmal. Examination finds no pseudomembrane. By diagnostic imaging, the foreign body can be detected, with confined emphysema or atelectasis.

7.9.3 Nasal Diphtheria

Nasal diphtheria should be differentiated from intranasal foreign body that the foreign body is commonly found in unilateral nostril. By rhinoscopy, the foreign body can be detected, but there is no pseudomembrane. Diagnostic imaging can also demonstrate the shadow of the foreign body.

Reference

Khodaei I, Sinha A, Dingle A. Diphtheria: a case report. J Laryngol Otol. 2008;122(12):1397–400.

Suggested Reading

Gu HX. Medical microbiology. Beijing: People's Medical Publishing House; 2006.
Li N. Oxford infectious diseases (translation into Chinese). Beijing: People's Medical Publishing House; 2011a.
Li LJ. Studies of infectious diseases. Beijing: Higher Education Press; 2011b.
Zhang LX, Zhou XZ. Modern studies of infectious diseases. Beijing: People's Military Medical Press; 2010.
Zhou Z. Studies of infectious diseases. Beijing: People's Medical Publishing House; 2008.

8 Epidemic and Endemic Typhus

Li Li and Guiying Li

Typhus is an acute infectious disease caused by *Rickettsia*. Clinically, it can be divided into two categories, including epidemic typhus and endemic typhus. Epidemic typhus is also known as louse-borne typhus which commonly occurs in winters and springs and causes severe systemic symptoms. It is caused by *Rickettsia prowazekii* and transmitted via human body louse. The clinical symptoms include sustained high fever, severe headache, skin rashes, and central nervous system symptoms, with an acute onset. The whole course of epidemic typhus lasts for 2–3 weeks, with most cases being self-limited. Endemic typhus, also known as flea-borne typhus or murine typhus, is caused by *Rickettsia mooseri* and transmitted via rat flea, with common occurrence in autumns and winters.

8.1 Etiology

Rickettsia prowazekii, the pathogen of epidemic typhus, is a gram-negative tiny bacillus, with a size of (0.3–1) μm × (0.3–0.4) μm. It has polymorphism in the intestinal wall cells of human body lice, with strong resistance to low temperature and dryness. However, it is sensitive to heat, ultraviolet rays, and common disinfectants and can be inactivated at 56 °C for 30 min.

Rickettsia mooseri, the etiologic agent of endemic typhus, shares similar biological properties with *Rickettsia prowazekii*.

L. Li (✉)
Department of Radiology,
Beijing You'an Hospital, Capital Medical University,
Beijing, China
e-mail: sycrbyxx@126.com

G. Li
Department of Radiology,
Beijing Fengtai Hospital of Integrated Traditional
and Western Medicine, Beijing, China

8.2 Epidemiology

8.2.1 Source of Infection

Patient infected with epidemic typhus is its only source of infection, with infectivity in the last 1–2 days of the incubation period. The infectivity is at its peak in the first week after the onset of the disease, which usually lasts for no more than 3 weeks. In extremely rare cases, the pathogen can incubate in the mononuclear phagocyte system for a long period of time causing relapse when the body's immune system is compromised; this occurrence is known as recurrent typhus.

House mouse is the major source of infection of endemic typhus, with *Rickettsia mooseri* transmitted between mice via mouse fleas. After the death of the infected mouse, mouse fleas leave the corpse of their host to sting or bite human. Therefore, human can be infected. In addition, the sources of infection also include patient, cattle, sheep, pig, horse, and mule.

8.2.2 Route of Transmission

Human body lice are carriers of *Rickettsia prowazekii* to transmit epidemic typhus, with body lice as the most common carriers, followed by head lice. After stings or bites of infected lice, *Rickettsiae* multiply in epithelial cells of lice intestinal wall and then are discharged along with feces. When lice carrying *Rickettsiae* sting or bite a healthy person, the feces with *Rickettsiae* are discharged on the skin, which enters the person's body via scratch or bite marks of the skin. Occasionally, the pathogens can also gain their access into the human body via the respiratory tract or conjunctiva. The high fever or death of the infected patient causes lice to transfer to a new host. In such a way, the disease spreads in humans.

Endemic typhus spreads with mouse flea as the carrier of the pathogen, with similar route of transmission to epidemic typhus. *Rickettsiae* gain their access into the human body

H. Li (ed.), *Radiology of Infectious Diseases: Volume 2*, DOI 10.1007/978-94-017-9876-1_8

after surviving in the cells of flea intestinal wall and replicates in large quantity. Mouse flea stings or bites cannot introduce *Rickettsiae* into the human body. However, as they discharge feces or vomits, *Rickettsiae* can then gain access into the human body via scrapes on the skin. The pathogen can also gain its access into the human body via the respiratory tract and conjunctiva.

8.2.3 Susceptibility

People are generally susceptible to typhus. Permanent immunity can be acquired after its infection. Cross immunity against epidemic typhus and endemic typhus does exist.

8.2.4 Epidemic Features

The prevalence of epidemic typhus is closely related to human lice, which commonly occur in winter. Occurrence and prevalence of epidemic typhus can be found during war and famine.

Endemic typhus is an infectious disease with natural focus and sporadically occurs worldwide. It is more common in tropical and subtropical areas. In China, the incidence rate is higher in north, southwest, and northwest areas, and the disease is more common in late summer and autumn. Epidemic typhus and endemic typhus can concur in one regional area.

8.3 Pathogenesis and Pathological Changes

8.3.1 Pathogenesis

The major pathogenesis of epidemic typhus is pathogen-induced vascular lesions, toxin-induced toxemia, as well as some immune and allergic reactions.

After invasion of the pathogen into the human body via skin defects, it first grows and replicates in local lymphatic tissues or endothelial cells of minor blood vessels and capillaries causing rupture of the cells and overflow of the pathogens. Initial rickettsemia consequently occurs. After that, the pathogens spread into endothelial cells of minor blood vessels in all organs establish new foci of infection. After a large quantity replication of the pathogen, secondary rickettsemia and various clinical symptoms occur. At the same time, the large quantity of pathogens causes swelling and rupture of the endothelial cells, causing blockage and embolism in vascular lumen with different severities. In addition, perivasculitis, tissue necrosis, and increased capillary permeability occur, causing hemorrhage, plasma extravasation, reduced effective blood volume, DIC, disturbed blood coagulation mechanism, oliguria, azotemia, and myocardiac lesions.

8.3.2 Pathological Changes

The basic pathological changes of epidemic typhus are located in vessels, with accompanying perivascular lesions in systemic parenchymal organs. Generally, the pathological changes of minor blood vessels are prominent, with proliferation, thrombus, and necrosis. The vascular endothelial cells proliferate in a large quantity to form thrombus. Periodical or round-shaped tissue necrosis can be found in vascular walls. Infiltrations of plasmacytes, monocytes, and lymphocytes can be found at vascular adventitia, which shows characteristic perivascular miliary typhus tubercles or granulomas. Such pathological changes can be found all over the body, which are especially obvious in skin dermis, myocardium, brain, meninges, liver, kidneys, and alveolar wall. Corresponding clinical symptoms occur, including skin rashes, cardiovascular disorders, psychiatric abnormalities, meningeal irritation sign, hepatic dysfunction, pneumonia, and shock.

The pathological changes of the central nervous system are commonly found in the cerebral gray matter, cerebellum, medulla oblongata, and basal ganglia. Their severity and diffusivity can greatly elongate the duration of psychiatric and neurological symptoms even after drop of body temperature.

The early manifestations of the disease include typhus tubercles and the toxemic symptoms, with no characteristic pathological changes. These early symptoms include bronchitis, meningoencephalitis, subarachnoid minor hemorrhage, and hepatorenal swelling. The spleen shows acute swelling, with proliferations of cells in the monocyte-macrophages system, lymphoblasts, lymphocytes, and plasmacytes. In addition, the kidneys show hemorrhage, edema, and degenerative changes of parenchymal cells.

Endemic typhus shares similar pathogenesis and pathological changes with epidemic typhus. However, the cases of endemic typhus have slight vascular lesions and rare occurrence of thrombus in minor vascular vessels and capillaries.

8.4 Clinical Symptoms and Signs

8.4.1 Epidemic Typhus

Epidemic typhus can be divided in to three types: typical typhus, mild typhus, and recurrent typhus.

8.4.1.1 Typical Typhus

The incubation period of epidemic typhus lasts for 10–14 days. In some cases, prodromal symptoms occur that persist for 2–3 days, such as fatigue, headache, dizziness, chills, and low fever. However, most cases show an acute onset, with accompanying chills, severe and persistent headache, systemic muscles pain as well as conjunctival and facial congestion.

Fever

The fever also has an acute onset, with a rapid increase of the body temperature to above 39 °C. Chills occur prior to occurrence of fever, which is continued fever with the high fever commonly persisting for 2–3 weeks. A consequent rapid decrease of body temperature to normal can be found within 3–4 days.

Skin Rashes

About above 90 % of epidemic typhus cases shows skin rashes, which is characteristically epidemic typhus. The skin rashes occur at 4–5 days after the onset of the disease, which spread concentrically to the whole body within 1–2 days. However, the face, palms, and soles are commonly not involved. The skin rashes are congestive maculopapules in bright red or hemorrhagic rashes, which persist for about 1 week and fade away with residual pigmentation.

Central Nervous System Symptoms

The central nervous system symptoms occur early, with severe headaches, accompanying dizziness, tinnitus and decreased hearing ability, slow response, delirium, shivering of both hands, and meningeal irritation sign. By examination of cerebrospinal fluid, only slight increases of protein and pressure can be found.

Hepatosplenomegaly

About 90 % of epidemic typhus cases have splenomegaly. Slight hepatomegaly is found in rare cases.

Other Symptoms

Digestive symptoms are common, including poor appetite, nausea, vomiting, abdominal distension, and constipation. In serious cases, symptoms of toxic myocarditis occur, such as rapid heart rate, low and blunt heart sounds, arrhythmia with gallop rhythm, and hypotension. Even circulatory failure or acute renal failure may occur.

8.4.1.2 Mild Epidemic Typhus

The cases with mild epidemic typhus commonly have a history of vaccination or a medication history of antibiotics in its early stage. The fever sustains for a short period of time, usually 8–9 days. The body temperature is commonly under 39 °C, showing remittent fever. The systemic toxic symptoms are mild, with obvious headache and general soreness and pain but rare neurological symptoms. The skin rashes are congestive, which can be rarely or hardly found and fade away in 1–2 days. Hepatomegaly and splenomegaly are rarely found in the cases of this type.

8.4.1.3 Recurrent Epidemic Typhus

The recurrent epidemic typhus is also known as Brill-Zinsser disease that is rarely found in China. The cases usually have a past history of epidemic typhus. After the initial onset, the pathogen, *Rickettsiae*, incubates in human body for a long period of time, commonly ranging from several years to several decades. When the immunity of such individuals is compromised, the pathogen can be reactive to replicate, causing relapse of epidemic typhus. Such cases commonly have mild clinical symptoms, with short duration of fever, no skin rashes, and rare complications. By Weil-Felix reaction, negative findings or low titer (lower than 1:160) can be found, with specific antibody IgG positive.

8.4.2 Endemic Typhus

The incubation period of endemic typhus usually lasts for 1–2 weeks, with similar clinical manifestations to epidemic typhus. However, endemic typhus has mild disease conditions, with short duration of the conditions and rare complications. Clinically, it commonly is manifested as acute onset, a body temperature of around 39 °C in a continued fever or remittent fever. The fever usually persists for about 9–14 days, with accompanying fatigue, obvious headache, general soreness and pain, other systemic toxic symptoms, and conjunctival congestion. About 50–80 % of endemic typhus cases have congestive skin rashes.

8.5 Typhus-Related Complications

Epidemic typhus can be complicated by bronchopneumonia, otitis media, myocarditis, parotitis, meningoencephalitis, and myelitis. It also can be complicated by infectious psychosis and gangrenes of fingers, toes, earlobe, and nasal tip. In some serious cases, endemic typhus can be complicated by renal or respiratory failure.

8.6 Diagnostic Examinations

8.6.1 Laboratory Tests

8.6.1.1 Weil-Felix Reaction

It has simple procedures but poor specificity that fails to differentiate epidemic typhus from endemic typhus. It may also have false-positive findings due to cross agglutination with pathogens of relapsing fever, tuberculosis, and brucellosis.

8.6.1.2 Complement Fixation Test

It can be applied for the diagnosis or epidemiological survey.

8.6.1.3 Rickettsia Agglutination Test

Agglutination test can be performed with particulate antigens of *Rickettsia prowazekii* and serum from patients, which has high specificity and early demonstration. In addition, it facilitates the differential diagnosis of epidemic from endemic typhus.

8.6.1.4 Indirect Hemagglutination Test (IHAT)

Particulate antigens can be used to detect specific antibodies, with high sensitivity and no cross-reactions with other infectious rickettsia. It is applicable for the early diagnosis, but does not facilitate the differential diagnosis of *Rickettsiae* infections.

8.6.1.5 Indirect Immunofluorescence Test

The test has simple procedures, with high sensitivity and specificity. It can distinguish specific IgG and IgG in blood samples for differentiation of acute infection from previous infection. It can be applied for the early diagnosis and differential diagnosis from other diseases caused by rickettsia.

8.6.1.6 Molecular Biology Assay

By DNA probe or PCT technology, the DNA of pathogen can be detected in blood samples, with high specificity and sensitivity. In addition, the result of assay can be harvested quickly. Such assay facilitates the early diagnosis.

8.6.1.7 Pathogen Isolation

Pathogen isolation is not applied in clinical practice. However, it can be clinically applied if necessary.

8.6.2 Diagnostic Imaging

8.6.2.1 Ultrasound

Ultrasound is commonly applied for the examination of abdominal organs and myocardiac lesions.

8.6.2.2 X-Ray, CT Scanning, and MR Imaging

These radiological examinations are commonly applied to examine various complications of typhus.

8.7 Imaging Demonstrations

8.7.1 Imaging Demonstrations of Typhus

8.7.1.1 Nervous System

Head CT scanning demonstrates diffusive low-density foci.

8.7.1.2 Cardiovascular System

The heart may be involved. Le et al. reported 1 case of typhus, with echocardiographic demonstrations of enlarged right atrium and ventricle and a little regurgitation in tricuspid valve, pulmonary artery, and bicuspid valve.

8.7.1.3 Abdomen

Ultrasound demonstrates slightly enlarged liver and spleen, with increased echo from the liver. It has been reported that liver is 1.5–2.0 cm inferior to the ribs and the spleen is 1–4 cm inferior to the ribs. There are also diffusive renal lesions and increased echo from renal cortex.

8.7.2 Imaging Demonstrations of Typhus-Related Complications

8.7.2.1 Pneumonia

Based on the chest X-ray demonstrations, typhus can be categorized into following four types.

Interstitial Type

Chest X-ray demonstrates thickened and blurry pulmonary markings in both lungs, which may be in a diffusive network of shadow.

Bronchopneumonia Type

Chest X-ray demonstrates thickened pulmonary markings in both lungs as well as spots and flakes of shadows along the pulmonary markings, which extensively involve middle and inner zone of both lungs. The shadows are in low density, with unclearly defined boundaries.

Lobar Pneumonia Type

Chest X-ray demonstrates large flakes of even density shadows distributing in the lung lobes or segments.

Enlarged Pulmonary Hilum Shadow Type

Chest X-ray demonstrates dense and enlarged shadow of pulmonary hilum, with unclearly defined structures and boundaries. CT scanning demonstrates pulmonary inflammation, pleural effusion, and thickened pleura.

8.7.2.2 Otitis Media

Acute Purulent Otitis Media and Mastoiditis

CT Scanning

The demonstrations include increased density of mastoid air cell, bone absorption of the air cell septum with decreased density, and empyema in the tympanum and mastoid sinus with increased density. In some cases, fluid level can be demonstrated.

MR Imaging

The demonstrations include middle ear effusion, air fluid level, and increased signal of mastoid air cell in spots and flakes of equal T1 and long T2 signals. In the cases of hematocele, T1WI and T2WI demonstrate high signals or uneven high signals.

Chronic Purulent Otitis Media

Based on pathological findings and clinical manifestations, it can be divided into simplex type, granuloma type, and cholesteatoma type.

CT Scanning

The demonstrations of simplex type include bone absorption and destruction of ear ossicles, thickened mucosa of tympanic cavity, and thickened mucosa of mastoid sinus or large air cell. Bone hyperplasia can be found at the septum of air cell and its peripheral structures, with demonstrations of thickened septum of air cell, increased density, and absence of bone destruction. The demonstrations of granuloma type include destructed auditory ossicles and even breakage and destruction of ossicular chain, bone destruction, and blurriness as well as increased density in the atticus, entrance of mastoid antrum, and breast antrum. The granulation tissues are demonstrated as soft tissue shadows with high density. Contrast CT scanning demonstrates enhancement due to abundant vascular vessels in the granulation tissues. The demonstrations of cholesteatoma type include mass shadows with soft tissue density in the atticus, entrance of mastoid antrum and mastoid antrum, bone destruction, dilated entrance of mastoid antrum, and tympanic cavity with smooth edges as well as bone hyperplasia and sclerosis. Contrast scanning demonstrates no enhancement of cholesteatoma and enhanced ring in its peripheral inflammatory granulation tissues. In some serious cases, sigmoid sinus wall, cover of tympanic mastoid antrum, semicircular canal, and facial nerve canal may be destructed.

MR Imaging

Compared to cerebral gray matters, inflammatory granulation tissues are demonstrated as equal or slightly high signals by T1WI and high signals by T2WI. Contrast imaging demonstrates enhancement. Cholesterol granuloma is demonstrated as high signals by T1WI and T2WI. Cholesteatoma is demonstrated as similar signals to muscles and lower signals than brain tissues, with commonly uneven signals, high signals by T2WI. Contrast imaging demonstrates no enhancement of cholesteatoma but ring-shaped enhancement of its peripheral granulation tissues.

8.7.2.3 Myocarditis

Ultrasound

Color Doppler ultrasound demonstrates bicuspid valve regurgitation and negative regurgitation spectrum in both left and right atrium, with predominantly slight regurgitation.

MR Imaging

By T2WI or by T1WI with contrast Gd-DTPA, myocardial inflammation is demonstrated as high signal of focal myocardium, with no changes by plain T1WI. This indicates that only T1WI demonstration has no diagnostic value for myocarditis. T2WI has a low positive rate, which may be related to its relatively less water content in the tissues. By contrast Gd-DTPA, T1WI is more sensitive than T2WI to the lesions, which is related to the effects of contrast agent including obviously shortened T1 relaxation time of the defective myocardium and increased signal intensity of the defective myocardium. By contrast imaging, images harvested by T1WI are more clear than those by T2WI. Therefore, contrast T1WI facilitates more in the diagnosis of myocardial inflammation.

8.7.2.4 Myelitis

CT scanning demonstrates swelling of spinal cord in the diseased area, which has uneven density. MR imaging demonstrates long T1 and long T2 signals of the lesions.

8.8 Basis for the Diagnosis

8.8.1 Diagnosis of Typhus

8.8.1.1 Epidemiological Histories

8.8.1.2 Clinical Manifestations

The clinical manifestations include fever and skin rashes.

8.8.1.3 Laboratory Test

By Weil-Felix test, a high titer (above 1:320) can define the diagnosis. Otherwise, by contrasting double serum samples, an increase of titer for more than four times can define the diagnosis.

8.8.2 Diagnosis of Typhus-Related Complications

8.8.2.1 Pneumonia

The cases commonly have a history of typhus, respiratory symptoms of coughing and expectoration, occasional moist, and dry rales of both lungs. In addition to routine blood test findings, thickened pulmonary markings and patches of shadows can be demonstrated by chest X-ray and CT scanning. In combination of the above findings, the clinical diagnosis can be made.

8.8.2.2 Myocarditis

Patients with typhus have accompanying symptoms of low and blunt heart sound, arrhythmia of gallop rhythm, and hypotension.

Changed ST-T by electrocardiography can be found. And myocardiac enzyme can be found with an increase.

T2WI and contrast T1WI of MR imaging demonstrate high signals of focal myocardium.

8.8.2.3 Otitis Media

Acute Otitis Media

Patients with typhus have middle ear effusion, with accompanying symptoms of fever, headache, ear pain, and vomiting. By physical examination, dragging pain of the auricle and decreased conductive hearing can be found.

By otoscopy, a series of symptoms can be found, including congestive and protruding eardrum or eardrum with tension in a color of dark red. Otherwise, absent visual marker, weakened movement of eardrum, yellowish pus after the eardrum, or eardrum perforation can be found.

By diagnostic imaging, increased density of the mastoid air cell, effusion of middle ear canal, and air-fluid level can be found.

Chronic Otitis Media

The cases have a previous history of typhus. The clinical manifestations include otorrhea, perforation of eardrum, and conductive deafness.

By diagnostic imaging, bone absorption and destruction of auditory ossicles, granuloma, and cholesteatoma can be found.

Myelitis

Patients with typhus patients have clinical manifestations of paraplegia and sensory disturbance.

By examination of cerebrospinal fluid, the pressure is normal, with slight increases of protein and cell count.

CT scanning demonstrates swelling of involved segmental spinal cord, with uneven density. MR imaging demonstrates long T1 and long T2 signals of the lesions.

8.9 Differential Diagnosis

8.9.1 Tuberculous Meningitis and Viral Meningitis

Typhus with neurological symptoms as its initial symptoms should be differentiated from tuberculous meningitis and viral meningitis.

Individuals with a history of contacts to patients with tuberculosis, PPD test positive, or children patients suffering from active tuberculosis are susceptible to tuberculous meningitis. The cases with temperament changes, fever, headache, vomiting, and intractable constipation, with no known causes, should be suspected as having tuberculous meningitis. Serum Weil-Felix reaction facilitates to distinguish tuberculous meningitis from viral meningitis.

Brain CT scanning demonstrations of typhus are similar to those of viral encephalitis. In addition, the cerebrospinal changes have no obvious difference between the cases of the two diseases. The differential diagnosis is mainly based on clinical case history and serum Weil-Felix reaction.

8.9.2 Pneumonia

For the cases of typhus complicated by pulmonary infection, only X-ray examination hardly has diagnostic value for its differential diagnosis from pneumonia induced by bacteria, virus, and mycoplasma infection. The diagnosis can be defined based on epidemiological histories, clinical manifestations, and findings by Weil-Felix reaction.

Suggested Reading

Childs H, Friedrich MG. Cardiovascular magnetic resonance imaging in myocarditis[J]. Prog Cardiovasc Dis. 2011;54(3):266–75.

Jiang C, Li L. Endemic typhus complicated by thoracic myelitis and arachnoiditis: report of 1 case. New Med. 2001;32(9):574.

Le Y, Yin ZL. Characteristic clinical manifestations of pediatric typhus. Chin J Infect Dis. 2002;20(6):368–9.

Li LJ. Studies of infectious diseases. Beijing: Higher Education Press; 2011.

Yu DZ. Infectious zoonosis. Beijing: Science Press; 2009.

Zhang LX, Zhou XZ. Modern studies of infectious diseases. Beijing: People Military Medical Press; 2010.

Epidemic Cerebrospinal Meningitis

9

Mengtian Sun and Jingliang Cheng

Epidemic cerebrospinal meningitis is a suppurative meningitis caused by *Neisseria meningitidis*. Its main clinical manifestations include sudden high fever, headache, vomiting, mucosal petechiae and ecchymosis, and signs of meningeal irritation. In some serious cases, explosive onset may occur, with septic shock and cerebral parenchymal damages. The disease is distributed worldwide that is prevailing sporadically or epidemically. Its occurrence is more common in winters and springs and is more commonly found in children.

9.1 Etiology

The pathogen of epidemic cerebrospinal meningitis is *Neisseria meningitides*, which can be categorized into the genus of *Neisseria*. It is a gram-negative diplococcus and can be detected from the nasopharynx of carriers and from the blood, cerebrospinal fluid, and the skin petechiae of patients. This bacterium is obligate aerobe and can release endotoxin by splitting, which contributes to its pathogenicity. According to the differences between the specific capsular polysaccharide, it can be divided into 13 serogroups, namely, A, B, C, D, X, Y, Z, 29E, W135, H, I, K, and L. The serogroups of A, B, and C are most common, accounting for above 90 % of all capsular polysaccharides. The serogroup C has the strongest pathogenicity, followed by serogroup B, and the serogroup Y has the weakest pathogenicity. Generally, the serogroup A causes pandemic prevalence, while the serogroups B and C cause sporadic and small-scaled epidemic prevalences. The prevailing strain varies in different regions during different periods of time. The cases caused by the serogroups B and C are commonly found in Europe and the United States, while the cases caused by the serogroups A and C are commonly found in Asia and Africa. In the recent 30 years, the prevailing strain in China is predominantly serogroups A, while the serogroups B and C cause sporadic prevalence. In addition, the prevalence of serogroup B is increasing.

9.2 Epidemiology

9.2.1 Source of Infection

Carriers of *Neisseria meningitides* and patients with epidemic cerebrospinal meningitis are the sources of infection, with a high rate of asymptomatic infection. During the epidemic period, the carrying rate of the bacteria is up to 50 %, with infection, but no symptoms. At the end of incubation period and during the acute phase of the disease, patients with epidemic cerebrospinal meningitis are capable of spreading the infection, and the infectious phase terminates within 10 days after the onset. The bacteria have a favorable response to therapies that can be inactivated soon. Therefore, carriers of the bacteria, as the source of infection, are of greater importance.

9.2.2 Routes of Transmission

Epidemic cerebrospinal meningitis is an airborne disease, and the bacteria spread along with droplets from coughing and sneezing. Infants and young children can also be infected by close contacts to patients, such as embracing, breast feeding, and kissing.

9.2.3 Susceptible Population

The susceptibility of epidemic cerebrospinal meningitis is closely related to the antibody level of populations, with

M. Sun • J. Cheng (✉)
Department of MRI,
The First Affiliated Hospital,
Zhengzhou University,
Zhengzhou, Henan, China
e-mail: cjr.chjl@vip.163.com

H. Li (ed.), *Radiology of Infectious Diseases: Volume 2*, DOI 10.1007/978-94-017-9876-1_9

more common occurrence of asymptomatic infection. Infants under the age of 6 months are rarely infected due to the acquired immunity from the mother, while the incidence rate in infants aged between 6 months and 2 years is the highest. Its infection by human being can produce persistent immunity against the bacteria.

9.2.4 Epidemiological Features

The disease occurs all year round but with obvious seasonal changes. It commonly occurs in the period from November to May of the next year, with a peak occurrence during March and April. The occurrence in the period from February to April accounts for 60–90 % of the annual total cases. Its infection by humans can produce specific immunity. However, along with the decreased immunity level in populations, the newly infected cases are increasing, which renders its periodic prevalence. Generally, the disease has a small-scaled epidemic every 3–5 years, while a large-scaled epidemic every 7–10 years. Due to the widespread practice of vaccination, such a periodic prevalence has not been obvious.

9.2.5 Present Prevalence

African epidemic zone of epidemic cerebrospinal meningitis is the high incidence area of the disease. In the past 20 years, its outbreak in the zone has caused over 1 million cases and nearly 90,000 cases of deaths, with serogroup A as the main pathogenic type of bacteria.

China is one of the countries with a high incidence rate of epidemic cerebrospinal meningitis. Along with the wide use of vaccination against serogroup A, its incidence has decreased year by year since the year of 1982. After the year of 1990, the incidence has been kept under 1/100,000. In the year of 2004, the incidence was 0.208/100,000, with a mortality rate of under 6 %. Due to both sources of infection and susceptible populations, the prevailing serogroup may be varied, and the frequent flow of personnel renders an epidemic of epidemic cerebrospinal meningitis possible.

9.3 Pathogenesis and Pathological Changes

9.3.1 Pathogenesis

Neisseria meningitides invade human body via respiratory tract, followed by their binding to the specific receptor on the respiratory mucosa and the surface of endothelial cells. Subsequently, they penetrate the mucosal barrier to cause inflammation via epithelial cells or between cells. The bacteria then travel along with blood flow to invade meninges, leading to cerebrospinal meningitis. Vascular endothelial cells in the cerebral and spinal meninges show pathological changes of necrosis, edema, congestion, hemorrhage, and increased permeability to cause purulent inflammation of cerebrospinal meninges and increased intracranial pressure. Patients may sustain symptoms of convulsion and coma. In some serious cases of encephaledema, cerebral herniation occurs to cause death rapidly.

9.3.2 Pathological Changes

Neisseria meningitides involve cerebrospinal meninges to cause suppurative cerebrospinal meningitis whose lesions predominantly locate in the pia mater and arachnoid membrane to cause suppurative inflammation. In the early stage, the pathological changes include vascular congestion, edema, serous exudates, and focal bleeding spots. In the advanced stage, there are large quantities of exudates of neutrophil, fibrin, and plasma in the cerebrospinal fluid (CSF), and the exudates show suppurative changes. Due to the sticky pus in the skull base and the direct invasion of the suppurative lesions, meningeal adhesion occurs. Purulent inflammation can involve the 2nd, 3rd, 6th, 7th, and 8th pair of cranial nerves. Fulminant meningoencephalitis is mainly induced by invasion of lipoidase endotoxin from *Neisseria meningitidis* toward cerebral blood vessels to cause spasmodic contraction of the cerebral arterioles. The vascular endothelial cells are thus impaired further to result in the increased vascular permeability, plasma exudation, cerebral edema, and increased intracranial pressure. In some serious cases, cerebral herniation occurs.

9.4 Clinical Symptoms and Signs

Based on the severity of conditions and the clinical manifestations, epidemic cerebrospinal meningitis can be divided into following for clinical subtypes.

9.4.1 Mild Type

The condition is slight, with clinical manifestations of low-grade fever, slight headache, pharyngodynia, and other symptoms of upper respiratory tract infection. Tiny hemorrhagic spots can be found on the skin.

9.4.2 Common Type

It is the most common type, accounting for above 90 % of all the cases of epidemic cerebrospinal meningitis. The whole illness course can be divided into four typical periods, and the respective clinical features are described as the following.

9.4.2.1 Prodromal Period (The Period of Upper Respiratory Tract Infection)

Its duration is about 1–2 days, with symptoms of upper respiratory tract infection such as low-grade fever, pharyngodynia, and coughing. Most patients do not experience this period.

9.4.2.2 Septicemic Period

After the sudden onset or after the prodromal period, toxemic symptoms such as high fever and chills, headache, muscular soreness, poor appetite, and mental fatigue occur, with occasionally found arthralgia and splenomegaly. In such a period, 70–90 % patients have petechiae or ecchymosis either on skin or mucosa. In some serious cases, ecchymosis rapidly extends to show necrosis due to thrombosis. Most cases progress into the meningitic period within 12–24 h.

9.4.2.3 Meningitic Period

Symptoms of meningitic period often concur with symptoms of septicemic period. Based on the symptoms of prodromal period, patients further sustain severe headache, frequent vomiting, mania, and signs of meningeal irritation. The blood pressure may increase with decreased rate of pulse. Some serious patients may experience delirium, mental problems, and convulsion. The meningitic period commonly lasts for 2–5 days, followed by the convalescent period.

9.4.2.4 Convalescent Period

After treatment, the body temperature gradually returns to normal, with absence petechiae and ecchymosis on the skin. The central necrotic areas in large petechiae show ulceration, with subsequent formation of scab and recovery. The symptoms gradually improve, with occurrence of herpetic lips in about 10 % of the patients. The patients can be cured within 1–3 weeks.

9.4.3 Fulminant Type

Some patients have an acute and sudden onset of symptoms that change rapidly. Death may occur within 24 h in the cases with inappropriate or delayed therapeutic intervention. Such a type is more common in children and can be divided into the following three subtypes:

9.4.3.1 Fulminant Type with Shock

Severe toxic symptoms occur, with acute onset of high fever and chills. But in some serious cases, the body temperature of patients is normal, with accompanying headache and vomiting. Within short period of time, extensive petechiae or ecchymosis on the skin and mucosa is present, which rapidly extends to fuse into large flakes with central necrosis. Circulatory failure is characteristic manifestation of the subtype, with pale complexion, cyanosis at ends of extremities and around lips, colored skin, limbs coldness, find and rapid pulses, and shortness of breath. Delayed emergency rescuing may result in rapid deterioration of the conditions, with deteriorating symptoms of peripheral circulation failure, obviously decreased blood pressure, decreased amount of urine output, and coma.

9.4.3.2 Fulminant Type with Meningoencephalitis

It is characterized by severely damaged cerebral meninges and parenchyma. Within 1–2 days after onset, serious neurological symptoms commonly occur, with more serious unconsciousness, rapid progress into coma, and frequent convulsions, in addition to the symptoms of high fever, headache, and vomiting. In some serious cases, patients may develop cerebral herniation, commonly cerebral tonsillar herniation, with manifestations of more serious coma, dilated pupils, increased muscular tension, internal rotation of upper limbs, rigidity of lower limbs, and rapid progress into respiratory failure.

9.4.3.3 Fulminant Type with Shock and Meningoencephalitis

Both the symptoms of fulminant type with shock and fulminant type with meningoencephalitis can be found in the patients.

9.4.4 Chronic Septicemic Type

It is rarely found, and the patients are commonly adults. The illness course commonly extends to several weeks or even several months. The clinical manifestations include intermittent coldness or fever. The episode usually lasts for about 12 h, with an interval of about 1–4 days. After the episode of coldness or fever, groups of skin rashes occur, sometimes even with petechiae, commonly accompanied by arthralgia and splenomegaly.

9.5 Epidemic Cerebral Meningitis-Related Complications

Epidemic cerebral meningitis-related complications mainly include secondary infection, purulent lesions caused by dissemination to other organs during septicemic period, and the impairments of meningitis to the brain and surrounding tissues.

9.5.1 Subdural Effusion

It occurs in infants with unclosed anterior fontanel who suffer from epidemic cerebral meningitis, commonly found within several hours or several days after occurrence of epidemic cerebral meningitis. Its occurrence is due to the invasion of the bacteria into the space between the dura and arachnoid along with blood flow during the septicemic period, with secondary exudation to form effusion. Otherwise, it is caused by inflammatory embolism of bridging veins in the subdural space due to access of plasma protein to the subdural space that results from obviously increased permeability of cerebrovascular wall.

9.5.2 Hydrocephalus

The rapidly increased intracerebroventricular effusion and adhesion-induced occlusion of cerebroventricular passages cause obstructed cerebrospinal fluid circulation. Therefore, the intracerebroventricular effusion further increases with enlarged lateral ventricle and malabsorption of arachnoidal granulations. Subsequently, hydrocephalus develops.

9.5.3 Pneumonia

It is commonly found in the elderly and infants, with clinical symptoms of fever, pharyngeal congestion, swelling of tonsils, and moist rales of lungs. The severity of serious hypoxia and the progressing rate of conditions fail to be positively related to the pulmonary signs.

9.6 Diagnostic Examinations

9.6.1 Laboratory Test

9.6.1.1 Routine Blood Test

The WBC count significantly increases to about $20 \times 109/L$. The neutrophil count also increases. The cases with the complication of DIC show decreased platelets.

9.6.1.2 Cerebrospinal Fluid (CSF) Examination

Cerebrospinal fluid examination is an important examination for a definitive diagnosis. During the typical meningitic period, the pressure of cerebrospinal fluid reaches above 1.96 kPa, with an appearance of turbidity or pus. The WBC count significantly increases, with a predominant increase of neutrophil count and an increase of protein content. The glucose and chlorides decrease significantly, sometimes even undetectable.

9.6.1.3 Bacteriological Examination

The tissue fluid from ecchymosis is harvested for smear, staining, and microscopy. Such an examination is simple and convenient, with a positive rate of over 80 %. After precipitation of the cerebrospinal fluid, the positive rate of the smear is about 60–70 %. Bacterial culture is the golden standard for clinical diagnosis, which should be performed prior to the medication of antibiotics. Bacterial culture with blood or cerebrospinal fluid has a low positive rate. Based on the positive finding, typing of bacterial strain and drug sensitivity test should be performed.

9.6.1.4 Serum Immunological Essay

It plays facilitative role in the diagnosis, which can be applied for the patients who have used antibiotics and negative findings by bacterial culture.

9.6.1.5 Nucleic Acid Detection

It can be applied to detect DNAs of serogroups A, B, and C in serum and cerebrospinal fluid in the early stage of the disease. The positive rate in cerebrospinal fluid examination is about 92 % and that of serum examination about 86 %.

9.6.2 Diagnostic Imaging

9.6.2.1 Ultrasonography

It is commonly applied for the diagnosis of serious epidemic cerebral meningitis complicated by cardiovascular diseases.

9.6.2.2 Chest X-Ray

It is commonly applied for the diagnosis of limbs purulent arthritis and for the exclusion of complicated pulmonary infections and other pulmonary lesions.

9.6.2.3 CT Scanning

It is commonly applied for the respiratory diseases and changes of central nervous system.

9.6.2.4 MR Imaging

It is commonly applied for the detection of lesions in the central nervous system.

9.7 Imaging Demonstrations

9.7.1 Central Nervous System (CNS)

9.7.1.1 CT Scanning

In the early stage, no abnormalities can be found. With the progress of the conditions, there may be enlarged cerebral ventricles, subdural effusion, focal or diffusive low-density shadows in the brain parenchyma, and increased density of cisterns. Enhanced scanning demonstrates obvious abnormal enhancement of the meninges.

9.7.1.2 MR Imaging

MR imaging has no specific demonstrations, with common findings of subdural effusion and supratentorial hydrocephalus. Due to purulent inflammations of cerebral pia mater and subarachnoid space, the subarachnoid space is filled with large quantities of inflammatory exudates, with demonstrations of blurry sulcus and subarachnoid space in the diseased area in medium to low T1WI signal. FLAIR sequence can more clearly demonstrate the shape and range of lesions, with demonstrations of filled sulci in the diseased area by linear or strip-liked medium to high or high signal. In the cases complicated by parenchymal inflammation, T2WI patchy slight high signal can be demonstrated in the brain parenchyma adjacent to the diseased area. For most patients, enhanced imaging demonstrates abnormal linear enhancement of meninges and arachnoid membrane (Fig. 9.1). Boos et al. reported that chronic epidemic cerebral meningitis in the elderly has no typical imaging demonstrations, possibly with cerebral infarction, but no obvious enhancement of meninges. O'Farrell et al. reported one case of transverse myelitis complicating epidemic cerebral meningitis, with demonstrations of high T2WI signal in the inferior part of medulla oblongata, the superior part of cervical cord, and cerebellar tonsil.

Case Study 1

An infant girl aged 8 weeks, with fever and diarrhea. Polymerase chain reaction of cerebrospinal fluid defined the diagnosis of epidemic cerebral meningitis. For case detail and figures, please refer to Yip K, et al. *Cases J*, 2009 2: 6335.

Case Study 2

A female patient aged 25 years, with complaints of headache and vomiting. The bacterial culture of cerebrospinal fluid defined the diagnosis of epidemic cerebral meningitis.

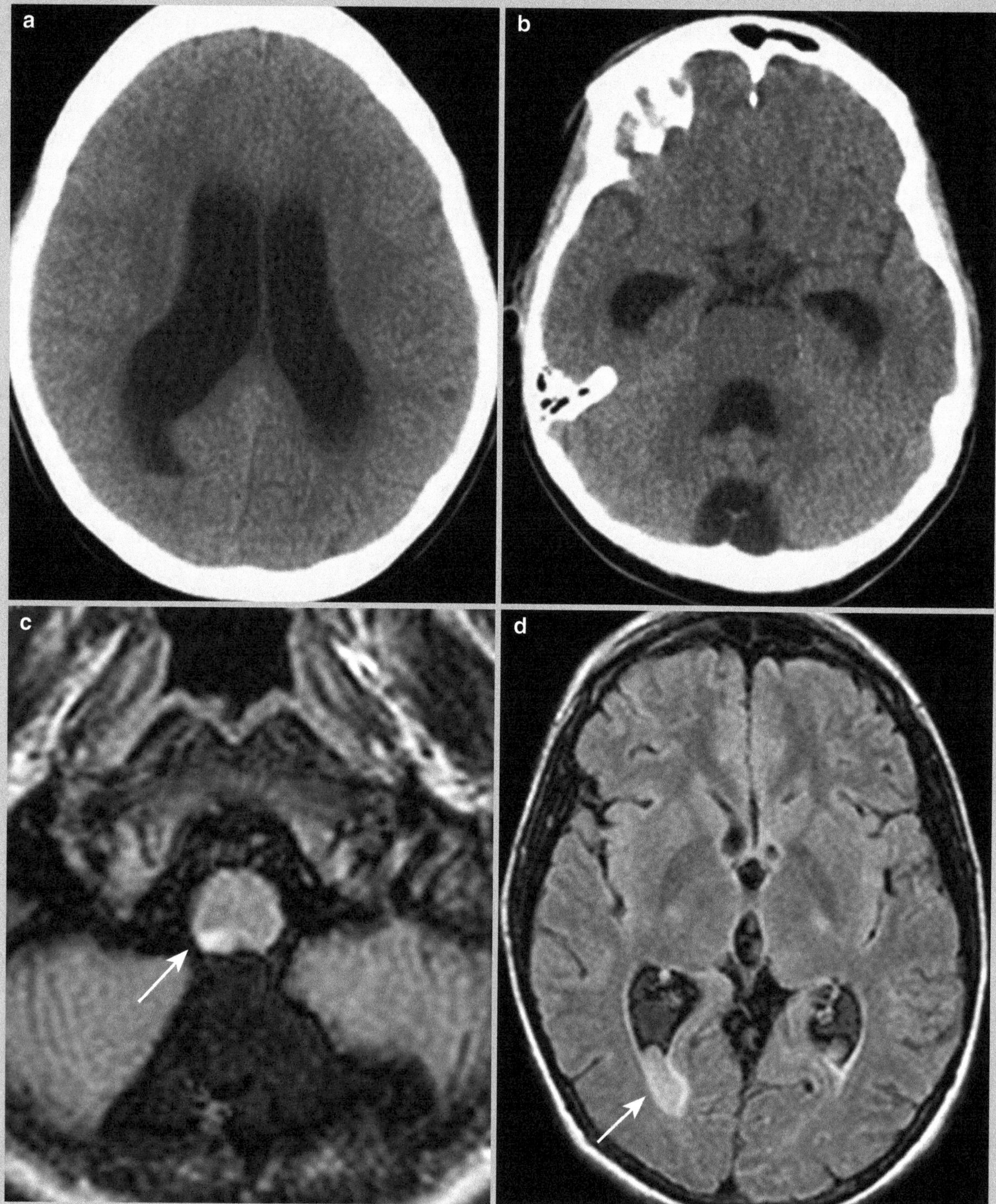

Fig. 9.1 Epidemic cerebrospinal meningitis. (**a**, **b**) Transverse CT scanning demonstrates obviously enlarged cerebroventricular system including the four ventricles and communicating hydrocephalus. (**c**) Transverse FLAIR sequence demonstrates patches of high signals at the right posterior part of medulla oblongata. (**d**) Patches of high signals surrounding the triangular area in the right lateral ventricles and suppurative ependymitis (pointed by *arrows*) (Reprint with permission from vandebeek D, et al. *Arch Neurol*, 2007, 64(9): 1350)

Case Study 3
A male patient aged 17 years, with complaints of fever, nausea, and headache. The laboratory tests defined the diagnosis of epidemic cerebral meningitis.
For case detail and figures, please refer to Kastenbauer S, et al. *Arch Neurol*, 2001, 58(5): 806.

9.7.2 Pulmonary Infection

By chest X-ray, the demonstrations are not specific, including patches of shadows as bronchopneumonia and lobar infiltration which are commonly found in the inferior lobe and the right middle lobe, with accompanying pleural effusion in about 20 % of the cases.

9.8 Basis for the Diagnosis

9.8.1 Diagnosis of Epidemic Cerebral Meningitis

The suspected cases are commonly found in winters and springs and in epidemic areas, with a history of close contacts to patients with epidemic cerebral meningitis. The suspected cases also have symptoms of sudden high fever, nausea, vomiting, deteriorating headaches, petechiae and ecchymosis on skin and/or mucosa, irritation, delirium, coma, and convulsions, with accompanying signs of meningeal irritation. The early diagnosis should be made based on the cerebrospinal fluid examination and serum immunological essay.

The cases with imaging demonstrations of enlarged supratentorial ventricles, subdural effusion, and abnormal enhancement of meninges should be suspected as having epidemic cerebral meningitis.

9.8.2 Diagnosis of Epidemic Cerebral Meningitis-Related Complications

9.8.2.1 Subdural Effusion

After treatments for meningitis, the cases with persistent fever or recurrent fever, repeated convulsions, persistent protrusion of anterior fontanel, or recurrent protrusion of anterior fontanel after treatment should be suspected as having secondary subdural effusion. By subdural puncture, the discharged slightly yellowish fluid exceeds 2 ml. Its protein quantification is usually above 0.04 g/dl.

The diagnostic imaging demonstrates stripes of fluid signal in the peripheral brain, thickened meninges, and obvious abnormal enhancement by enhanced imaging.

9.8.2.2 Hydrocephalus

It has clinical manifestations of intracranial hypertension. By diagnostic imaging, the demonstrations include symmetrically enlarged supratentorial ventricles.

9.8.2.3 Pneumonia

The patients have clinical manifestations of fever, pharyngeal congestion, enlarged tonsils, and moist rales of lungs. By laboratory tests, the affinity of hemoglobin, blood platelet, and carbon dioxide rapidly decreases, with increased leukocytes. By pharyngeal smear, a large quantity of *Neisseria meningitides* can be found. Diagnostic imaging shows demonstrations of bronchopneumonia.

9.9 Differential Diagnosis

9.9.1 Suppurative Meningitis Caused by Other Bacteria

Based on the route of bacterial invasion, they can be preliminarily distinguished. *Streptococcus pneumoniae* infection is common in adults and mostly occurs secondary to pneumonia, otitis media, and craniocerebral trauma. *Haemophilus influenza* infection is common in infants and young children. Infections caused by *Staphylococcus aureus* are mostly secondary to skin infections. *Pseudomonas aeruginosa* meningitis is secondary to lumbar puncture, anesthesia, radiography, or surgical operation. Gram-negative bacilli infection often occurs after craniocerebral operation. In addition, the occurrence of above bacterial infections is sporadic rather than seasonal, with no petechiae or ecchymosis on the skin or mucosa. The definitive diagnosis should be based on bacteriologic examinations.

9.9.2 Tuberculous Meningitis

Patients with tuberculous meningitis commonly have a history of tuberculosis or a history of close contacts to patients with tuberculosis. The disease has a chronic onset and a long course of illness, with symptoms of low-grade fever, night sweating, and emaciation. The neurological symptoms occur late, and there are no ecchymosis and petechiae. By examinations of cerebrospinal fluid, there are decreased leukocytes that are predominantly monocytes, increased protein as well as decreased glucose and chlorides. By the smear of cerebrospinal fluid and acid-fast staining, the acid-fast bacilli can be found positive, based on which it can be differentiated from epidemic cerebral meningitis.

9.9.3 Epidemic Encephalitis B

It is commonly found in children from July to September, with serious lesions in cerebral parenchyma. The symptoms of coma and convulsion are commonly found, with no petechiae on the skin. Clinically, there are acute onset, high fever, awareness disturbance, convulsions, tonic spasms, and meningeal irritation signs. The cerebrospinal fluid is clear, with WBC count of (0.05–0.5) × 109/L, normal or slightly increased levels of glucose and protein, and normal level of chlorides. The immunological essay such as specific IgM is facilitative for the differential diagnosis.

References

Kastenbauer S, Winkler F, Fesl G, et al. Acute severe spinal cord dysfunction in bacterial meningitis in adults: MRI findings suggest extensive myelitis. Arch Neurol. 2001;58(5):806–10.

van de Beek D, Patel R, Wijdicks EF. Meningococcal meningitis with brainstem infarction. Arch Neurol. 2007;64(9):1350–1.

Yip K, Gosling RD, Jones V, et al. An unusual case of meningococcal meningitis complicated with subdural empyema in a 3 month old infant: a case report. Cases J. 2009;2:6335.

Suggested Reading

Boos C, Daneshvar C, Hinton A, et al. An unusual case of chronic meningitis. BMC Fam Pract. 2004;6:21.

Brandtzaeg P, van Deuren M. Classification and pathogenesis of meningococcal infections. Methods Mol Biol. 2012;799:21–35.

Li LJ. Studies of infectious diseases. Beijing: Higher Education Press; 2011.

Sabra A, Benger J. Meningococcal disease in children: a clinical review. Turk J Pediatr. 2011;53(5):477–88.

Trivedi K, Tang CM, Exley RM. Mechanisms of meningococcal colonisation. Trends Microbiol. 2011;19(9):456–63.

O'Farrell R, Thornton J, Brennan P, et al. Spinal cord infarction and tetraplegia–rare complications of meningococcal meningitis. Br J Anaesth. 2000;84(4):514–7.

Wang YM. Studies of infectious diseases. Beijing: People's Health Publishing House; 2010.

Gonorrhea

10

Xiaodan Wang and Yanqing Gao

Gonorrhea is a suppurative inflammation of the urogenital system caused by *Neisseria gonorrhoeae* or briefly gonococcus, which also includes infections of the eye, pharynx, and rectum and disseminated gonococcus infection. It is one of the most common sexually transmitted infections with a relatively short incubation period. Symptoms and signs of gonorrhea commonly appear within 3–5 days after infection.

10.1 Etiology

Neisseria gonorrhoeae is categorized into the genus of *Neisseria*, which was firstly isolated from urethral secretion of a patient by *Neisseria* in 1879. *Neisseria gonorrhoeae* is in oval or kidney-like shape that is often arranged in pairs with the contact surface being flat or slightly depressed. Its diameter is about 0.6–0.8 μm, and it is gram negative with no spores and no flagellum.

The exterior membrane of the cell wall of gonococcus is composed of lipopolysaccharide, outer membrane protein, and pili. The lipopolysaccharide may be related to its toxicity, pathogenicity, and immunogenicity. The outer membrane protein acts as the first weapon for its attack into the serosa of epithelial cells. Pili play a role in mediating and adhering, which is related to its pathogenicity. The antigenic chromosome of pili can produce their variants without pili to avoid antibody response of the host. It can also adhere to various kinds of epithelial cells to suppress the phagocytosis of neutrophils in the host. Most of the gonococcus contains plasmid, whose encoding and regulating functions are related to β-lactamase, chromosome mutations and its drug-resistance.

X. Wang • Y. Gao (✉)
Department of Dermatology, Beijing You'an Hospital, Capital Medical University, Beijing, China
e-mail: gyqing2001bj@sina.com

Gonococcus has weak tolerance to external environment and is intolerant to dryness and coldness. It can grow favorably in an environment with a temperature of 35–36 °C and a pH value of 7.2–7.5 containing 5–7 % CO_2. In a dry environment, it dies within 1–2 h. In an inadequately dried environment and pus fluid, it keeps its infectivity for more than 10 h or even several days. Gonococcus is sensitive to common disinfectants, which can be killed in 1:4,000 silver nitrate solution within 7 min or in 1 % phenol within 1–3 min.

10.2 Epidemiology

Gonorrhea can be found worldwide with the highest incidence rate in sexually transmitted diseases. The CDC in China has reported that the incidence of gonorrhea ranks sixth in sexually transmitted diseases in China, with a decrease from 1998 to 2005. The occurrence of gonorrhea is related to age, gender, race, educational background, sexual behaviors, and immunity. In addition, it varies in different regions. It can occur in any age group and has higher incidence in young male adults.

Gonorrhea mainly spreads via sexual contacts. Asymptomatic patients and patients with mild symptoms are the main source of infection. And the patients in incubation period are also contagious. Gonorrhea can also spread via nonsexual contacts such as contact to secretions from patients with gonorrhea, contaminated utensils including clothes, towel, bath tub, and toilets. Vertical transmission occurs during delivery of an infected woman to cause gonococcal conjunctivitis, pneumonia, and even infection of vulva and vagina in neonates. Infected pregnant woman can involve amniotic cavity to spread the infection to fetus. In addition, the disease can spread via hands of medical staff and healthcare appliances, which is known as nosocomial infection.

H. Li (ed.), *Radiology of Infectious Diseases: Volume 2*, DOI 10.1007/978-94-017-9876-1_10

10.3 Pathogenesis and Pathological Changes

Humans are the only natural host of gonococcus, which has affinity to simple columnar epithelium and transitional epithelium such as male urethra, cervix, and bladder mucosa. Gonococcus reproduces at the surface of columnar epithelial cells after adherence of its pili to the cell via adhering factors. After that, it moves upward along the genital tracts into the target cells via phagocytosis of columnar epithelial cells for further reproduction. The cells are then damaged and disrupted. Gonococcus can also move from mucosal cell space into submucosa to cause necrosis by the coordinative effect of endotoxin, oligosaccharide, and complements. It can also induce aggregation and phagocytosis of neutrophil granulocytes to cause local acute inflammation with symptoms of congestion, swelling, suppuration and pain, and erosion and shedding of mucosa, which is typical for purulent inflammation of urethra. Without prompt and appropriate treatment, gonococcus may further attack urethral glands and crypt to cause chronic lesions. Otherwise, it may gain its access into posterior urethra or cervix and spreads upward to cause inflammations of urogenital tracts and neighboring organs such as skenitis, anteprostatitis, prostatitis, vesiculitis, endometritis, and salpingitis. In some severe cases, gonococcus can disseminate all over the body along with blood flow.

10.4 Clinical Symptoms and Signs

The clinical manifestations after infection of gonococcus are dependent on the site, severity, and time of the infection as well as the virulence of bacterial strain, susceptibility of the organism, and existence of prior disease. Its incubation period is relative short, generally lasting for about 2–5 days.

10.4.1 Acute Gonorrhea in Males

Its onset generally occurs 3–5 days after sexual contact, with typical initial symptoms of redness and swelling of urethral meatus that is mildly itchy or slight stabbing pain, and discharge of thin mucus. The conditions aggravate after 24 h with manifestations of yellowish purulent and more secretions, odynuria, dysuresia, frequent urination, urgent urination, as well as general upset (Fig. 10.1). By physical examination, large quantity of purulent secretions can be found at urethral meatus with redness and swelling. In some severe cases, urethral mucous eversion can also be found.

10.4.2 Gonorrhea in Females

About 50 % of the female patients with gonorrhea are asymptomatic or slightly affected and, therefore, tend to be neglected. Its onset in females is commonly at the cervix and may also be found at the vagina, urethra, or rectum.

Gonococcal cervicitis is clinically characterized by increased and abnormal vaginal secretions that are initially mucous and then purulent. There are also mild odynuria, urgent urination, and difficult urination. By routine examination, swelling and tenderness are found at the cervical opening with yellowish purulent secretions. Gonococcal urethritis is characterized by redness and swelling at the urethral meatus. Pus can be pressed out from the paraurethral gland in patients with skenitis. Gonococcal bartholinitis is characterized by unilateral

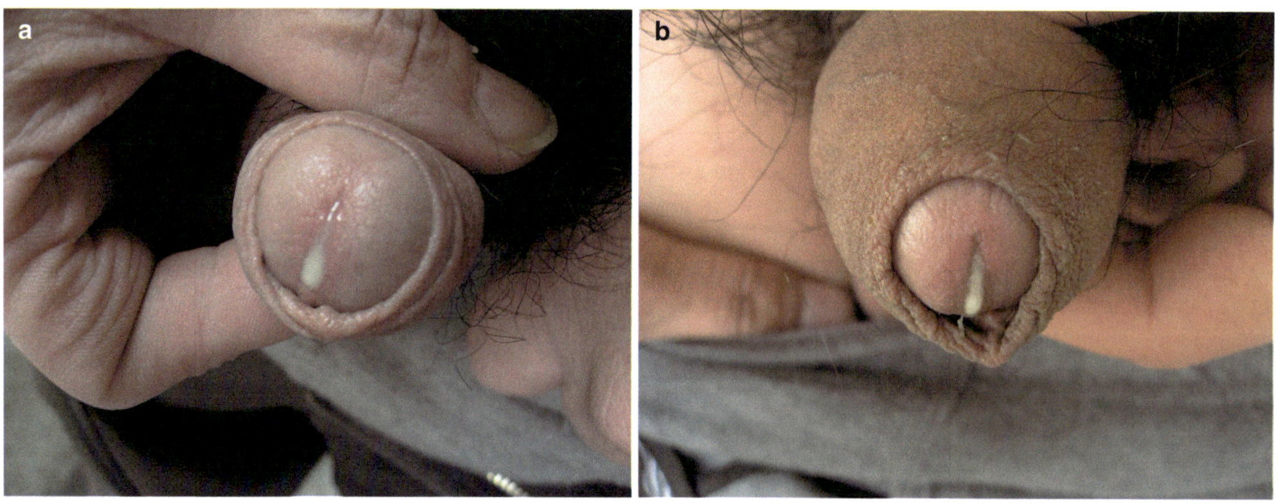

Fig. 10.1 Gonorrhea in male. (**a**, **b**) Purulent secretions at urethral meatus (Note: The figures were provided by Sun X at the Department of Dermatology, You'an Hospital, Beijing, China.)

redness, swelling, and pain of the greater vestibular gland, abscess caused by occluded duct, and fever.

Vagina of girls is composed of columnar epithelial cells, and, therefore, they are vulnerable to infection of gonococcus. Infection commonly occurs after close contacts to or sharing the same bathroom appliances with infected parents. In some rare cases, the infection is caused by sexual abuse. Clinically, it is characterized by swelling and burning pain of vulva as well as purulent secretion in vagina.

10.4.3 Gonococcal Anorectitis

The disease is more common in homosexual males (accounting for 40 %), and female patients are often self-infected by vaginal secretions (accounting for 5 %). About 50 % of the patients are asymptomatic, and others may experience anal pruritus and burning sensation. In severe cases, the patients experience tenesmus, bloody purulent stool, and constipation. By examination of anus and rectum, the mucosa can be found with congestion, edema, and purulent secretion.

10.4.4 Gonococcal Pharyngitis

Its occurrence is comparatively common after oral sex, with manifestations of acute pharyngitis or acute tonsillitis. Clinically, it is characterized by dry and sore throat, odynophagia, sometimes accompanying fever, and cervical lymphadenectasis.

10.4.5 Gonococcal Conjunctivitis

Its autoinfection is common in adult patients, which is usually unilateral. Neonates are commonly infected when they are delivered through the birth canal of the infected mother; their symptoms develop 2–3 days after the delivery and are usually bilateral. The initial symptom is usually purulent conjunctivitis, which may, if without prompt appropriate treatment, rapidly develop into destructive keratitis and corneal opacity, even blindness.

10.4.6 Disseminated Gonococcal Infection

It is a systemic infection of gonococcus caused by dissemination of the bacteria all over the body along with blood flow. And its incidence is 1–3 %, more common in females (accounting for about 2/3) during menstrual period and middle and late gestation periods. It also can be found in individuals with deficiency of complement components C5–C9 (accounting for less than 5 %). It may be manifested as gonococcal septicemia, arthritis, peritendinitis, myocarditis, endocarditis, and meningitis.

10.5 Gonorrhea-Related Complications

10.5.1 Gonorrhea-Related Complications in Males

Gonococcal urethritis in males, if without prompt appropriate treatment, can develop upward to involve the posterior urethra, causing posterior urethritis, prostatitis, cystospermitis, and epididymitis. Scars formed after repeated attacks of inflammation can cause urethral stenosis. In some cases, stricture or obstruction of seminiferous duct occurs, with secondary sterility.

10.5.1.1 Gonococcal Prostatitis

The occurrence of acute gonococcal prostatitis is more common at the third week after the onset of gonorrhea with manifestations of fever, shiver, perineal pain, and dysuria. Rectal examination demonstrates prostate enlargement with tenderness which may cause abscess if left untreated. Patients with chronic prostatitis are mild and their secretions are often found around the urethral opening in the morning. Rectal examination can touch relative harshness of prostate and node with tenderness. And examination of prostatic fluid bears the findings of the epithelial cells, few pus cells, and a decrease of lecithin-b.

10.5.1.2 Gonococcal Vesiculitis

During acute phrase of the disease, patients have manifestations of fever, frequent micturition, dysuria, terminal cloudy urine with blood, and sometimes accompanying semen retention. Rectal examination can reach the swollen seminal vesicle with severe tenderness. No obvious subjective symptoms are found in patient with chronic vesiculitis, while sometimes accompanying hematospermia. Rectal examination can reach the hard part of vesiculitis.

10.5.1.3 Gonococcal Epididymitis

The occurrence of gonococcal epididymitis commonly follows acute gonococcal urethritis. It is usually unilateral with manifestations of fever, scrotal swelling, epididymal swelling, and pain. Initially, there is ill-defined area with testicles which gradually become indistinct, reflective throbbing pain in contralateral groin and hypogastrium, and commonly cloudy urine. At the same time, there are often accompanying prostatitis and vesiculitis.

10.5.1.4 Urethral Stenosis

Patients with persistent symptoms may cause urethral stenosis. Individual cases may sustain stricture or obstruction of the vas deferens with dysuria. In severe cases, urinary retention is also found. The disease also can secondary to stricture of vas deferens, cystis vesiculae seminalis, and sterility.

10.5.2 Gonorrhea-Related Complications in Females

The disease is commonly caused by non-prompt treatment of gonococcal cervicitis with uplink infection of the inflammation.

10.5.2.1 Gonococcal Pelvic Inflammation

The factors that contribute to pelvic abscess and peritonitis include acute salpingitis, endometrial inflammation, secondary tubal ovarian abscess, and rupture. The occurrence of the disease often follows menstruation with the incidence of 10–20 %. The clinical manifestations are various and dominant pictures include fever, shiver, hypogastralgia, increased purulent leucorrhea, and thickness of bilateral adnexa with tenderness. Repeated outbreak can cause stenosis or obstruction of the ovarian ducts as well as ectopic pregnancy and sterility.

10.5.2.2 Fitz-Hugh-Curtis Syndrome (FHCS)

FHCS is a kind of capsule inflammation which is caused by pelvic infection delivering to hepatic layer via right paracolic sulci with manifestation of right upper quadrant pain syndrome. Clinically, according to pathological changes of FHCS, the disease can be divided into two types, acute FHCS and chronic FHCS. Acute FHCS has symptoms of slightly exudative inflammation on the liver surface, congestion and edema of liver capsula, spots of hemorrhages, and fibrous exudation. While in chronic phrase, zonary adhesion between liver surface and abdominal wall, thickness of liver capsula are visible.

Acute episode of right upper quadrant pain is the typical manifestation of FHCS which may radiate into the back; the pain gets worse when patients breathe deeply or cough accompanying fever, nausea, vomiting, sudden increased secretion of nearby vagina. Physical examination demonstrates obvious tenderness in right upper quadrant. Pelvic adnexal tenderness and abscess may be found or are absent.

10.6 Diagnostic Examinations

10.6.1 Laboratory Test

10.6.1.1 Smear Examination

Gram stain of vaginal discharge demonstrates gram-negative diplococcus in polymorphonuclear leukocyte. It is suitable for the diagnosis of patients with acute urinary-tract infection with sensitivity and specificity both over 95 %. The examination is not recommended for the diagnosis of oropharynx and rectum which are infected and gonococcal cervicitis.

10.6.1.2 Culture Examination

Cultivation method is sensitive to both male and female patients with mild symptoms or asymptomatic carriers. The diagnosis can be defined when cultivation is positive. Before the introduction of genetic diagnosis, cultivation method is the only method for the screening of gonorrhea recommend by the World Health Organization.

10.6.1.3 Drug Sensitive Test

Drug sensitive test was operated after positive culture. The application of disk diffusion for drug sensitive test or agar dilution method can detect the minimum inhibitory concentration for the purpose to guide clinical medication.

10.6.1.4 Gene Diagnosis

Gene Probe Diagnosis

The probes applied include plasmid DNA probe, chromosomal gene probe, and rRNA gene probe.

Gene Diffusion Test

PRC can further improve the accuracy to detect gonococcus with advantage of rapidity, sensitivity, specificity, and simplicity. And it can directly detect trace amounts of pathogens in clinical specimens.

10.6.2 Imaging Examination

10.6.2.1 Ultrasound

Ultrasound can be used for the examination and diagnosis of gonorrhea-related complications for its noninvasiveness, practicability, and relative high accuracy.

10.6.2.2 CT Scanning

CT scanning is unsuitable for the examination of scrotum or testes for the radiation damage to gonad caused by X-ray, but it is appropriate for the diagnosis of pelvic inflammation and hepatitis externa.

10.6.2.3 MRI

MRI is often used for the examination of gonorrhea-related complications especially for pelvic organs and gonad.

10.7 Imaging Demonstrations

10.7.1 Acute Prostatitis

10.7.1.1 Ultrasound

Two-Dimensional Ultrasonography

1. Prostate enlarges slightly or obviously featuring bilateral symmetric or asymmetry.
2. The echo of envelope is clear and complete. There may be an exception to individual patients with prostatic abscess rupture.
3. Inter echo is a little low and uneven. The occurrence of suppuration accompanies low echo or uneven enhancement, and small no echo area is visible. Typical prostatic abscess has manifestations of ill-defined interstructure of parenchyma, irregular low echo, and anecho area with indication of liquid flow.
4. The disease is often accompanied by the enlargement of seminal vesicle with increased tension, poor echo, or anecho in the inner structure (Fig. 10.2).

Case Study 1

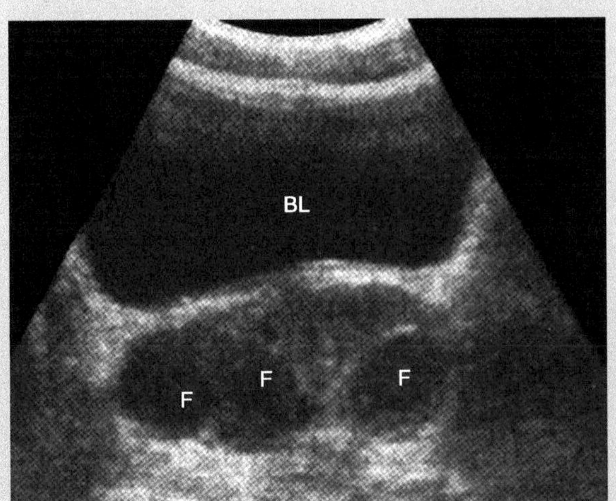

Fig. 10.2 Prostatic abscess. Ultrasound demonstrates prostatic abscess. Note: *BL* is bladder, *F* is abscess

CDFI

CDFI demonstrates circumscribed or diffuse increase of blood flow signal with pulsation which indicates the occurrence of inflammatory congestion. There is no blood supply in pus cavity in patients with abscess, while there is rich blood signal in the tissue around the abscess cavity.

10.7.1.2 CT

In acute prostatitis, plain CT scan demonstrates diffuse enlargement of the prostate with smooth edge and decreased density and low-density focus following liquefaction necrosis, while in chronic prostatitis, CT scan demonstrates no obvious abnormality; the prostate is changeable in size with regular contour, sometimes accompanying patchy slightly hypodense shadow which may have uneven density after enhancement. Prostatic abscess has manifestations of irregular single cavity or multilocular low-density lesions which may allocate dispersedly. And larger abscess may wear through the envelope causing diffuse inflammatory infiltration and fluid retention of the near structures. Typical patients with enhanced scan have manifestations of edge enhancement with unchangeable density in central necrosis area.

10.7.1.3 MRI

The patient with acute prostatitis has symptoms of diffuse enlargement of the prostate, inhomogeneous signal on T_1WI and T_2WI, and longer T2 shadow in hyperintense signal on T_2WI which indicates the formation of false abscess. Inhomogeneous hypointense signal is visible in peripheral zone T_2WI. Uneven signal in prostate and inhomogeneous decreased signal in peripheral zone T_2WI are found in cases with chronic prostatitis. No obvious enhancement in early stage of enhancement scan. DWI demonstrates more isointensity in prostatitis.

10.7.2 Vesiculitis

10.7.2.1 Ultrasound

Transrectal ultrasonography demonstrates ill-defined seminal vesicle with increased short diameter and uneven inner echo, duct dilation and thickness, coarse wall, and reciprocating flow of punctate fluid echo in inner structure. CDFI bears the findings of obvious flow signals in or around the seminal vesicle with high flow velocity in cases of acute vesiculitis. In chronic cases, flow signals in or around the seminal vesicle slightly increase with higher or unconspicuous flow velocity. Besides, the occurrence of cystis vesiculae seminalis is more common in acute vesiculitis, while spermatic calculus and calcification are common in chronic ones.

10.7.2.2 CT

In acute vesiculitis, seminal vesicle enlarges symmetrically with thickened wall and ragged edge. Uneven content density of seminal vesicle has shadows which are honeycombed, mottled, and stripy. Neighboring thick-walled bladder is also visible. In chronic vesiculitis, seminal vesicle enlarges symmetrically or asymmetrically with uneven density.

10.7.2.3 MRI

Acute Cystospermitis

Seminal vesicle enlarges symmetrically with increased tension in elliptical-like shape. Equisignal or hypointensity on T_1WI, relative hyperintense signal on T_2WI, often complicate with hemorrhage. Hypointensity may occur in fibrous hyperplasia. There are interface faintness between seminal vesicle and peripheral adipose tissue.

Chronic Cystospermitis

The disease has manifestations of atrophy of seminal vesicle with tube wall thickness, obvious decrease of seminal vesicle fluid, and decreased signal on T_2WI.

10.7.3 Epididymitis

10.7.3.1 Ultrasound

Acute Epididymitis

Epididymis enlarges in a limited or diffuse way which has irregular shape and ill-defined margin. There is decreased echo in epididymis, sometimes with anecho by abscess, and commonly accompanying ipsilateral hydrocele testis and cirsocele. CDFI and power Doppler show sufficient abnormal color flow in epididymis lesion which is arranged in dendritic or colorful flower clump. Flow grade is II and III dominant. Annular color blood flow signal is visible around the abscess, with absence of flow signal in anecho area. After the disease is cured, the epididymis shows obvious decrease in size or restores to its normal size. Blood signal decreases and is flow grade II based.

Chronic Epididymitis

Commonly, the epididymis enlarges in a confined way which is common in tail or head (tail is more common), but less significant than the increase in the cases of acute epididymitis. There is inhomogeneous echo, commonly complicating abscess of epididymis and hydrocele testis, and some cases may sustain cirsocele. CDFI demonstrates no obvious blood abnormality of the epididymis in most cases of epididymitis. Few cases may have slight increase in blood signal in part of the enlarged epididymis.

10.7.3.2 CT

CT examination is unremarkable or only demonstrates epididymitis enlarging asymmetrically or the formations of abscess. In the cases complicated by didymitis and the formation of hydrocele, CT examination often demonstrates corresponding signs.

10.7.3.3 MRI

Diffuse epididymitis enlarges asymmetrically with neighboring scrotal-skin thickening and swelling. Homogeneous or inhomogeneous hyperintense signal on T_2WI in epididymitis often complicates by hydrocele. Hypointense signal on T_2WI occurs commonly in chronic phrase. In case of the formation of pus, epididymitis is irregular with local swelling with hypointense signal on T_1WI and high-low mixed signal on T_2WI. Enchantment of MRI demonstrates uneven enchantment of neighboring abscess.

10.7.4 Pelvic Inflammation

10.7.4.1 Ultrasound

Limited effusion in pelvic cavity was found. The occurrence of pelvic abscess has manifestations of single or multiple masses around the uterus or other structures. The formation of hypoecho or liquidus anecho area may contain strong echo or zonal separated echo; the wall is relatively thick and coarse. Hypoechoic mass may contain sufficient blood signal, while it is absent after the formation of abscess (Figs. 10.3 and 10.4).

Case Study 2

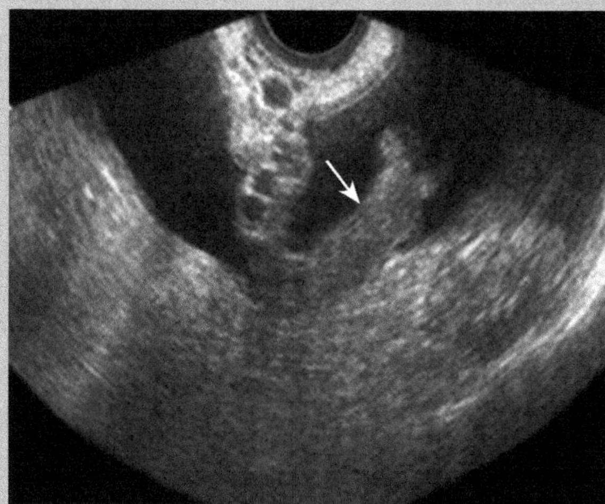

Fig. 10.3 Pelvic inflammation. Ultrasound finding of pelvic fluid and thickening of oviduct (indicated by *arrow*)

Case Study 3

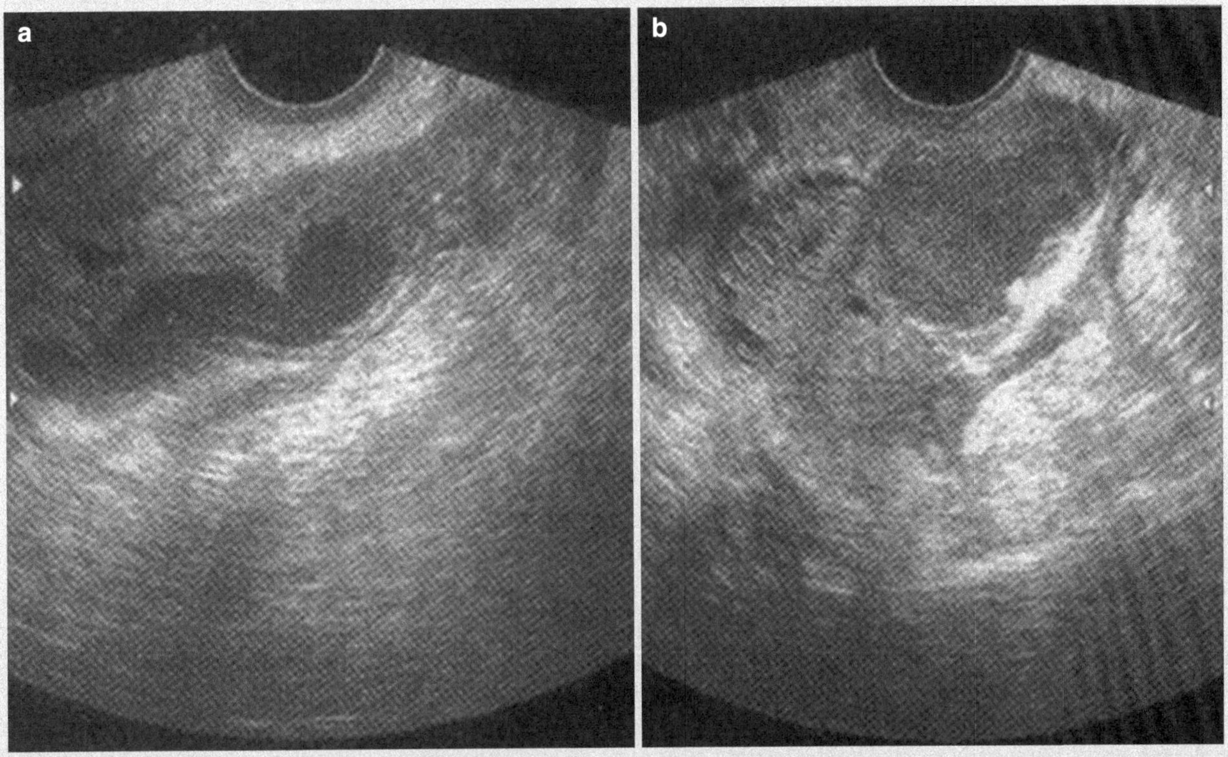

Fig. 10.4 Pyosalpinx. (**a**, **b**) Pyosalpinx by ultrasound

10.7.4.2 CT

There are no characteristic manifestations in early stage of pelvic inflammation. The formation of encapsulated effusion has ill-defined masses with irregular thickened wall and uneven edges with watery density in inner structure. Cyst wall enhancement is inhomogeneous while hydatid fluid is non-enhancing (Fig. 10.5).

Case Study 4

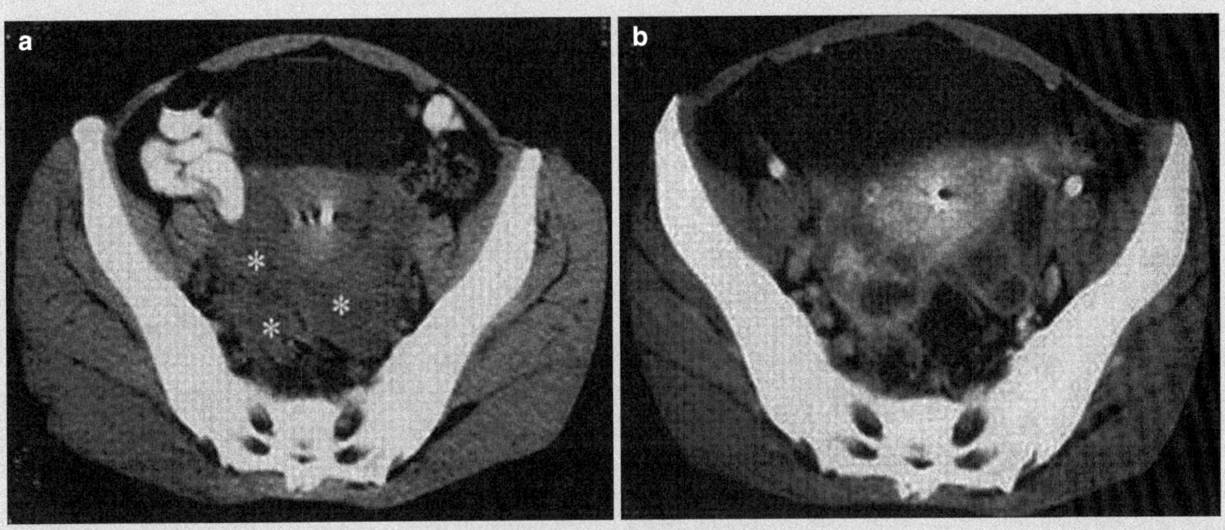

Fig. 10.5 Pelvic inflammation. (**a**) CT plain scan demonstrates ill-defined masses with inhomogeneous density around the uterus (indicated by *asterisk*) in which contains obscured low density. (**b**) Contrast scan demonstrates obvious enhancement in the edge and spacing of mass. Non-enhancement in hydatid fluid was found

10.7.4.3 MRI

Commonly, pelvic inflammation in early stage is unremarkable. The occurrence of pelvic abscess has manifestations of single or multiple, round or ellipse lesions in the pelvic cavity with masslike long T_1 and long T_2 signals on MRI. Gas bubble in some abscess is also visible. Enchantment examination demonstrates obvious ring-shaped enchantment in the wall of an abscess.

10.7.5 Hepatitis Externa

10.7.5.1 Ultrasound

Commonly, no abnormality was found. In individual cases, thickness of limited liver capsula and few seroperitoneum without characteristic are found.

10.7.5.2 CT

CT plain scan demonstrates the shape, the site, and the density of the liver are normal. Homogeneous or unhomogeneous thickness of liver capsula is occasional. Linear or zonal low-density shadow is visible when complicating seroperitoneum. There are characteristic manifestations on enhanced CT scanning. During arterial phase, enchantment in varying degree and obvious thickness of liver capsula are visible, which are commonly located on the lateral and ventral right hepatic lobe, follow on ventral the left hepatic lobe with homogeneous or unhomogeneous high-density shadow in linear or zonal appearance. Plaque-like or wedge-shaped enchantment is found when local liver parenchyma is involved. In portal vein phase, there is obvious decrease in density with faint enchantment. Non-enhancement by delayed scan is also visible. Some patients may suffer from pleural effusion.

10.7.5.3 MRI

Thickened liver capsula shows linear or zonal signal on T_1WI and relative hyperintense signal on T_2WI. The involvement of subcapsule accumulating effusion and liver parenchyma are hypointense signal on T_1WI and hyperintense signal on T_2WI. Enhanced MRI demonstrates linear or zonal liver capsula enchantment and plaque-like or wedge-shaped enchantment of liver parenchyma involved.

10.8 Diagnostic Basis

10.8.1 The Diagnosis of Gonorrhea

10.8.1.1 Contact History

The patients have extramarital contact, spouse infection history, or contact with secretions from a patient with gonorrhea. The mother of a newborn baby with gonorrhea is also included.

10.8.1.2 Clinical Manifestations

The male has symptoms of urethritis, while the female has symptoms of urethral discomfort and increased vaginal secretions. The patients also suffer from gonococcal conjunctivitis, pharyngitis, and disseminated gonorrhea.

10.8.1.3 Laboratory Test

Primary diagnostic value can be established when smear of acute urethritis in male with gram stain demonstrates gram-negative diplococcus in cells. The diagnosis can be defined based on the findings of positive gonococcus culture.

10.8.2 Imaging Diagnosis of Gonorrhea-Related Complications

10.8.2.1 Prostatitis

1. The diagnosis of gonorrhea is clear.
2. The patient has clinical manifestations of dysuria. Rectal examination demonstrates prostate enlargement and tenderness.
3. Imagine examination demonstrates prostate enlargement with uneven echo/density/signal of the prostate.
4. Prostatic fluid examination bears the findings of increased lecithin corpuscle, leukocytosis, smear positive, and cultivation of *Neisseria gonorrhoeae* positive.

10.8.2.2 Vesiculitis

1. Patients with gonorrhea have clinical manifestations of hemospermia, odynuria, and hypogastralgia. Rectal examination demonstrates swollen seminal vesicle with tenderness.
2. Imagine examination demonstrates acute seminal vesicle enlargement, thickening of cystic wall. CDFI bears the findings of sufficient blood in seminal vesicle. Chronic seminal vesicle enlarges or atrophies with obvious decrease of liquid and uneven echo or density.
3. Route examination of semen demonstrates large number of erythrocytes and leukocytes. Cultivation of gonococcus from semen is positive.

10.8.2.3 Epididymitis

1. Patients with gonorrhea have symptoms of redness, swelling, fever, pain of the scrotum, and enlargement of epididymis with tenderness.
2. Ultrasonography demonstrates seminal vesicle enlargement with deceased uneven echo. CDFI can indicate abnormal blood in epididymal lesions with varying degrees of hydrocele of tunica vaginalis. The diagnosis of acute epididymitis can be defined by the course of disease within 1 month. And the diagnosis of chronic epididymitis

can be established when the course stretches out over 1 month with uneven echo and no obvious blood abnormality in epididymis by CDFI.

10.8.2.4 Pelvic Inflammation

1. Patients with gonorrhea have clinical manifestations of fever, hypogastralgia, and increased purulent leucorrhea. Physical examination bears the findings of the thickness of bilateral adnexa with tenderness.
2. The diagnosis of pelvic inflammation can be defined by imagine examination with the formation of abscess. However, only by the demonstrations by imagine examination, inflammatory masses without the formation of abscess often cannot differentiate from other pelvic masses. Definitive diagnosis can be defined on the base of the clinical manifestations of short-term review.

10.8.2.5 Hepatitis Externa

1. Patients with gonorrhea have clinical manifestations of sudden severe right low abdominal pains and increased secretion of vagina. Physical examination demonstrates pelvic adnexa tenderness with mass.
2. Plain scanning of MRI and CT scan demonstrates thickness of liver capsula, subcapsule accumulating fusion. Enhancement scanning shows linear or zonal enhancement of liver capsula.
3. Abdominoscopy demonstrates violin string-like adhesion.

10.9 Differential Diagnosis

10.9.1 Differential Diagnosis of Gonorrhea

10.9.1.1 Disease Should Be Differentiated from Gonorrhea in Males

Nonspecific Urethritis

There are usually obvious precipitating factors such as trauma and mechanical irritation.

Nongonococcal Urethritis

The patient has sexual contact history with an incubation period of 7–12 days. The symptoms are mild or asymptomatic with few mucus or mucous purulent secretions.

10.9.1.2 Disease Should Be Differentiated from Gonorrhea in Females

Nonspecific Vaginitis

The precipitating factors include trauma, foreign body. Clinical manifestations include vaginal burning, fall bilge feeling, and increased purulent or mucus secretions.

The Infection of Bedsonia Trachomatis

The patient has sexual contact history with no obvious or asymptomatic symptoms. Cervical edema, easy hemorrhage. There are also purulent or mucus secretions.

Monilial Vaginitis, Trichomonas Vaginitis, and Bacterial Vaginitis

Pseudohypha, spore, and trichomonad are found, respectively, in the secretion of vagina of the above three diseases. The diagnosis can be defined by increased gram-negative bacillus brevis.

10.9.2 Differential Diagnosis of Gonorrhea-Related Complication

10.9.2.1 Tuberculosis of Prostate

Prostatitis should be differentiated from tuberculosis of prostate. They both have similar clinical manifestations. However, tuberculosis of prostate commonly presents with history of urinary tuberculosis, and rectal examination demonstrates irregular tuber of the prostate. Imaging examination can render demonstration of ill-defined irregular enlargement of the prostate. Necrosis and liquefaction are the chief manifestations of the disease with uneven density and signal.

10.9.2.2 Tuberculosis and Abscess of Seminal Vesicle

Vesiculitis should be differentiated from tuberculosis and abscess of seminal vesicle. Tuberculosis of seminal vesicle is often secondary to upper tract planting, prostate, tuberculosis of epididymis, among which necrosis and calcification are visible. The history has a diagnostic value. Abscess of seminal vesicle is rare and CT or MRI demonstrates the formation of pus cavity and the wall of abscess. Enhanced scanning bears the findings of marked homogenous enhancement. The clinical manifestations of fever, shiver, and increased leukocytes have differential diagnostic value for the disease.

10.9.2.3 Tuberculosis of Epididymis

Epididymitis should be differentiated from tuberculosis of epididymis. The disease often has history of tuberculosis with relative long course, mild symptom, the formation of scrotal sinus, and toruloid seminal duct. Ultrasound and CT often demonstrate the enlargement of epididymis with uneven echo/density, sometimes calcification. CDFI can indicate weakening blood flow signal. However, epididymitis often has manifestations of acute or repeated episodes, relative remarkable localized pain, no scrotal sinus formation, and toruloid seminal duct. Imaging examination often demonstrates no calcification formation. CDFI can indicate sufficient blood.

10.9.2.4 Carcinomatous Peritonitis, Tuberculous Peritonitis, and Cholecystitis

Hepatitis externa should be differentiated from carcinomatous peritonitis and tuberculous peritonitis. Enhanced scanning of carcinomatous peritonitis and tuberculous peritonitis by CT and MRI can also demonstrate strengthening liver capsula. The scanning is not just limited for liver capsula enchantment, but for extensive enchantment of enterocelia. In addition, nodular or cloddy mass enchantment is visible in enterocelia.

10.9.2.5 Others

Pelvic inflammation in the acute phase should be differentiated from acute appendicitis, acute pyelonephritis, torsion of ovarian abscess, and exfetation.

Suggested Reading

Cho HJ, Kim HK, Suh JH, et al. Fitz-Hugh-Curtis syndrome: CT findings of three cases. Emerg Radiol. 2008;15(1):43–6.

Jia PZ, Li LJ. Studies of infectious diseases. Nanjing: Jiangsu Science and Technology Press; 2010.

Li SN, Tang GJ. Modern general diagnostics by CT. Beijing: China Medical Science Press; 2007.

Ma YL. Studies of infectious diseases. Shanghai: Shanghai Science and Technology Press; 2011.

Wang CL, Guo XJ, Yuan ZD, et al. Radiologic diagnosis of Fitz-Hugh-Curtis syndrome. Chin Med J (Engl). 2009;122(6):741–4.

Yang J. Ultrasound diagnostics. Lanzhou: Lanzhou University Press; 2010.

Zhang XJ. Dermatology and sexually transmitted diseases. Beijing: People's Medical Publishing House; 2008.

11 Human *Streptococcus suis* Infection

Ning He, Hongjun Li, and Xinhua Zhang

Human *Streptococcus suis* infection is a zoonosis caused by *Streptococcus suis*. Populations engaging in pig slaughtering and processing are high-risk groups. The bacteria gain their access into the human body via skin wound to cause the infection. Its clinical manifestations include common bacterial infection symptoms such as fever, chills, headaches, and poor appetite. In severe cases, it can be complicated by toxic shock syndrome (TSS) and streptococcus meningitis syndrome (SMS).

11.1 Etiology

Streptococcus suis was firstly isolated by De Moor in 1963 from specimens collected during the outbreak of piglet septicemia in the Netherlands. At that time, it was categorized into group R α-hemolytic streptococcus. In the year 1968, based on capsular typing, Elliot nominated it as capsular type 2 *Streptococcus suis*. Based on the polysaccharide antigen typing of *Streptococcus suis*, it can be further divided into 35 serotypes (1–34 and 1/2) with serotype 2 being the most virulent, followed by serotype 1. Serotype 2 is the most common pathogen isolated from infected pigs or patients. According to classification by Lancefield, *Streptococcus suis* can be categorized into group R, group S, and group T, with group R (serotype 2) and group S (serotype 1) being the most common. *Streptococcus suis* isolated from human specimens is virtually serotype 2. Therefore, specific antiserum against group R can be used for precipitation test. In such a way, the strain of serotype 2 *Streptococcus suis* can be identified.

N. He • H. Li (✉) • X. Zhang
Department of Radiology, Beijing You'an Hospital, Capital Medical University, Beijing, China
e-mail: lihongjun00113@126.com

11.1.1 Physical and Chemical Properties

Streptococcus suis is categorized into the family of *Streptococcaceae*, which is a Gram-positive, spherical-shaped, or oval-shaped bacteria. The bacteria have no spore but have capsules, which grow into small colorless semi-transparent colonies on blood plate with raised regular smooth edges and with a diameter of 0.5–1.0 mm. Based on the hemolytic classification, *Streptococcus suis* is α-hemolytic on sheep blood plate but β-hemolytic on horse blood plate. The appropriate conditions for its culture include blood culture bottle and blood plate as the medium at a temperature of 37 °C for 18–20 h. The newly isolated *Streptococcus suis* has a typical morphology, with its chain length being up to above 20 thallus. After the second generation, its morphology is no longer typical and may even be Gram-negative coccobacillus without the shape of a chain. *Streptococcus suis* has poor intolerance to its surrounding physical and chemical factors and is sensitive to common disinfectants.

11.1.2 Factors Determining Its Virulence

Currently, it is believed that the important factors determining the virulence of *Streptococcus suis* includes the following.

11.1.2.1 Capsular Polysaccharide

So far, it is the only proved and the most important factor that determines the virulence of *Streptococcus suis*.

11.1.2.2 Lysozyme Released Protein and Extracellular Protein Factor

In addition to capsular polysaccharides, the two proteins are the more commonly used indicators to assess the virulence of *Streptococcus suis*.

H. Li (ed.), *Radiology of Infectious Diseases: Volume 2*, DOI 10.1007/978-94-017-9876-1_11

11.1.2.3 Hemolysin of *Streptococcus suis*

Hemolysin is believed to be a major factor indicating the virulence of several bacteria. It may facilitate *Streptococcus suis* to invade and decompose cells.

11.1.2.4 Protein of 44,000, IgG Binding Protein, and Other Factors

Protein of 44,000 is a protein in the bacterial cell wall of serotype 2 *Streptococcus suis*. IgG binding protein is heat shock protein, which is reported to be associated with its virulence. In addition, pili and adhesion factors are also common factors determining the bacterial virulence.

11.1.3 MLST Analysis

Multilocus sequence typing (MLST) was performed for the strains isolated during outbreaks of human *Streptococcus suis* infection in provinces of Jiangsu and Sichuan in China. The pathogenic strains are proved to be MLST type 7.

11.2 Epidemiology

11.2.1 The Source of Infection

Sick and deceased pigs with *Streptococcus suis* infection are the main source of infection. It has been reported that serotype 2 *Streptococcus suis* can be isolated from deceased deer, sheep, chickens, ducks, horses, cats, dogs, and ruminants. But the evidence is not sufficient to define them as the source of infection.

There has been no evidence to prove that human *Streptococcus suis* infection can spread from person to person.

11.2.2 Route of Transmission

Human *Streptococcus suis* infection spreads via contact with pigs and unprocessed pork products infected by *Streptococcus suis*. The bacteria gain their access through skin wound or conjunctiva to cause the infection.

11.2.3 Population Susceptibility

People are generally susceptible. Populations with direct contact to sick or deceased pigs or pork products are high-risk populations. In them, individuals with skin wounds are especially vulnerable to be infected. Most foreigner scholars believe that human *Streptococcus suis* infection is an important occupational disease with sick animals as its source of infection. Infection of *Streptococcus suis* by people with immune deficiency is more serious.

11.2.4 Epidemic Features

The epidemiological features of the disease are still not fully understood. It is highly sporadic along with the outbreak of swine *Streptococcus* infection, which is more commonly found in summers. The spread of swine *Streptococcus* infection in pigs may be closely related to the hot and humid environment. Therefore, hotness and humidity are most likely to indirectly contribute to the increased occurrence of human *Streptococcus suis* infection in summers. This disease is not necessarily related to gender or age, but has a close relationship to occupation. Populations engaging or involving in pig breeding, slaughter, processing, delivery, sales, and cooking are high-risk groups, especially those who slaughter sick and deceased pigs.

In 1968, scholars from Denmark firstly reported three cases of human *Streptococcus suis* infection that leads to meningitis and is complicated by septicemia. In 1975, sporadic cases were reported in the Netherlands. Thereafter, the cases of human *Streptococcus suis* infection have been continually reported in Chinese Hong Kong, the United Kingdom, Canada, Germany, France, the United States, Australia, Belgium, Brazil, Spain, Japan, Thailand, Sweden, and mainland China. By the year 2000, more than 200 cases of human *Streptococcus suis* infection had been reported across the world. Countries or regions with more reported cases are generally characterized by developed industry of livestock breeding or by a common lifestyle of eating pork, with highly sporadic prevalence. In China, human *Streptococcus suis* infection was reported in Jiangsu province in 1998, with 25 cases of occurrence and 14 cases of death. From June to August 2005, an outbreak of human *Streptococcus suis* infection occurred in Sichuan province, which has been the most serious outbreak of human *Streptococcus suis* infection in the world, with 204 cases of occurrence and 38 cases of death.

11.3 Pathogenesis and Pathologic Changes

11.3.1 Pathogenesis

Human *Streptococcus suis* infection mainly spreads via skin wound after direct contact. The *Streptococcus suis* gains its access into the human body via wounds of skin or mucosa, which rapidly grows and reproduces in the blood after spreading into the blood flow to cause septicemia. The bacteria then gain their access into organs and tissues along with blood flow to cause pathological changes in multiple organs and tissues. Meanwhile, the bacteria release toxins to cause severe toxic reactions of the body, with following occurrence of toxemia. Under the effects of bacterial toxins, severe patients experience vascular endothelial lesions and disseminated intravascular coagulation (DIC) that leads to systemic microcirculatory disorder and multiple organ failure.

11.3.2 Pathological Changes

The severe clinical manifestations of human *Streptococcus suis* infection can be divided into two types: SMS and TSS.

The main pathological changes of SMS include purulent meningitis, obvious meningeal vascular congestion, infiltration of a large quantity of neutrophils, and slight pathological changes in other organs.

TSS is characterized by septicemic shock complicated by DIC. The pathological changes include cellular degeneration and necrosis of multiple organs and tissue parenchyma, varying quantities of neutrophil infiltration, interstitial vascular congestion and leakage hemorrhage, and formation of capillary microthrombus (hyaline thrombus). The involved organs have pathological changes of (1) petechiae and ecchymosis in the skin, mucosa (of gastrointestinal tract, respiratory tract, and urogenital tract), and serosa; bleeding of heart, liver, kidney, adrenal gland, esophagus, and intestines with incoagulable bright red blood; and varying quantities of microthrombus (hyaline thrombus) in capillaries of some organs (like lung and kidney) which are PTAH-positive fibrin thrombus; (2) pulmonary congestion and edema, focal and flakes of hemorrhage, and formation of microthrombus in capillaries; (3) acute pneumonia; (4) slight hepatomegaly as well as spots and focal or flakes of necrosis of hepatocytes; (5) renal congestion and hemorrhage and varying quantities of microthrombus in glomerular capillaries; (6) myocardial degeneration, spots of myocardial necrosis and infiltration of inflammatory cells, and interstitial vascular congestion with multifocal hemorrhage; (7) serous cavity effusion such as pleural, pericardial, and abdominal cavities; more lesions in the lung, kidney, and heart but not obvious lesions in the brain and cerebral meninges; and (8), in some cases, a skin wound that is commonly found on the arms and feet.

Severe human *Streptococcus suis* infection can be complicated by DIC. The pathological changes include intracapillary microthrombus in multiple organs and tissues and leakage hemorrhage, incoagulable blood, and secondary multiple organ failure and shock.

Patients with SMS have highly dilated and congested meningeal vascular vessels, widened subarachnoid cavity, and leakage of neutrophils, fibrin, and fluids in large quantities. Therefore, the patients sustain intracranial hypertension due to increased quantity of cerebrospinal fluid. And the patients complain of headache, projectile vomiting, and positive pathological signs. Due to the involved cranial nerves, patients may experience different degrees of hearing impairment or even permanent deafness.

11.4 Clinical Symptoms and Signs

The incubation period ranges from several hours to 7 days, commonly 2–3 days. The duration of the incubation period is related to the virulence and quantity of pathogenic bacteria as well as the immunity of the infected human. Generally, the shorter period of incubation predicts the more serious conditions. According to the clinical manifestations, it can be divided into the following types:

11.4.1 Common Type

It commonly has an acute onset, with manifestation of fever, chills, headache, dizziness, general upset, and fatigue. Some patients may experience nausea, vomiting, abdominal pain, and diarrhea. No shock or coma occurs in the common type of the disease.

11.4.2 Shock Type

Based on the systemic infection, the shock type has manifestations of hypotension with adult systolic pressure lower than 90 mmHg and pulse pressure lower than 20 mmHg, with accompanying two or more conditions: (1) renal dysfunction, (2) coagulation disorder or disseminated intravascular coagulation, (3) hepatic dysfunction, (4) acute respiratory distress syndrome, (5) petechiae and ecchymoses in skin and mucosa of the whole body or conjunctival congestion, and (6) soft tissue necrosis, fasciitis, myositis, and gangrene.

11.4.3 Meningitis Type

The clinical manifestations include fever, chills, general upset, fatigue, headache, and vomiting. In severe cases, coma occurs, with positive meningeal irritation sign and purulent changes of the cerebrospinal fluid.

11.4.4 Mixed Type

The manifestations of both shock type and meningitis type can be found in such type of cases.

11.5 Human *Streptococcus suis* Infection-Related Complications

11.5.1 Meningitis

About 85 % of cases with human *Streptococcus suis* infection have typical manifestations of meningitis. *Streptococcus suis* meningitis is characterized by higher incidence of hearing loss (54–80 %) than other bacterial meningitis, which commonly occurs within 24 h after the onset (1–14 days). In some cases, the onset of *Streptococcus suis* meningitis begins with occurrence of deafness. Bilateral deafness is more common than unilateral deafness. In some cases, the deafness is characterized by subclinical high-profile hearing loss. Other dysfunctions related to the 8th pair of cranial nerves are also common, with 30–50 % of cases with meningitis showing dizziness and ataxia. The patients may also experience palsy of the 3rd pair of cranial nerves, with unilateral or bilateral facial paralysis.

11.5.2 Toxic Shock Syndrome (TSS)

TSS is commonly caused by group A streptococcus and rarely caused by group B and group C streptococcus. *Streptococcus suis* is a rare pathogen of TSS, but commonly causes outbreak of TSS, with high rate of mortality. TSS has a short period of incubation, with an average incubation period of 2–3 days ranging from several hours to 7 days. The manifestations commonly include sudden high fever (in 100 % of TSS cases) with the highest body temperature of 42 °C and accompanying headache (in 56.25 % of TSS cases), diarrhea and other gastrointestinal symptoms (in 68.75 % of TSS cases), and skin petechiae and ecchymoses (in 81.25 % of TSS cases) that are commonly distributed in the face, limbs, and head with no protrusion higher than the skin surface and no ulceration. The outcomes of TSS include shock (in 100 % of TSS cases), oliguria (in 81.25 % of TSS cases), and death (in 81.25 % of TSS cases). There may be also blood coagulation dysfunction, renal insufficiency, hepatic insufficiency, acute respiratory distress syndrome, soft tissue necrosis, and fasciitis. By autopsy, the findings commonly include bleeding in multiple parts and multiple organs with different degrees and ranges and visceral capillary diffuse coagulation. The autopsy findings are similar to those findings by autopsy of dead pigs infected by *Streptococcus suis*.

11.5.3 Other Related Complications

Streptococcus suis has been isolated from patients with endocarditis and septicemia who have no diagnosis of meningitis and toxic shock. The patients may suffer from fulminant ecchymosis and rhabdomyolysis. Vilaichone et al. reported two cases of serotype 2 *Streptococcus suis* infection complicated by peritonitis. Robertson et al. reported their findings after detecting titer of antibodies against *Streptococcus suis* in pig-feeding workers, with a positive rate of 21 %, which indicated that subclinical infection of *Streptococcus suis* is common in certain vocations. They believe some cases of *Streptococcus suis* infection have only a manifestation of moderate fever.

11.6 Diagnostic Examinations

11.6.1 Laboratory Tests

11.6.1.1 General Laboratory Tests

Routine Blood Test

WBC count increases, but in some serious cases, WBC count may be normal or decreased in the early stage. The percentage of neutrophils increases. Some severe patients also have thrombocytopenia. The cases with secondary DIC have serious thrombocytopenia.

Routine Urine Test

There is positive finding of protein and positive finding of ketone in some cases.

Biochemical Detection

In some patients, ALT, AST, and TBil levels increase; albumin decreases; and Cr and BUN levels increase.

Cerebrospinal Fluid Examination

The cases of purulent meningitis have intracranial hypertension, significantly increased WBC count that is commonly above 0.5×10^6/L and mainly multinucleated cells, increased protein, and decreased glucose and chloride.

Blood Gas Analysis

The severe cases commonly have metabolic acidosis, respiratory alkalosis, and type I respiratory failure, with findings of decreased $PaCO_2$, decreased HCO_3, and decreased PaO_2. In the advanced stage, there are also respiratory acidosis and type II respiratory failure, with findings of increased $PaCO_2$, decreased HCO_3, and decreased PaO_2.

DIC Indicators

Patients with DIC have findings of positive 3P test, increased D-dipolymer, and thrombocytopenia.

11.6.1.2 Etiological Identification

The laboratory tests for *Streptococcus suis* include biochemical identification, serotyping, and specific gene detection after isolation of the strain following bacterial culture. So far, there has been no mature examination for its specific antibody.

Biochemical Identification

Manual identification by Api20-step of API biochemical identification system can be applied for the isolated strain. Otherwise, VITEK 2 Compact or other biochemical identification system can be applied to identify the isolated strain. In such ways, the species of the isolated strain can be defined.

Serotyping

The defined species by biochemical identification can be further defined for its serotype by using 1–34 serotypes of *Streptococcus suis* or monoclonal antibody.

PCR Gene Identification

The isolated and purified colonies or suspected moist colonies on the plate should be firstly chosen. Specific primers are then applied for PCR amplification. The specific primers (tuf) of *Streptococcus* genus, specific *Streptococcus suis* species, type 2 capsular polysaccharide gene (cps2j) of *Streptococcus suis*, related protein encoding gene fragments released by *Streptococcus suis* lysozyme (mrp), and hemolysin gene of *Streptococcus suis* (sly) should be subsequently detected. For those patients who have given large doses of antibiotics, the collected specimens should be directly examined by PCR to detect the specific genes of swine streptococcus species (16SrRNA) as well as specific virulence genes. The cases with positive findings can be defined as human *Streptococcus suis* infection.

11.6.2 Imaging Examinations

11.6.2.1 Ultrasound

Color Doppler ultrasound of the heart is indicated for patients with infective endocarditis.

11.6.2.2 X-Ray

Chest X-ray is indicated for patients with secondary acute respiratory distress syndrome.

11.6.2.3 CT and MRI

Cranial and brain CT scanning and MR imaging are indicated for cases of human *Streptococcus suis infection* complicated by meningitis. Radiological examinations have limited value for the diagnosis and differential diagnosis. However, their applications clinically facilitate understandings about the range, location, and severity of the lesions as well as early finding of complications. Although the radiological examinations lack direct specificity to pathogens of intracranial infections, the imaging demonstrations facilitate to define the diagnosis of various complications. Especially for clinically suspected cases of brain abscesses, intracranial hypertension, and focal signs, MR imaging should be the examination of choice to define the diagnosis.

11.7 Imaging Demonstrations

11.7.1 The Nervous System

In the cases with the nervous system involved, typical purulent meningitis can be demonstrated.

11.7.1.1 CT Scanning

In the early stage, plain CT scanning demonstrates lesions in the interface between gray and white matters that are in low-density or low–high-mixed-density area with poorly defined boundary. However, the lesions have a higher density than their adjacent areas, with spots of bleeding foci inside them. Contrast CT scanning demonstrates no enhancement of the low density area. In some other cases, contrast CT scanning demonstrates irregular spots or gyrus-like enhancement. The adjacent sulci are demonstrated with faded color or to be absent, and there are cerebral edema and space-occupying effect in different degrees around the foci. In the cerebral abscess stage, plain CT scanning demonstrates low-density area with well-defined boundary, intact or not intact abscess wall, and regular or irregular ring-shaped shadows with equal or slightly higher density. Contrast MR imaging demonstrates intact abscess wall in ring-shaped enhancement with thinness and even thickness that are not specific. In the cases with small abscesses, nodular enhancement can be demonstrated. The distribution of foci is not consistent to that of blood vessels.

11.7.1.2 MR Imaging

In the acute inflammation stage of purulent meningitis, a large quantity of exudates fills up the subarachnoid space. MR imaging demonstrates abnormally increased T2WI signals of the cerebral convex and cistern as well as thickened meninges. The early meningeal lesions mainly involve the top cerebral convex and the anterior interhemispheric fissure. The meningeal inflammation often involves the dura mater to cause subdural effusions or empyema. In the advanced stage of meningitis, the subarachnoid space and basilar brain thicken and adhere to block the circulation of the cerebrospinal fluid. Therefore, communicating or obstructive hydrocephalus occurs. Purulent meningitis often involves adjacent brain parenchyma to cause meningoencephalitis. The early manifestations include vascular congestion, brain cells edema, and infiltration of perivascular inflammatory cells. At this time, MR imaging demonstrates plump gyrus, shallow or absent sulci, and local or diffuse long T1 and long T2 signals in the cortex and subcortex. In the advanced stage of meningoencephalitis, there are capillary hyperplasia and aggravated extracellular edema. MR imaging demonstrates similar findings to tumor but with no tumor body. Therefore, the space-occupying lesions of tumor can be excluded. In the cases of meningitis, meningeal exudates accumulate in the basilar brain to cause vascular inflammation, fiber hyperplasia, luminal stenosis, or even occlusion. Therefore, cerebral infarction occurs. Cerebral abscess is commonly divided into two stages, encephalitic stage and capsular stage. The demonstrations of encephalitic stage include irregular long T1 and long T2 signals with poorly defined boundaries that fuse with the surrounding cerebral edema. The demonstrations of capsular stage include central liquefaction and necrosis of the abscess cavity in long T1 and long T2 signals and extensive edema in the peripheral cerebral parenchyma. Contrast imaging demonstrates ring-shaped enhancement with thin wall and well-defined boundary and no nodular shadows protruding inwards on the abscess wall.

11.7.2 The Respiratory System

In the cases with the respiratory system involved, secondary acute respiratory distress syndrome may occur. Chest X-ray demonstrates increased and blurry pulmonary markings in both lung fields, extensive interstitial infiltration, pleural reaction, and a small quantity of pleural effusion. In severe cases, pulmonary infiltrative shadows fuse into large flakes which may even develop into white lung.

11.7.3 The Circulatory System

In the cases with the circulatory system involved, infective endocarditis may occur. Color Doppler ultrasound of the heart demonstrates enlarged left ventricle and enlarged left atrium, suspected neoplasm on the mitral valve, as well as small quantities of regurgitation via the mitral valve and tricuspid valve. During hospitalization a reexamination was done after 8 weeks therapy, and findings include still enlarged left ventricle and left atrium, absence of neoplasm on the mitral valve, small to moderate quantity of regurgitation via the mitral valve, and small quantity of regurgitation via the tricuspid valve.

11.8 Diagnostic Basis

11.8.1 Human *Streptococcus suis* Infection

In combination with the epidemiological history, clinical manifestations, and laboratory tests findings, the diagnosis can be defined. Other diseases with similar manifestations should be excluded.

11.8.1.1 Diagnostic Evidence

Epidemiological History

The patients have a history of direct contact to diseased or deceased pigs or other livestock within 7 days before the onset. Especially, the patients have defective skin mucosa with a history of slaughtering diseased or deceased pigs, processing or selling pork products prepared from diseased or deceased pigs, and burying diseased or deceased pigs.

Clinical Manifestations

The disease has an acute onset, with chills, fever, and other systematic infectious toxic symptoms. Concurrent TSS and/or SMS can be found.

Laboratory Tests

The peripheral WBC count increases which is mainly neutrophils. Bacterial culture is positive or specific gene detection is positive.

11.8.1.2 Diagnostic Criteria

Suspected Cases

The patients who have a history of direct contact to diseased or deceased pigs or other livestock within 7 days before the onset and have manifestations of acute systemic infective toxicity should be suspected as the cases of human *Streptococcus suis* infection. Otherwise, the suspected cases should have an abovementioned epidemiological history as well as increased peripheral total WBC count and increased percentage of neutrophils.

Clinically Diagnosed Cases

The patients have an abovementioned epidemiological history, with manifestations of TSS and/or SMS.

Definitively Diagnosed Cases

Definitive diagnosis can be made after *Streptococcus suis* is isolated by bacterial culture of specimen collected from suspected or clinically diagnosed cases. Otherwise, the definitive diagnosis can be made based on a positive finding by a specific gene detection of specimen collected from suspected or clinically diagnosed cases.

11.8.2 Human *Streptococcus suis* Infection-Related Complications

11.8.2.1 Purulent Meningitis

The cases with diagnosis of human *Streptococcus suis* infection have clinical manifestations of headache, fever, irritation, consciousness disturbance, coma, and meningeal irritation sign.

Plain CT scanning demonstrates increased density of sulci and cisterns and poorly defined borderline between gyri.

Contrast CT scanning demonstrates enhancement of the brain surface. MR imaging demonstrates deformed subarachnoid space and high T2WI signal with enhancement. In the advanced stage of the disease, cerebral abscess may be demonstrated.

Cerebrospinal fluid examination following lumbar puncture demonstrates cerebrospinal hypertension, increased WBC count, and increased protein.

11.8.2.2 Acute Respiratory Distress Syndrome

The cases with human *Streptococcus suis* infection have respiratory symptoms.

Chest X-ray demonstrates increased and blurry pulmonary markings in both lung fields and extensive interstitial infiltration in both lungs. In severe cases, pulmonary infiltrative shadows fuse into large flakes which may even develop into white lung.

11.8.2.3 Infective Endocarditis

The cases with human *Streptococcus suis* infection have circulatory symptoms.

Color Doppler ultrasound of the heart demonstrates enlarged left ventricle and left atrium, neoplasm on the mitral valve, and regurgitations via the mitral valve and tricuspid valve.

11.9 Differential Diagnosis

Human *Streptococcus suis* infection should be differentiated from other diseases that have manifestations of fever, petechiae, ecchymoses, shock, and multiple organ dysfunction. It should especially be differentiated from the following diseases.

11.9.1 TSS Caused by Other Streptococcus

Group A streptococcus and its produced streptococcal pyrogenic exotoxins (SPE) such as SPE-A, SPE-C, and SPE-F can cause serious TSS. *Streptococcus mitis* infection caused by group B, C, or G streptococcus as well as *Streptococcus viridans* can also cause TSS. In combination with the epidemiological history of direct contact to diseased or deceased pigs within 7 days before the onset, other streptococcus-induced TSS can be differentiated from human *Streptococcus suis* infection. Detection of SPE-A by PCR or immunological assays facilitates the diagnosis. Identification of group A streptococcus or other streptococcus based on specimen collected from the infective position or based on blood culture can differentiate the diagnosis.

11.9.2 TSS Caused by Staphylococcus

TSS caused by staphylococcus is induced by *Staphylococcus aureus* which produces toxic shock syndrome toxin I (TSST-I) and enterotoxins. Its clinical manifestations are similar to those of human *Streptococcus suis* infection. It can be divided into menstrual-related TSS (mTSS) and nonmenstrual-related TSS (nmTSS). The manifestations of sudden onset of the symptoms during menstrual period in young women with a history of using vaginal tampon during menstruation facilitate the diagnosis of mTSS. The cases of TSS after focal infection, trauma, and invasive operations should be suspected as nmTSS. The differential diagnosis should be made based on successful isolation of *Staphylococcus aureus* from clinical specimens or a positive finding of specific TSST-I or enterotoxin A, B, C, D, or G.

11.9.3 Other Diseases

Human *Streptococcus suis* infection should also be differentiated from Gram-positive bacterial septicemia, septic shock, fulminant type of epidemic cerebrospinal meningitis, epidemic hemorrhagic fever, systemic inflammatory response syndrome, and other diseases. In its advanced stage, human *Streptococcus suis* infection should also be differentiated from other serious infections caused multiple organ dysfunction syndrome or multiple organ failure.

Suggested Reading

Chuang SK. Fact sheet on Streptococcus suis infection. 2005. Obtained from http://www.chp.gov.hk.

Du YP, Qian WJ, Xu GB. Serotype 2 Streptococcus suis infection by human complicated by purulent meningitis: report of 8 cases. Chin J Prevent Med. 2000;34(5):305.

Hu XS, Zhu FC, Wang H, et al. Human Streptococcus suis infection syndrome. Chin J Prevent Med. 2000;34(3):150–2.

Ministry of Health of the People's Republic of China, Clinical guideline for human Streptococcus suis infection [EB/OL]. [2006-12-31]. http://www.moh.gov.cn/newshtml/17110.Htm.

Suankratay C, Intalapaporn P, Nunthapisud P, et al. Streptococcus suis meningitis in Thailand. Southeast Asian J Trop Med Public Health. 2004;35(4):868–76.

Sun XM. MR imaging and its sequence selection for the diagnosis of acute purulent meningitis: report of 43 cases. J South Med University. 2007;27(5):745–6.

Vilaichone RK, Mahachai V, Nunthapisud P. Streptococcus suis peritonitis: case report. J Med Assoc Thai. 2000;83(10):1274–7.

Wei G. The diagnostic value of MR imaging for pediatric purulent meningitis. Med Innov China. 2009;6(24):127.

Yao KH, Yang YH. Human Streptococcus suis infection. Chin J Infect Dis. 2006;24(1):64–6.

Zhang SQ, Chen ZS. CT scanning demonstrations and its diagnostic value for purulent meningitis, tuberculous meningitis and viral encephalitis. Hebei Med. 2004;10(6):537–8.

Zhang DH, Peng CX, Lu WL, et al. Infective endocarditis caused by human Streptococcus suis infection: report of 1 case. Chin J Infect Dis. 2009;27(5):320.

Legionnaires' Disease

12

Cuiyu Jia, Dawei Zhao, and Jianan Yu

Legionnaires' disease is an acute infectious disease caused by *Legionella pneumophila* (LP). It is mainly a lung infection, with complications involving extrapulmonary multiple systems. Since the first prevalence of LP infection was reported in the United States in 1976, LP infection has been continually reported for many times worldwide. LP-induced *Legionella* pneumonia and Pontiac fever are known as Legionnaires' disease, which can have sporadic prevalence or epidemic outbreak.

12.1 Etiology

LP is aerobic Gram-negative bacterium that is parasitic in human mononuclear cells and macrophagocytes. After LP was firstly isolated and proved to be the pathogenic bacteria of Legionnaires' disease in 1977, its scientific classification was established in 1979 and was categorized into the species of *L. pneumophila*, the genus of *Legionella*, and the family of Legionellaceae. The species of *L. pneumophila* can be further divided into different serogroups or serotypes. Currently, 50 species of *Legionella* have been discovered, with more than 70 serotypes. In them, at least 20 serotypes are related to human diseases. LP has been identified to be the most closely related to human diseases and is an important pathogenic bacterium that causes epidemic and sporadic community-acquired pneumonia and hospital-acquired pneumonia. LP has 16 serotypes and LP serotype 1 (LP1) is the main pathogenic bacterium of *Legionella* pneumonia and LP serotype 6 (LP6) commonly causes Pontiac fever.

C. Jia (✉) • D. Zhao • J. Yu
Department of Radiology, Beijing You'an Hospital, Capital Medical University, Beijing, China
e-mail: jiacuiyu@sina.com

LP has a width of 0.3–0.9 μm and a length of 2–20 μm. It has a slim thallus, with no formation of inner spores or follicles, no capsule, and no production of acids. With the help of 1–2 or more polar flagella or lateral flagella, it can move. Akinesis bacterial strains are occasionally found. The growth of LP needs amino acid and ferric salt, with methionine and cysteine as the most important substances for its growth. The environment for growth of LP should contain 2.5–5 % CO_2, with an optimum temperature of 35–36 °C and an optimum pH value of 6.0–8.0. LP has strong resistance to the external environment. In addition, other microorganisms in the external environment might affect the virulence and infectivity of LP.

12.2 Epidemiology

12.2.1 The Source of Infection

Currently, the source of LP infection remains unknown. In scientific literature, it has been reported that the source of LP infection is believed to be contaminated water sources and soil. The cooling towers for air conditioning and drinking water supply system carrying LP are the important source of LP infection for its outbreaks and prevalence. The infected animals and humans as the sources of LP infection remain controversial.

12.2.2 Route of Transmission

LP infection spreads mainly via the respiratory tract, and aerosol is an important carrier for spreading LP. Protozoon is another carrier of LP for its spreading. Contaminated water is also a significant route of its transmission. In addition, it has been reported that the contaminated surgical incision also causes LP infection. So far, no human-to-human transmission has been reported.

H. Li (ed.), *Radiology of Infectious Diseases: Volume 2*, DOI 10.1007/978-94-017-9876-1_12

12.2.3 Susceptible Populations

People are generally susceptible to Legionnaires' disease, whose occurrence is more common in middle-aged adults and the elderly. In addition, male patients with Legionnaires' disease are more commonly found than female patients. In the sporadic cases, LP infection in hospital accounts for 5 %, and hospital-acquired pneumonia accounts for more than 20 %. Patients with chronic diseases, patients receiving long-term blood purification or kidney transplant, patients with tumors, patients using immunosuppressor, and people addicted to smoking and alcohol are more susceptible to this disease.

12.2.4 Epidemiological Features

Legionnaires' disease occurs worldwide, with report of cases in recent years from North America, Europe, Oceania, Asia, and Africa. According to documentary records, the prevalence of Legionnaires' disease occurred at least ten times in the United States with hundreds of thousands of reported cases. In 1982, the first case in China was reported from Nanjing. After that, multiple outbreaks and prevalence occurred in Beijing and Shanghai. Afterward, sporadic cases were reported in various regions. Legionnaires' disease can be prevalent epidemically or sporadically and can be found all year round, with more common occurrence in summers and autumns.

12.3 Pathogenesis and Pathological Changes

12.3.1 Pathogenesis

The destructive effects of LP on human body can be divided into indirect effects and direct effects. The indirect effects begin from its destructive effects on the alveolar macrophages (MØ). Studies have demonstrated that after LP is phagocytized by MØ, it can inhibit the integration of phagosome into the lysosome and regulate the pH value within the mononuclear macrophages for an appropriate condition for its survival and reproduction. By interfering the depolarization of cells, LP captures MØ to successfully escape the immune defense of the human body. It can also utilize the nutrients of MØ to continue its survival and multiplication, followed by splitting of the MØ to cause acute lesions of the alveolar epithelium and endothelium with accompanying edema and fibrin exudation. LP can cause damage effects through inducing cell apoptosis as well. And its direct destructive effects are due to its production of hemolysin, cytotoxin, and enzymes. The inhaled pathogenic bacteria are phagocytized by MØ and multiply in phagocytic vesicles to produce cytotoxin. The MØ is then killed and other MØ are invaded. The existence of antibody seems unable to terminate the reproduction of pathogenic bacteria, and cell-mediated immunity plays an important role in anti-infection. The lymphocytes are stimulated by antigens to produce cytokines that can inhibit the reproduction of bacteria in MØ. Afterward, antibody, complements, and multinuclear granulocytes can kill the bacteria. In addition, studies have demonstrated that flagella and some virulence factors contribute to the pathogenesis of the disease.

12.3.2 Pathological Changes

Pathological changes of Legionnaires' disease involve the lungs, liver, kidneys, muscles, and the central nervous system. Among all the pathological changes, pulmonary lesions are the most prominent.

12.3.2.1 Lungs

In the acute stage, it is fibrinous suppurative pneumonia, and in the advanced period of the acute stage, it is organizing pneumonia. The pathological changes of the lungs in the acute stage can be divided into mainly two types: type I of acute fibrinous suppurative pneumonia (95 %) that is characterized by a large quantity of fibrin exudation, neutrophil disintegration, cell debris, and macrophage infiltration and type II of acute diffuse alveolar damage, with alveolar epithelium hyperplasia, desquamation, and formation of hyaline membrane. It is different from common lobar pneumonia in the aspects of concurrence of fibrinous suppurative bronchitis and obvious mononuclear cells and MØ in the inflammatory exudates. By silver staining, the Bacillus brevis in alveolar lumen can be stained dark brown, with a length of 2–4 μm. Especially in the alveolar MØ, it can be observed that many bacteria that have been phagocytized are multiplying within the cells. The lesions usually have a mixed distribution in lobes and lobules. In the advanced stage, the lesions are demonstrated as the organization of exudates and hyaline membranes as well as interstitial fibrosis. In some severe cases, honeycomb lung can be found. The pulmonary vascular lesions mainly invade pulmonary muscular arteries, with lesions focally distributed. Non-necrotizing vasculitis, with infiltrations of plasma cells, lymphocytes, and histocytes, and intimal fibrosis or aneurysm may occur.

12.3.2.2 Pleura

The pathological changes of the pleura can be serous pleurisy, serous fibrinous pleurisy, or suppurative pleurisy. About one third of the cases have pleural involvement.

12.3.2.3 Other Pathological Changes

Other pathological changes include inflammation, infectious toxic changes, and secondary changes. Centrilobular fatty changes can be found in the liver. Renal biopsy demonstrates interstitial nephritis. The disease is often accompanied by rhabdomyolysis that further deteriorates renal lesions to cause acute renal failure. The neurological changes are currently believed to be caused by toxins. Cerebrovascular microthrombogenesis and spots of bleeding in the brain tissues occur.

The above-mentioned pathological changes can disappear after the disease is cured. But the pathohistological changes are not absolutely specific in the cases of *Legionella* pneumonia. Therefore, the diagnosis should be based on the pathohistological changes and etiological examinations.

12.4 Clinical Symptoms and Signs

The clinical symptoms of *Legionella* infection mainly include two types: *Legionella* pneumonia and Pontiac fever.

12.4.1 *Legionella* Pneumonia

The incubation period lasts for 2–10 days, with an average of 5–6 days. Clinical symptoms are hardly distinguishable from those of pneumonia caused by pneumococcus and other bacteria. The conditions have different severities. And the prodromal symptoms include fatigue, low-grade fever, and poor appetite.

12.4.1.1 Respiratory Symptoms

At the early stage after onset, dry cough is common, while at the later stage, half of the patients may cough up thin or thick phlegm and one third of the patients can have hemoptysis in small quantity with accompanying chest pain and dyspnea. In some serious cases, cyanosis occurs. In rare cases, pulmonary consolidation signs can be found, with dry or moist rales and even pleural effusion and pleural friction sound. Patients using immunosuppressor like glucocorticoid are likely to have pulmonary cavity and abscess. Clinically, it is often misdiagnosed as pulmonary infarction based on the finding of severe chest pain. In some severe cases, death occurs due to respiratory failure.

12.4.1.2 Gastrointestinal Symptoms

Some patients may experience nausea, vomiting, and abdominal pain. About 25–50 % of the patients have abdominal distension, diarrhea, and watery stool. In some severe cases, gastrointestinal bleeding or even gastric perforation occurs.

12.4.1.3 Symptoms of the Central Nervous System

Half of the patients have manifestations of central nervous system involvement including disturbance of consciousness, disorientation, slow responses, and even coma.

12.4.1.4 Cardiac Symptoms

The symptoms include bradycardia, infectious endocarditis, pericarditis, and cardiac failure.

12.4.1.5 Urinary Symptoms

Patients may rarely experience proteinuria, hematuria, and even renal failure in some serious cases.

12.4.1.6 Other Symptoms

Patients may rarely experience thrombocytopenia, DIC, and septic shock.

12.4.2 Pontiac Fever

The incubation period lasts for only 1–2 days, with an acute onset. It is a self-limited febrile disease, with major manifestation of flulike symptoms such as aversion to cold, fever, headache, muscular pain, fatigue, nausea, and dry cough. No pneumonia or shock occurs and no organ lesions in the liver or kidneys. The course of the disease is very short, lasting for about 1 week. Patients can be cured without receiving any therapy, with favorable prognosis.

12.5 Legionnaires' Disease-Related Complications

In the early stage of Legionnaires' disease, the manifestations of extrapulmonary multisystem involvement can be found. The extrapulmonary infection accompanying pneumonia can involve the brain, intestines, kidneys, liver, spleen, peritoneum, prostate, pericardium, bone marrow, skin and fascia, rectum, myocardium, peripheral lymph nodes, thyroid, pancreas, testicles, and muscles. The extrapulmonary infection with no accompanying pneumonia may involve the blood, intestines, nasal sinus, endocardium, peritoneum, pericardium, and skin and fascia.

12.6 Diagnostic Examinations

12.6.1 Laboratory Tests

12.6.1.1 Routine Laboratory Tests

In most cases, erythrocyte sedimentation rate speeds up, with increased WBC count. In some cases, left shift of the neutrophilic nucleus is found. Lactic dehydrogenase, serum glutamic-oxaloacetic transaminase, and bilirubin may rise. Or proteinuria, hyponatremia, and hypophosphatemia may be found. Hyponatremia is one of the characteristic laboratory findings of Legionnaires' disease.

12.6.1.2 Bacteriologic Examinations

Bacterial Isolation and Culture

Bacterial isolation and culture is the most reliable examination for the diagnosis of Legionnaires' disease. The sensitivity was internationally reported to be 50–80 %. The successful isolation of LP from airway secretions, phlegm, pleural effusion, or lung tissues is a reliable evidence to define the diagnosis.

Direct Fluorescent Antibody Test

Direct fluorescent antibody test has a high specificity to LP and, therefore, has favorable diagnostic value. This test is simple, convenient, and rapid but with a lower sensitivity.

12.6.1.3 Immunological Examinations

Antigen Detection

After the infection of LP serotype 1, the antigen can be detected in the urine within several hours. But this examination fails to distinguish acute infection from previous infection.

Serologic Examination

About 1 week after LP infection, specific IgM antibody can be detected. The IgG antibody begins to increase 2 weeks after the onset and peaks in about 1 month. Indirect immunofluorescence is the most commonly used examination for the diagnosis of Legionnaires' disease. In acute and convalescence stages, the antibody titer increases as high as at least four times. In the cases with a titer not lower than 1:128 or with single serum titer not lower than 1:256, the diagnosis of Legionnaires' disease can made.

PCR Detection

PCR detection is quick, efficient, and sensitive. It has been extensively valued in clinical practice but with certain rate of false positive.

12.6.2 Diagnostic Imaging

X-ray and CT scanning can be applied for the diagnosis and differential diagnosis of *Legionella* pneumonia. MR imaging can be applied for the diagnosis and differential diagnosis of neurological disorders complicating Legionnaires' disease.

12.7 Imaging Demonstrations

12.7.1 Chest Lesions

12.7.1.1 X-Ray Radiology

Chest X-ray of *Legionella* pneumonia mainly includes pulmonary parenchyma infiltration shadows, which are commonly found in unilateral pulmonary segments or lobes. The shadows may further enlarge to extend to the contralateral lung.

Diverse Morphology of X-Ray Demonstrations

In addition to large flakes of shadows, the shadows may be in patches, nodular, cord-like, and reticular.

The Early Stage

In 1–2 days after the onset, infiltrative shadows can be found in the inferior lung field, which may be in morphologically large flakes or patches. In some cases, pleural effusion is found.

The Progressive Stage

The lesions rapidly spread to multiple lobes and segments and even to the contralateral lung. The lesions are large flakes of pulmonary consolidation, with an incidence rate of pulmonary cavity being about 10 %. The changes resemble those in *Staphylococcus aureus* pneumonia.

Pleural Effusion

Pleural effusion is common, with an incidence rate of about 40 %. The lesion is commonly unilateral, in small to medium quantity. In rare cases, it is accompanied by a small quantity of pericardial effusion. Sometimes, pleural effusion occurs prior to pulmonary parenchyma infiltration.

Pulmonary Abscess

The incidence rate of pulmonary abscess is up to 17 %, with rare formation of cavity. It is commonly found in patients with compromised immunity and using cortical hormone. Cavities occur rapidly but with a slow closure.

X-Ray Demonstrations and Clinical Symptoms

At both the onset and convalescence stage, X-ray changes lag behind the clinical symptoms. In some cases, chest X-ray infiltrative shadows are found 3 days after the onset. And in some cases, after effective therapies, X-ray infiltrative shadows temporarily continue to progress or are slowly absorbed in 2 weeks or even several months. Macfarlane et al. reported that in about half of the patients with *Legionella* pneumonia, lung infiltrative shadows have been completely absorbed after 10 weeks and sometimes even after 1 year. The absorption is slower than that of other bacterial pneumonia. Therefore, only chest X-ray demonstrations are insufficient for the assessment of the therapeutic efficacy for *Legionella* pneumonia. Some scholars indicated that the clinical manifestations and prognosis of *Legionella* pneumonia are insignificantly related to lung infiltrative range (unilateral lung or multiple lung lobe) demonstrated by chest X-ray. However, they are related to the quantity of bacteria in the sputum (Fig. 12.1).

Prognosis

After medication of erythromycin, the clinical symptoms rapidly improve. But the radiologically demonstrated lesions completely disappear after 1–2 months. In rare cases, cord-like or linear shadows still remain after several months (Fig. 12.2).

Case Study 1
A male patient aged 51 years, with a case history of alcoholism.

For case detail and figures, please refer to Dietrich PA, et al. 1978, 127 (3): 577.

Case Study 2
A female patient aged 39 years, with chronic renal failure.

For case detail and figures, please refer to Dietrich PA, et al. 1978, 127 (3): 577.

Case Study 1

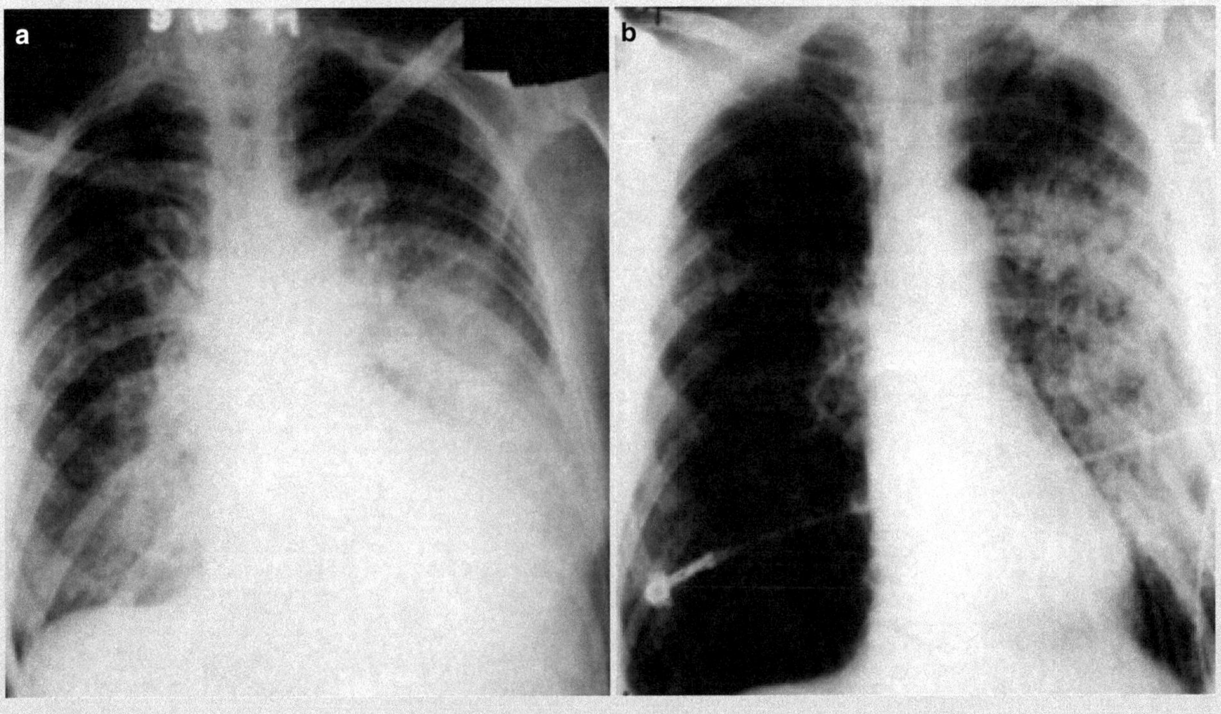

Fig. 12.1 Legionella pneumonia. (**a**) At day 4 after the onset, chest X-ray demonstrates congestive heart failure. (**b**) At day 9 after the onset, chest X-ray demonstrates obvious flakes of shadows in the left lung after treatment for congestive heart failure.

Case Study 2

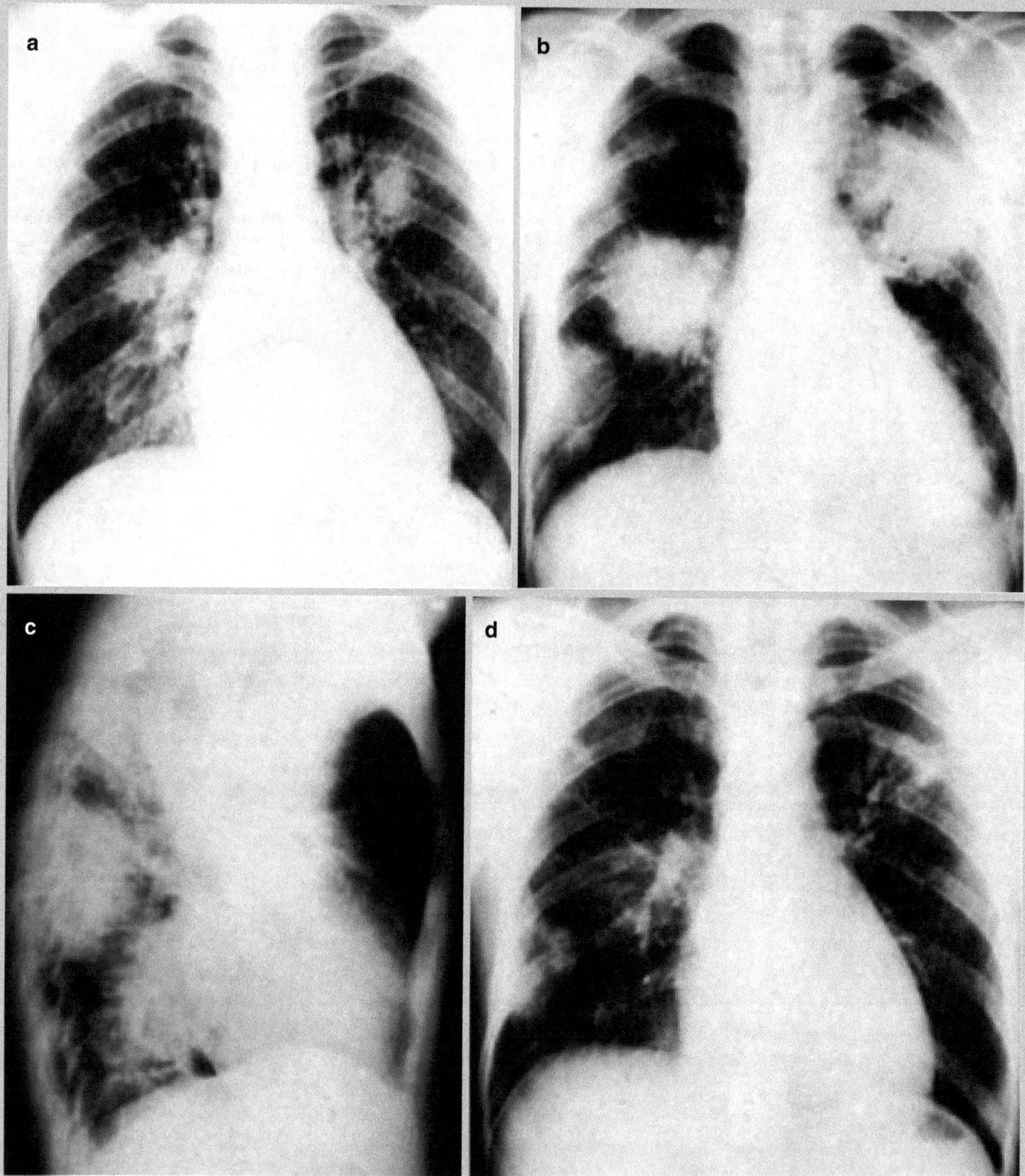

Fig. 12.2 Legionella pneumonia. (**a**) At the day 4 after the onset, chest X-ray demonstrates blurry shadows around bilateral pulmonary hilum. (**b, c**) At the day 8 after the onset, chest X-ray demonstrates obviously enlarged lesion range with consolidation shadows. (**d**) At the convalescence stage, chest X-ray demonstrates flakes of shadows in both lungs

12.7.1.2 CT Scanning

CT scanning demonstrations of *Legionella* pneumonia are diverse, which is characterized by multiple lobe and segment involvement. Large flakes and patches of shadows are the most common, with accompanying pleura lesions. Cavities can be found, with irregular thick wall or regular thin wall. No fluid level is found, with commonly accompanying large flakes or small patches of shadows. Occasionally, multiple air sacs in different sizes can be found in both lungs, which resemble those seen in *Staphylococcus aureus* pneumonia. Chest CT scanning demonstrates more lesions and more clearly defined lesions than chest X-ray. Therefore, chest CT scanning provides more reliable evidence for the diagnosis and therapeutic assessment.

Case Study 3

A female patient aged 60 years. She complained of chest distress, shortness of breath, dyspnea, cough without phlegm, and no obvious chest pain for 5 days. There is also fever, with the highest body temperature of around 37.4 °C, with subjective fatigue. Chest X-ray and CT scanning in a local hospital indicated pulmonary inflammation. Pulmonary function test indicated severe restrictive pulmonary ventilation and severe impaired function of pulmonary diffusion. By laboratory test, IgM antibody against LP serotype 1 is positive.

Case Study 3

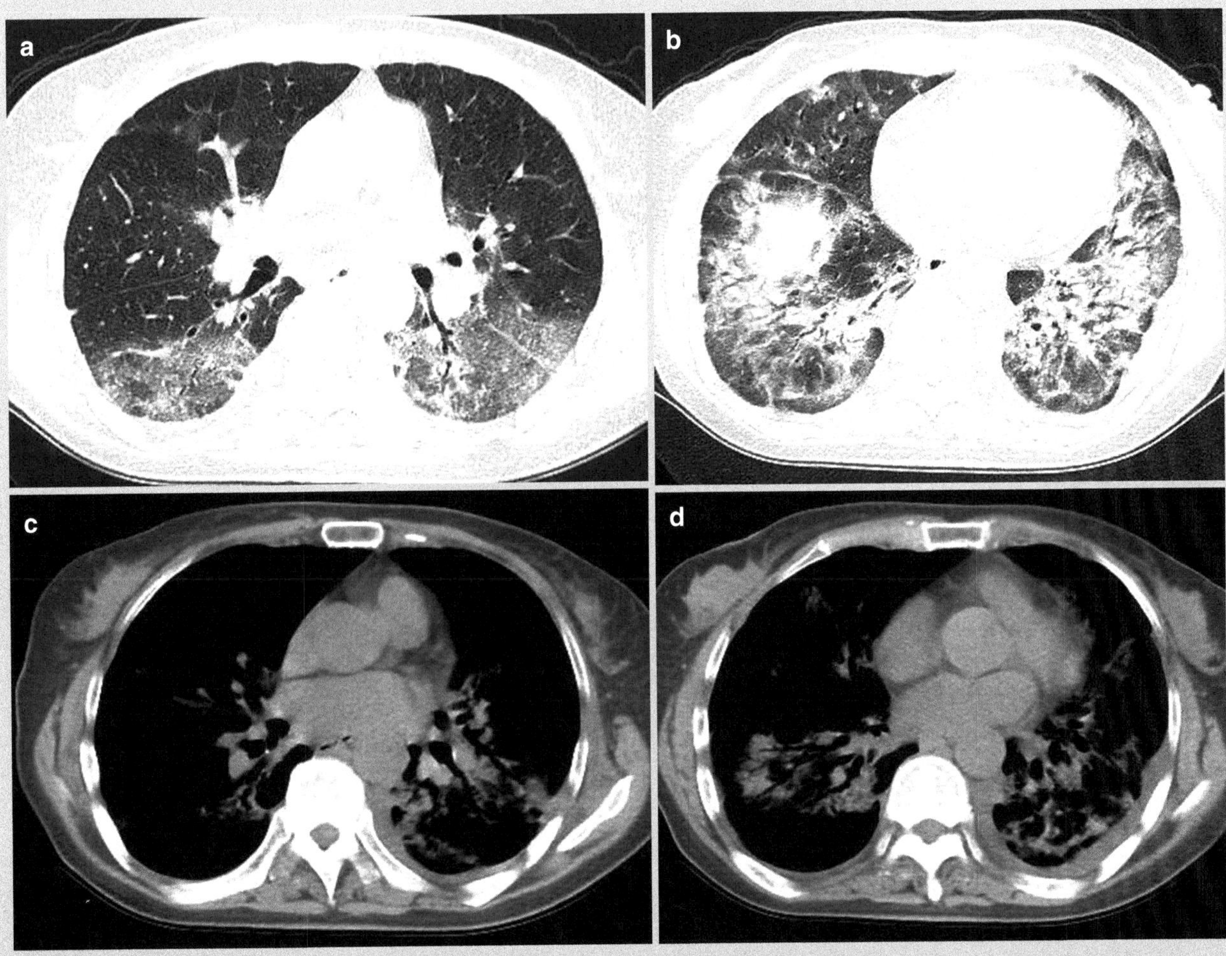

Fig. 12.3 Legionella pneumonia. (**a–b**) HRCT demonstrates multiple flakes of ground-glass opacities and consolidation shadows in both lungs, with internal air bronchogram sign. (**c–d**) Mediastinal window demonstrates both lung consolidation and a small quantity of arc-shaped liquid density shadows in both thoracic cavities. (**e–f**) Reexamination after 2 weeks treatment, HRCT demonstrates obviously absorbed lesions, with scattering patches and consolidation shadows in both lungs. (**g**) Reexamination after 2 months treatment, CT scanning still demonstrates ground-glass opacities in both lungs

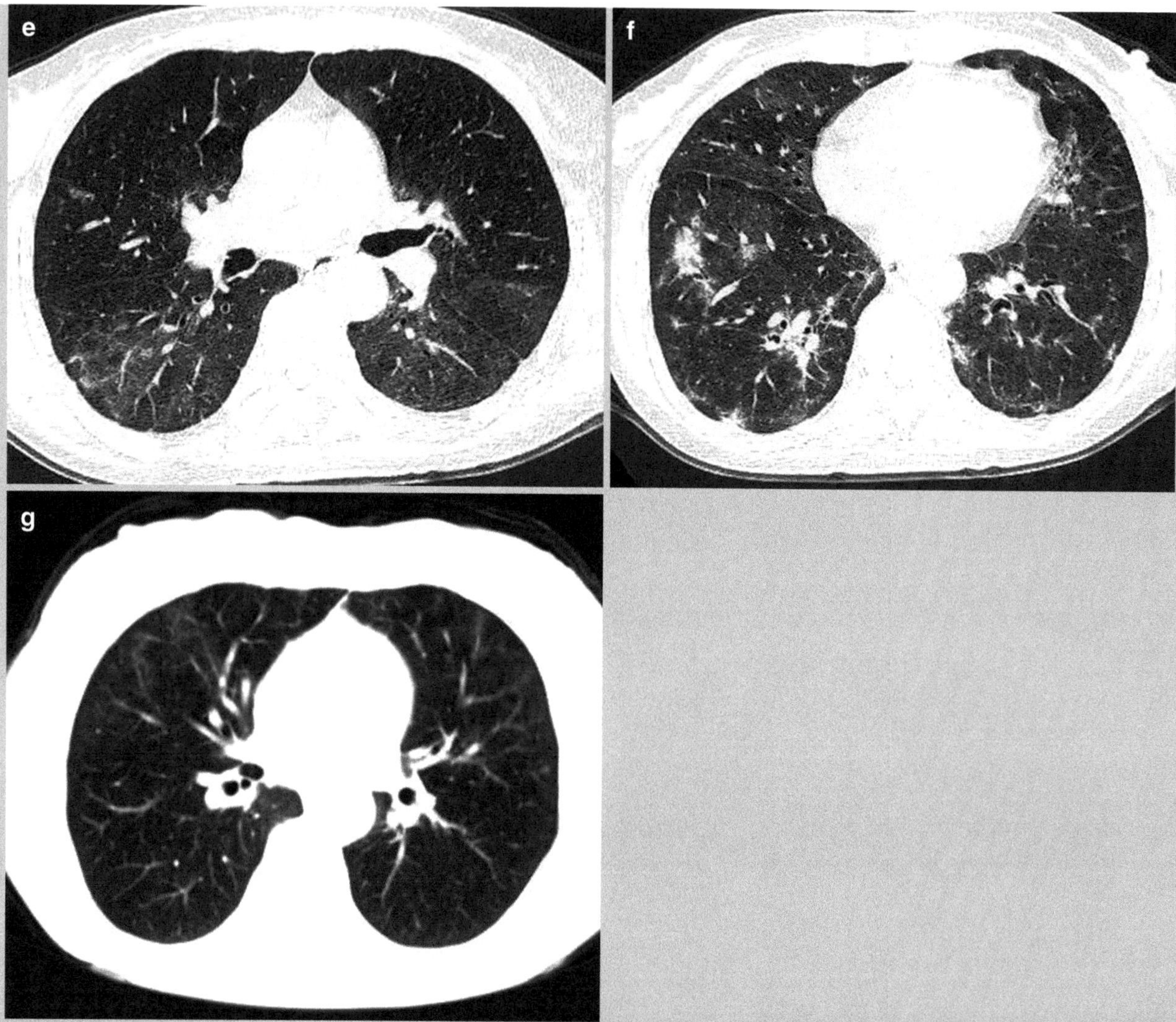

Fig. 12.3 (continued)

Case Study 4
Legionella pneumonia.
For case detail and figures, please refer to Lei, ZD. et al. *Chinese Medical Imaging Technology*, 2006, 22 (11): 1668.

12.7.2 Central Nervous System

Legionnaires' disease is a systemic infectious disease. Currently, the lesions of the central nervous system are believed to be caused by *Legionella* toxin, with diverse clinical manifestations. In mild cases, flulike symptoms occur, while in severe cases, the symptoms include drowsiness, vomiting, headache, disorientation, limb dyskinesia, disturbance of consciousness, and limb and facial paralysis, with typical pathological reflex and meningeal irritation sign. CT scanning demonstrates low-density shadows in the cerebrum or brainstem and small lesions of hemorrhage. MR imaging demonstrates encephalitis. And FLAIR MRI demonstrates high signal. MR imaging and SPECT demonstrate abnormal brain perfusion. Functional imaging facilitates the diagnosis of *Legionella* encephalopathy.

Case Study 5
Legionella disease complicated by central nervous system lesions.
For case detail and figures, please refer to Morgan JC, et al. *J Neurol Neurosurg Psychiatry*, 2004, 75 (4): 651.

12.8 Diagnostic Basis

12.8.1 Diagnostic Basis

12.8.1.1 Epidemiological Data

Legionnaires' disease occurs in summers and autumns, and patients commonly have a history of using air-conditioning humidification system or shower bathing. Those aged above 40 years, who habitually smoke, who have chronic pulmonary disease or heart disease, who are on adrenocortical hormone therapy, and who have been hospitalized or used respiratory therapeutic equipment should be suspected of having Legionnaires' disease.

12.8.1.2 Clinical Data

Patients with at least one of the following conditions should be suspected as having Legionnaires' disease: pneumonia with initial symptoms of diarrhea, severe systemic symptoms but mild respiratory symptoms, pneumonia and accompanying neurological symptoms, pneumonia and negative routine culture of respiratory sections, and pneumonia ineffectively treated by β-lactam antibiotic therapy.

12.8.1.3 Laboratory Tests

Etiological examinations and immunological assays are the main examinations to define the diagnosis.

12.8.1.4 Diagnostic Imaging

Changes in pulmonary parenchyma infiltrative shadows, pulmonary abscess, pleural effusion, encephalitis, cerebral infarction, and hemorrhage lesions can be demonstrated by radiological examinations. And X-ray demonstrations commonly lag behind the clinical symptoms.

12.8.2 Diagnostic Criteria

1. Clinical symptoms of respiratory tract infection, such as fever, chills, cough, and chest pain.
2. Chest X-ray demonstrates shadows of pulmonary inflammation.
3. LP growth is demonstrated by culture of respiratory secretions, phlegm, blood, or pleural effusion on BCYE or other special medium.
4. Positive finding by DFA of the respiratory secretions.
5. Antibody titer after serum IFA increases as high as four times than before serum IFA, reaching 1:128 or higher.
6. Antibody titer after serum tube agglutination test increases as high as four times than before serum tube agglutination test, reaching 1:80 or higher.

Patients with items 1 and 2, plus either item 3 or 4, can be diagnosed as having *Legionella* pneumonia. Patients with items 1, 2, and 5 should be suspected as having *Legionella* pneumonia. If IFA is considered to be a definitive diagnostic indicator, the diagnostic criteria can be changed as the following: patients with either item 1 or 2, plus one from items 3, 4, and 5 can be diagnosed as having *Legionella* pneumonia.

12.9 Differential Diagnosis

Legionella pneumonia should be differentiated from the diseases showing wide distribution, polymorphous changes, and concurrent pulmonary fibrosis. The most common diseases include idiopathic interstitial pneumonia, pneumonia-type carcinoma, and viral pneumonia. Idiopathic interstitial pneumonia usually develops from the peripheral lower lung to the central and the upper lung. Most cases of idiopathic interstitial pneumonia have no symptoms of fever. Hormone therapy is effective for ground-glass opacities and consolidation shadows in the acute stage. In addition, traction bronchiectasis is common. However, fibrosis of *Legionella* pneumonia mainly occurs around the lesions, which rarely tracts the central bronchi. Patients with pneumonia-type carcinoma usually experience no fever, with dead tree sign, lump shadow, and even lymphatic metastasis. Viral pneumonia is also commonly accompanied by fibrosis but mostly with mild symptoms and early radiological demonstrations of no abnormality or only non-segmental ground-glass opacity. By laboratory test, WBC count and differential counts generally show no increase. In rare patients with severe symptoms, the imaging demonstrations are also obvious and the lesions are sensitive to hormone therapy.

References

Dietrich PA, Johnson RD, Fairbank JT, et al. The chest radiograph in legionnaires' disease. Radiology. 1978;127(3):577–82.

Lei ZD, Feng KQ, Jia WL, et al. Imaging demonstrations of Legionella pneumonia and their diagnostic value. Chin Med Imaging Technol. 2006;22(11):1668–71.

Morgan JC, Cavaliere R, Juel VC. Reversible corpus callosum lesion in legionnaires' disease. J Neurol Neurosurg Psychiatry. 2004;75(4):651–4.

Suggested Reading

Chen Y. The present prevalence of legionnaires disease and its therapeutic and preventive strategies. Shanghai J Prev Med. 2001;13(2):54–5.

Codony F, Alvarez J, Oliva JM, et al. Factors promoting colonization by legionellae in residential water distribution systems: an environmental case–control survey. Eur J Clin Microbiol Infect Dis. 2002;21(10):717–21.

Hu DL, Liao JK, Yang G. Legionnaires disease. Foreign Med Sci (Sect Prev Med). 2003;30(4):391–4.

Liu SC, Yang PJ, Guo XH, et al. Chest radiology of legionnaires disease: report of 20 cases. Chin J Coal Ind Med. 2012;15(9):1392–3.

Wu SM, Zhang ZY, Zhang ZQ. Newly emerging infectious diseases and re-emerging infectious diseases. Shanghai: Shanghai Science and Technology Education Press; 2010.

13 Leprosy

Zhiyan Lu, Jingwei Wu, and Guangyuan Cheng

Leprosy is a chronic infectious disease caused by *Mycobacterium leprae*. It mainly invades the skin and peripheral nervous system. In patients with compromised immunity, deep tissues and organs can be involved. And in severe cases of leprosy, disfiguration and disability of extremities occur.

13.1 Etiology

Mycobacterium leprae is categorized into the genus of mycobacterium, which is a slender bacillus with a length of 2–7 μm and a width of 0.4 μm. It resembles mycobacterium in aspects of shape and staining. After patients receive therapy, it commonly turns into multimorphism including short rod and particle-like. The unevenly stained granular thallus is the dead bacterium with ruptured cell membrane and overflow of cytoplasm. The bacterium has no spore, capsule, and flagella, with both positive Gram staining and acid-fast staining and being stained red by acid-fast staining. *M. leprae* is a typical intracellular parasitic bacterium, and infected cells containing large quantities of *M. leprae* can be observed in the specimen of exudates from patients with certain type of leprosy. The cytoplasm of these infected cells is foamy, and these infected cells are known as foam cells or leprosy cells. The existence of these cells constitutes a major difference between leprosy and mycobacterium tuberculosis infection.

M. leprae has certain tolerance to external environment. It can survive for 9 days in exosomatic dry nasal secretions, and its optimum growth temperature is 27–30 °C. Accordingly, it mainly grows in surface tissues of human body with low body temperature, mucous membrane, and superficial peripheral nerves. *M. leprae* can be completely inactivated under ultraviolet radiation for 30–60 min, direct sunlight for 2 h, or at the temperature of 60 °C for 10–30 min. The growth of *M. leprae* is extremely slow, with its generation time of logarithmic growth phase being 11–13 days. However, its in vitro culture has not yet achieved success.

13.2 Epidemiology

13.2.1 Source of Infection

Epidemiologic studies have confirmed that the patients with leprosy are still the only source of infection. Particularly those untreated patients with lepromatous leprosy or borderline leprosy who carry more quantities of bacteria have stronger infectivity. The bacteria are discharged mainly via the mucous membrane and the skin. The patients with lepromatous leprosy are the main source of infection. In recent years, wild armadillo, black vervet, and some other animals have been found to show the infection similar to human lepromatous leprosy infection. However, epidemiological studies have demonstrated that animals are unlikely to be the source of infection.

13.2.2 Route of Transmission

The exact route of transmission remains unknown. Currently, it is believed that the routes of transmission include the respiratory tract, close skin contact, and indirect contacts. *M. leprae* is generally believed to invade the human body via the respiratory tract and skin. In addition, it can also be transmitted via the placenta from mother to fetus. It has been demonstrated that *M. leprae* is present in the placenta and cord blood.

13.2.3 Susceptible Population

Humans have different levels of naturally acquired immunity against *M. leprae*, and people in good health are hardly

Z. Lu (✉) • J. Wu • G. Cheng
Department of Radiology, Zhongnan Hospital, Wuhan University, Wuhan, Hubei, China
e-mail: 13377870857@189.cn

H. Li (ed.), *Radiology of Infectious Diseases: Volume 2*, DOI 10.1007/978-94-017-9876-1_13

susceptible to leprosy. The population susceptibility is related to the status of cellular immunity. Children and persons with weak immunity to *M. leprae* are the susceptible populations. And males are more susceptible to leprosy than females, with an incidence ratio of (2–3):1.

13.2.4 Epidemic Features

In the year 2010, a total of 228,474 cases of leprosy have been reported worldwide. By the end of 2010, a total of 192,246 cases of leprosy have been registered all over the world (Table 13.1).

In China, a total of 1,324 cases of leprosy have been newly reported in 2010, with a discovery rate of 0.099/100,000 (Table 13.2). Compared to the year 2009, the newly reported cases decreased by 17.1 % in 2010. By the end of 2010, a total of 6,032 cases of leprosy have been registered in China, with an incidence of 0.45/100,000, including 2,886 cases receiving combined chemotherapy. According to the basic criteria about eradicating leprosy in China with an incidence of lower than 1/100,000, there had been four provinces in China with an incidence of leprosy above that level by the end of 2010, namely, Yunnan, Guizhou, Tibet, and Sichuan. By the end of 2004, there had been 605 hospitals and villages across mainland China with 555 inpatients receiving therapies and totally 18,175 affected cases that had been cured.

13.3 Pathogenesis and Pathological Changes

13.3.1 Pathogenesis

The pathogenesis of *M. leprae* after its invasion into human body is similar to that of mycobacterium tuberculosis. The onset of the disease after invasion of the bacteria, the development of conditions after onset, and the clinical manifestations are all dependent on the immunity of the invaded human body against *M. leprae*. After its invasion, *M. leprae* is firstly swallowed by macrophages. After being processed, some antigens are thoroughly expressed on the surface of cell membrane of macrophages, which then collaborate with HLA II type of antigens (DR, DP, and DQ) on the cell membrane of macrophages. And then its recognition by T cells triggers immune responses. In the cases of normal immune responses, T lymphocytes are activated to induce immune responses, with macrophages playing their role to eliminate *M. leprae* and form the epithelioid cells and Langerhans cells. In the cases of compromised immunity or the cases with changed expressing locus of HLA-DR antigen due to the infection of *M. leprae* and even expressing impairment, the failed recognition by T cells induces weak immune responses that are unable to eliminate the bacteria. Therefore, the lesions are diffusive and widespread but with slight immune impairments. Leprosy cells containing large quantities of *M. leprae* form at the site of lesions, which are derived

Table 13.1 Total registered cases and newly reported cases in 2010 in 130 WHO-defined regions (Europe not included)

WHO-defined regions	Total registered cases by 2010 (1/10,000)	Newly reported cases in 2010 (1/100,000)
Africa	27,111 (0.38)	25,345 (3.53)
America	33,953 (0.38)	37,740 (4.25)
Southeast Asia	113,750 (0.64)	156,254 (8.77)
East Mediterranean	9,046 (0.17)	4,080 (0.67)
West Pacific	8,386 (0.34)	5,055 (0.28)
Total	192,246 (0.34)	228,474 (3.93)

Table 13.2 Regional prevalence of leprosy in mainland China in 2010

	Newly reported cases				
Epidemic region	Total cases	Incidence (1/100,000)	National percentage (%)	Compared to 2009 (%)[a]	Compared to 2005 (%)
North China	6	0.004	0.5	−25.0	−25.0
Northeast	2	0.002	0.2	−33.3	−66.7
East China	216	0.055	16.3	−13.9	−9.2
Middle South	291	0.078	22.0	−23.6	−26.7
Southwest	766	0.389	57.8	−16.6	−19.8
Northwest	43	0.044	3.2	22.9	−20.4
National	1,324	0.099	100.0	−17.1	−20.1

The data is from Sun, PW. Yu, MW. Yan, LB. et al. Epidemiological analysis of leprosy in China in 2010. *Journal of Nanjing Medical University (Natural Science Edition)*, 2012, 32(2): 155–159

[a]The values are calculated by the following formula: newly reported cases in 2010 firstly minus newly reported cases in 2009, and the results are divided by the newly reported cases in 2009

from infected macrophages by large quantities of *M. leprae* containing lipids. In recent years, scholarly studies about immunological pathogenesis of leprosy indicated that the status of immunity and histocompatibility antigens have direct impacts on the onset of leprosy and its clinical type.

13.3.2 Pathological Changes

13.3.2.1 Tuberculoid Leprosy (TL)

This type commonly occurs in patients with a strong immunity. *M. leprae* has affinity to nerve tissues, and its invasion causes infiltration of lymphocytes and macrophages around nerve tissues. The infiltrated macrophages may turn into fixed epithelioid cells whose clusters form Langerhans cells cause tuberculoid granuloma. The nerve myelin is often destroyed, with hyperplasia and thickening of neurolemma.

13.3.2.2 Borderline Leprosy (BL)

This type of BL includes three subtypes: borderline tuberculoid leprosy (BTL), mid-borderline leprosy (MBL), and borderline lepromatous leprosy (BLL). The common manifestation of the three subtypes is a narrow subcutaneous non-infiltrative strip. But BTL is characterized by formation of granuloma by intradermal epithelioid cells, rare surrounding lymphocytes, swelling dermic nerves due to infiltration of histiocytes and epithelial cells, as well as a possible small quantity of bacteria in the dermic nerves. MBL is characterized by intradermal extensive granuloma, intradermal histiocyte-based infiltration, slight swelling and cell infiltration of the dermic nerves, and moderate quantities of bacteria at the lesions. BLL is characterized by subdermal macrophagic granulomas, intradermal foam cell-based infiltration, and perineurium in onionskin-like appearance with large quantities of bacteria.

13.3.2.3 Lepromatous Leprosy (LL)

In the cases of LL, the patients lack immunity to fight against *M. leprae*, and the pathogens spread all over the body along with lymph and blood flows. LL is characterized by extensive atrophy of the skin, thinner epidermis, destructed collagen fibers, and non-infiltrative strip in the subcutaneous papillary layer. Additionally, there is typical leproma in deep dermis, containing histiocytes, macrophages, rare lymphocytes, and rare plasma cells. Macrophages that contain fragmented or granular *M. leprae* forming a foamy appearance are known as foam cells, namely, leprosy cells, which are a characteristic change of LL. Endothelial cell proliferation in minor vascular vessels containing abundant bacteria commonly develops into necrotic vasculitis in the skin, resulting in ulceration. Characterized by onionskin-like appearance, dermal perineurium has infiltration of histiocytes and plasma cells, with mild swelling of nerve tracts.

13.3.2.4 Other Undifferentiated Leprosy

The cases of this type have no specific manifestations, which occurs commonly in the early stage of leprosy and can be healed by itself or develops into another type of leprosy. The pathological changes include nonspecific inflammation and lymphocytic infiltration around the dermic neurovascular bundles. The detection of *M. leprae* in the nerve tracts can define the diagnosis.

13.4 Clinical Symptoms and Signs

Leprosy has a chronic onset, with no obvious symptoms in the early stage. The incubation period lasts averagely for 2–5 years, and in some cases, it may be up to above 10 years. The severity of clinical manifestations varies, including self-healed asymptomatic skin rashes in mild cases and progressively destructive conditions in severe cases. The three basic characteristic manifestations of leprosy include loss of skin sensation, edema of peripheral nerves, and the presence of acid-fast bacilli by smear test of tissues at skin lesions. The early symptoms of the disease are nonspecific low-grade fever, general upset, muscular soreness and pain, and strange skin sensation. Advanced lepromatous leprosy commonly involves the eyes, testes, ovaries, bones, liver, spleen, and other tissues and organs.

13.4.1 Main Clinical Manifestations

13.4.1.1 Skin Lesions

Most patients sustain skin lesions of different severity, and the skin lesions are diverse, including macula, papule, node, ulcer, and atrophy. Skin appendages such as hairs, eyebrows, and lanugo may shed off; sweat glands and sebaceous glands may be destroyed causing perspiration stagnation and dry skin. And *M. leprae* can be detected in skin lesions.

13.4.1.2 Symptoms of Peripheral Nerves

Almost all patients sustain peripheral nerve impairments in different severity. The cases with only neurological symptoms but no skin lesions are defined as simplex neuritis leprosy, which mainly involve terminal nerves and superficial nerve trunks such as ulnar nerves, median nerves, common peroneal nerves, and facial nerves. The nerves are spindle-like, nodular, or evenly thick in shape. In the early stage, superficial sensory dysfunction occurs, followed by sensation loss of consecutively warmth, pain, and touch. The conditions further develop into nerve paralysis or muscle atrophy, resulting in impaired vascular dilation and constriction. Consequently, insufficient blood supply causes malnutrition of limbs, with manifestations of chapped skin, blister, ulcer, cyanosis of fingers and/or toes, swelling, and decreased body temperature.

13.4.2 Clinical Typing

13.4.2.1 Tuberculoid Leprosy (TL)

TL is the most common clinical type, accounting for 60–70 % of leprosy cases. The host of this type has a strong immunity to confine the infection. The main clinical manifestations are skin lesions and peripheral neurological lesions, which are commonly unilateral with a small range and no involvement of organs and mucosa. Therefore, patients of this type have stable conditions. The examinations for *M. leprae* usually show negative results, but the lepromin test usually shows strongly positive result. This type of leprosy tends to self-heal, with no infectivity and favorable prognosis.

13.4.2.2 Borderline Tuberculoid Leprosy (BTL)

The host of this type has strong immunity that is capable of partly resisting the growth of *M. leprae*. The skin lesions are in a large quantity and distribute extensively but asymmetrically, with multiple shapes. Many peripheral nerves are involved, with lesions distributing asymmetrically. BTL is usually accompanied by deformities of hands and feet and unilateral numbness of limbs with sole ulcer, burning, or infection of fingers. The examination of skin lesions for bacteria shows positive results. The lepromin test may be weakly positive, suspected positive, or negative. BTL type has a favorable prognosis, which can turn into TL type after standard therapies. Otherwise, due to effects of adverse factors, it may also turn into BL type or LL type.

13.4.2.3 Borderline Leprosy (BL)

BL is characterized by multiple skin lesions in various complex shapes. The nerve lesions are multiple and soft and are moderately swelling. This type of condition can be accompanied by mucosa lesions, lymph node lesions, testis lesions, and organ lesions. The examination of the lesions for *M. leprae* shows positive result, but the lepromin test is negative. Due to unstable cellular immunity, leprosy reactions and transformation into another type occur.

13.4.2.4 Borderline Lepromatous Leprosy (BLL)

The manifestations of this type are similar to those of lepromatous leprosy, but with a mild severity. In the early stage, the mucosa can be involved, and in the late stage, organs can be involved, with occurrence of saddle nose, ulcer of nasal mucosa, and enlarged lymph nodes. Routine bacteria examination for *M. leprae* shows strongly positive result, but the lepromin test is negative. The patient has cellular immunity compromised. Due to the unstable immunity of the patients with this clinical type of leprosy, it can develop into TL type or LL type.

13.4.2.5 Lepromatous Leprosy (LL)

This is another immunocompromised extremity of clinical leprosy. The lesions are diffusive and widespread, with slight damages to tissues. The skin lesions are small and multiple, distributing extensively and symmetrically, with light color. The lesions involve thick nerves with no obvious lesions. However, the cases in middle and advanced stages may develop serious muscular atrophy and deformity due to extensive symmetric involvement of nerve trunks (Figs. 13.1 and 13.2). Its occurrence in the face may lead to the formation of typical lion face. The commonly found ulcers in the limbs can hardly be healed. One of the important features of LL is the shedding of eyebrows. The nasal mucosa can be

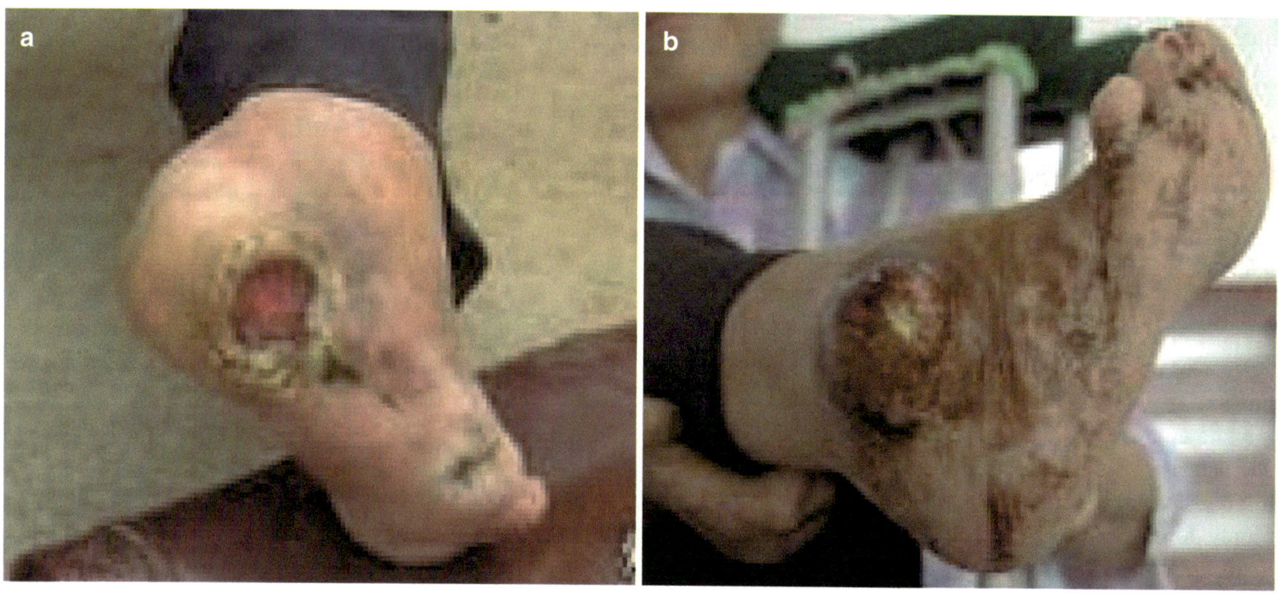

Fig. 13.1 Foot ulceration in a patient with leprosy

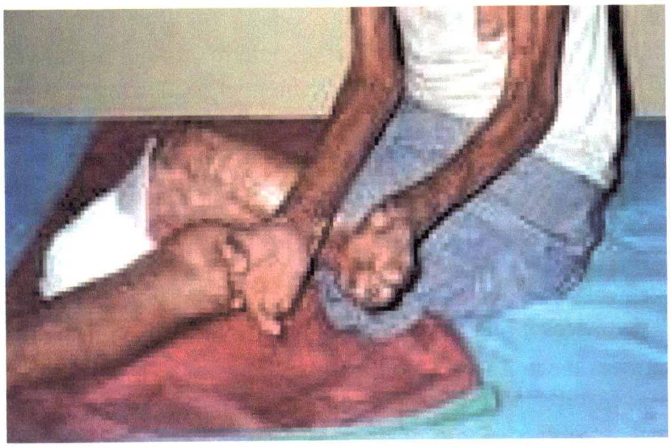

Fig. 13.2 Deformities of fingers and toes in patients with leprosy

involved early and saddle nose occurs in the advanced stage. The most common ocular lesions are cornea and iris lesions, which may result in permanent vision decrease or blindness. The liver, spleen, testis, and breasts can also be involved. Bone lesions are mainly found at the short bones in the hands and feet, commonly bone destruction and absorption due to involved blood circulation and malnutrition. The above organ lesions are more common in patients in advanced lepromatous leprosy, especially in untreated patients. Generally, immediate death rarely occurs.

13.5 Leprosy-Related Complications

In the chronic course of leprosy, the immune responses to antigen of *M. leprae* can be triggered to cause acute allergic symptoms, which are known as leprosy reactions. Based on the immunological features and clinical manifestations, the leprosy reactions can be categorized into type I allergic reactions and type II allergic reactions. The clinical manifestations include reddish swollen skin lesions or erythema nodules as well as swollen and painful peripheral nerves and commonly accompanying rapid loss of nerve functions. These symptoms should be immediately managed to avoid permanent disabilities.

13.5.1 Type I Leprosy Reactions (Delayed-Type Hypersensitivity)

This type is commonly found in patients with borderline leprosy who have unstable immunity, which is also known as reverse response. The manifestations include nodule and erythema of original skin lesions with accompanying elevated edema or newly developed skin lesions with redness, swelling, and pain and disturbance of sensation and movement due to progressive neuritis. Type I leprosy reaction gradually occurs with a duration of several weeks.

13.5.2 Type II Leprosy Reactions (Humoral Immunity)

Type II leprosy reactions, also known as erythema nodosum leprosum reaction, is found in treated or untreated patients with multibacillary leprosy. The manifestation includes painful skin nodules at the face and limbs in a diameter of 2–5 mm. In the cases with severe leprosy reactions, the skin lesions are multimorphic and erythematous with accompanying systemic symptoms, including fever, fatigue, painful limbs, and even iridocyclitis, orchitis, neuritis, arthritis, and enlarged lymph nodes. The natural course of the reaction lasts for 1–2 weeks, and many patients may experience repeated onsets of the reaction.

13.6 Diagnostic Examinations

13.6.1 Laboratory Tests

13.6.1.1 Lepromin Test

The test result provides important reference for typing and prognosis of leprosy, but does not contribute to its diagnosis.

13.6.1.2 ELISA

ELISA is applied to detect PGL-1 IgM antibody in serum of patients. The result facilitates monitoring of patients with multibacillary infection and thus is valuable in clinical treatment. However, the detection rate of the antibody is low in patients with paucibacillary infection.

13.6.1.3 Human Neuron Antibody Test

The result provides reference for early diagnosis of various types of leprosy.

13.6.1.4 Antigen Detection

The PGL-1 monoclonal antibody is applied to detect the specific antigen in pathological sections of the patient. Such a detection is expected to be a new specific diagnostic examination for leprosy.

13.6.2 Diagnostic Imaging

13.6.2.1 Ultrasound

It is commonly applied for the examination of the abdomen, including hepatic lesions and splenic lesions.

13.6.2.2 X-Ray Radiology

It is commonly applied for the examination of the limbs, spinal column, and bone lesions of the pelvis.

13.6.2.3 CT Scanning

It is commonly applied for the examination of the lungs, liver, spleen, as well as bone and joints.

13.6.2.4 MR Imaging

It is commonly applied for the diagnosis of lesions in the peripheral nerves.

13.7 Imaging Demonstrations

13.7.1 Bones and Joints

Based on the pathological changes of bones and joints, the X-ray demonstrations can be categorized into specific lesions and nonspecific lesions. The nonspecific lesions are more commonly found by X-ray radiology.

13.7.1.1 Specific Lesions

The invasion of *M. leprae* into the bone tissues usually involves only distal metaphysis of phalanges. The metaphysis of tubular bones has the richest nutrients and blood supply, where the capillaries are in a circular curved arrangement with slow blood flow. Therefore, *M. leprae* is more likely to be stagnated and multiply at this location to produce leprosy-related neoplastic granuloma, erosive and destructive bone with the formation of cystoid lesions or extensive osteoporosis, and destructive vascular branches.

> **Case Study 1**
> A female patient aged 58 years had a history of mixed leprosy for 15 years.
> For case detail and figures, please refer to Faget and Mayoral. *Radiology*, 1944, 42 (1): 1.

> **Case Study 2**
> A female patient aged 37 years had a history of nodular leprosy for 10 years.
> For case detail and figures, please refer to Faget and Mayoral. *Radiology*, 1944, 42 (1): 1.

Bone Cystic Changes

It is the destructive reactions of granulation tissues in patients with bone leprosy, which are commonly found in the metaphysis of phalanges or metacarpus. The lesion is a confined small round osteoporosis area with thin and poorly defined boundary that is possibly sclerotic. The bone trabecula is deranged or absent.

Bone-Expansive Changes

The diseased bone has extensively decreased density and the bone trabecula has osteoporosis or is absent. The bone marrow cavity is dilated and enlarged to cause a thicker and irregular appearance of the bone. The bone cortex is thin, which is more common in long bones of limbs and trunk.

According to the course of the disease, Paterson divided bone lesions into three stages: the reaction stage, the healing stage, and the healed stage.

1. *The reaction stage.* This stage is characterized by poorly defined osteoporotic region, reticular bone trabecula, and small round osteolytic defects. The lesions are commonly located in the phalangeal distal center and develop into multiple cystic bone inflammation, which resembles to tubercular phalangitis.
2. *The healing stage.* The small osteolytic defect area is more clearly defined with no sclerotic edge.
3. *The healed stage.* The small osteolytic defect area is absent, and residual osteolytic lesion can be found in large defect, with sclerotic edge, endosteal hyperplasia, and medullary canal occlusion.

13.7.1.2 Nonspecific Lesions

Enlarged Bone Nutrient Artery Hole

It often occurs in the distal end of first hand phalanx, with localized narrow or cystic bone defects whose diameter can be up to 0.5 cm (normally 0.1 cm) and edges are slightly irregular. Such a condition is commonly found in cases of lepromatous leprosy. These signs are relatively fine and can be found in early stage.

> **Case Study 3**
> A male patient aged 64 years had a history of lepromatous leprosy for 6 years.
> For case detail and figures, please refer to Enna CD et al. *Radiology*, 1971, 100 (2): 295.

Case Study 4
A male patient aged 34 years had a history of lepromatous leprosy for 4 years.

For case detail and figures, please refer to Enna CD et al. *Radiology*, 1971, 100 (2): 295.

Osteolysis and Bone Absorption

Osteolysis and bone absorption are main reasons for limb disabilities in patients with leprosy, which can be divided into two types, common bone absorption and intensive bone absorption.

Common Bone Absorption

Phalangeal absorption commonly begins from the distal fingertip, with a V-shaped defect or sharpened fingertip. The fingertip is then flattened, and the bone absorption extends upwards to cause lysis, shedding, and absence of most part of the distal phalanx. Otherwise, rare irregular bone fragments remain. Consequently, irregular osteolysis and bone absorption occur in the middle phalanx and then the first phalanx. Such changes rarely involve the metacarpus and carpal bones. Foot bone absorption begins at the distal phalanx and metatarsophalangeal joint, and the whole course of bone absorption resembles to hand phalangeal absorption. The absorption of metatarsophalangeal joint has early manifestations of blurry and erosive joint surface and narrowed space, possibly with dislocation or incomplete dislocation. The bone absorption continues to spread upwards to the middle phalange and proximal metatarsal bone, possibly with the tarsal bone involved.

Intensive Bone Absorption

The short bone shaft gradually becomes thin evenly, with increasingly narrowed marrow cavity and thickened bone cortex. The involved bone ends remain normal. In other words, the whole bone shaft becomes pointy and slender in appearance, which is commonly found in phalanges and metacarpal bones.

Case Study 5
Bone inflammation in a patient with leprosy

For case detail and figures, please refer to Enna CD et al. *Radiology*, 1971, 100 (2): 295.

Case Study 6
Bone inflammation in a patient with leprosy

For case detail and figures, please refer to Enna CD et al. *Radiology*, 1971, 100 (2): 295.

Case Study 7
Periostitis in a case of leprosy, with clinical manifestation of red legs

For case detail and figures, please refer to Enna CD et al. *Radiology*, 1971, 100 (2): 295.

Secondary Infection

The infection of skin soft tissues can spread to involve adjacent bones and joints and cause leprosy periostitis, osteitis, and osteomyelitis. The X-ray demonstrations of leprosy osteomyelitis are the same as those of common purulent osteomyelitis. However, leprosy osteomyelitis is characterized by chronic bone destruction and accompanying bone absorption. Leprosy arthritis commonly occurs in interphalangeal joints, metatarsophalangeal joints, and ankle joints, with manifestations of bone absorption, bone atrophy, joint destruction and depression, joint bone lysis, or accompanying joint dislocation and deformity, with possible messy existence of small bone fragments. The manifestations resemble to those of Charcot arthrosis.

For case detail and figures, please refer to Enna CD, et al. *Radiology*, 1971, 100 (2): 295.

Osteoporosis

The X-ray demonstrations include sparse and blurry bone markings, widened space or even absent space, rough and sparse bone structure, decreased bone density, and thin bone cortex. In addition to traumatic infection and nerve malnutrition, osteoporosis due to immobilization and limbs deformity also contributes to occurrence of leprosy osteoporosis.

Fracture

Comminuted fracture is more common in patients with leprosy. The callus forms at the site of breakage with favorable healing, which is different from those of common pathological fractures.

It has been reported that in the early stage of tuberculoid leprosy, the manifestations include claw hand deformity, articular changes, atrophy and absorption of bones, as well as osteolytic defects. And it has been also reported that in the cases of lepromatous leprosy, bone cystic changes, enlarged nutrient vessel holes, and osteoporosis are more common.

Case Study 8
A male patient aged 22 years had a history of lepromatous leprosy for 5 years. By smear examination of the suctions from hand cysts, sphere-like acid-tolerant bacteria are found.

For case detail and figures, please refer to Faget and Mayoral. *Radiology*, 1944, 42 (1): 1.

Case Study 9
A male patient aged 22 years had a history of lepromatous leprosy for 17 years and then developed into mixed leprosy.

For case detail and figures, please refer to Faget and Mayoral. *Radiology*, 1944, 42 (1): 1.

Case Study 10
A male patient aged 42 years had a history of mixed leprosy for 7 years.

For case detail and figures, please refer to Faget and Mayoral. *Radiology*, 1944, 42 (1): 1.

13.7.2 Neurotrophic Osteoarthrosis

Neurotrophic osteoarthrosis, also known as Charcot joint, is an osteoarthrosis caused by multiple factors. The manifestations include central or peripheral nerve lesion-induced sensory disturbance, joint swelling, bone destruction and absorption, and deranged joint structures.

13.7.2.1 X-Ray

The X-ray demonstrations are divided into three types: absorptive type, hyperplastic type, and mixed type. It is generally believed that bone absorption is the primary pathological change of the disease, followed by bone hyperplasia, periosteal reaction, and ectopic ossification. Therefore, bone absorption is the early X-ray demonstration, while secondary hyperplastic and mixed changes can be demonstrated by X-ray in the middle and advanced stages.

The early X-ray demonstrations of Charcot joint include widened articular interspace, clearly defined joint surface, and increased density of soft tissues. The early stage can last for a long period of time. With further development of the conditions, the articular cartilages are destructed to narrow down the joint interspace. Meanwhile, the subchondral bone is destructed and absorbed to cause irregular joint surface and loss of articular stability. Therefore, the sign of dislocation can be found. After that, the bone destruction occurs under the joint surface, while the bone and periosteum show compensatory hyperplasia and sclerosis. At the same time, lysis and rupture occur at the joint surface, with deposition of many irregular bone fragments in the joint and the soft tissues surrounding the joint. In addition, ectopic depositions of calcified substances further increase local density that causes varying densities. In this stage, typical X-ray demonstrations can be found including swelling of articular soft tissues, articular dislocations or incomplete dislocations, bone absorption, bone hyperplasia and sclerosis, joint lysis and rupture, multiple multimorphic bone fragments in the joint and its surrounding soft tissues, and calcification opacities.

For different locations of lesions, the X-ray demonstrations are also different. The lesions of the knee and ankle joints can be demonstrated as rupture and lysis of bone ends, many bone fragments in the articular interspace, and obvious bone hyperplasia at the margin. The lesions of hip joint are demonstrated as acetabular destruction with shallow and enlarged acetabula, bone absorption of femoral head, no increased density of bone ends, and articular free bodies. The lesions of shoulder joint are characterized by flattened and shallow glenoid cavity, atrophy of humeral head, and accompanying ligament calcification. The lesions of phalangeal joint are characterized by obvious bone destruction and accompanying inflammatory changes of local soft tissues).

13.7.2.2 CT Scanning and MR Imaging

In demonstrating early lesions and small bone fragments, CT scanning is superior to X-ray radiology. MR imaging can demonstrate more details. In addition to destructed bone structure, MR imaging can demonstrate earlier about swelling of soft tissues, articular effusion, joint cartilage destruction, edema of bone marrow, and small bone fracture.

Case Study 11
A male patient aged 36 years had a history of mixed leprosy for 20 years, with complication of syphilitic infection.

For case detail and figures, please refer to Faget and Mayoral. *Radiology*, 1944, 42 (1): 1.

Case Study 12
For case detail and figures, please refer to Faget and Mayoral. *Radiology*, 1944, 42 (1): 1.

Case Study 13
A female patient aged 49 years had a history of mixed leprosy for 17 years.

For case detail and figures, please refer to Enna CD et al. *Radiology*, 1971, 100 (2): 295.

Case Study 14
Leprosy hand deformity

For case detail and figures, please refer to Ankad Balachandra S. et al. *Journal of Clinical and Diagnostic Research*, 2011, 5 (4): 703.

Case Study 15
A female patient aged 38 years had a history of mixed leprosy for 13 years.

For case detail and figures, please refer to Faget and Mayoral. *Radiology*, 1944, 42 (1): 1.

13.7.3 Lesions of Nerves and Skin

13.7.3.1 Ultrasound

High-resolution ultrasonography and color Doppler ultrasound can be applied to detect nerve lesions of patients with leprosy via demonstrations of slow blood supply increase, abnormal echo signal, and thickened nerves. Blood flow signal of increased blood supply can be detected at inflammation involved endoneurium and epineurium in patients with leprosy. The peripheral nerves in patients with leprosy are usually thickened, which are more commonly found at median nerves and ulnar nerves. The thickened nerves are more commonly found in patients with type I and type II reactions whose impaired nerves and their distal nerves are displayed with increased blood supply. Studies have demonstrated that thickened nerves with the enlarged sites being close to the compressive side of median nerves and ulnar nerves, occasionally abnormal length of nerves, and decreased body temperature at the thickened end indicate possible infection of *M. leprae*.

Case Study 16
Ultrasound demonstrations of normal peripheral nerves

For case detail and figures, please refer to Jain S. et al. *PLoS Negl Trop Dis*, 2009, 11, 3 (8): e498.

Case Study 17
Changes of peripheral nerves in a patient with leprosy

For case detail and figures, please refer to Jain S. et al. *PLoS Negl Trop Dis*, 2009, 11, 3 (8): e498.

13.7.3.2 MR Imaging

MR imaging can detect early neuritis with demonstrations of thickened peripheral nerves and inflammation. Ankad et al. reported that MRI can be applied to detect inflammation of the ulnar nerve, edema of the soft tissues, and changes of bone marrow.

For case detail and figures, please refer to Slim FJ et al. *Lepr Rev*, 2009, 80 (4): 373.

13.7.4 Tropic Ulcer

Ulceration in the acute or chronic stage indicates vascular leakage with accompanying early venous backflow, which is consistent with arteriovenous fistula. In the ulceration area, a typical vascular vessel usually appears, and the intravascular contrast agent passes through this vessel more rapidly than that through other vascular vessels. Therefore, angiography of lower limbs can effectively examine the vascular vessels in the areas with ulceration.

13.7.5 Lesions of the Liver and Spleen

In the advanced stage of *M. leprae* infection, reticular endothelial system is commonly impaired, including impaired liver, spleen, and bone marrow, especially in the cases of lepromatous leprosy. Doppler ultrasound demonstrations of the lesions can be divided into following two types.

13.7.5.1 Normal Type

The morphology and size of both the liver and spleen are normal. There is no pathological echo from the internal parenchyma of the liver and spleen, and both organs have clearly defined vascular network.

13.7.5.2 Swelling Type

The morphology of the liver and spleen is quite normal with their core diameters being longer than normal levels. The parenchymal echogenic dots are thickened and denser and changes can be found in the vascular network.

13.7.6 Others

Borderline lepromatous leprosy can also cause enlarged lymph nodes, skin rashes, and other lesions. By diagnostic imaging, corresponding demonstrations can be found (Fig. 13.3).

Case Study 18

A female patient aged 64 years. In 2008, the patient suffered from systemic sporadic erythema nodosa with no known causes. Erythema nodosa are occasionally itchy, with no effusion, suppuration, and desquamation, and the skin rashes mainly occurred in her face. The skin pathology indicated inflammatory granuloma and PAS staining negative, with subsequent diagnosis of sarcoidosis. After treatment, the skin rashes gradually improved. She withdrew the medications of prednisone and thalidomide 2 years ago. In the year 2012, she began to experience systematic widespread skin rashes that are more obvious in the face with accompanying itch and slight pain. In a local hospital, she was given anti-infectious and anti-allergic therapies with no obvious effectiveness. By physical examination, she had scattering infiltrative erythema and nodules in different sizes in the face, ulceration based on erythema; scattering ring-shaped dark red spots at the trunk; and soybean-sized nodules at the lower limbs that are hard and painless. Ultrasonography indicated enlarged right supraclavicular, bilateral axillary, and bilateral inguinal lymph nodes. In May 2012, the skin biopsy indicated inflammatory granuloma and PAS staining negative that cannot exclude the possibility of leprosy. The finding of positive *M. leprae*, in combination to skin biopsy, indicated the diagnosis of borderline lepromatous leprosy.

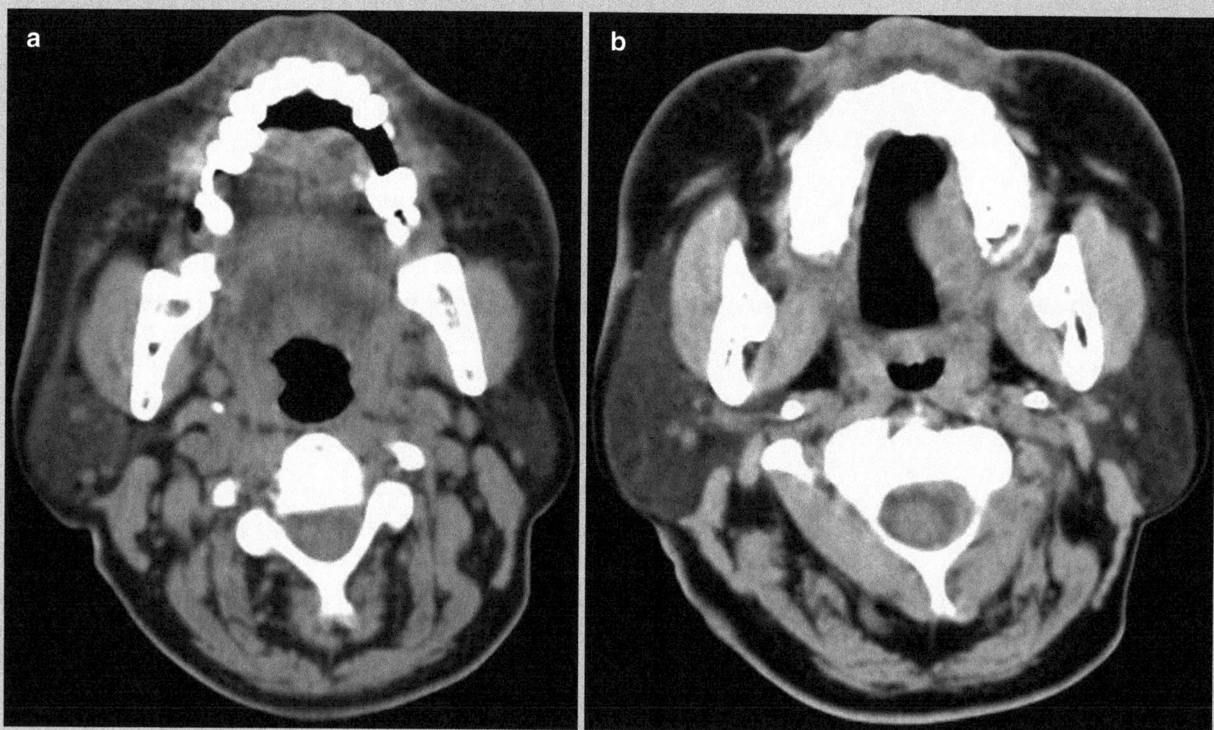

Fig. 13.3 Facial changes of the patient with borderline lepromatous leprosy. (**a**, **b**) Cervical CT scan demonstrates multiple irregular lesions with low-density and clearly defined boundaries

Note: the case and image are provided by Tang, YH. at Rui Jin Hospital, Shanghai, China.

13.8 Diagnostic Basis

13.8.1 The Diagnosis of Leprosy

The diagnosis of leprosy can be established based on comprehensive analysis of the epidemiological history, clinical manifestations, bacteriological examination, and pathology. The diagnostic basis is as the following: (1) a history of contact, living in an epidemic area, or close contact to patient with leprosy; (2) early occurrence of skin lesions with accompanying superficial sensory disturbance and perspiration stagnation, or area of sensory numbness; (3) thick peripheral nerve trunk or cutaneous branch nerves; (4) the finding of *M. leprae* in skin lesion or tissue sections; and (5) special pathological changes by histopathological examinations.

Among the abovementioned (1–4), the diagnosis for the cases with only one item of findings should be cautious. The diagnosis for the cases with two or the above two items of finding commonly can be established. The diagnosis for the cases with (5) and detection of *M. leprae* can be defined.

13.8.2 Neurotropic Osteoarthrosis

Patients with leprosy have clinical manifestations of swollen and deformed joints that are painless, as well as normal articular movements.

X-ray radiology demonstrates swollen tissues, articular bone absorption as well as bone hyperplasia and sclerosis, deranged articular structures as well as articular lysis and deformity, multiple multimorphic fragments, and calcification in the joints and their surrounding soft tissues.

13.9 Differential Diagnosis

13.9.1 Differential Diagnosis of Leprosy

Leprosy should be differentiated from various skin diseases and various types of neuritis. The differential diagnosis can be made based on the findings of leprosy manifestations including superficial sensory disturbances, perspiration stagnation, thick nerves, and other tests findings. The cases of leprosy commonly have multimorphic skin lesions with concurrent peripheral nerve involvements, which can be the basis for its differentiation from simplex skin diseases. In combination to skin scrapings for bacteriological examination and pathological examination, correct diagnosis can be established.

13.9.2 Differential Diagnosis of Neurotropic Osteoarthrosis

13.9.2.1 Osteoarthritis

Osteoarthritis has manifestations of movement disorders and pain, but with no decreased or absent sensation. X-ray radiology demonstrates sclerosis of the articular surface, intact bone of the articular surface, no bone lysis and absorption, no soft tissue swelling, and no joint dislocation.

13.9.2.2 Synovial Osteochondroma of the Joint

Synovial osteochondroma of the joint has manifestations of intact bone of the articular surface with no bone lysis, regular shape of synovial osteochondroma, and clearly defined boundary and the tumor in size of a pomegranate seed.

13.9.2.3 Gouty Arthritis

The cases of gouty arthritis have a history of intermittent onset, with increased blood and urine acid. It commonly involves toes and metatarsophalangeal joints. The gouty tophus in the soft tissues adjacent to involved joint may cause eccentric swelling and marginal penetrating destruction of bone ends. X-ray commonly fails to demonstrate gouty tophus, which is different from multiple bone fragments surrounding the joint.

13.9.2.4 Hemophilic Arthritis

The cases of hemophilic arthritis have an apparent bleeding history, with hematocele in joint capsule-induced articular swelling and increased density. Erosion may occur in the osseous articular surface. Subcartilaginous trabecular bone absorption and collapse may also occur in osseous articular surfaces. However, deranged articular structures rarely occur and free bone fragments are rarely found.

13.9.2.5 Rheumatoid Arthritis

The lesions commonly involve proximal interphalangeal joints and distal joints of limbs, with no destructive bone absorption at bone ends. The cases have a history of migratory articular swelling and pain, with serum rheumatoid factor positive.

References

Sun PW, Yu MW, Yan LB, et al. Epidemiological analysis of leprosy in China in 2010. J Nanjing Med Univ (Nat Sci Ed). 2012;32(2):155–9.

Jain S, Visser LH, Praveen TL, et al. High-resolution sonography: a new technique to detect nerve damage in leprosy. PLoS Negl Trop Dis. 2009;3(8), e498.

Enna CD, Jacobson RR, Rausch RO. Bone changes in leprosy: a correlation of clinical and radiographic features. Radiology. 1971;100(2):295–306.

Slim FJ, Faber WR, Maas M. The role of radiology in nerve function impairment and its musculoskeletal complications in leprosy. Lepr Rev. 2009;80(4):373–87.

Ankad Balachandra S, Hombal A, Sudhakar R, et al. Radiological changes in the hands and feet of Leprosy patients with deformities. J Clin Diagn Res. 2011;5(4):703–7.

Faget GH, Mayoral A. Bone changes in Leprosy: a clinical and roentgenologic study of 505 cases. Radiology. 1944;42(1): 1–13.

Suggested Reading

Ma YL. Studies of infectious diseases. Shanghai: Shanghai Science and Technology Press; 2011.

Zhang LX, Zhou XZ. Modern studies of infectious diseases. Beijing: People's Military Medical Press; 2010.

Li N. (translator), Oxford studies of infectious diseases. Beijing: People's Medical Publishing House; 2011.

Prevalence of leprosy in 2010 by WTO. Leprosy update, 2011. Wkly Epidemiol Record. 2011; 86(36):389–99.

Johnson AC, Reddy R, Johnson S, et al. Lower limb angiography in leprosy. Radiology. 1978;126(2):327–32.

14 Leptospirosis

Ruili Li, Hongjun Li, and Aidong Zhang

Leptospirosis, also known as field fever, is an acute infectious zoonosis with natural focus caused by various pathogenic leptospiras. Rodents and pigs are the major sources of its infection, which has an acute onset. At its early stage, the symptoms include high fever, fatigue and weakness, systemic pain soreness, conjunctival congestion, calf tenderness, as well as swelling of superficial lymph nodes. At its middle stage, it is clinically characterized by diffuse pulmonary bleeding and apparent lesions at the liver, kidneys, and the central nervous system. At its advanced stage, most patients can be cured, but some rare patients may further develop fever, ocular uveitis, and occlusive cerebral arteritis. Leptospirosis is a globally distributed disease, more commonly affecting the tropical and subtropical areas.

14.1 Etiology

Leptospira is categorized into the order of Spirochaetales, the genus *Leptospira*, and the family of Treponema. Currently, the genus *Leptospira* is divided into two species: *Leptospira interrogans* and *Leptospira biflexa. Leptospira interrogans* is pathogenic to humans and animals while *Leptospira biflexa* leads a free life. The pathogen of leptospirosis, belonging to the genus *Leptospira,* is pathogenic to humans, livestock, and wild animals. The pathogenic *Leptospira* is slender and cylinder shaped, with 12–18 fine treponemas twining delicately and regularly around. The appearance is just like a watchband with regularly arranged coils. With no flagella, the thallus is curved in a C or S shape, since either or both of its ends bend like a hook. The length of thallus varies from 4 to 20 μm, with a mean length of 6–10 μm and a mean diameter of 0.1–0.2 μm. The leptospira has active movements, which rotates steadily around the long axis with both soft ends and rigid middle part. And the penetrating strength is strong. *Leptospira*, composed of the type-specific antigen and the group-specific antigen, has a complex antigenic structure.

Leptospira is Gram negative. In the past, the bacteria were stained black by the silver staining and light red by the Giemsa staining. Currently, the bacteria can be observed after immunofluorescence and immunoenzyme staining. *Leptospira* has a strong resistance to the environment and can be survive in a cold, humid, and weak base environment for a long period of time. It is very sensitive to dryness, heat, acid, alkali, and disinfectants.

14.2 Epidemiology

14.2.1 Distribution

Leptospirosis affects many areas around the world, mainly prevailing in tropical and subtropical areas. It can be found in 31 provinces, cities, and autonomous regions in mainland China, especially the southwestern area and the southern area of mainland China.

14.2.2 Source of Infection

Rodents and pigs are two major sources of its infection. And they can excrete the bacteria along with urination for a long period of time.

14.2.3 Route of Transmission

There are three major routes of its transmission. In most cases, contract to leptospira-contaminated water is the most important route of its transmission.

R. Li • H. Li (✉) • A. Zhang
Department of Radiology, Beijing You'an Hospital,
Capital Medical University, Beijing, China
e-mail: lihongjun00113@126.com

H. Li (ed.), *Radiology of Infectious Diseases: Volume 2*, DOI 10.1007/978-94-017-9876-1_14

14.2.3.1 Contact Transmission

Leptospiras can survive in the body of wild animals for a long period of time. It can spread from livestock to humans and from livestock via wild animals to humans. The urine carrying leptospiras discharged by rats and pigs can contaminate their external environment (e.g., water and soil). Humans with common contacts to the contaminated water or soil are at a high risk of invasion by the bacteria via wounded skin.

14.2.3.2 Transmission via the Nasal Mucosa and Gastrointestinal Mucosa

Leptospiras can be transmitted via mucosa at the gastrointestinal tract, respiratory tract, and reproductive system.

14.2.3.3 Others

Leptospira can infect humans via breast feeding and congenital infection. Humans are rarely infected by bacteria-containing urine from patients.

14.2.4 Susceptible Population

Populations are generally susceptible. Farmers, fishermen, drainage workers, slaughterhouse workers, and animal raisers have higher occurrence of infection due to their common contacts to contaminated water. The persons traveling in the epidemic area are more susceptible than local residents due to their weak immunity. After the infection, the immunity against the same type of pathogens can be acquired. Sporadic cases can be found all year round in high-temperature areas, slaughterhouses, and mining areas.

14.2.5 Epidemic Features

14.2.5.1 Age of Onset

Leptospirosis commonly occurs in young and middle-aged adult farmers, with a peak incidence in the group aged 10–39 years. Male patients account for above 80 % due to their increased chances of infection.

14.2.5.2 Prevailing Season

Leptospirosis commonly prevails in July, August, and September, with a peak incidence in August and September.

14.2.5.3 Types of Prevalence

Prevalence with Rainfall

During the rainy seasons, water tends to deposit both inside and out of the villages. In addition to overflow of feces and urine containing the bacteria discharged by animals, the environment is contaminated with the following possible occurrence of outbreak.

Prevalence in Rice Field

Rats are the major sources of the disease in this prevailing type. When rats eat the rice in the rice field, they may urinate in the field. Thus, farmers working then in the field are more likely to contract the disease via their contact with the contaminated water.

Prevalence with Flood

Flood may wash away the livestock sheds with leptospiras and therefore be contaminated for spreading of the disease. In such prevailing type, outbreak commonly occurs with pigs as the major source of infection.

Sporadic Prevalence

As a variety of animals carrying leptospiras are distributed widely, many areas and places may be contaminated by the bacteria.

14.3 Pathogenesis and Pathological Changes

Leptospira can be divided into several types, all of which have both variant-specific surface antigen and common internal antigen. Different variants have different pathogenicity to humans, with different human organs involved. The relationship between its variants and clinical typing is complex. The same variant may cause different types of clinical symptoms, while the same clinical type of symptoms can be induced by different variants.

14.3.1 Pathogenesis

After invading the organism via skin or mucosa, the leptospiras grow and reproduce rapidly in the blood. In the first week of after onset, the pathogens can be found in the peripheral blood, which are then eliminated by the reticular endothelial system. In the organism, endothelial injuries develop in the small blood vessels and cause vascular bleeding and migration of the leptospiras into the tissues, resulting in relative hypoxia of the tissues. The incubation period usually lasts for 1–2 weeks, followed by the onset of systemic symptoms caused by the toxins released after the reproduction and disintegration of the bacteria.

14.3.1.1 Route of Invasion, Reproduction in the Organisms, and Systemic Toxic Symptoms

After invading into human body via skin wound or mucosae at the oral cavity, nose, intestinal tract, and eye conjunctiva, the leptospiras spread into the blood circulation and different organs (including the cerebrospinal fluid and eyes) via the lymph vessels and small blood vessels, resulting in bacteremia after rapid reproduction.

14.3.1.2 Organ Damages

The severity of the organ damages depends on the type and virulence of leptospiras as well as the body reactions. Clinically, the conditions are characterized by different clinical types due to prominent symptoms of one certain organ, such as diffuse pulmonary bleeding, icteric bleeding, renal failure, and meningoencephalitis.

14.3.1.3 Nonspecific and Specific Responses at the Middle and Late Stages

The initial response of human body to invasion of leptospiras is characterized by an increased count of neutrophils in the blood and mild inflammatory responses, with no infiltration of white blood cells and no suppuration. The reticular endothelial cells are subject to apparent proliferation with a distinct phagocytic ability. The swelling of superficial lymph nodes can be observed in the groin and other parts of the body. And these responses are nonspecific.

About 1 week after the onset, specific antibodies can be detected, firstly IgM and following IgG. The titers of specific antibodies peak in the first month of the whole illness course. After the emergence of specific antibodies, the symptoms of leptospiremia gradually disappear. However, leptospiras can still survive, reproduce, and be excreted along with urination without being affected by the specific antibodies in the blood. After the immune response is triggered to decrease or eliminate the pathogens in the human body, some patients may experience late-onset fever and late-onset symptoms of the eyes and the nervous system. These manifestations are possibly related to hypersensitivity or the pathogen itself, leptospiras. Some scholars believe that these manifestations are symptoms of remnant infection.

14.3.2 Pathological Changes

The changes of leptospirosis are pathologically categorized into acute systemic toxic lesions, mainly affecting the systemic capillaries and resulting in bleeding and circulatory disturbance of different levels. Meanwhile, severe functional disturbance is caused by extensive degeneration of parenchymal organs and necrosis. The inflammatory responses are commonly mild, with following organ lesions.

14.3.2.1 Lung

Bleeding is the major lesion of the lungs, which is mainly diffusive bleeding with common occurrence in the subpleural area. During recent years, it constitutes the main cause of death in the cases of anicteric leptospirosis. At the surface of lungs, spots and flakes of bleeding can be observed, with mucosal bleeding at the tracheae and bronchi and even interstitial and alveolar bleeding as well as apparent pulmonary edema. Diffuse pulmonary bleeding primarily occurs in the capillaries, which develops gradually from spots to patches and masses. Histological examination demonstrates that intact capillaries in the lung tissues are subject to serious congestion and bleeding. The bronchial lumen and alveolus are filled by red blood cells. In some cases, some alveoli may contain air, possibly with a small quantity of serous fluid exudation. With a purplish-black color, the infected lung is twice or three times as heavy as the normal lung. The section surface is dark red, with overflow of bubble-shaped or dark red bloody fluid.

14.3.2.2 Kidney

The changes of kidneys are pathologically characterized by interstitial nephritis, with swollen kidneys, widened renal cortex, and medullary congestion. Bleeding spots can be observed at the renal pelvis and subcapsular cortex of the kidneys, with blood clots in the renal pelvis in some cases. By microscopy, the main lesions are found at the renal tubules, mostly at the distal convolution and the ascending branch of Henle loop. The epithelial cells at the renal tubules are subject to degeneration and necrosis, with some shedding in the lumen. Lumen obstruction of the renal tubules occurs due to basilar membrane rupture of some renal tubules, dilated renal tubules, and filling of blood cells or hyaline casts in the lumen. By electron microscopy, no changes can be observed in the endothelial cells of the glomerulus, with immune complexes and complement depositing at the basilar membrane of the glomerulus. Edema can be found in the interstitial tissue around the renal tubules, with accompanying infiltration of large monocytes, lymphocytes, as well as rare eosinophils and neutrophils. Leptospiras can be detected in most renal tissues.

14.3.2.3 Liver

The damages to hepatic tissue can vary from mild to severe. The long illness course results in serious damages. In the cases with mild lesions, no apparent changes can be found from the appearance of the liver. By microscopy, mild interstitial edema and vascular congestion as well as sporadic focal necrosis can be observed. In some serious cases, jaundice, bleeding, hepatomegaly, and even hepatic failure occur. Under a microscope, cell infiltration (mainly the neutrophils), swollen hepatocytes, fatty degeneration, and deranged hepatocytes can be observed around the portal area, with accompanying focal necrosis of hepatocytes. Some changes of the liver are pathologically characterized by excretion disturbance of the bile, with hepatocytic necrosis as the less serious lesion. In such cases, slight elevation of serum transaminase can be detected. The occurrence of jaundice may be caused by hepatic inflammation and necrosis as well as obstructed capillary bile ducts and hemolysis.

14.3.2.4 Heart

Myocardial damage is believed to be the major lesion of leptospirosis. Rare bleeding spots and focal necrosis can be observed at the pericardium of patients. By examinations, the myocardium can be demonstrated with hyaline or granular degeneration of the myocardial fibers, usually hydropic degeneration of the myocardial fibers as well as sometimes focal myocardial necrosis and fibrolysis of myocardial fibers. The conditions are commonly accompanied by interstitial inflammation and edema. Electron microscopy demonstrates swollen and empty myocardial mitochondria, with absence of the cristae, blurry and broken muscular filament fibers, as well as absence of the intercalated disk. Vascular damages mainly involve systemic capillaries.

14.3.2.5 Other Organs

Spleen

Generally, the spleen has a normal size but commonly with congestion and small spots or patches of bleeding. The normal structure of the spleen is commonly destroyed.

Adrenal Gland

Bleeding lesions can be frequently observed in the cortex, occasionally with infarct lesions. In most cases, the cortex lipids may be subject to decrease or even absence. Focal or diffuse inflammatory infiltration can be observed at the cortex and medulla.

Pancreas

In the pancreas, necrosis possibly occurs, with surrounding infiltration of neutrophil cells and lymphocytes.

Lymph Nodes

Congestion or bleeding can be discovered in the cervical, supraclavicular, inaugural, and mesenteric lymph nodes, with apparent phagocytosis.

Bone Marrow

The bone marrow can be demonstrated with proliferation of granulocytic system.

Reproductive System

Apparent bleeding can be found at the endometrium, and a small quantity of bleeding is observed at the testis and prostate glands.

Bladder and Ureteral Wall

Spots of bleeding can be observed.

Gastrointestinal Tract

Bleeding occurs at the mouth mucosa, with diffuse congestion and bleeding at the mucosa of the stomach and intestines.

Meninges and Brain Parenchyma

There are congestion, edema, bleeding, infiltration of inflammatory cells, and degeneration of the neurocytes. In addition, cerebral arteritis, infarction, and atrophy may occur.

Skeletal Muscle

The gastrocnemius is observed with swelling, absence of striations, and bleeding, with accompanying sarcoplasmic vacuolation and fusion, only remnant fine particles in the myoplasm, as well as absence of myoplasm and myofibril. The only remained sarcolemma has changed contour due to lytic necrosis. Bleeding and leptospiras can be found in the muscular interstitial tissues. Electron microscopy can demonstrate well-defined structure of the myofilaments as well as swollen mitochondria.

14.4 Clinical Symptoms and Signs

The incubation period generally lasts for 2–20 days, commonly 7–12 days. The clinical symptoms of leptospirosis are extremely complex, ranging from mild with no apparent symptoms to severe with occurrence of death. Factors affecting clinical manifestations include not only the bacterial types or the strain virulence of a same bacteria type but also individual difference as well as immunity of the infected patients. According to Edward and Domm, leptospirosis can be divided into two stages: the septic stage and the immune response stage. In China, Cao divided the illness course into three stages: the early stage, the middle stage, and the advanced stage. The staging of the disease is important to guide the clinical practice, especially the early diagnosis and treatment.

14.4.1 The Early Stage (The Leptospiremic Stage)

The early stage is usually within 3 days after the onset, with the following clinical manifestations.

14.4.1.1 Fever

Its onset is sudden and acute, with accompanying aversion to cold and chills. The body temperature can increase up to 39 °C in a short period of time. Remittent fever is common at this stage.

14.4.1.2 Headache

Headache is apparent, with accompanying systemic myalgia. Gastrocnemius is the most commonly involved muscle.

14.4.1.3 Systemic Upset

Feebleness of legs is commonly observed at this stage.

14.4.1.4 Conjunctival Congestion

Conjunctival congestion is characterized by no secretion, pain or photophobia, and persistent congestion which may persist even after the body temperature returns to normal.

14.4.1.5 Systemic Superficial Lymphadenectasis

It is commonly observed at the groin and armpit. The enlarged lymph nodes are commonly in a size of soybean or horsebean, with tenderness but no congestion, inflammation, and suppuration.

14.4.1.6 Symptoms of the Digestive System

The symptoms include nausea, vomiting, anorexia, and diarrhea.

14.4.2 The Middle Stage (The Organ Lesion Stage)

During days 3–14 after the onset, organ lesion-induced clinical manifestations can be found, including hemoptysis, diffuse pulmonary bleeding, jaundice, extensive bleeding of the skin mucosa, proteinuria, hematuria, cylindruria, renal insufficiency, and meningoencephalitis. The clinical manifestations at this stage constitute the main basis for typing of leptospirosis, which is categorized into pulmonary bleeding type, hemorrhagic icterus type, renal type, and meningitis type.

14.4.2.1 Influenza and Typhoid Type

About 60–80 % of the cases of leptospirosis can be categorized into this type, which is mostly characterized by systemic symptoms. With an acute and sudden onset, the patients experience chills, fever (38–39 °C), headache, conjunctival congestion, and systemic myalgia that is prominently gastrocnemius soreness and pain. There are also symptoms of nasal obstruction, pharyngalgia, and coughs. The clinical manifestations resemble the symptoms of influenza, upper respiratory infection (URI), or typhoid fever. The natural course is usually 5–10 days.

14.4.2.2 Pulmonary Bleeding Type

In addition to the symptoms of leptospiremia, the patients experience coughs, bloody sputum, and hemoptysis. This clinical type can be further divided into common pulmonary bleeding and diffuse pulmonary bleeding according to the range and severity of lesions demonstrated by X-ray radiology as well as the cardiopulmonary manifestations.

Common Pulmonary Bleeding

The clinical symptoms resemble those of leptospiremia, with accompanying hemoptysis and bloody sputum of different degrees. The physical signs of the chest are inapparent. X-ray radiology demonstrates increased pulmonary markings.

Diffuse Pulmonary Bleeding (Massive Pulmonary Hemorrhage)

After invasion of leptospiras into human body, the infected individuals commonly experience an incubation period and a transient period of early infection that commonly lasts for 2–3 days. After that, the patients sustain sudden onset of facial paleness, accelerated heart and breath rate, palpitation and irritation. The conditions may further develop into circulation failure and respiratory failure. At this time, moist rales are overwhelmingly heard at both lungs, and hemoptysis progressively deteriorates. In recent years, they are the common causes of death in the cases of anicteric leptospirosis. X-ray radiology demonstrates diffuse spots and flakes of shadows in both lungs.

14.4.2.3 Hemorrhagic Icterus Type

Most cases are caused by the icterohemorrhagic serotype of leptospira. The clinical manifestation is characterized by hemorrhagic icterus and its mortality rate is high. Jaundice commonly occurs at days 3–7 after the onset and accompanying bleeding of different degrees occurs in 80 % of the cases. This type also features renal and hepatic lesions, with 70–80 % of the cases experiencing involvement of the kidneys. The renal lesions vary from mild symptoms including proteinuria, hematuria, as well as a small quantity of WBC and casts in the urine to severe symptoms including renal insufficiency, oliguria or anuria, acidosis, uremic coma, and even death. Renal failure is the common cause of death in the cases of this type.

14.4.2.4 Renal Failure Type

The clinical symptoms are characterized by prominent renal damages, with manifestations of proteinuria, hematuria, cylindruria, oliguria, anuria, azotemia of different levels, and acidosis. As icterus does not occur in the cases of this type, renal failure in this case can be differentiated from that in the cases of hemorrhagic icterus type. In severe cases, death occurs due to renal failure.

14.4.2.5 Meningoencephalitis Type

The clinical symptoms are characterized by encephalitis or meningitis, with severe headache, systemic pain and soreness, vomiting, gastrocnemius pain, diarrhea, irritation, unconsciousness, neck rigidity, and Kernig sign positive. Before the immune responses, the cell count in the cerebrospinal fluid is not subject to increase, commonly varying from ten to several hundreds per cubic millimeter. In some rare cases, the cell count can reach 1,000/mm^3. In addition, the CSF is also demonstrated with weakly positive protein response and normal levels of sugar and chlorides. The clinical manifestations resemble those of aseptic meningitis.

14.4.3 The Convalescence or Late-Onset Symptoms Stage

After the body temperature returns to normal, various symptoms gradually regress. However, in some rare cases, fever recurs after several days to 3 months to show symptoms, which are known as late-onset symptoms.

14.4.3.1 Late-Onset Fever

After the body temperature returns to normal for 1–5 days, fever may recur, with a body temperature of 38–38.5 °C. In about 50 % of the cases, the count of eosinophil granulocytes in peripheral blood is subject to increase. After being treated or untreated, the patients experience return of the body temperature to normal within 1–3 days.

14.4.3.2 Ocular Late-Onset Symptoms

Such symptoms are commonly found in the cases in northern regions of China. Ocular symptoms commonly occur 1 week to 1 month after the onset of disease and are mainly characterized by uveitis, iridocyclitis, and choroiditis. In addition, episcleritis and retrobulbar neuritis may also occur.

14.4.3.3 Neurological Late-Onset Symptoms

Reactive Meningitis

In some rare cases, the patients experience late-onset fever concurrently with meningitis. However, the cerebrospinal fluid examination bears normal findings. And the symptoms may be self-cured.

Occlusive Cerebral Arteritis

Occlusive cerebral arteritis, also known as moyamoya disease, can be observed in the cases caused by *Leptospira pomona*. It is one of the most common and the most severe neurological complications of leptospirosis. And the cases account for 0.57–6.45 % of all the leptospirosis cases. About 90 % of the patients are children aged below 15 years, and about 10 % of the patients are young and middle-aged adults. The incidence has no significant gender difference, with a delayed incidence peak for more than 3 months after local prevalence of leptospirosis. The symptoms occur within 9 months after the onset of leptospirosis, including hemiplegia, aphasia, and repeated transient paralysis.

Pretibial Fever

In some extremely rare cases, nodular erythema occurs in the convalescence stage at the skin of bilateral anterior tibia, with accompanying fever that regresses within 2 weeks. Its occurrence is closely related to the immune responses.

14.5 Leptospirosis-Related Complications

Generally, complications occur in the early or middle stage of a disease, while late-onset symptoms occur in the advanced stage. The complications of leptospirosis are characterized by ocular and long-term neurological complications.

Uveitis is the most common ocular complication of leptospirosis, mostly anterior uveitis (iridocyclitis) with manifestation of vitreous opacity and white precipitates at the surface of the iris. The second common complication includes retina lesions and optic nerve lesions. Some patients may also experience complications of sclera, pupil, and ocular muscle. Most symptoms occur within 2–8 weeks of the illness course, with favorable prognosis in most cases. However, some rare cases have prolonged illness course or repeated occurrence.

The neurological complications are characterized by advanced cerebropathies, whose occurrence is probably related to disturbance of blood supply to brain tissues caused by narrowed or occlusive cerebral vascular lumen due to anaphylactic reactions. The patients may experience persistent headache, dizziness, and limb numbness after the acute stage. The neurological symptoms, characterized by central nerve-related paralysis and motor language impairment, may occur 2–5 months after the onset. Some patients may experience psychiatric symptoms.

14.6 Diagnostic Examinations

14.6.1 Routine Test and Blood Biochemical Test

14.6.1.1 Routine Blood Test

In the cases with no jaundice, the WBC count and the neutrophil granulocyte count are normal or increase slightly. However, in the cases with jaundice, the WBC count mostly increases, about 50 % of the cases being $(10–20) \times 10^9/L$ and the highest level being $70 \times 10^9/L$. In some rare cases, leukemoid reactions occur, such as increased neutrophil granulocyte count, mostly at a level of 81–95 %. The patients with bleeding may experience anemia and thrombocytopenia, which may have the lowest level of $15 \times 10^9/L$. Accelerated erythrocyte sedimentation rate (ESR) is a characteristic laboratory finding of the disease, which may persist for 2–3 weeks.

14.6.1.2 Liver Function Test

In the cases with jaundice, the bilirubin level increases, which fluctuates with the severity of jaundice. In about 2/3 of the cases, the bilirubin level is lower than 342 μmol/L, and the highest level of bilirubin can be up to 1,111 μmol/L. Generally, the bilirubin level continues to increase at week 1 and 2 of the illness course, with following decrease at week 3 and 4. The serum transaminase level may be found with an increase, whose degree is not parallel to the severity of the conditions. Therefore, the increase of serum transaminase level fails to be a direct indicator for assessment of liver damages. In addition, about 50 % of the cases are demonstrated with increased CPK, whose average value is five times as high as the normal level.

14.6.1.3 Urine Test and Renal Function Test

As leptospiras cause common and severe damages to the kidneys, renal dysfunction of different severities is demonstrated in most patients. By routine urine test, 70 % of the cases is demonstrated with mild proteinuria, RBC, WBC, or casts.

14.6.2 Specific Detection

14.6.2.1 Pathogen Isolation

As leptospiras can be hardly stained, they cannot be directly observed via common microscope. Instead, dark field illumination can be applied for their detection. At week 1 of the illness course, pathogen can be detected in the blood. During this period of time, the blood specimen can be collected from the patient to inoculate in Korthof medium for the culture of pathogens. In such a way, leptospiras are more likely to be detected. Since week 2, the antibodies are gradually produced in the infected human body, with absence of pathogens in the blood. Therefore, detection of pathogen at this time in the blood is almost impossible. However, since week 2, along with gradual increase of the antibody titer in the blood, the positive rate by serological test is increasing. During this period of time, the pathogens are excreted along with urination, which can, therefore, be detected in the urine. Recently, pathogens are directly detected by direct microscopy, immunofluorescence, silver staining, and toluidine blue staining after the bacteria are concentrated by ultracentrifugation. In such ways, fast diagnosis can be achieved, with a positive rate of 50 %, which facilitates the early diagnosis.

Animal inoculation is another reliable way to isolate the pathogens. The blood or other body fluid specimens can be collected from the patient, with following inoculation into the abdominal cavity of experimental animals, such as young guinea pigs or golden hamsters. For the cases at the advanced stage, the urine specimens can be inoculated into subcutaneous area of the abdomen of the experimental animals. Three to five days after the inoculation, the peritoneal fluid should be collected for dark field examination. Otherwise, the blood specimens should be collected from the heart of animals for examination. The positive rate by animal inoculation is comparatively high. However, such an examination needs more time and is costly.

14.6.2.2 Serological Test

Agglutination Lysis Test

Despite high specificity and sensitivity, the agglutination lysis test requires different types of living bacteria for its operation. Generally, lectin occurs 7–8 days after the onset and increases gradually then. A titer of above 1:400 as positive, it can persist for several months to years. The cases with a titer of paired sera every 2 weeks with above four times increase are defined positive.

ELISA

A positive finding by ELISA is earlier than that by the agglutination lysis test, indicating a higher sensitivity. The total consistent rate of agglutination lysis test and ELISA reaches 86.2 %. In recent years, the leptospira-specific IgM antibody technique has been commonly applied, which is characterized by its high specificity.

Indirect Hemagglutination Test (IHT)

IHA has genus specificity for pathogen detection, but with no group or serotype specificities. Compared to the agglutination lysis test, IHT has an earlier positive result. In addition, IHT requires simple operation and no complicated equipment, and it is appropriate to be widely adopted in community-oriented hospitals.

Indirect Hemolysis Test

Indirect hemolysis test has a higher sensitivity than IHA.

Indirect Immunofluorescence

Compared to hemagglutination test, both the detection of antibody and the negative conversion are earlier, which is more valuable for the early diagnosis.

Since the known antigens of leptospiras are applied to detect the corresponding antibodies in the blood specimens, the early diagnosis cannot be defined by these examinations. The following techniques can be applied for the early diagnosis.

DNA Probe for Leptospiras

In 1984, Schoone et al. have demonstrated that DNA probe is a highly sensitive way for the early diagnosis of the disease. Thereafter, it has been clinically applied. The probe is prepared with DNA of Wijnberg strain, Copenhagen type, and icterohemorrhagic group of leptospiras; the homologous DNA of 2 pg can be detected at cellulose nitrate membrane, with cross hybridization to pathogenic leptospiras of Patoc I strain of different serogroups.

Gene Amplification Technique (GAT)

In 1989, VanEys et al. examined bovine urine specimens after their infection by Hardjo leptospiras with PCR amplification technique. Their conclusion was that PCR DNA amplification technique by PCR is a novel method for the diagnosis of leptospirosis. Such a way has simple operations and is appropriate for large-scale epidemiological investigations.

14.6.3 Diagnostic Imaging

14.6.3.1 Ultrasound

Ultrasound is appropriate for the detection of hepatic, splenic, and renal lesions as well as the examination of heart, lymph nodes, and gastrocnemius.

14.6.3.2 X-Ray Radiology and CT Scanning

X-ray radiology and CT scanning are commonly applied to assess pulmonary lesions.

14.6.3.3 MR Imaging

MR imaging is clinically applied to assess abdominal and neurological lesions.

14.7 Imaging Demonstrations

14.7.1 Lung

14.7.1.1 X-Ray Radiology

In the cases of leptospirosis being classified as pulmonary bleeding type, chest X-ray demonstrates variant lesions at different clinical stages. The lesions are demonstrated chronologically as thickened lung markings, miliary shadows, nodular shadows, patches of shadows, and flakes of fused shadows.

The Early Stage

X-ray demonstrates no obvious abnormalities, with only increased and blurry lung markings and occasional scattered small nodular blurry lesions (Fig. 14.1).

The Middle and Advanced Stages

X-ray demonstrates miliary and nodular shadows diffuse in both lungs, mainly in the middle and lateral parts of the middle and lower lung fields. Most shadows are densely contributed at the lateral parts. The lung apex is commonly well defined. Along with progress of the conditions, pulmonary bleeding increases and the nodular shadows fuse together to form small and large flakes of high-density shadows with extremely blurry boundaries. The lesions may involve the lung apex (Fig. 14.2).

In some cases, pleural effusion is demonstrated as unilateral pleural effusion in a large quantity or bilateral pleural effusion in small quantities. The lesions are symmetrically distributed, with concurrent shallow bilateral costophrenic angles. In some cases, interlobar fissure effusion can be demonstrated as long stripes of shadows.

The Convalescence Stage

Reexamination by X-ray after 1 week medication of sensitive penicillin, the patients demonstrated with spots and flakes of hemorrhagic lesions absorbed.

The summary of imaging demonstrations is as follows:

1. Lesions are more likely to be distributed in the lateral parts of both lungs than in the middle and medial parts, namely, positive splay sign.
2. Multiple nodular shadows can fuse into flakes of shadows. And the primary nodular shadows (the bleeding spots) can be defined via the uneven flakes of shadows.
3. The lung apex and base are well defined, and the lesions are rarely distributed around the hilum.
4. In most cases, the transparency of both lung fields is evenly decreased to produce ground glass opacities, which are caused by pulmonary bleeding due to toxic damages of the pulmonary capillaries induced by toxins produced by leptospiras or direct damages from leptospiras.
5. The development and absorption of the lesions are rapid, with daily changes.
6. In some cases, X-ray demonstrations are inconsistent with severity of clinical symptoms.

Case Study 1

A male patient aged 53 years experienced high fever with a body temperature of 40 °C, coughing up little sputum, myalgia, and headache. After hospitalization, he experienced septic shock and respiratory failure. Serological test demonstrated leptospira positive, with a leptospira titer of 1:1,600.

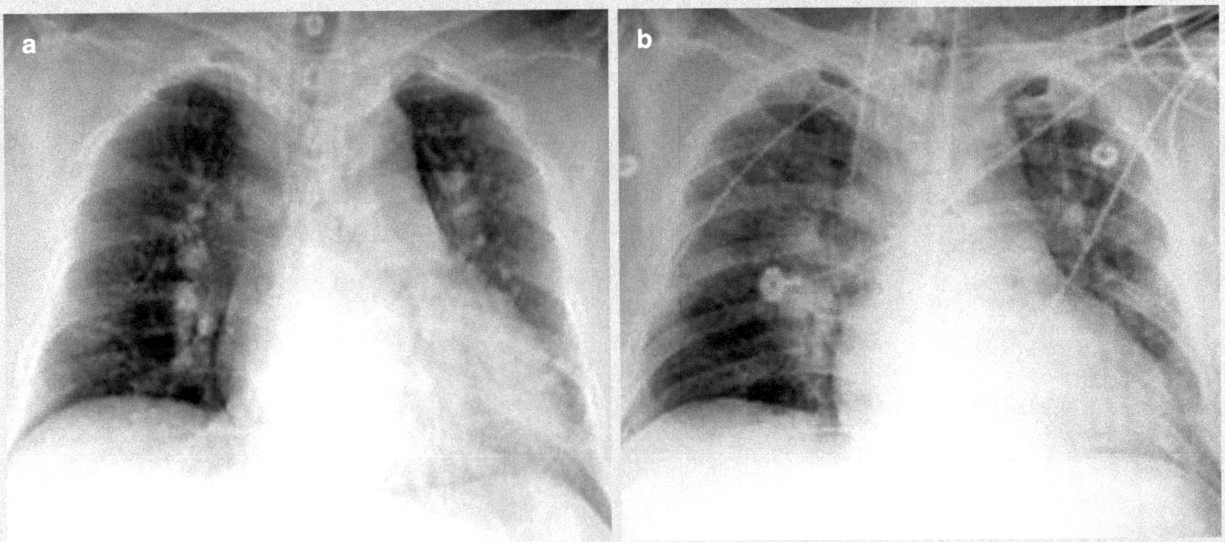

Fig. 14.1 Leptospirosis with pulmonary bleeding. (**a**) X-ray at day 1 of hospitalization demonstrates enlarged heart shadow and small patches of shadows in the left upper lung. (**b**) X-ray at day 2 of hospitalization demonstrates development of the conditions, with patches of blurry shadows in both lungs (Reprint with permission from Wei YF, et al. *J Microbiol Immunol Infect*, 2012, 45 (3): 251)

Case Study 2

A 46-year-old male vagrant reported a history of sleeping in a forest and eating food bitten by rats 5 days ago. He experienced nausea, diarrhea, myalgia, dizziness, headache, hemoptysis, and high fever with a body temperature of 39 °C. Leptospira was detected in his blood.

For case detail and figures, please refer to Luks AM, et al. *Chest*, 2003, 123 (2): 639.)

Case Study 3

Two cases of adult males were diagnosed with leptospirosis with pulmonary bleeding.

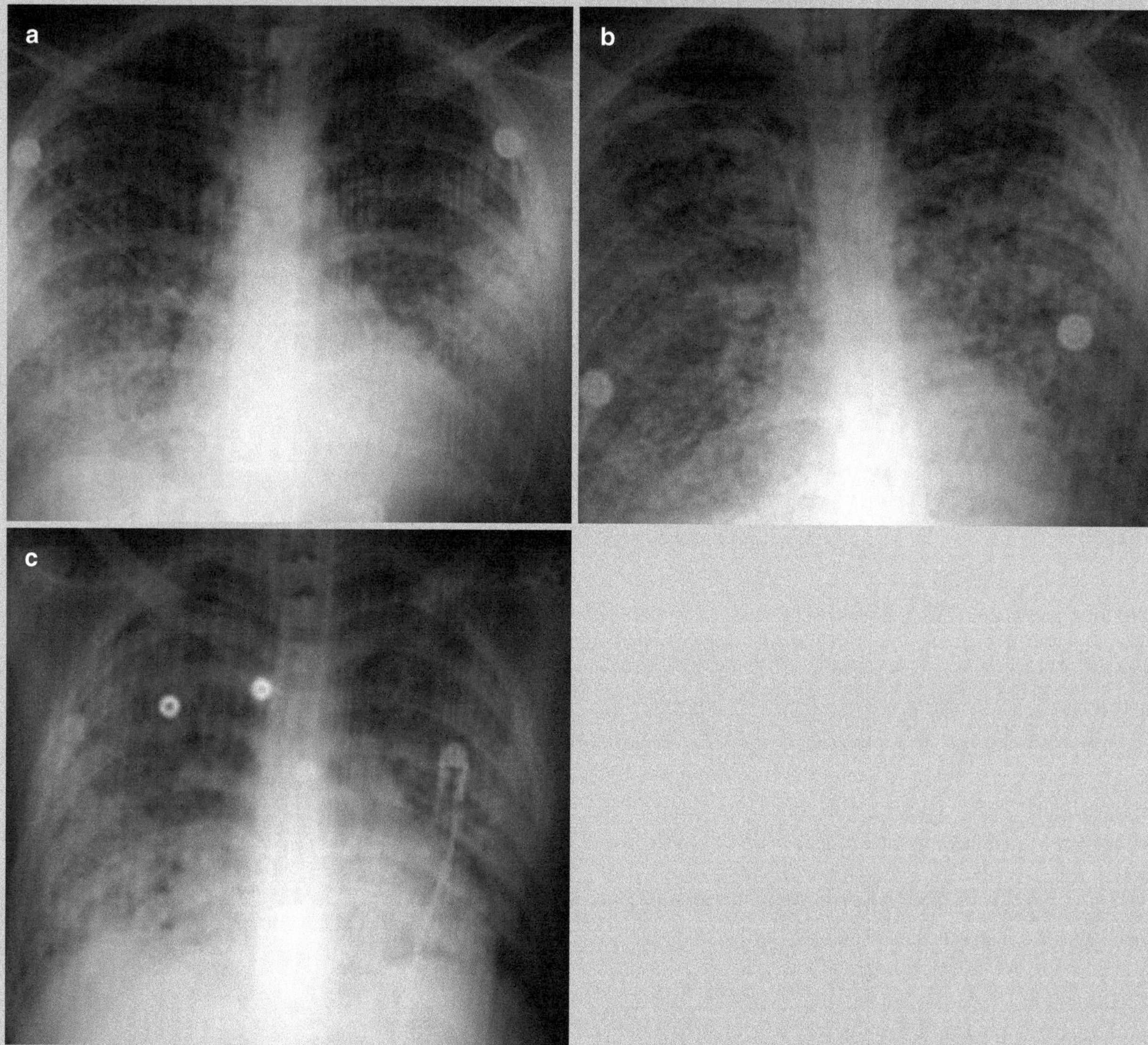

Fig. 14.2 Leptospirosis with pulmonary bleeding. (**a**) X-ray demonstrates nodular shadows with poorly defined boundaries in the lateral parts of both lower lungs. Some nodular shadows are demonstrated with fusion and the lung apex is comparatively well defined. (**b**) At the development stage, both lungs are demonstrated with diffuse nodular shadows. (**c**) Another case of leptospirosis with pulmonary bleeding at the middle or advanced stage. The nodular shadows are demonstrated with fusion in both longs to form diffuse patches of shadows (Reprint with permission from Ketai L, et al. *Thorac Imaging*, 2006, 21 (4): 265)

14.7.1.2 CT Scanning

CT scanning is superior to X-ray in demonstrating bleeding lesions. By CT scanning, the bleeding lesions are demonstrated as fine spots of shadows due to small volume of bleeding. Along with the increased volume of bleeding, the fine spots of shadows gradually fuse and are enlarged to form small patches, cotton-like, mass-like, and even patches of shadows with extremely blurry boundaries (Figs. 14.3 and 14.4). Meanwhile, in the cases with larger range of bleeding but rare intra-alveolar bleeding, CT scanning demonstrates lesions as ground glass opacities. As bleeding is dynamic and progressive, early demonstrations by radiology may be shadows with uniform morphology. However, in the advanced stage, shadows of various morphologies are demonstrated with mixed existence.

Case Study 4

A male patient aged 19 years experienced headache, neck pain, muscular pain, fever, nausea, vomiting, hemoptysis, and respiratory failure.

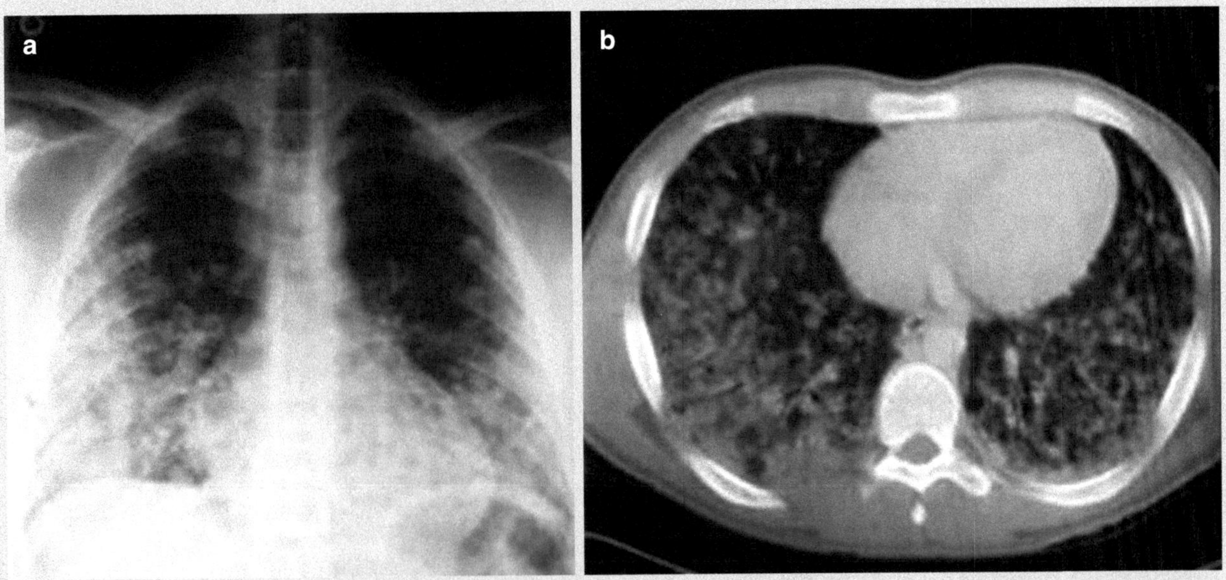

Fig. 14.3 Leptospirosis with pulmonary bleeding. (**a**) X-ray demonstrates patches of blurry shadows in bilateral middle and lower lung fields. (**b**) CT scanning demonstrates alveoli and interstitium of both lungs with infiltrative inflammation (Reprint with permission from Kishimoto M, et al. *Am J Med Sci*, 2004, 328 (2): 116)

Case Study 5

A male patient reported a history of contact to contaminated water by infected rats. He experienced high fever, headache, myalgia, hemoptysis, and jaundice. Bronchoalveolar lavage (BAL) demonstrated pulmonary bleeding. Serological test demonstrated positive.

For case detail and figures, please refer to Marchiori and Müller. *J Thorac Imaging*, 2002, 17 (2): 151.)

Case Study 6

A male patient reported a history of contact to contaminated water by infected rats. He experienced high fever, headache, myalgia, hemoptysis, and icterus. Autopsy demonstrated the diagnosis of leptospirosis.

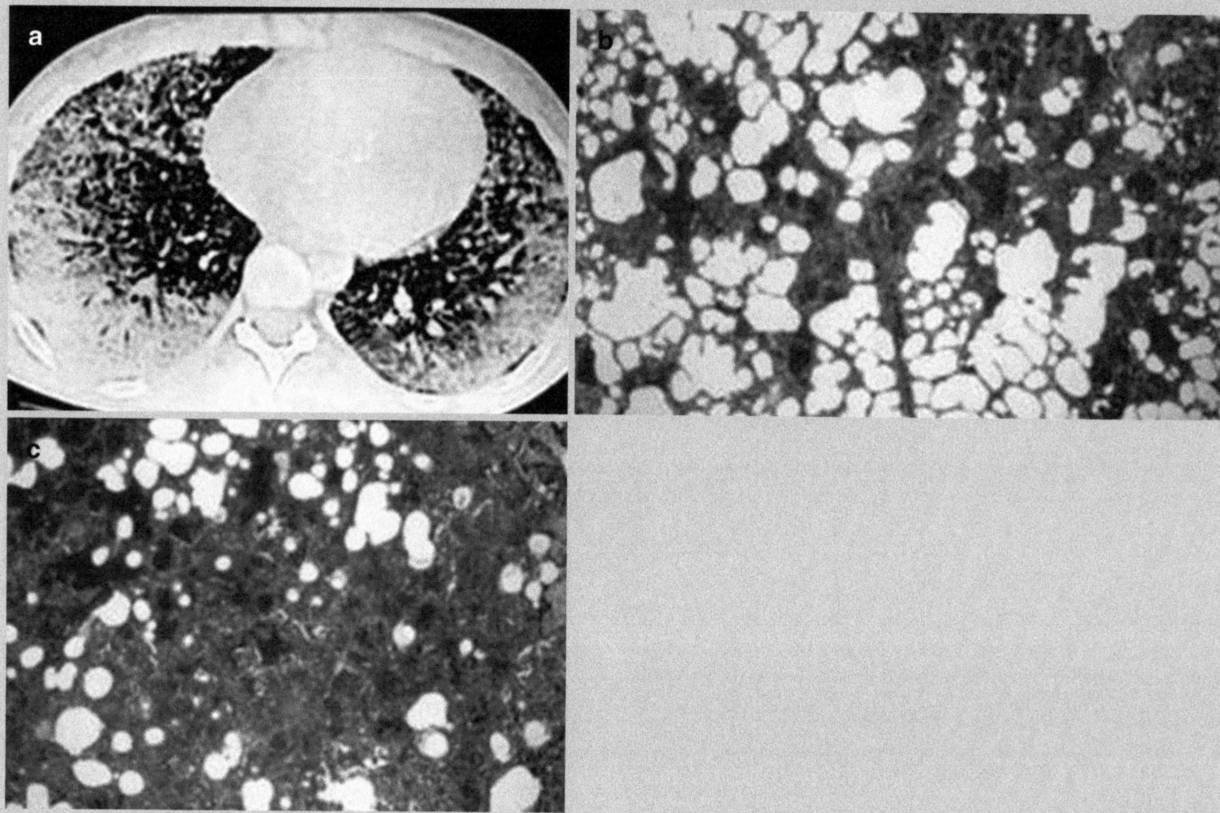

Fig. 14.4 Leptospirosis with pulmonary bleeding. (**a**) HRCT demonstrates ground-glass and nodular shadows in both lungs and consolidation shadows in the subpleural area. (**b**) Autopsy under low-power microscope demonstrates extensive pulmonary bleeding (Reprint with permission from Marchiori and Müller, J *Thorac Imaging*, 2002, 17 (2): 151)

14.7.2 Liver

14.7.2.1 Color Doppler Ultrasound

Color Doppler ultrasound demonstrates mild to moderate hepatomegaly, smooth liver capsule, and weakened and unevenly distributed echoes from the liver, with quite clearly defined vascularization.

14.7.2.2 CT Scanning

CT scanning demonstrates enlarged liver and multiple low-density lesions in the liver (Fig. 14.5).

Case Study 7
A 61-year-old male farmer experienced fatigue, right upper abdominal pain, and hepatomegaly. Endoscopy demonstrated ulceration at the transverse and ascending colon. Abdominal CT scanning demonstrated multiple low-density lesions in the liver, with slight ring-shaped enhancement. The initial diagnosis was hepatic metastasis of colon carcinoma. However, no malignancies were detected by biopsy of colon and liver tissue. Thereafter, the patient reported a history of close contacts to pigs. The antibody titer of leptospiras was then detected high.

For case detail and figures, please refer to Granito A, et al. *World J Gestroenterol*, 2004, 10 (16): 2455.

Case Study 8
A male patient aged 62 years experienced fever with a body temperature of 39 °C, icterus, nausea, vomiting, fatigue, and dizziness. By dark field microscopy, leptospiras were observed.

For case detail and figures, please refer to Kaya E, et al. *World J Gestroenterol*, 2005, 11 (28): 4447.

Case Study 9
A boy aged 10 years complained of headache, fever with a body temperature of 37 °C, abdominal pain, and fatigue for 10 days as well as language impairment for 6 days. Physical examination demonstrated hepatosplenomegaly. He was also detected leptospira positive.

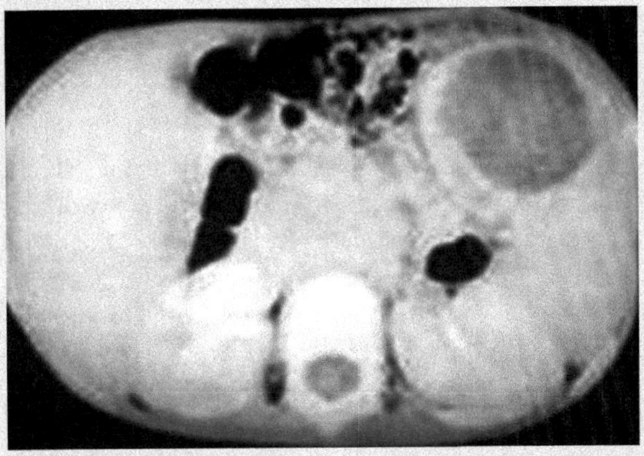

Fig. 14.5 Leptospirosis with hepatic and splenic lesions. CT scanning demonstrates the swelling of spleen, with a size of 6 cm × 4 cm

14.7.3 Brain

Cerebral leptospirosis is a series of clinical symptoms with manifestations of neurological damages caused by leptospiras. The illness course can be divided into the organ lesion stage (the middle stage or complications stage, hereinafter referred to as the cerebral lesions in the complications stage) and the convalescence stage (the late-onset symptoms stage, hereinafter referred to as the cerebral lesions in the late-onset symptoms stage). The lesions of these two stages may coexist, and their clinical manifestations can be hardly distinguished. The relationship between the imaging demonstrations and clinical symptoms is analyzed as the following.

14.7.3.1 Cerebral Lesions at the Complications Stage

The clinical manifestations are characterized by symptoms of encephalitis and meningitis, with severe headache, vomiting, irritation, unconsciousness, neck rigidity, and Kernig sign positive. The imaging demonstration features diffuse cerebral lesions. CT scanning demonstrates normal density, slightly low density, or diffuse cerebral edema. MR imaging demonstrates diffuse multiple spots and flakes of low or equal T1WI signal and high T2WI signal. The signs of demyelination are sometimes demonstrated.

14.7.3.2 Cerebral Lesions in the Late-Onset Symptoms Stage

The symptoms are clinically characterized by reactive meningitis or occlusive cerebral arteries, with manifestations of hemiplegia, aphasia, and multiple repeated transient paralysis. Cerebral angiography demonstrates stenosis of the involved vascular vessels. The imaging demonstrations feature diffuse or focalized lesions. Multiple diffuse lesions are commonly distributed in different areas of unilateral blood vessels, with equal or low T1WI as well as high T2WI signals. Occasionally, the lesions can be found at the interface of cortico-white matters, with typical manifestation of infarction. Local lesions are mostly characterized by signs of cerebral infarction (Fig. 14.6).

Case Study 10
A female patient aged 13 years complained of headache and irritation for 7 days as well as unconsciousness for 3 days. Her body temperature was 36.9 °C. Leptospira was detected positive.

For case detail and figures, please refer to Kurtoğlu MG, et al. *Tohoku J Exp Med*, 2003, 201 (1): 55.

Case Study 11
A male patient aged 43 years experienced gradual progressive instability, respiratory tract infection (RTI), ataxia, and dysarthria. He reported to have a working environment close to ditch. Examinations of the blood and cerebrospinal fluid demonstrated leptospira positive and he was clinically diagnosed with chronic leptospiral vasculitis.

For case detail and figures, please refer to Brinar and Habek. *Clin Neurol Neurolsurg*, 2010, 112 (7): 625.

Case Study 12
A male patient aged 51 years experienced fever with a body temperature of 38 °C.

For case detail and figures, please refer to Babamahmoodi and Babamhmoodi. *Casereport Med*, 2011, 2011: 504308.

Case Study 13
A male patient aged 17 years experienced multiple organ failure and hematemesis. ELISA demonstrated leptospira IgM positive.

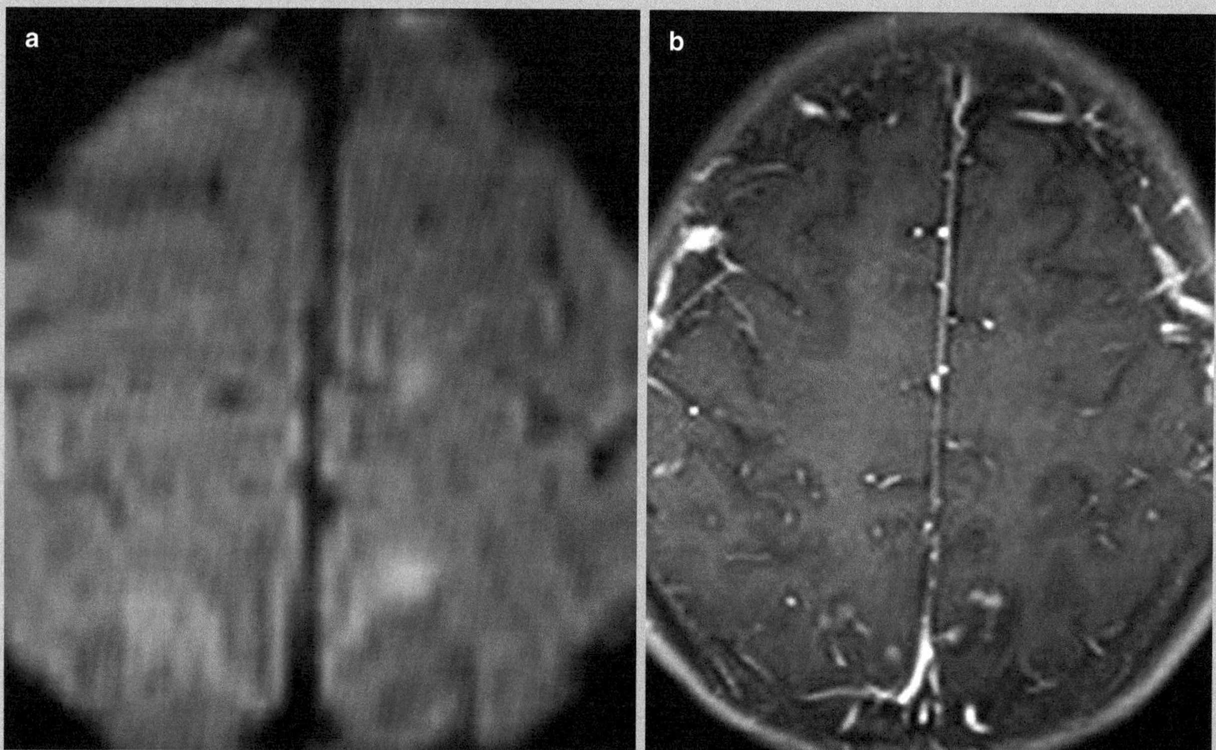

Fig. 14.6 Leptospirosis with cerebral lesions. (**a**) DWI demonstrates strips of high signals at the bilateral parietal lobes, suggesting restricted diffusion and subacute infarction. (**b**) Contrast imaging demonstrates gyri-like enhancement. (**c–d**) SWI demonstrates multiple spots of low signals at the supratentorial white matter, basal ganglia, callosum, pons, and cerebellum, suggesting slight bleeding (Reprint with permission from Naphadeps, et al. *J Infect*, 2012, 64 (5): 538

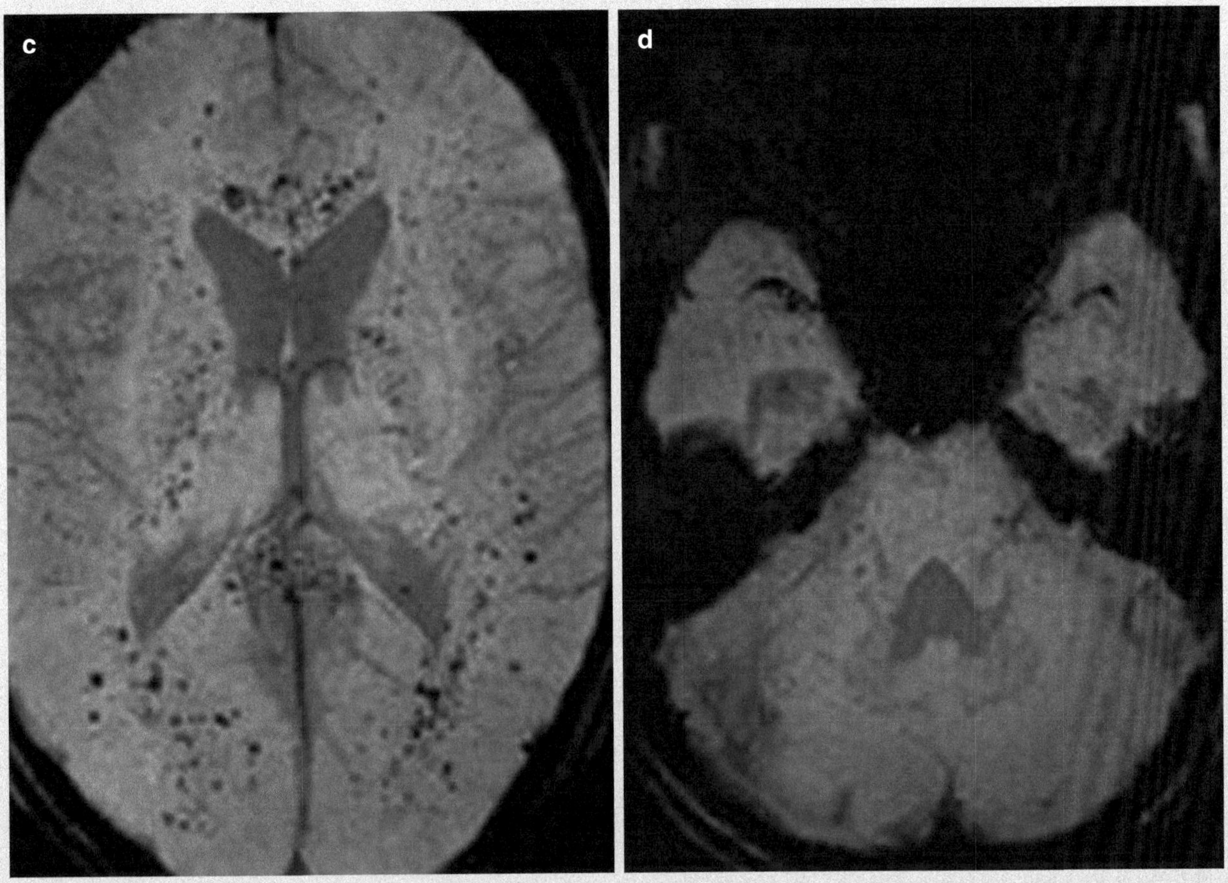

Fig. 14.6 (continued)

Case Study 14

A patient was diagnosed with neurological leptospirosis. He/she experienced acute fever, aversion to cold, headache, and vomiting. Serological test demonstrated leptospira antibody positive.

For case detail and figures, please refer to Matthew T, et al. *Indian J Med Res*, 2006, 124 (2): 15.

14.7.4 Imaging Demonstrations of Lesions at Other Organs

14.7.4.1 Spleen

Color Doppler ultrasound demonstrates enlarged spleen with weakened and even echoes. The splenic artery and vein are subject to slight thickness, with increased blood flow volume. More vascular distributions can be observed in the spleen.

14.7.4.2 Kidney

Color Doppler ultrasound demonstrates bilaterally enlarged kidneys with intact capsule and thickened cortex. The echoes from cortex are weakened with uneven distribution, which can be hardly distinguished from those of the medulla. Less vascular distributions can be observed in both kidneys, with increased resistance at the renal artery.

14.7.4.3 Myocardium

Color Doppler Ultrasound

Color Doppler ultrasound demonstrates enlarged left cardiac ventricle. The activities of the left ventricular wall and interventricular septum diffusively decrease, with shrunk and thickened myocardium. The heart rate decreases and the myocardium is demonstrated with uneven echoes. The range of mitral valve motion is decreased. CDFI demonstrates slight regurgitation signals at each valve orifice, with decreased velocity of the blood flow.

X-Ray Radiology

X-ray demonstrates enlarged heart shadow and existence of cardiac arch. The enlarged heart shadow can also be flask shaped, with absence of cardiac arch.

14.7.4.4 Superficial Lymph Node

Color Doppler ultrasound demonstrates inaugural and subaxillary swollen lymph nodes, with multiple round- or oval-shaped low-echo nodules that have clearly defined boundaries. The enlarged lymph nodes are demonstrated with thickened cortex, central location of the medulla, and more vascular distributions.

14.7.4.5 Gastrocnemius

Color Doppler ultrasound demonstrates thickened bilateral gastrocnemius and poorly defined running course of the striated muscle. The weakened echoes are unevenly distributed.

14.8 Diagnostic Basis

14.8.1 Epidemiology

In epidemic regions during summers and autumns, the acute infectious cases with similar clinical manifestations and a history of contact to contaminated water in recent 1–2 weeks should be suspected as leptospirosis. In non-epidemic regions, sporadic occurrence may be reported due to contact to secretions by infected rats and other host animals.

14.8.2 Clinical Manifestation

At the early stage, the disease is characterized by acute infection, with chills and fever, pain and soreness, fatigue, conjunctival congestion, myalgia, and lymphadenalgia. At the early stage, the patients may also experience digestive symptoms, respiratory symptoms, and bleeding tendency.

14.8.3 Laboratory Test

14.8.3.1 Peripheral Blood

The total count of WBC and the count of neutrophil granulocytes slightly increase, with accelerating ESR.

14.8.3.2 Serum Agglutination Test

The serum agglutination test is positive.

14.8.3.3 Blood Culture

The pathogen grows slowly by blood culture.

14.8.3.4 Urine Test

Urine test demonstrates mild proteinuria. Microscopic urinalysis demonstrates WBC, RBC, and casts. Most patients experience accompanying azotemia.

14.8.4 Radiology

14.8.4.1 X-Ray Radiology and CT Scanning

Patient with pulmonary bleeding is demonstrated with ground-glass opacities at both lungs. Otherwise, diffuse spots, flakes, or fused flakes of shadows are demonstrated at both lungs.

14.8.4.2 Ultrasound and CT Scanning

Patient is demonstrated with enlarged liver, multiple low-echo or low-density lesions in the liver, enlarged spleen, and enlarged kidneys.

14.8.4.3 CT Scanning and MR Imaging

CT scanning demonstrates normal-density, slight low-density, or diffuse cerebral edema. MR imaging demonstrates multiple diffuse spots and flakes of abnormal signals at the gray and white matters, which are low T1WI signals in most cases, equal signals in some rare cases, and high T2WI signals of all the cases. Demyelination can be occasionally observed.

14.9 Differential Diagnosis

As the clinical manifestations are complex, its early diagnosis is challenging and the disease tends to be misdiagnosed. Its clinical diagnosis requires positive result by etiological or serological test in combination to epidemiological data, early clinical manifestations, laboratory tests findings, and imaging demonstrations. The disease should also be differentiated from other diseases.

14.9.1 Fever

It should firstly distinguished from other diseases with acute fever, such as typhoid fever, influenza, upper respiratory infection, acute schistosomiasis, scrub typhus, pneumonia, epidemic hemorrhagic fever, and sepsis. In addition to the clinical symptoms, the epidemiological history commonly provides hint for the differential diagnosis. The occurrence of proteinuria and azotemia provides important basis for the differential diagnosis. For the cases of bronchopneumonia, chest X-ray demonstrates spots of shadows distributing in the middle and medial parts of bilateral middle and lower lungs along the lung markings, with poorly defined structure of the hilum, which facilitate the differential diagnosis.

14.9.2 Icterus

The disease should also be differentiated from icteric hepatitis. Generally, the cases of icteric hepatitis have a chronic onset, with prominent digestive symptoms such as poor appetite, but with no conjunctival congestion and gastrocnemius tenderness. The body temperature is usually normal or shows low-grade fever, with slightly low or normal WBC count in most cases and no accelerated ESR. ALT and AST levels indicating the hepatic function are obviously abnormal, with no increase of serum creatine kinase. However, leptospirosis has reverse manifestations. The epidemiological history and serological test also provide valuable evidence for the differential diagnosis. Concerning obstructive icterus, it commonly has no development course of acute infectious diseases with fever. CT scanning and MR imaging mainly demonstrate dilated biliary duct system above the obstruction or accompanying cholecystectasis. The diagnostic criteria include dilation of the intrahepatic bile duct by at least 3 mm or the diameter of common bile duct exceeding 10 mm, with acknowledged causes of obstruction such as neoplasm, calculus, and inflammation. Routine urine test and blood nonprotein nitrogen (NPN) test also facilitate the differential diagnosis from other icteric diseases. Renal changes commonly occur in the cases of leptospiral icterus, while the patients with other types of icteric diseases seldom experience renal changes.

14.9.3 Nephritis

For the cases of leptospirosis that show renal lesions but no icterus, it should be differentiated from nephritis. Leptospirosis has similar development course with other acute infectious diseases with fever, with conjunctival congestion, apparent myalgia, normal blood pressure, and no edema.

14.9.4 Myalgia

Myalgia should be differentiated from acute rheumatic fever (ARF). ARF features migrating joint pain, while leptospirosis features myalgia, prominently gastrocnemius.

14.9.5 Bleeding or Hemoptysis

Leptospirosis with bleeding should be differentiated from upper gastrointestinal bleeding, hematuria, as well as hemorrhagic hematosis such as leukemia, thrombocytopenia, and aplastic anemia via peripheral blood test, bone marrow examination, and GI examination. Other hemorrhagic sepsis commonly have severe illness course and a high mortality rate, which can be epidemiologically distinguished from leptospirosis. Leptospirosis with hemoptysis should be differentiated from tuberculosis, bronchiectasis, and tumors via chest X-ray radiology and CT scanning.

The key points for the differential diagnosis of pulmonary bleeding by X-ray radiology are as follows.

14.9.5.1 Acute Hematogenous Disseminated Pulmonary Tuberculosis

Acute hematogenous disseminated pulmonary tuberculosis has a long illness course, with mild symptoms and slow progress. In the cases of acute miliary tuberculosis, X-ray demonstrates three evens, even and wide distribution of the miliary lesions in both lungs, with even density and even size. In the cases of subacute hematogenous disseminated pulmonary tuberculosis, chest X-ray demonstrates widely distributed lesions with different sizes, which are mainly miliary lesions and mostly distributed in the middle and upper lungs.

14.9.5.2 Diffuse Alveolar Carcinoma

Alveolar carcinoma usually occurs in an elderly age group, which originate from bronchiolar epithelium. Chest X-ray demonstrates miliary nodules with different sizes that distribute diffusely in both lungs, with poorly defined boundaries and uneven density. Vacuoles can be observed between the nodules.

14.9.6 Meningoencephalitis

Both leptospirosis with meningoencephalitis and epidemic encephalitis B prevail in summers and autumns and can be hardly distinguished. With severe conditions, epidemic encephalitis B commonly occurs in children, with more obvious cerebral symptoms than leptospirosis, such as convulsion and comma. Patients with epidemic encephalitis B experience no apparent conjunctival congestion or gastrocnemius tenderness. The WBC count is relatively high, with normal findings by routine urine test and liver function examination. The patients usually have no case history of contact to contaminated water. Epidemic encephalitis B has characteristic CT demonstrations of low-density lesions at bilateral basal ganglia and hypothalamic area. In addition, the cerebral peduncle is commonly involved, but rare involvement of the cerebral cortex, brain stem, and callus. MR imaging demonstrates long T1 and long T2 signals at the corresponding positions, with slightly high FLAIR signals, mostly high DWI signals, and rarely slightly high DWI signals.

References

Babamahmoodi F, Babamhmoodi A. Recovery from intracranial hemorrhage due to leptospirosis. Case Rep Med. 2011;2011:504308.

Brinar VV, Habek M. Rare infections mimicking MS. Clin Neurol Neurosurg. 2010;112(7):625–8.

Granito A, Ballardini G, Fusconi M, et al. A case of leptospirosis simulating colon cancer with liver metastases. World J Gastroenterol. 2004;10(16):2455–6.

Kaya E, Dervisoglu A, Eroglu C, et al. Acute pancreatitis caused by leptospirosis: report of two cases. World J Gastroenterol. 2005;11(28):4447–9.

Ketai L, Currie BJ, Alva Lopez LF. Thoracic radiology of infections emerging after natural disasters. Thorac Imaging. 2006;21(4):265–75.

Kishimoto M, Brown JD, Chung HH, et al. Leptospirosis misdiagnosed as pulmonary-renal syndrome. Am J Med Sci. 2004;328(2):116–20.

Kurtoğlu MG, Tuncer O, Bozkurt H, et al. Report of three children with leptospirosis in rural area of the east of turkey. Tohoku J Exp Med. 2003;201(1):55–60.

Luks AM, Lakshminarayanan S, Hirschmann JV. Leptospirosis presenting as diffuse alveolar hemorrhage: case report and literature review. Chest. 2003;123(2):639–43.

Marchiori E, Müller NL. Leptospirosis of the lung: high-resolution computed tomography findings in five patients. J Thorac Imaging. 2002;17(2):151–3.

Mathew T, Satishchandra P, Mahadevan A, et al. Neuroleptospirosis-revisited: experience from a tertiary care neurological centre from south India. Indian J Med Res. 2006;124(2):155–62.

Naphade PS, Raut AA, Pai BU. Microhaemorrhages in leptospirosis on susceptibility weighted imaging. J Infect. 2012;64(5):538–9.

Wei YF, Chiu CT, Lai YF, et al. Successful treatment of septic shock and respiratory failure due to leptospirosis and scrub typhus coinfection with penicillin, levofloxacin, and activated protein C. J Microbiol Immunol Infect. 2012;45(3):251–4.

Suggested Reading

Lei BJ. Leptospirosis. Beijing: People's Medical Publishing House; 2007.

Wagenaar JF, Goris MG, Partiningrum DL, et al. Coagulation disorders in patients with severe leptospirosis are associated with severe bleeding and mortality. Trop Med Int Health. 2010;15(2):152–9.

Habek M, Brinar VV. Central sleep apnea and ataxia caused by brainstem lesion due to chronic neuroleptospirosis. Neurology. 2009;73(22):1923–4.

15 Lyme Disease

Shi Qi and Feng Chen

Lyme disease (LD), also known as Lyme spirochetosis, is a tick-borne spirochetosis caused by *Borrelia burgdorferi* (Bb). It may involve multiple organs and systems, especially skin, joints, heart, and central nervous system.

15.1 Etiology

Borrelia burgdorferi is categorized into the genus *Borrelia* in the family Spirochaetaceae. Based on the genetic variance of the isolated pathogens, it can be further divided into several subspecies. Bb is a Gram-negative bacterium, and it can be favorably stained by Wright or Wright-Giemsa staining, which can be directly observed under a dark field microscope or a phase contrast microscope. With a length of 11–38 μm, Bb, which usually has 7–12 flagella, is a microaerophilic bacterium. At the temperature of 34–37 °C, Bb can grow slowly in the Barbour Stoenner-Kelly medium. Bb is sensitive to heat, dryness, and common chemical disinfectants but survives well at the conditions of low temperature and high humidity.

15.2 Epidemiology

Lyme disease is nominated after its first outbreak in Lyme town of the United States in 1975, which causes juvenile arthritis in a group of people.

S. Qi (✉) • F. Chen
Department of Radiology, Beijing You'an Hospital, Capital Medical University, Beijing, China
e-mail: sw0510@126.com

15.2.1 Source of Infection

The sources of infection include diseased or infected wild and domestic animals. Generally, the patients with Lyme disease do not constitute its source of infection.

15.2.2 Route of Transmission

Lyme disease is commonly transmitted via ticks. In addition, it can also be transmitted via some blood-sucking arthropods such as deerfly and horsefly.

15.2.3 Susceptible Population

Populations are generally susceptible to Lyme disease, especially fieldworker working in forests.

15.2.4 Epidemic Features

15.2.4.1 Regional Distribution

Lyme disease occurs worldwide, especially widespread in the northern hemisphere. So far, in more than 50 countries in the world, cases of Lyme disease have been reported, with the most cases reported in the United States. The cases of Lyme disease have been reported in 49 states of the United States. In China, the first case of Lyme disease was reported in the province of Heilongjiang in 1985. So far, the cases of Lyme disease have been reported in 27 Chinese provinces (cities, districts), and there are natural epidemic focus of Lyme disease in 18 provinces (cities, districts). The main epidemic areas include the northeast forest area, the northwest forest area, and Inner Mongolia forest area.

H. Li (ed.), *Radiology of Infectious Diseases: Volume 2*, DOI 10.1007/978-94-017-9876-1_15

15.2.4.2 Temporal Distribution

Lyme disease has seasonal prevalence, with 2 peak periods of infection each year, namely, June and October. And its occurrence in June is more common.

15.2.4.3 Population Distribution

Most patients with Lyme disease are young adults and its occurrence is related to the occupation. Fieldworkers working in forest have a high risk of infection. Outdoor activities like hunting, fishing, and travelling may increase the risk of infection.

15.3 Pathogenesis and Pathological Changes

15.3.1 Pathogenesis

Borrelia burgdorferi mainly exists in the midgut diverticulum of ticks. When a person is bitten by an infected tick, the spirochetes in the diverticulum are regurgitated from the salivary gland to the sucking mouthpart. Then, the spirochetes gain their access into the microvessels in the human skin and invade the organs and systems along with blood flow. However, the pathogen causes a short bacteremic period and the quantity of spirochetes in the blood is also small. However, multiple organs and systems are impaired, indicating multiple factors underlying its pathomechanism.

15.3.2 Pathological Changes

Several days after the access of the spirochetes into the skin, the first infection period (localized skin primary lesion) begins. There are perivascular infiltrations of plasma cells and lymphocytes of both superficial and deep blood vessels in the affected skin, with the manifestation of erythema chronicum migrans (ECM). The LPS component of the spirochetes can cause systemic symptoms and hepatosplenomegaly. The tissue sections of ECM show thickened epithelium, mild keratosis with accompanying mononuclear cells infiltration, as well as epidermis edema, but with no pyogenic reaction and granuloma reaction. After the spirochetes invade organs and tissues along with blood flow, the second infection period (dissemination period) follows, mainly with lesions of the central nervous system (especially cranial nerves) and heart. There are perivascular mononuclear cell infiltration in the brain cortex, in the cranial nerves (especially facial nerve, oculomotor nerve, and abducent nerve), and in heart tissue. Several months after the onset of Lyme disease, the third infection period (persistent infection period) begins, mainly with joint lesions, skin lesions, and advanced nerve lesions. There are proliferative erosive synovitis of the joint, accompanying vascular hyperplasia, synovial villi hypertrophy, fibrin deposition, and mononuclear cell infiltration as well as erosive lesions in bones and cartilages. The skin lesions include skin atrophy and decoloration or thickened collagen fibrous tissue bundles with tight arrangement like scleroderma lesion and atrophic acrodermatitis. The nervous system is involved with progressive encephalomyelitis, axonal demyelination, perivascular lymphocyte infiltration, thickened vascular wall, and collagen fiber hyperplasia.

15.4 Clinical Symptoms and Signs

The incubation period of Lyme disease ranges from 3 to 32 days. Clinically, Lyme disease is divided into three stages, which consecutively occurs or consecutively occurs with overlapping.

15.4.1 Skin Lesion Period

This period is characterized by erythema chronicum migrans (ECM) whose occurrence is commonly found at the thigh, armpit, and groin. The period lasts averagely for 7 days. Even if untreated, the skin lesions can heal by themselves.

15.4.2 Dissemination Period

15.4.2.1 Manifestations of the Nervous System

Lyme disease damages both terminal nerves and central nerves. The typical neurological symptoms generally occur after the absence of ECM, including meningitis, encephalitis, chorea, cerebellar ataxia, cranial neuritis, sensorimotor radiculitis, and myelitis. Among these conditions, meningitis, cranial neuritis, and radiculitis are more common.

15.4.2.2 Cardiac Manifestation

Atrioventricular conductive blockage is the most common cardiac manifestation, which is more common in males. In some rare cases, pericarditis and myocardial lesions can be found. The cardiac lesions of LD are generally mild, with no obvious lesions in cardiac valves. These lesions persist for a short period of time, with favorable prognosis.

15.4.2.3 Bone and Joint Manifestation

In the early period of LD, migratory pains may occur in joints, tendons, synovial bursas, and muscles, which may persist for several hours or even several days. The knee joint is the most commonly involved joint.

15.4.2.4 Other Manifestations

There are also cases with ocular lesions. The early manifestation is mainly conjunctivitis, which later develops into uveitis, keratitis, and hyalitis. There are also reports about urinary system manifestations such as urgent urination, odynuria, and urinary incontinence. By biopsy of bladder tissues, Bb can be detected at the bladder wall.

15.4.3 Persistent Infection Period

In this period, the common manifestations include arthritis, chronic atrophic acrodermatitis, and advanced neurological symptoms such as chronic progressive meningitis, transverse myelitis, paralysis, and dementia. Other manifestations during this period include benign skin lymphocytosis, hepatitis-like symptoms, deep myositis, and splenomegaly.

15.5 Lyme Disease-Related Complications

15.5.1 Congenital Lyme Disease

The pathogen can spread via vertical transmission from mother to fetus, causing congenital infection. The further outcomes may include premature delivery, stillbirth, symphysodactylia, and central blindness.

15.5.2 Double Infections

In some cases, patients with Lyme disease may be coinfected by forest encephalitis.

The other complications have been described in Sect. 15.4 of this chapter.

15.6 Diagnostic Examinations

15.6.1 Laboratory Tests

15.6.1.1 Etiological Detection

Direct Detection or Detection After Staining

Tissues of the skin, synovium, lymph node, or specimen of cerebrospinal fluid are collected for dark field microscopy or sliver staining to detect Bb. In such a way, the pathogen can be rapidly detected, but with a low detective rate. The application of specific direct fluorescent antibody staining can increase the detection rate.

Pathogen Isolation

The pathogens can be isolated from the samples of the skin, lymph nodes, blood, and cerebrospinal fluid from the patients. The positive rate (86 %) of skin tissues around the lesions is relatively higher.

PCR Technique

PCR can be applied to detect the DNA of Bb in the blood, urine, cerebrospinal fluid, and skin from the patients, with a high sensitivity. Meanwhile, the genotype of the infected strain can also be identified.

15.6.1.2 Serological Test

Currently, the serologic test for specific antibody of Lyme disease lacks of standardized reagent and procedure. The test result is sometimes false-negative or false-positive.

15.6.2 Diagnostic Imaging

Diagnostic imaging is commonly applied to assess and diagnose cardiac dysfunctions, neurological impairments, and arthritis caused by Bb.

15.7 Imaging Demonstrations

15.7.1 Ultrasound

In the cases with Lyme disease complicated by cardiac impairments, ultrasound may reveal pericarditis and left cardiac dysfunction.

15.7.2 X-Ray

X-ray is commonly applied for the examination of joint lesions that complicate Lyme disease. Several weeks to several months after the onset, chronic arthritis may occur, with manifestations of joints swelling, articular effusion, thin articular cartilage, and articular marginal bone erosion. The characteristic manifestation is infrapatellar bursa edema. The X-ray reveals joints swelling, the disappearance of the fat density in the knee-joint capsule, narrowed articular space, and cystic degeneration under articular surface. In the cases of chronic conditions, X-ray reveals linear calcification of the tendon.

15.7.3 MR Imaging

MR imaging is mainly applied to examine neurological lesions and joint lesions that complicate Lyme disease.

15.7.3.1 Neurological Lesions

Early neurological lesions have no specific imaging demonstrations. Generally, several weeks or months after the onset, MR imaging reveals meningitis, usually with accompanying headache and fever. The condition may turn into chronic.

In some cases, contrast imaging demonstrates meningeal enhancement. The intracranial changes mainly include multiple patches of long T1 and T2 signals with a diameter of 2–3 mm surrounding the bilateral ventricles and/or under the cortex and enhancement of some lesions. Water and fat suppression T2WI demonstrates high signals, with no accompanying space-occupying effect. Some lesions may be located in the basal ganglia and brainstem. As for the spinal cord, it seldom has transverse myelitis but has multiple focal lesions in high T2WI signal. Contrast imaging demonstrates enhanced nerve roots with radiculitis. In the advanced stage, the patient may also have nonspecific encephalatrophy (Fig. 15.1).

Case Study 1

A female patient aged 41 years, with a medical history of epilepsy.

For case detail and figures, please refer to Agarwal R, et al. *Radiology*, 2009, 253 (1): 167.

Case Study 2

A male patient aged 71 years, with headache, fatigue, fever and diplopia.

For case detail and figures, please refer to Hildenbrand P, et al. *AJNR*, 2009, 30(6): 107.

Case Study 3

A female patient aged 77 years, with positive blood IgM for Lyme disease.

Note: The case and images are provided by Tang, YH. at Rui Jin Hospital, Shanghai, China

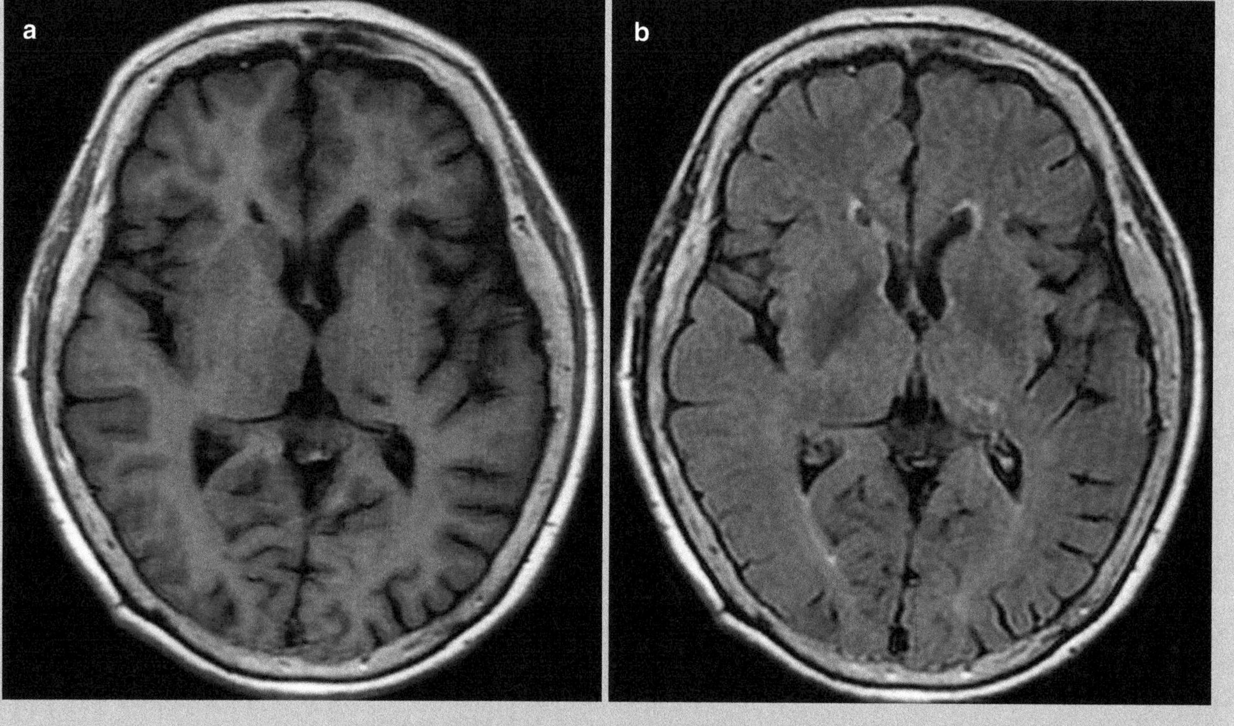

Fig. 15.1 Lyme disease complicated by neurological lesions. (**a**) T1WI demonstrates strips of low signal in the left thalamus. (**b**) T2WI FLAIR demonstrates stripes of high signal in the left thalamus

15.7.3.2 Joint Lesions

For joint lesion, MR imaging is superior in demonstrating lesions of the soft tissues and joint cartilages. The main findings include bone erosion around the major joints, multiple cystic degenerations under the bone cortex, osteophyte formation, absent joint cartilage, and articular effusion. In some pediatric cases, there are also enlarged lymph nodes in the soft tissues surrounding the joints, myositis, and fasciitis. Contrast T1WI demonstrates enhanced enlarged lymph nodes (>1 cm), flakes of enhancement in the muscles around the joints, and edema around superficial and deep fascia.

Case Study 4

A male patient aged 16 years.

For case detail and figures, please refer to Ecklund et al. *AJR Am J Roentgenol*, 2005, 184 (6): 1904.

15.7.3.3 Myocarditis

In the acute stage, delayed contrast MR imaging demonstrates stripes of enhancement in the myocardium (Fig. 15.2).

Case Study 5

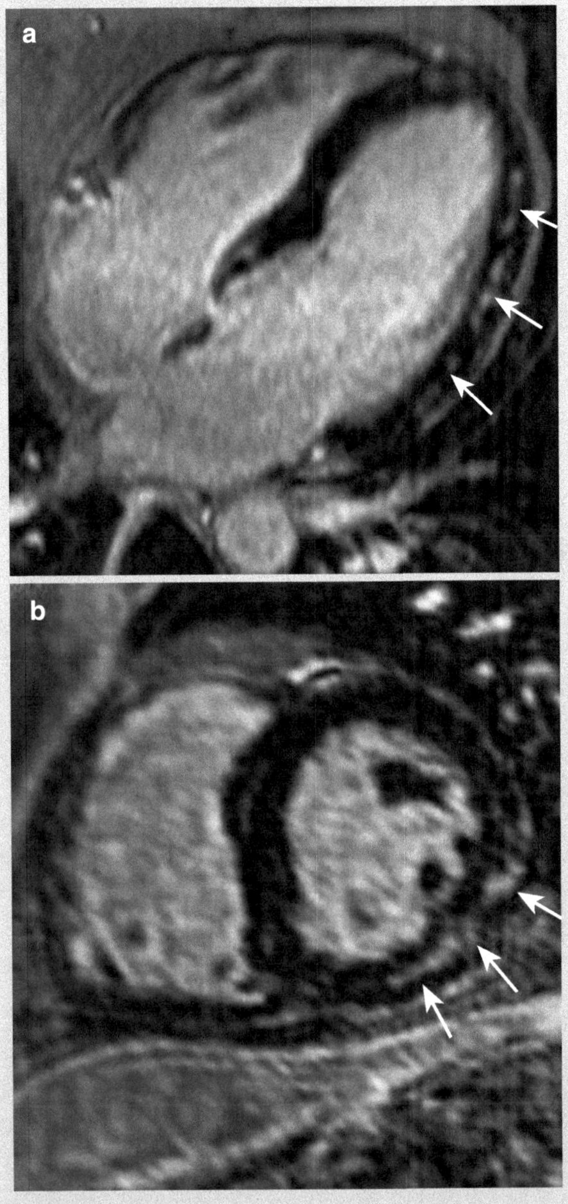

Fig. 15.2 Lyme disease complicated by cardiac lesions. (**a**) Contrast imaging of the four cardiac chambers in the advanced stage demonstrates moderate enhancement in the left ventricular wall (*arrows*). (**b**) Short-axis imaging demonstrates stripes of enhanced lesions in the left ventricular wall (*arrows*) (Reproduced with permission from Maher B, et al. *Heart.* 2012, 98 (3): 264)

15.7.4 Nuclear Medicine

Generally, assessment and diagnosis of Lyme disease do not necessarily require nuclear medicine examination. And it fails to demonstrate abnormalities for early neurological lesions. The advanced neurological lesions are usually demonstrated as decreased cerebral cortex perfusion and increased radioactive uptake by the affected joint.

For case detail and figures, please refer to Sumiya H, et al. *J Nucl Med*, 1997, 38 (7): 1120.

15.8 Diagnostic Basis

The diagnosis of the Lyme disease should be based on the epidemiologic history, clinical manifestations, and laboratory tests.

15.8.1 Epidemiology

The patient has a history of visit or living in an epidemic area in the epidemic season, with an experience of being bitten by a tick.

15.8.2 Clinical Manifestations

The characteristic erythema chronicum migrans and the skin lesions being above 10 cm in diameter highly indicate Lyme disease.

15.8.3 Laboratory Tests

Bb can be isolated from the tissue fluid or body fluid of the patient. One month after the infection, IgG positive supports the diagnosis of Lyme disease. IgG positive alone is likely to be false-positive.

15.8.4 Imaging Demonstrations

The imaging demonstrations include encephalitis, cranial granuloma, pericarditis, myocarditis, facial nerve radiculitis, joint swelling, articular effusion, bone destruction, and hyperplasia.

15.9 Differential Diagnosis

The neurological diseases complicating Lyme disease should be differentiated from other encephalitis or poliomyelitis. The LD joint lesions should be differentiated from rheumatic fever and rheumatoid arthritis. The diagnostic imaging has no specific demonstration for joint lesions. In combination to clinical history and laboratory tests, their diagnosis can be defined.

References

Agarwal R, Sze G. Neuro-lyme disease: MR imaging findings. Radiology. 2009;253(1):167–73.

Ecklund K, Vargas S, Zurakowski D, et al. MRI features of Lyme arthritis in children. AJR Am J Roentgenol. 2005,184(6):1904–1909.

Hildenbrand P, Craven DE, Jones R, et al. Lyme neuroborreliosis: manifestations of a rapidly emerging zoonosis. AJNR Am J Neuroradiol. 2009;30(6):1079–87.

Maher B, Murday D, Harden SP. Cardiac MRI of Lyme disease myocarditis. Heart. 2012;98(3):264.

Sumiya H, Kobayashi K, Mizukoshi C, et al. Brain perfusion SPECT in Lyme neuroborreliosis. J Nucl Med. 1997;38(7):1120–2.

Suggest Reading

Biesiada G, Czepiel J, Leśniak MR, et al. Lyme disease: review. Arch Med Sci. 2012;8(6):978–82.

Blanc F, Ballonzoli L, Marcel C, et al. Lyme optic neuritis. J Neurol Sci. 2010;295(1):117–9.

Brown SJ, Dadparvar S, Slizofski WJ, et al. Triple-phase bone image abnormalities in Lyme arthritis. Clin Nucl Med. 1989;14(10):730–3.

Donta ST, Noto RB, Vento JA. SPECT brain imaging in chronic Lyme disease. Clin Nucl Med. 2012;37(9):e219–22.

Holmgren AR, Matteson EL. Lyme myositis. Arthritis Rheum. 2006;54(8):2697–700.

Jia FZ, Li LJ, Ding YX, et al. Studies of infectious diseases. Nanjing: Jiangsu Science and Technology Press; 2010.

Karadag B, Spieker LE, Schwitter J, et al. Lyme carditis: restitutio ad integrum documented by cardiac magnetic resonance imaging. Cardiol Rev. 2004;12(4):185–7.

Lawson JP, Rahn DW. Lyme disease and radiologic findings in Lyme arthritis. AJR Am J Roentgenol. 1992;158(5):1065–9.

Li MD, Wang YM, Niu JQ, et al. Practical studies of infectious diseases. Beijing: People's Medical Publishing House; 2004.

Naik M, Kim D, O'Brien F, et al. Lyme carditis. Circulation. 2008;118(18):1881–4.

Nau R, Christen HJ, Eiffert H. Lyme disease-current state of knowledge. Dtsch Arztebl Int. 2009;106(5):72–81.

16 Neonatal Tetanus

Yinglin Guo, Lili Tang, and Bailu Liu

Neonatal tetanus is an acute infectious disease characterized by trismus as well as systemic muscular rigidity and spasm caused by tetanospasmin, which is produced after *Clostridium tetani* (C. tetani) invade the navel.

16.1 Etiology

C. tetani is a rod-shaped Gram-positive bacillus, with a length of 2–18 μm and a width of 0.5–1.7 μm. It is strictly anaerobic, with surrounding flagella but no capsule. *C. tetani* is characterized by forming wider round-shaped spore at the top of the thallus, producing a drumstick appearance microscopically. Filmlike spreading growth emerges after an incubation period of 24 h at 37 °C on blood plates, with accompanying β hemolysis. It performs neither carbohydrate fermentation nor proteolysis. Spores can be damaged at 100 °C and can survive in the dry soil and dusts for decades.

C. tetani plays a pathogenetic role primarily by producing two types of exotoxins, tetanospasmin, and tetanolysin. Tetanospasmin is plasmid encoding. As a neurotoxin, it constitutes the major pathogenic substance to cause tetanus, with high affinity to brainstem nerve cells and the anterior horn cell nucleus of spinal cords. The toxin can be absorbed by local never cells or travels along with lymph and blood flow to invade the central nerve system, with strong toxicity which is just weaker than botulin. Chemically, it is a heat-sensitive protein that can be dissolved at 65 °C for 30 min or be destructed by digestive proteinases in intestinal tract. Tetanolysin is sensitive to oxygen whose function and antigenicity resemble to streptolysin O, but its pathogenesis underlying the occurrence of tetanus remains elusive.

Y. Guo (✉)
Department of Radiology, Taiping People's Hospital, Daowai District, Harbin, Heilongjiang, China
e-mail: guoyinglinhmu@126.com

L. Tang • B. Liu
CT Department, The Second Affiliated Hospital, Harbin Medical University, Harbin, Heilongjiang, China

16.2 Epidemiology

C. tetani is ubiquitous in soil, dusts, and stool of animals and humans. Neonatal tetanus occurs commonly when umbilical cord is cut during delivery, caused by invasion of *C. tetani* into the navel due to unsterilized or incompletely sterilized hands of midwives, scissors, or gauze.

16.3 Pathogenesis and Pathological Changes

The major pathogenesis of neonatal tetanus is that *C. tetani* invade the navel. It occurs often 4–7 days after delivery, caused by invasion of *C. tetani* into the navel due to unsterilized or incompletely sterilized hands of midwives, scissors, or gauze and unawareness of the navel sterilization. The bandaging of navel provides an oxygen-insufficient environment facilitative to the reproduction of *C. tetani*, which consequently produce tetanotoxin. The tetanospasmin it produces travels along the nerve cord and lymph flow into anterior horn cells of spinal cord and the brainstem motoneuron. Consequently, it binds to ganglioside in central nervous tissues, where it blocks the release of inhibitory neurotransmitters, glycine, and γ-aminobutyric acid, to interfere the coordinative role of inhibitory neurons. Therefore, the afferent stimulation of the motor nervous system is strengthened, causing sustained strong contraction of the muscles all over the body. The toxin can also excite sympathetic nerves, leading to tachycardia, hypertension, and profuse perspiration. Tetanolysin can cause necrosis of local tissues and impairments to the myocardium.

16.4 Clinical Symptoms and Signs

The incubation period of neonatal tetanus commonly lasts for 3–14 days, and its occurrence is usually at 4th–7th day after delivery. Therefore, it is commonly referred to as

H. Li (ed.), *Radiology of Infectious Diseases: Volume 2*, DOI 10.1007/978-94-017-9876-1_16

tetanus of the 7th day. Generally, the cases with a shorter period of incubation sustain more serious conditions and higher mortality rate. Clinically, the disease is divided into two types, mild type and serious type. The whole course of illness includes incubation period, pre-spasm stage, spasm stage, and convalescent stage.

The serious type of neonatal tetanus occurs within a week after delivery. The baby patients commonly experienced traditional mode of delivery, and the serious type generally has an incubation period of no more than 7 days, a pre-spasm stage of no more than 24 h, a body temperature of no lower than 39 °C or a normal body temperature, spasm stage persisting for no less than 30 s, and interval between spasm episodes no longer than 5 min, with complications of pneumonia and septicemia. The mild type of neonatal tetanus occurs after the first week of delivery, with an incubation period no shorter than 7 days, a pre-spasm stage no less than 24 h, trismus, spasms no longer than 10 s, and interval between spasms no less than 15 min.

The period from the onset of symptoms to the initial convulsion is known as the pre-spasm stage. During the spasm stage, there are feeding refusal, trismus, facial muscular tension and pulled up mouth corners in appearance of forced smile, accompanying paroxysmal clenched fists, excessive flexion of upper extremities, and extension of lower extremities in posture of opisthotonos. During the episodes of spasm, the disease is characterized by favorable consciousness of the baby patients and convulsion induced by slight stimulation. During the early stage with no obvious convulsion, the baby patients keep crying and the mouth fails to be wide open. The spatula test that touches the oropharynx with a spatula or tongue blade can cause an immediate trismus, which facilitates the diagnosis.

16.5 Neonatal Tetanus-Related Complications

Neonatal tetanus can be complicated by many conditions, and the complications are commonly secondary to the serious type of neonatal tetanus. Serious complications are the main cause of death in cases of neonatal tetanus. The baby patients sustain spasms and increased secretions in the airway to cause apnea or respiratory failure, and secondary infections. Frequent convulsions may cause cerebral ischemia and cerebral hypoxia that further progress into encephaledema and cerebral hemorrhage. Due to the episodes of convulsion, the baby patients consume more energy and experience metabolic disturbance that lead to hypoglycemia and disturbances of electrolytes and aid-base balance.

16.6 Diagnostic Examinations

16.6.1 Laboratory Tests

16.6.1.1 Routine Blood Test

In the cases with secondary pulmonary infections, peripheral WBC count significantly increases.

16.6.1.2 Bacteria Culture

Pyogenic aerobic bacteria can be isolated from secretions of wound, and *C. tetani* can also be isolated by anaerobic culture. As clinical manifestations of neonatal tetanus are specific, the diagnosis presents no challenges, especially for the cases with typical symptoms. Therefore, evidence from bacteria culture is not required for its diagnosis.

16.6.2 Diagnostic Imaging

For the cases with respiratory disorders, such as pneumonia, pulmonary atelectasis and pulmonary embolism, chest X-ray, and CT scanning are recommended. For the cases with complications of central nervous system, such as encephaledema, cerebral hemorrhage, and cerebral herniation, cerebral CT scanning or MR imaging is recommended to define the diagnosis.

16.7 Imaging Demonstrations

16.7.1 Respiratory System

Due to laryngospasm and paroxysmal convulsion, unsmooth respiration and stasis of respiratory secretions occur. In addition to the use of respirator, the baby patients are susceptible to pulmonary infections, aspiratory pneumonia, and pulmonary atelectasis.

16.7.1.1 Chest X-Ray

Chest X-ray may demonstrate no abnormal findings. Otherwise, it demonstrates only increased, thickened, and blurry pulmonary markings. When the conditions progress, chest X-ray can demonstrate patchy blurry shadows in the inner and middle zones of middle and lower pulmonary fields in both lungs that distribute around the pulmonary markings. It can also demonstrate the fusion of lesions into large flakes of shadows or parenchymal changes and dense shadows of pulmonary hilum. In the cases with pulmonary atelectasis, chest X-ray demonstrates triangle shape or narrow strips of dense shadows, with their apex pointing to the pulmonary hilum.

Case Study
A newborn baby girl aged 5 days after full-term birth has a body temperature of 40 °C and a WBC count of $22.8 \times 10^9/L$ (Fig. 16.1).

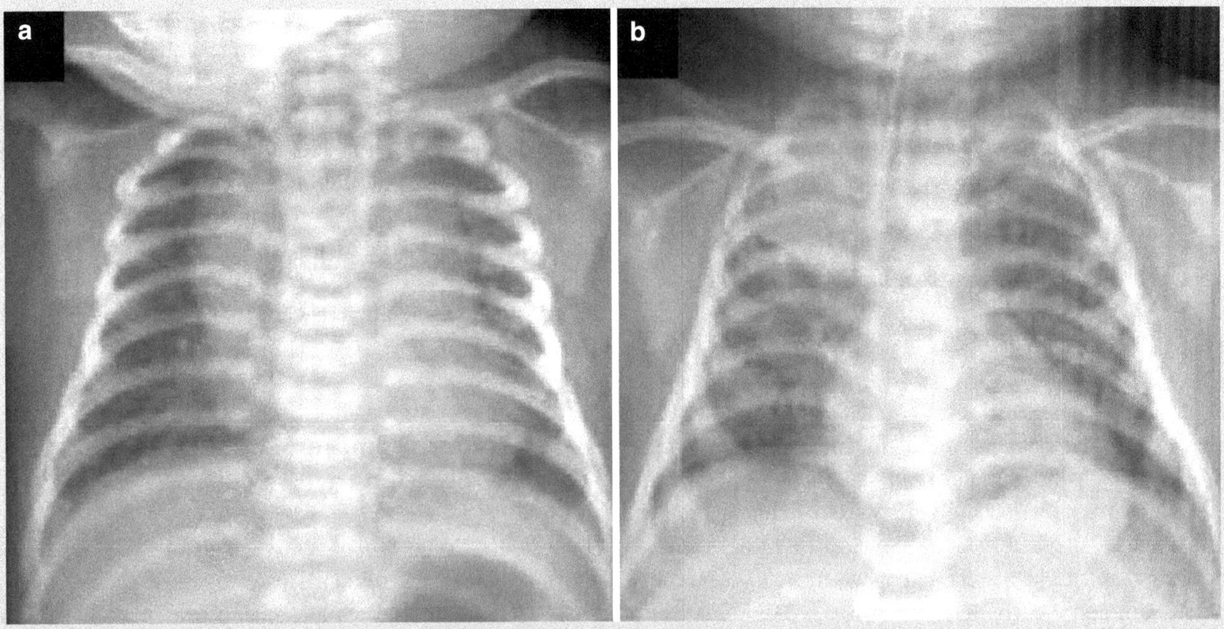

Fig. 16.1 Neonatal tetanus complicated by pulmonary atelectasis (**a**) Chest X-ray demonstrates no obvious abnormality when hospitalized. (**b**) By reexamination after 8 days, chest X-ray demonstrates atelectasis of the upper lobe in the right lung (Reprint with permission from Chang SC, et al. *Pediatr Neonatol*, 2010, 51(3): 182)

16.7.1.2 CT Scanning

CT scanning demonstrates thickened and blurry bronchovascular bundle in the middle and lower fields of both lungs. The lesions are mostly small patches of cloudy shadows, with some fusing into large flakes or triangular parenchymal shadows. In the cases with pulmonary atelectasis, the demonstrations also include lobular, segmental, or lobar atelectasis.

16.7.2 Central Nervous System

16.7.2.1 CT Scanning

Encephaledema has CT demonstrations of low-density shadows in cerebral parenchyma with unclearly defined boundaries, unclearly defined borderline between the gray and white matters, and absence of some sulci. In the case of cerebral parenchymal hemorrhage, CT scanning demonstrates spots, patches, round or roundlike-shaped shadows in high density, with surrounding flakes of low-density shadows due to encephaledema. In the cases of subarachnoid hemorrhage, CT scanning demonstrates absent sulci and cisterns and increased destiny. And the CT demonstrations of subdural hematoma include crescent-shaped high-density shadows under bone lamella and migration of brain parenchyma inwards due to compression.

16.7.2.2 MR Imaging

MR imaging of cases with acute encephaledema demonstrates flakes of high T1 and high T2 signals. The cases of cerebral hemorrhage show spots or flakes of equal/high signal by T1WI and high or mixed signal by T2WI.

16.8 Basis for Diagnosis

16.8.1 Neonatal Tetanus

Based on the history of delivery mode, the diagnosis can be made for the cases choosing traditional mode of delivery or possible incomplete sterilization when the umbilical cord was severed. The disease has typical symptoms and etiological examinations by bacteria culture are not necessary for the diagnosis.

16.8.2 Neonatal Tetanus-Related Complications

16.8.2.1 Respiratory System

The slight type of neonatal tetanus shows mild respiratory symptoms, whereas the serious type shows pathological changes such as pulmonary parenchymal changes and pulmonary atelectasis.

16.8.2.2 Central Nervous System

Infants with neonatal tetanus may show pathological changes of encephaledema and cerebral hemorrhage.

16.9 Differential Diagnosis

16.9.1 Prepharyngeal or Retropharyngeal Abscess

Patients with tetanus can develop clinical symptoms such as difficulties in opening mouth and sucking milk; however, these symptoms rarely occur in infants with neonatal tetanus, with no muscular spasms. X-ray shows diffuse thickening of prevertebral soft tissues at the retropharyngeal wall possibly with smooth and clearly defined surface and possible findings of air-fluid level. CT scanning demonstrates diffusive thickening of anterior cervical or pharyngeal soft tissues, accompanying absence of fat spaces, and possible heterogeneous density. These findings indicate formation of abscess. When the disease is caused by mycobacterium tuberculosis, the accompanying demonstrations include calcification or bone tuberculosis. MR imaging demonstrates anterior cervical or pharyngeal abscesses as low signal by T_1WI and high signal by T_2WI.

16.9.2 Purulent Meningitis

Clinical manifestations include fever and repeated spasms. However, in the intervals of repeated spasms, muscular tension and trismus are absent, but unconsciousness and abnormal cerebrospinal fluid are present. Therefore, the differential diagnosis can be made based on these clinical manifestations. In the early stage of purulent meningitis or mild cases of purulent meningitis, both CT scanning and MR imaging demonstrate no obvious abnormality. Plain CT scanning demonstrates increased density or obstruction in the basal cistern, possibly with accompanying encephaledema and hydrocephalus. Enhanced CT scanning demonstrates curve-like or gyrus-like enhancement. MR imaging demonstrates asymmetrically bilateral subarachnoid cavities by T1WI with inside equal or slightly short T_1 signal, while the cases of gyrus edema are demonstrated as having focal or diffusive multiple flakes of long T_1 and long T_2 signals. By enhanced Gd-DTPA scanning, the gyrus and ependyma are demonstrated as having linear and gyrus-like enhancement, while the cases with subdural effusion are demonstrated as having crescent-like lesions under the inner lamina of skull.

16.9.3 Hypocalcemia and Neonatal Convulsion

Hypocalcemia and neonatal convulsion can also cause spasms of the extremities. However, these diseases fail to show trismus, forced smile, and no muscular tension, and opisthotonos occurs during intervals between spasms.

References

Chang SC, Wang CL. Neonatal tetanus after home delivery: report of one case. Pediatr Neonatol. 2010;51(3):182–5.

Suggested Reading

Hasil Sensus Penduduk. Maternal and neonatal tetanus elimination in Bali and Java, Indonesia, 2010. Wkly Epidemiol Rec. 2010;46(26): 473–88.

Jia WX. Medical microbiology. Beijing: People's Health Publishing House; 2008.

Wang GQ, Deng YX. Neonatal tetanus complicated by intracranial hemorrhage: a report of 2 cases. J Clin Pract Pediatr. 2009;24(10):782.

Yao L. Pediatrics. Beijing: People's Health Publishing House; 2008.

Other Infectious Diarrhea

17

Li Li, Mingxiao Sun, and Jing Zhao

Other infectious diarrhea, with cholera, bacillary and amebic dysentery, typhoid, and paratyphoid fever excluded, is a group of infectious diseases with diarrhea as the main symptom caused by pathogenic microorganisms and their products or parasites. It has been legally listed as Class C infectious diseases in China. This disease prevails all over the world and has been one of the global public health issues. According to the announced epidemics of the legally listed infectious diseases by the Ministry of Health in the People's Republic of China in 2009, the reported cases of infectious diarrhea account for 27.33 % of the total reported cases of Class C infectious diseases and 11.11 % of the total reported cases of all legally listed infectious diseases.

17.1 Etiology

Infectious diarrhea can be caused by bacteria, viruses, fungi, and parasites. The bacterial and viral infections are more common, especially viral infection. In the cases of bacterial infection, the more common pathogens include diarrheic *Escherichia coli* (including enterohemorrhagic *Escherichia coli*, enteropathogenic *Escherichia coli* and enterotoxigenic *Escherichia coli*), *Salmonella, Campylobacter*, and *Yersinia*. Concerning the viral infection, the more common pathogens include rotavirus, norovirus, calicivirus, astrovirus, and enteral adenovirus. And the common pathogens of parasitic infection are cryptosporidium, giardia, and amoeba, while the common pathogens of fungal infection include candida, aspergillus, and mucor.

L. Li (✉) • J. Zhao
Department of Radiology, Beijing You'an Hospital, Capital Medical University, Beijing, China
e-mail: sycrbyxx@126.com

M. Sun
Department of Orthopedics, City Development District Hospital, Yantai, Shandong, China

17.1.1 Bacterial Infection

17.1.1.1 Diarrheic *Escherichia coli* Infection

E. coli, as normal bacterial colony at the intestinal tract of human or animal, are generally nonpathogenic. It is a Gram-negative and facultative anaerobic bacteria in short rod shape with no spore. The antigenic structure of *E. coli* is relatively complex, mainly including three types: thallus antigen (O antigen), envelope antigen (K antigen), and flagellar antigen (H antigen). O antigen is the foundation for serotyping, based on which more than 160 serotypes have been found. Certain serotypes are pathogenic, and those, as pathogen of human diarrhea, are known as diarrheic *E. coli*.

17.1.1.2 *Vibrio Parahaemolyticus* Infection

Vibrio parahaemolyticus (VP) is a pathogenic bacteria causing zoonosis and was firstly isolated in Japan in 1950. It is one of the main pathogenic bacteria causing foodborne diarrhea, which has been categorized into the family of Vibrionaceae, the genus of *Vibrio parahaemolyticus* and is a Gram-negative rod-shaped or arch-shaped bacteria with flagella but no spore. It is morphologically various, with halophilic growth. Its antigenic structure is complex, and, so far, with known 13 O antigens and 71 K antigens. In China, the main antigens of the bacteria are O_3 and K_6.

17.1.1.3 Salmonellosis

Salmonellosis, also known as nontyphoidal salmonellosis, is an umbrella term referring to infection caused by Salmonella, with typhoid and paratyphoid A, B, and C excluded. Salmonella is a Gram-negative and aerobic or facultative anaerobic short rod-shaped bacillus, with no capsule and spore. Most of them have dynamic flagella and pili. Salmonella has a relatively strong tolerance to the external environment but is intolerant to heat and high temperature.

17.1.1.4 Campylobacterial Infection

According to the latest bacterial classification rules, campylobacter is categorized into the family of campylobacteraceae,

H. Li (ed.), *Radiology of Infectious Diseases: Volume 2*, DOI 10.1007/978-94-017-9876-1_17

which includes 18 species and several subspecies. Among them, *Campylobacter jejuni* and *Campylobacter coli* can cause human diarrhea. Campylobacterium is a Gram-negative microaerophilic and polymorphous bacteria with flagella but no spore. O antigen and H antigen are its main antigens. They can trigger local immunity in the affected intestinal tract, while IgG, IgM, and IgA antibodies against O antigen are produced in the blood to play certain protective role. Campylobacter has a weak resistance to external environment and is sensitive to heat as well as physical and chemical disinfectants.

17.1.1.5 *Yersinia Enterocolitica* Infection

Yersinia enterocolitica (Y. e.) is a Gram-negative aerobic or facultative anaerobic bacillus, which is dynamic and cold resistant. However, it is sensitive to damp heat and chemical disinfectants.

17.1.2 Virus Infection

Viral infection plays an important role in acute infectious diarrhea, with the most common diarrheic viruses of rotavirus and *Norovirus*. Rotavirus commonly causes sporadic infantile diarrhea in autumns and winters, while *Norovirus* can cause large-scale outbreak and epidemic of diarrhea in children and adults.

17.1.2.1 Rotavirus Infection

Rotavirus is categorized into the family of reoviridae, which is a double-stranded RNA virus. Its diameter is approximately 70–75 nm whose center is a dense core with a diameter of 36–45 nm containing the viral nucleic acid. Since rotavirus has double layers of capsid and is arranged in a radiating style from the inside outwards, under an electron microscope, it appears like a wheel and was therefore nominated as rotavirus. The virus is stable at external environment, which can survive for 7 months at room temperature. In addition, it is tolerant to acid and alkali. At a temperature of 55 °C for 30 min, it can be inactivated.

17.1.2.2 Norovirus Infection

Norovirus is a single-stranded positive RNA virus with no envelope. It has a diameter of 26–35 nm, replicating in the nucleus of host cells. Under an electron microscope, it can be found with a spherical or polyhedral shape. Up to now, at least three basic serotypes have been identified. The virus is tolerant to ether, acid, and heat. At a temperature of 60 °C for 30 min, the virus cannot be completely inactivated.

17.1.2.3 Enteric Adenovirus Infection

Enteric adenovirus (EAdV), namely, adenovirus types 40 and 41, is the main pathogen causing adenovirus intestinal infection and the second common pathogen of pediatric viral diarrhea. Under an electron microscope, EAdV has the same morphology as other common adenovirus. Exposure of EAdV to ultraviolet ray for 30 min can deprive of its infectivity.

17.1.3 Parasitic Infection

It has been known that above 50 kinds of parasites can cause diarrhea, and the most common diarrhea inducing parasites include cryptosporidium, *Giardia lamblia* Stile, and amoeba.

17.1.3.1 Cryptosporidium Infection

Cryptosporidium is one of the obligate intracellular parasites. It has a spherical shape with a diameter of 2–4 μm. Its life history is composed of schizogony, sporogony, and gametogony, with all the three periods occurring within the same host. Currently, eight species of zoonotic cryptosporidia and one genotype have been identified. *Cryptosporidium parvum* is related to diarrhea of human and most mammals. Cryptosporidium has an oocyst that has a relatively strong resistance to many common disinfectants and chemicals. The oocyst can stay alive in a damp and cold environment for several months or even about 1 year.

17.1.3.2 *Giardia lamblia* Stile Infection

Giardia lamblia Stile (1915), or shortly *Giardia*, commonly parasitizes of the duodenum or the upper small intestine of human or animals to cause abdominal pain, diarrhea, and malabsorption, namely, giardiasis. Giardiasis has been defined as one of the top 10 severe parasitosis in the world by WHO. Since its common prevalence in travelers, it is also known as travelers' diarrhea. The life cycle of *Giardia* can be divided into two phases: trophozoite (vegetative phase) and oocyst (transmitting phase). Trophozoites usually survive at the duodenum or the upper small intestine of human or animals, but sometimes at the biliary tract or pancreatic duct. The oocyst has strong survival ability in the external environment. It can remain alive in chlorinated water (0.5 %) for 2–3 days, while it is able to live in the feces for more than 10 days.

17.2 Epidemiology

17.2.1 Source of Infection

The main sources of infection are affected patients, including patients at the acute and chronic stages, and pathogen carriers (including patients at the convalescence stage and healthy pathogen carriers). In addition, affected animals, including poultry, livestock, beasts, and fish, can also act as sources of its infection.

17.2.2 Route of Transmission

Infectious diarrhea is mainly transmitted via fecal-oral route. In other words, people can be infected via intake of contaminated water or food, daily life contacts, or flies carrying pathogens.

17.2.3 Susceptible Population

Regardless of age and gender, people are generally susceptible to infectious diarrhea. However, rotavirus mainly invades infants aged from 6 months to 5 years, while adult infectious diarrhea caused by rotavirus is mainly found in juveniles and adults. Bacterial infection is related to the risk of infection, the severity of infection, and the immunity of organism. The immunity acquired after the infection is transient and unstable. Therefore, repeated infections are highly possible.

17.2.4 Epidemiological Features

17.2.4.1 Regional Distribution

Though infectious diarrhea occurs worldwide, the incidence rate has great regional variance, which is related to health care facilities, health care knowledge of common people, and their life style. Different pathogens are distributed in different regions. For instance, *Vibrio parahaemolyticus* tends to more commonly affect the coastal regions. The main sources of salmonella are animals, which spread the disease via meat, eggs, organs, and dairy products carrying the bacteria.

17.2.4.2 Seasonal Distribution

Infectious diarrhea can occur all year round but has obvious seasonal prevailing peak. Bacterial infectious diarrhea occurs more commonly in summers and autumns, while viral infectious diarrhea (such as rotavirus diarrhea and *Norovirus* diarrhea) and *Yersinia enterocolitica* diarrhea occur more commonly in winters.

17.3 Pathogenesis and Pathological Changes

17.3.1 Pathogenesis

17.3.1.1 Bacterial Infectious Diarrhea

According to bacterial toxins and bacterial invasiveness to the intestinal mucosa, the pathogenesis of bacterial infectious diarrhea can be divided into three types: enterotoxic, invasive, and adhesive types.

Enterotoxic Type

It has been known that after pathogenic bacteria gain their access into the intestinal tract, they do not invade the intestinal epithelial cells but only reproduce themselves at the small intestine and adhere to the intestinal mucosa to release pathogenic enterotoxins. As an exotoxin, the enterotoxin can trigger secretory reaction at the intestinal tract to increase the mucosal secretion via cytotoxic or noncytotoxic mechanism. Not all the toxic mechanisms of enterotoxins produced by various bacteria are the same. Noncytotoxic enterotoxins (cell activating enterotoxins) act on the adenylyl cyclase at the cytomembrane, thus interfering the cyclic nucleotide system.

Invasive Type

According to the bacterial invasiveness to the intestinal mucosa, the pathogenesis can be further divided into three subtypes.

1. *Invasion and destruction of epithelial cells*
   Facilitated by the invasiveness, the pathogenic bacteria directly invade the epithelium of colon and terminal ileum where they reproduce themselves. Then they induce the production of some cytokines like IL-8, which may result in excessive inflammatory responses to impair the colonic epithelial cells and cause histopathological lesions of the colon tissue. Consequently, exudative diarrhea occurs. The typical pathogenic bacteria include *Shigella* and enteroinvasive *E. coli*.
2. *Invasion of the lamina propria and mesenteric lymph nodes*
   The pathogenic bacteria invade the intestinal epithelial cells, which then penetrate the cells along with pinocytotic vesicles into the lamina propria of the intestinal wall where they reproduce themselves rapidly. Therefore, local microvilli degeneration occurs, with chemotactic response and inflammatory lesions due to aggregation of a large quantity of polymorphonuclear leucocytes at the lamina propria. Consequently, exudative diarrhea occurs.
3. *Penetration of the lamina propria to cause systemic dissemination*
   Some enteric pathogenic bacteria like typhoid bacillus can penetrate the mucosal epithelium to invade the lymphoid tissue at the intestinal wall, especially the aggregated lymphoid nodules and solitary lymph nodules at the inferior ileum. After that, the bacteria may reach the mesenteric lymph nodes along with lymph flow for further reproduction. The access into the systemic circulation via the portal vein or the thoracic duct can cause bacteremia or migrating lesions, with mild lesions at the intestinal epithelial cells.

Adhesive Type

This type of pathogenesis has been recently put forward. According to it, the pathogens just adhere to the intestinal mucosa, with no invasion to the epithelium, no impairments to the intestinal mucosa, and no production of enterotoxins. However, some of these pathogens like adhesive *Escherichia coli*, with the help of colonization factors of their fimbrial antigens, adhere to the brushlike border of the epithelial cells and decompose the microvilli. The microvilli are then subject to bluntness, twists, degeneration, and even liquefaction, which leads to decreased absorption area of the intestinal mucosa. The decrease of surface enzyme at the brushlike border can cause malabsorption, which further leads to malabsorptional diarrhea or osmotic diarrhea.

17.3.1.2 Viral Infectious Diarrhea

After invasion of various viruses into the intestinal tract, they replicate themselves at the columnar epithelial cells on the top of intestinal villi. The cells are then subject to vacuolar degeneration and necroses. Consequently, the basal cells at the crypt accelerate to migrate upwards to replace the destructed cells. Due to too rapid migration, the basal cells are not well developed to cause transformation of epithelial cells from columnar to cubic.

17.3.1.3 Parasitic Infectious Diarrhea

After the access of parasites into the intestinal tract, they invade the mucosa where they mainly release proteolytic enzymes to cause histolysis, which further causes ulceration as well as abdominal pain and diarrhea. Its pathogenesis is related to parasitic sites, mechanical injury, toxic effects of metabolites, or secretions produced by parasites as well as the triggered allergic reactions in organisms.

17.3.2 Pathological Changes

17.3.2.1 Bacterial Infectious Diarrhea

The invasiveness of EPEC includes plasmid-mediated cell adhesion and chromosome-mediated microvilli injury. The pathogens enter intestinal tract via mouth, and they survive and reproduce at the duodenum, jejunum, and superior ileum. They firmly adhere to the surface of intestinal epithelial cells or embed themselves in the depression at the surface of intestinal epithelial cells to cause local microvilli atrophy and thin intestinal mucosa. The lamina propria is then subject to inflammation, with hypertrophy of crypt cells as well as necrosis and ulceration at the intestinal mucosa. Such invasiveness can cause bowel dysfunction and diarrhea. Organs in the human body may be subject to nonspecific congestion and edema, especially obvious at the heart, liver, kidneys, and the central nervous system.

After EHEC gains its access into the intestinal lumen, it adheres to epithelial cells at the cecum and colon depending on the plasmid-mediated adhesive factors. The intestinal mucosa is then subject to necrosis of epithelial cells as well as congestion and edema of intestinal mucosa to further cause inflammatory hemorrhagic diarrhea. By naked-eye observation, diffuse hemorrhage and ulceration occur at the intestinal mucosa. VT can also gain its access into the blood flow and pass through the blood-cerebrospinal fluid barrier to cause toxemia. The vascular endothelial cells are subject to injury to cause thrombotic microangiopathy. In the cases with the lesions mainly at the kidneys, hemolytic uremic syndrome may occur. Due to the toxic effect, the parasympathetic nerves are subject to increased excitement, leading to sinus bradycardia and convulsion.

The changes caused by *Vibrio parahaemolyticus* are pathologically characterized by acute intestinal inflammation, which may involve stomach, jejunum, and ileum. The histological changes include submucosal edema, mild erosion, and cell necrosis. In severe cases, the patients experience different degrees of blood stasis at the liver, spleen, lung, and other organs.

The pathological changes of salmonella infection can be varied due to different pathogenic strains and clinical types. The changes of enterogastritis type are pathologically characterized by gastric mucosa congestion and edema, possibly spots of hemorrhage, and enlarged collecting lymph nodes at the intestinal tract. The changes of dysentery type are pathologically characterized by extensive inflammation and ulceration at the colonic mucosa and submucosa, resembling the lesions of bacillary dysentery. The pathological changes of septicemia type resemble changes caused by other bacteria, with suppurative lesions at any organ or tissue.

Campylobacter jejuni can cause local lesion at the intestinal mucosa, usually with no invasion into the blood stream. The intestinal lesions can be found at the jejunum, ileum, and colon, which are mainly nonspecific inflammatory response, and accompanying infiltration of neutrophils and plasmocytes. In addition, there are also intestinal mucosal edema, spots of hemorrhage, superficial ulceration, and crypt abscess.

17.3.2.2 Viral Diarrhea

The pathological changes of rotavirus infection are commonly confined at the small intestine, with manifestations of degeneration and necrosis of the villi epithelial cells as well as reactive hyperplasia of necrotic and lacunar cells. Within 24 h after the infection, the columnar intestinal epithelial cells are transformed into cubic intestinal epithelial cells. The microvilli are blunt and shortened, with or with no infiltration of monocytes in the lamina propria. In severe cases, the intestinal epithelial cells are subject to vacuolar degeneration, necrosis, and shedding off.

The main lesions of *Norovirus* infection are located at the duodenum and the superior jejunum, with manifestations of shortened microvilli at the intestinal epithelial cells, enlarged crypt, intracellular vacuolation, and infiltration of mononuclear cells in the lamina propria. Generally, there are no necrosis of intestinal epithelial cells and no submucosal inflammatory cell infiltration.

Enteric adenovirus mainly infects the jejunum and ileum. The intestinal mucosal villi of affected segment are shortened. In the infected cells, there are intranuclear inclusion bodies, with following cell degeneration and cytolysis, which further lead to intestinal absorption dysfunction and osmotic diarrhea. Infiltration of mononuclear cells can be found at the lamina propria of intestinal mucosa, with enlarged crypt.

17.3.2.3 Parasitic Diarrhea

Cryptosporidium mainly parasitizes at the brushlike border of intestinal epithelial cells in the vacuoles formed by the host cells. The proximal jejunum is the most common position to be parasitized by *Cryptosporidium*. In some severe cases, parasites may be found all over the digestive tract. The villi at the lesion of small intestine are subject to atrophy, shortness, and even absence. Hyperplasia of crypt epithelial cells occurs simultaneously with deepening of the crypt. The epithelial cells at the mucosa surface are in short columnar shape, with irregular arrangement of the nucleus. The villi epithelial cells and the lamina propria witness infiltrations of mononuclear cells and polynuclear granulocytes. The pathological changes of colonic mucosa resemble those of small intestine. Once the patients are cured, the above changes are all absent. In the cases with the infection involving the gall bladder, acute and necrotic cholecystitis may occur, with thickened and hardened gall bladder wall, flattened mucosal surface, and ulceration. Under a microscope, necrosis of gall bladder wall and accompanying infiltration of polynuclear cells can be observed. In the cases with cryptosporidial infection of the lungs, lung tissue biopsy demonstrates active bronchitis, focalized interstitial pneumonia, and other diseases. The parasites can also be found at the lungs, tonsils, pancreas, and gall bladder.

Jejunum biopsy indicates patients with giardiasis and diarrhea; different changes of jejunum are morphologically demonstrated. In some cases, the jejunum mucosa is normal, while in some other cases, mucosal proliferation occurs, with atrophy or absence of some villi. There are still some cases with mucosal edema. Other findings include ulceration and coagulative necrosis, presence of acute inflammatory cells (polymorphonuclear granulocytes and eosinophilic granulocytes) and chronic inflammatory cell infiltration at the lamina propria, and increased mitotic count of epithelial cell nuclei. All of the above pathological changes are reversible, and in other words, the patients can be completely cured.

17.4 Clinical Symptoms and Signs

17.4.1 Bacterial Diarrhea

Due to different virulence, invasiveness, and invading positions of different types of *Escherichia coli* as well as the individual differences in immunity, the clinical symptoms are accordingly different. Generally based on the symptoms, the cases can be classified into mild, moderate, and severe types. The mild-type symptoms include no fever, poor appetite, and diarrhea. The patients of moderate type experience the symptoms of mild type, nausea, vomiting, frequent diarrheas, mild dehydration, and acidosis. The patients of severe type experience, in addition to intestinal symptoms, mostly moderate to severe dehydration, electrolyte disturbance, and acidosis. The patients with watery stool may develop cholera-like symptoms and even acute renal failure. The patients with EIEC may experience symptoms of toxic bacillary dysentery, while cases of EHEC may be complicated by acute hemolytic uremic syndrome and thrombocytopenic purpura. Death may occur in cases with delayed treatment, especially infants and young children.

Salmonella infection can also be classified into three types, gastrointestinal, typhoid, and septicemic. The incubation period of gastrointestinal type mostly lasts for 6–24 h, and the patients experience an acute onset, with nausea, vomiting, abdominal pain, and diarrhea. The patients of infants and young children are more likely to experience dehydration and electrolyte disturbance. The patients excrete yellowish or greenish watery stool, possibly with mucus and blood.

The average incubation period of campylobacter infection is 3–5 days. The patients mainly experience fever, diarrhea, abdominal pain, and rarely vomiting. The patients excrete yellowish watery stool, possibly with mucus or pus and blood. In typical cases, the patients experience spasmodic colic around the navel.

The incubation period of *Yersinia enterocolitica* infection lasts for 4–10 days. The main symptoms include sudden fever, abdominal pain, and diarrhea. Some patients may experience symptoms resembling appendicitis, chronic reactive arthritis, erythema nodosum, septicemia, and exophthalmic goiter. They excrete watery stool, possibly with mucus and rarely with pus and blood.

17.4.2 Viral Diarrhea

Viral diarrhea is also called viral gastroenteritis. The incubation period of acute viral gastroenteritis usually lasts for 1–2 days. After the incubation period, the patients experience sudden onset of diarrhea and watery stool that persist for 4–7 days, and accompanying vomiting and different degrees of dehydration. More than one-third of child patients with rotavirus infection experience fever with a body temperature above 39 °C. In children with immunodeficiency, rotavirus or adenovirus can cause chronic intestinal infection, and the virus can be persistently released for several weeks or even months.

17.4.3 Parasitic Diarrhea

Cryptosporidium infection is clinically manifested as diarrhea, abdominal pain, nausea, vomiting, anorexia, fatigue, and loss of body weight, possibly with accompanying low-grade fever. The patients with immunodeficiency, especially patients with AIDS, experience chronic onset and persistent diarrhea. The stool may be watery or mucous, with no pus and blood but an unpleasant smell. Microscopy demonstrates leukocytes and pyocytes in the stool. In patients with immunodeficiency, cryptosporidium infection can be complicated by extraenteral diseases such as respiratory tract infection or biliary tract infection.

The incubation period of *Giardia lamblia* infection lasts for 7–14 days. The patients mostly experience self-limited diarrhea, chronic diarrhea, and related malabsorption and loss of body weight. Otherwise, the patients are asymptomatic carriers of *Giardia lamblia*. The stool is stinky watery, paste-like or mass-like. With delayed treatment, the patients may develop chronic cases.

17.5 Other Infectious Diarrhea-Related Complications

17.5.1 Respiratory Complications

17.5.1.1 Pneumonia

So far, it has been known that some pathogenic bacteria causing other infectious diarrhea can also cause pulmonary infection, and such pathogenic bacteria include *Escherichia coli*, *Yersinia*, rotavirus, adenovirus, and salmonella. The pathogenesis of pulmonary infection caused by these pathogenic bacteria is as follows: (1) Most importantly, diarrhea-induced disturbances of water and electrolyte compromise the immunity of the organisms, which increases the risk of pulmonary infection. (2) After intestinal infection by the pathogenic bacteria, the intestinal mucosa is subject to congestion, edema, inflammatory cells infiltration, ulceration, and exudation. The pathogenic bacteria, therefore, are provided with chances to enter into the blood flow to invade lungs, which further leads to pneumonia. (3) Intestinal bacterial translocation and colonization have been currently believed to be the leading cause of enterogenic infection. Normally, the stomach tends to be aseptic due to the acidic barrier, but changes of intragastric environment provide chances for bacterial colonization and translocation at the pharynx, which migrate downward into the lower respiratory tract causing pneumonia.

17.5.1.2 Bronchitis

Bronchitis is mostly caused by enteric adenovirus or rotavirus.

17.5.2 Neurological Complications

17.5.2.1 Viral Encephalitis

Rotavirus enteritis can be complicated by lesions at the central nervous system, which is possibly related to viremia, microangitis, and metabolites of NO. The main manifestations include encephalitis and benign convulsion.

17.5.2.2 Guillain-Barre Syndrome (GBS)

Guillain-Barre syndrome (GBS) is an autoimmune inflammatory demyelinating neuropathy. It is clinically characterized by symmetrical sensory, motor, and voluntary nerve dysfunction at the distal limbs. Pathologically, the changes are characterized by demyelination of peripheral nerves and nerve roots as well as inflammatory responses of lymphocytes and macrophages around the minor vascular vessels.

17.5.3 Gastrointestinal Complications

17.5.3.1 Intussusception

Enteric adenovirus enteritis is mostly complicated by intussusception, which more commonly occurs in infants aged 6 months to 2 years. After the infection of enteric adenovirus, the intestinal wall is subject to proliferation of lymph follicle, with enlarged mesenteric lymph nodes and thickened intestinal wall, which compress or pull the intestinal lumen to cause poor coordination of intestinal canal peristalsis or spasm of local intestinal canal. Therefore, affected intestinal canal is invaginated into the adjacent intestinal canal. In addition, after the viral infection, the child patients experience obvious increase of the serum gastrin, which strengthens small intestinal peristalsis and sphincter relaxation at the ileocecum. Therefore, the affected small intestine tends to be pushed into the colon to cause intussusception. And ileac intussusception is the most common in this group of patients. In addition, *Escherichia coli* enteritis and rotavirus enteritis can also be complicated by intussusception, which mostly occurs in severe type of patients with a low incidence rate.

17.5.3.2 Cholecystitis and Cholangitis

In the cases with *Giardia* parasitizing at the biliary tract, the patients may develop cholecystitis or cholangitis, occasionally with gallstone with *Giardia* as the core. In the cases of AIDS complicated by cryptosporidium infection, about 10–30 % shows involvement of the biliary tract to cause acalculous cholecystitis or sclerotic cholangitis. The symptoms include right upper quadrant pain and fever. In the cases complicated by campylobacter infection, the patients may also experience biliary tract infection and cholecystitis, which rarely occur.

17.5.3.3 Appendicitis

In the cases with *Giardia* parasitizing at the appendix, 10 % of such patients experience acute or chronic appendicitis.

17.5.4 Other Related Syndromes

17.5.4.1 Reye Syndrome

Encephalopathy-liver fatty metamorphosis syndrome, also known as Reye syndrome that was firstly reported by Reye in 1963, is a clinical syndrome characterized by acute encephalopathy complicated by organ (mostly liver) fatty degeneration. The syndrome may also involve kidneys and myocardium. The patients mostly experience frequent vomiting and severe headache after prodromic infection (commonly viral infections such as influenza virus infection, measles virus infection, and rotavirus infection). The conditions may rapidly develop into disturbance of consciousness, with liver dysfunction but no hepatomegaly. The patients are subject to hepatic mitochondria degeneration, decreased enzymatic activity, low fatty acid β-oxidation, increased blood ammonia, positive antiphospholipid antibodies, intracranial hypertension, as well as degeneration or swelling of neurons and astrocytes, with a high mortality.

17.5.4.2 Hemolytic Uremic Syndrome

Hemolytic uremic syndrome (HUS) is a syndrome that is clinically characterized by capillary hemolytic anemia, thrombocytopenia, and acute renal insufficiency, with or without accompanying neuropsychiatric symptoms. HUS occurs more commonly in infants, which is the leading cause of infantile acute renal failure. The occurrence of HUS is closely related to infection of *E. coli* O_{157}: H_7, whose incidence rate in children with hemorrhagic diarrhea for about 1 week is 9–30 %.

After Shiga toxin (Stx) gains its access into the kidney to impair the endothelial cells at the glomerulus capillary, it activates the thrombocytes to cause blood coagulation and hyperfunction of fibrinolytic system (thrombotic microvascular lesion). At the same time, some inflammatory cytokines like Gram-negative lipopolysaccharide (LPS and endotoxin), TNFα, and IL-1β promote the damages to the endothelial cells. In addition, physical damages to the erythrocytes that pass through microvessels can lead to hemolytic anemia.

About 25 % of patients with HUS experience neurological symptoms, including headache, psychiatric symptoms, hemiplegia, epilepsy, and coma. The possible pathogenesis includes damaged vascular endothelial cells as well as activated platelets and blood coagulation, which further lead to hyperfunction of blood coagulation, with strengthened adhesive and aggregative abilities of the platelets. The following formation of microthrombus blocks the vascular vessels, in addition to accompanying cerebral angiospasm, to cause ischemic injuries to tissues and organs. Pathological examinations indicate that the core of its pathogenesis is impairments to microvascular endothelial cells and the formation of microthrombus.

17.6 Diagnostic Examination

17.6.1 Laboratory Test

17.6.1.1 Stool Examination

Accurate isolation and identification of the pathogen from the stool of patients with diarrhea are the key for its definitive diagnosis. The positive rate of stool culture is 20–70 %, which is low. And the culture needs a long period of time.

17.6.1.2 Serological Test

1. After the infection of *Vibrio parahaemolyticus*, the serum antibody titer generally does not increase and persists transiently, which has limited diagnostic value. At the convalescence stage, the thermostable hemolysin antibody test commonly shows an increase, which can be applied for epidemiological investigation.
2. Indirect hemagglutination test can be performed with paired sera obtained, respectively, at the early stage and at the convalescent stage. An at least four times increase of the antibody titer indicates a diagnosis of *Campylobacter jejuni* infection.
3. By serum agglutination test after infection of Yersinia at the convalescence stage, at least four times increase of the antibody titer, compared to the acute stage, or a ratio of at least 1:160 has the diagnostic value. Serum antibodies IgA and IgG test against outer membrane protein of Yersinia has a higher specificity than serum agglutination test.
4. Double sera can be detected at the acute and convalescence stages for rotavirus antibody titer. The antibody titer with at least four times increase or the antibody titer at the convalescence stage above 1:64 has diagnostic value. However, this examination should not be applied for early diagnosis.

17.6.1.3 Immunological Assay

Antigen Detection

ELISA is the most commonly applied detection for antigen, which has advantages of high specificity and sensitivity, rapid results, and simple operations. In particular, monoclonal antibody enzyme-immunoassay has a higher specificity and sensitivity than conventional detections, and thus, it is applicable for large-scale clinical test and epidemiological investigation of serological typing.

Antibody Detection

By using ELISA, purely cultured *Giardia* antigens can be applied to detect the specific IgG antibody in serum and the specific IgA antibody in saliva, with favorable sensitivity and specificity. The detection of specific IgG antibody can be applied for facilitative diagnosis of giardiasis, while the detection of specific IgA antibody can be applied for epidemiological investigation.

17.6.1.4 Molecular Biological Examination

PCR

PCR is a practical technique with simple operations for rapid diagnosis. Its sensitivity and specificity in detection of *Campylobacter* are, respectively, 91 % and 97 %. PCR can facilitate to define cryptosporidium-infected patients with mild symptoms and even the asymptomatic cryptosporidium carriers. In addition, it can be applied to distinguish the species of parasites and their genotypes.

Nucleic Acid Hybridization and Reverse-Transcription PCR

Nucleic acid hybridization and reverse-transcription PCR can be applied to detect the virus RNA. Its application is intended both for clinical diagnosis and assessment of virus-contaminated environment. The examination of feces samples collected within 48 h after onset has comparatively high positive rate, which facilitates the early diagnosis.

17.6.2 Diagnostic Imaging

17.6.2.1 Ultrasound

Ultrasound can be applied for the diagnosis of other infectious diarrhea-related complications such as intussusception.

17.6.2.2 X-Ray

X-ray is often applied to diagnose other infectious diarrhea-related chest diseases.

17.6.2.3 CT Scanning

It is the most commonly applied radiological examination.

17.6.2.4 MR Imaging

MR imaging is mainly applied for the diagnosis of other infectious diarrhea-related neurological complications.

17.7 Imaging Demonstration

17.7.1 Respiratory Complications

X-ray and CT scanning can demonstrate bronchopneumonia, lobar pneumonia, or interstitial pneumonia.

Escherichia coli bronchopneumonia is demonstrated as multilobar diffuse patches of infiltration shadows mostly at the lower lungs as well as lesions of pyothorax and pleural effusion. Unilateral pyothorax at the more seriously ill side occurs in 40 % of the patients. Rotavirus bronchopneumonia is demonstrated as increased and thickened pulmonary markings at both lungs as well as patches of shadows. The early demonstrations of rotavirus pneumonia include thickened and blurry lung markings, with following consolidated lesions in both lungs, with different sizes and fusion. The lesions may invade multiple pulmonary segments or lobes whose density increases along with the development of the conditions.

17.7.2 Neurological Complications

17.7.2.1 Rotavirus Encephalitis

CT Scanning

CT scanning demonstrates most cases with no abnormalities, with occasional demonstration of absent sulci.

MR Imaging

As for MR imaging, in most cases, the demonstrations of T1WI, T2WI, and FLAIR are normal. T1WI may demonstrate low signals at the splenium of corpus callosum. Both T2WI and FLAIR demonstrate slightly high or high signals. After treatment, reexamination by MR imaging often demonstrates diffuse or focal brain atrophy, commonly broadened sulci, and normal or atrophic cerebellum.

DWI mainly demonstrates high signals at the splenium of corpus callosum, cerebellar dentate nucleus, cerebellar vermis, and cerebellar hemisphere. The lesions can be found at the splenium of corpus callosum and/or cerebellum (Figs. 17.1 and 17.2). After treatment, reexamination by DWI demonstrates absence of the high signals, but occasionally high signals at the cerebellar cortex.

Kubota et al. reported a case with demonstrated high signals at the cerebral hemisphere and the white matter of bilateral frontal lobes. After treatment for 14 weeks, the patient received MR imaging. FLAIR demonstrated high signals at the white matter of the left frontal lobe, slightly broadened sulci, and diffuse cerebellar atrophy. Shiihara et al. reported a case with demonstrated absence of the sulcus interface. The follow-up examination after 6 months demonstrated expanded fourth cerebral ventricle and broadened sulci.

Case Study 1

An infant boy aged 18 months was hospitalized due to vomiting and diarrhea for 2 days. Consequently, he experienced cyanotic lips, cold limbs, transient unconsciousness, and accompanying sursumversion and apnea. By physical examination, his trunk and limbs were subject to hypotonia, with no focal neurological signs. Rotavirus antibody was detected from his stool specimens. By cerebrospinal fluid examination, cell counts were normal, with mononuclear cells count of 4×10^6/L, protein 0.2 g/L, and glucose 4.5 mmol/L. Cranial and brain CT scanning demonstrated no abnormity. At day 2 after hospitalization, EEG during sleep demonstrated δ waves at the bilateral frontal lobes, which was more obvious at the left frontal lobe.

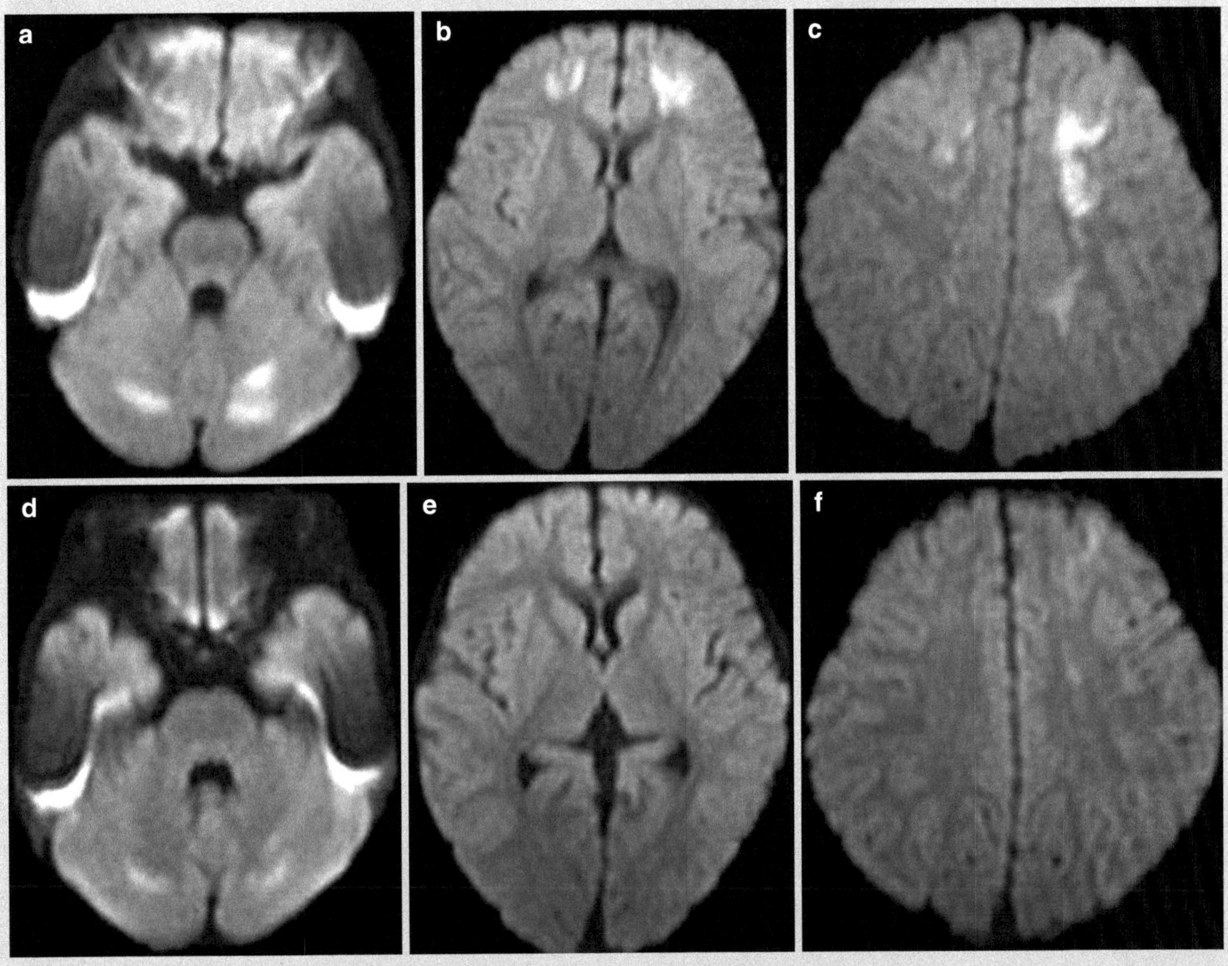

Fig. 17.1 Rotavirus encephalitis. (**a–c**) At day 3 after hospitalization, DWI demonstrates obvious high signals at the left cerebral hemisphere, the white matter of bilateral frontal lobes, and dental nucleus. (**d–f**) At day 10 after the onset, DWI demonstrates absence or shrinkage of the above lesions, with no newly formed lesions (Reproduced with permission from Kubota T, et al. *Brain Dev*, 2011, 3 (1): 21)

Case Study 2

A boy aged 4.5 years experienced vomiting and diarrhea for 2 days. Following examinations demonstrated rotavirus antibodies in the stool specimens. At days 3–4 after the onset, the boy experienced loss of consciousness for 10–20 s with accompanying sursumversion and following influent speech. At day 7 after the onset, the cerebrospinal fluid examination demonstrated protein 0.25 g/L, glucose 3.28 mmol/L, and rotavirus antibody negative, while MR imaging demonstrated no abnormality.

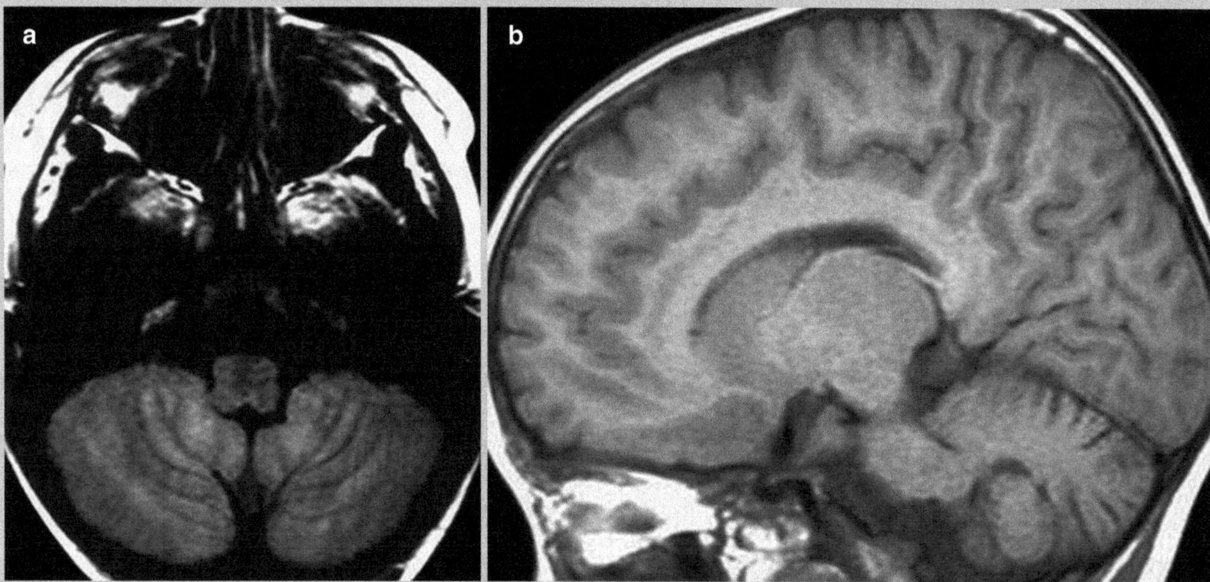

Fig. 17.2 Rotavirus encephalitis. (**a**) At day 29 after the onset, coronal T2WI demonstrates increased signals at the bilateral cerebellar cortex. (**b**) At day 93 after the onset, sagittal T1WI demonstrates broadened cerebellar sulci (Reproduced with permission from Shiihara T, et al. *Brain Dev*, 2007, 29 (10): 670)

Case Study 3

A boy aged 2 years was hospitalized due to sudden disturbance of consciousness after diarrhea and vomiting for 2 days. Rotavirus antibody was detected in the stool specimens. By laboratory tests, Na was 56.55 mmol/L and Cl was 91 mmol/L. EEG demonstrated intracerebral diffuse slow waves. Both cerebrospinal fluid examination and brain CT scanning demonstrated no abnormality.

For case detail and figures, please refer to Fukuada S, et al. *Pediatr Neurol*, (2009), 40 (2): 131.

17.7.2.2 Guillain-Barre Syndrome

MR neuroimaging demonstrates lesions at the nerve roots, ganglia, and nerve trunk area. Coronal imaging demonstrates typical cases with bilaterally symmetrical frog sign. The sign is possibly related to neural inflammatory edema and inflammatory cell infiltration, especially macrophage infiltration, demyelination, and angiopathies (including congestion at the intraneural vessels and perineural vertebral venous plexus, hyperplasia of small vessels, and inflammatory cell infiltration). The pathogenesis of the frog sign still needs to be clarified based on scientific studies.

Plain imaging demonstrates the cases of acute GBS with different degrees of thickening of involved spinal nerves and cauda equina. In some cases, the thickening is demonstrated as thickened both anterior and posterior roots, while in some other cases, thickening is demonstrated only as thickened anterior root. T1WI demonstrates moderate signals, while T2WI demonstrates moderate or slightly high signals. Contrast imaging usually demonstrates slight or obvious enhancement, with different degrees of enhancements for the same one patient. Coronal imaging demonstrates cord-like enhancement of the involved cauda equina. Transverse imaging demonstrates round, oval, or aggregated patches of enhancement. Sagittal imaging demonstrates backward aggregation of cauda equina, which is located at the middle and posterior lumbar spinal canal.

Based on the different ways of enhancements of the nerve roots, Ali Yikilmaz et al. classified these enhancements into four types: no enhancement, more obvious enhancement of the anterior root than the posterior root, same enhancement of the anterior root as the posterior root, and only enhancement of the anterior root.

17.7.3 Intussusception

17.7.3.1 Ultrasound

Transverse ultrasonography demonstrates high and low alternatively mixed echo area and its surrounding ring-shaped low-echo area. Otherwise, round-shaped center (liquid dark area) with homogeneous high echo is demonstrated, namely, the concentric ring sign or target ring sign. Vertical ultrasonography demonstrates similar signs to transverse ultrasonography, with the invaginated segment in round headlike structure and its surrounding low-echo area, namely, the sleeve sign. The thicker outer layer is demonstrated with lower echo, indicating more severe edema at the intestinal wall of the intussusception part. The ileum-type intussusception or ileocolon-type intussusception can be demonstrated as typical triple-ring sign with the intestinal cavity liquid as the background. The inner ring is the proximal intussusceptum segment; the middle ring is the distal intussusceptum segment; and the outer ring is the distal intestinal segment. Due to special features of pediatric small intestinal intussusceptions, small intestinal pneumatosis occurs. Therefore, high-frequency ultrasonography should be performed to improve the resolution power and achieve favorable demonstration of the small intestinal intussusception. And the diagnostic rate can thus be improved.

17.7.3.2 X-Ray

Abdominal X-ray for erect and supine positions is an essential routine examination before enema for children with intussusception. Its use facilitates the observation of pneumoperitoneum, intestinal obstruction, abdominal effusion, and preoperative gas distribution, which guide air enema diagnosis and reduction of the small intestine. Only about 10 % of the cases can be directly demonstrated with intracolonic soft tissue lump.

17.7.3.3 CT Scanning

CT scanning can demonstrate the characteristic sleeve sign and sausage sign as well as the particular stripe-shaped mass-like thickening at the mesenteries. CT scanning plays an important role in defining the occurrence of intussusception, location and degree of intussusception, as well as the complications of intestinal ischemia, necrosis, and strangulation. In particular, CT scanning can accurately define the diagnosis of small intestinal intussusception.

17.7.3.4 Electronic Colonoscopy

By electronic colonoscopy, after the gas injection, semi-spherical or cervix-shaped intussusceptal head can be demonstrated in the colonic cavity, which moves along with the pressure of gas injection. It can also be performed to observe the mucosa in the enteric cavity as well as to assess intestinal ischemia and necrosis.

17.7.4 Other Related Syndromes

17.7.4.1 Reye Syndrome

CT Scanning

CT scanning demonstrates mostly diffuse cerebral edema as low-density lesions at the basal ganglia, brainstem, and cerebellum. The density of the periventricular white matter is demonstrated with obvious decrease, which extends bilaterally towards the frontal lobe and the temporal lobe in a butterfly shape. After that, the low-density areas bilaterally penetrate into the cortex from the frontal lobe and temporal lobe like a deer horn. The cerebral ventricle is subject to deformity due to compression.

MR Imaging

In addition to diffuse cerebral edema, T1WI, T2WI, and FLAIR all demonstrate no abnormality. Otherwise, T2WI demonstrates high signals at the basal ganglia, brainstem, and cerebellum. For some patients, special changes can be radiologically demonstrated. It has been reported that some of the low-density lesions at the brainstem and thalamus demonstrated by CT scanning were in high signals by T1WI and T2WI. It has also been reported that MR imaging demonstrated diffuse changes at the cortex and white matter, which were laminar high T2WI signal along cortex at the acute stage, with enhancement by contrast imaging; diffuse cortical high T1WI signals at the chronic stage. Meanwhile, changes of white matter and cerebral atrophy can be demonstrated.

Mao YL et al. reported MR imaging demonstrations at the acute stage. The cases with high T1WI, T2WI, and FLAIR signals of scattering spots of lesions at the cortex and subcortex, with enhancement of the lesions by contrast imaging, are suspected to be intracerebral adipose deposition. The cases with equal T1WI signals as well as high T2WI and FLAIR signals of scattering flakes of lesions at the cortex and subcortex are suspected as cellular edema. By contrast imaging, marginal enhancement of the lesions is demonstrated, which supports the diagnosis of destructed blood-cerebrospinal fluid barrier caused by mitochondrial dysfunction of local vascular endothelial cells. The above two types of demonstrations may be found overlapping.

DWI is more sensitive to cerebral lesions than routine MR imaging, and, therefore, DWI can detect those cerebral lesions that routine MR imaging fails to demonstrate. DWI demonstrates most cases with high signal lesions at the whiter matter of thalamus, midbrain, and cerebellum (Fig. 17.3). DWI occasionally demonstrates high signal lesions at the whiter matter of subcortex and nearby sagittal sinus.

Case Study 4
A boy aged 5.5 years complained of altered mental status after vomiting and respiratory tract infection for 2 days. Laboratory tests demonstrated decreased blood glucose, AST 7125–9893 U/L, blood ammonia 204 μmol/L, and prolonged prothrombin time. Head CT scanning demonstrated mild cerebral edema.

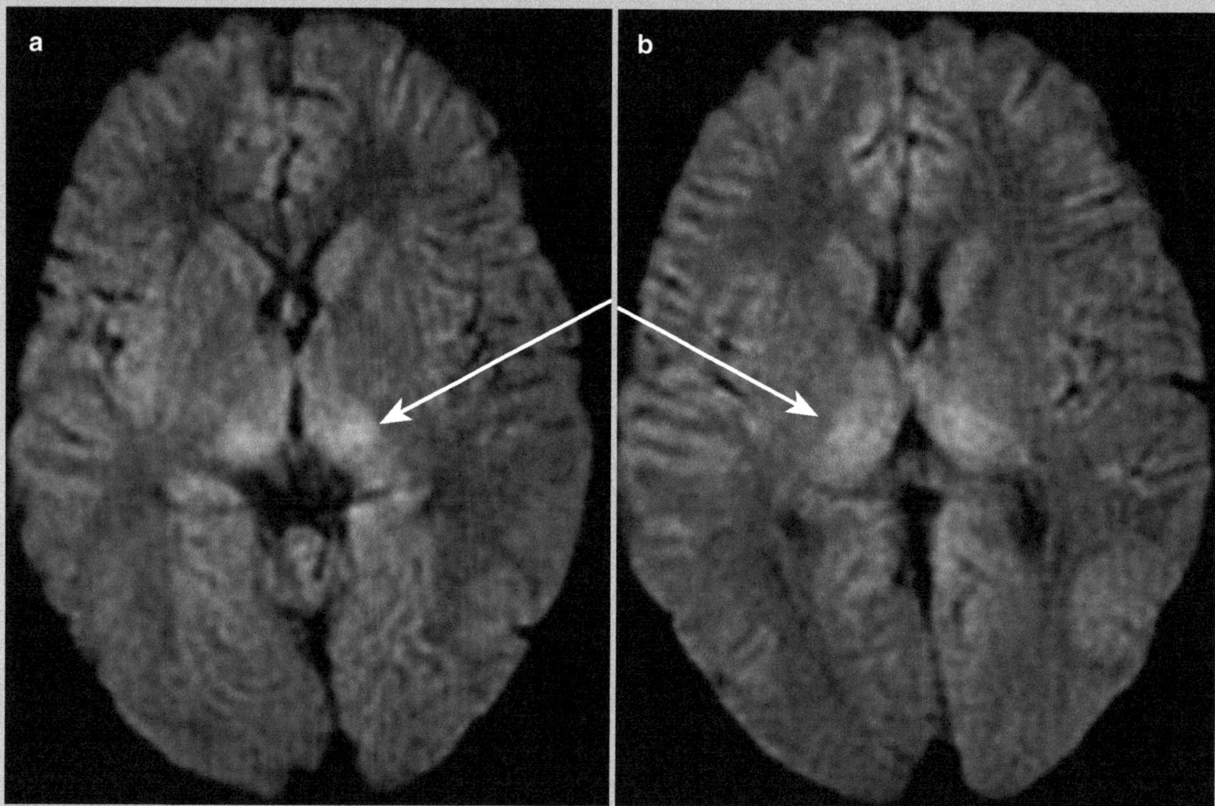

Fig. 17.3 Reye syndrome. (**a**, **b**) MR imaging of T1WI, T2WI, and FLAIR demonstrates no abnormality, while DWI demonstrates symmetrical limited diffusion at bilateral thalamus (indicated by *arrows*) (Reproduced with permission from Johnsen and Bird *Pediatr Neurol*, 2006, 34 (5): 405)

17.7.4.2 Hemolytic Uremic Syndrome

CT Scanning

CT scanning demonstrates no abnormality or low-density lesions at the basal ganglia and brainstem. Contrast scanning demonstrates enhancement of the lesions.

MR Imaging

T1WI demonstrates most lesions as low signals, while T2WI and FLAIR demonstrate slightly high or high signals. Most of the lesions are bilaterally symmetrical, possibly with accompanying bleeding at the acute stage. Otherwise, MR imaging demonstrates no abnormality. The lesions can be found at the basal ganglia, thalamus, cerebellum, brainstem, periventricular white matter, hippocampus, insular lobe, and capsula externa. Among these lesions, the lesions at the basal ganglia are the typical manifestations of involved central nervous system in the cases of HUS. Contrast imaging demonstrate enhancement of some lesions (Figs. 17.4 and 17.5). The lesions are reversible. By following up examinations, the lesions can be demonstrated to be absent or shrunk, with decreased signal. However, secondary bleeding has also been reported. At the acute phase, ADC values of periventricular white matter, basal ganglia, thalamus, and centrum semiovale can be increased or decreased, while the ADC values of cerebellum and brainstem can be decreased.

Case Study 5

A boy aged 4 years.

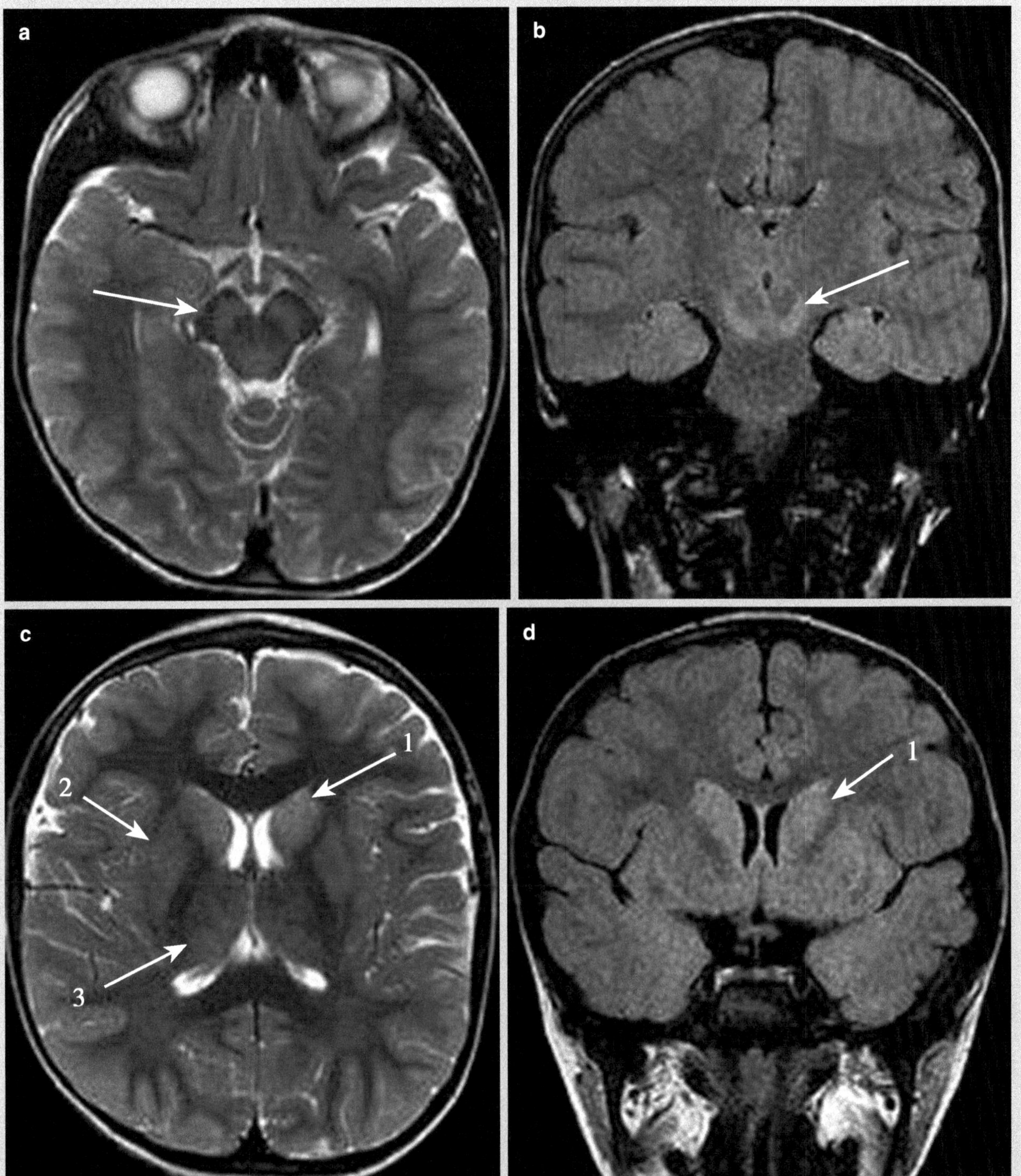

Fig. 17.4 Hemolytic uremic syndrome. (**a**, **c**) Transverse T2WI demonstrations. (**b**, **d**) Coronal FLAIR demonstrations. (**a**, **b**) High signals are demonstrated at the bilateral pedunculus cerebri (indicated by *arrows*) . (**c**, **d**) Slightly high signals are demonstrated at the *1* bilateral caudate nuclei, *2* putamen, and *3* thalamus (indicated by *arrows*) (Reproduced with permission from Koehl B, et al. *Pediatr Nephrol*, 2010, 25 (12): 2539)

Case Study 6
An infant girl aged 20 months was hospitalized due to generalized tonic-clonic seizures and drowsiness. The patient experienced bloody stool 3 days ago and anuria 1 day ago. Laboratory tests indicated acute renal failure, metabolic acidosis, and severe hemolytic anemia based on the findings of Scr 433.2 μmol/L, BUN 59.78 mmol/L, ALB 0.22 g/L, Ph 7.26, bicarbonate 12 mmol/L, WBC 30.4×10^9/L, GR% 79.1 %, HGB 1.05 g/L, PLT 125×10^9/L, Na 129 mmol/L, K 5.7 mmol/L, Ca 1.9 mmol/L, and P 3 mmol/L.

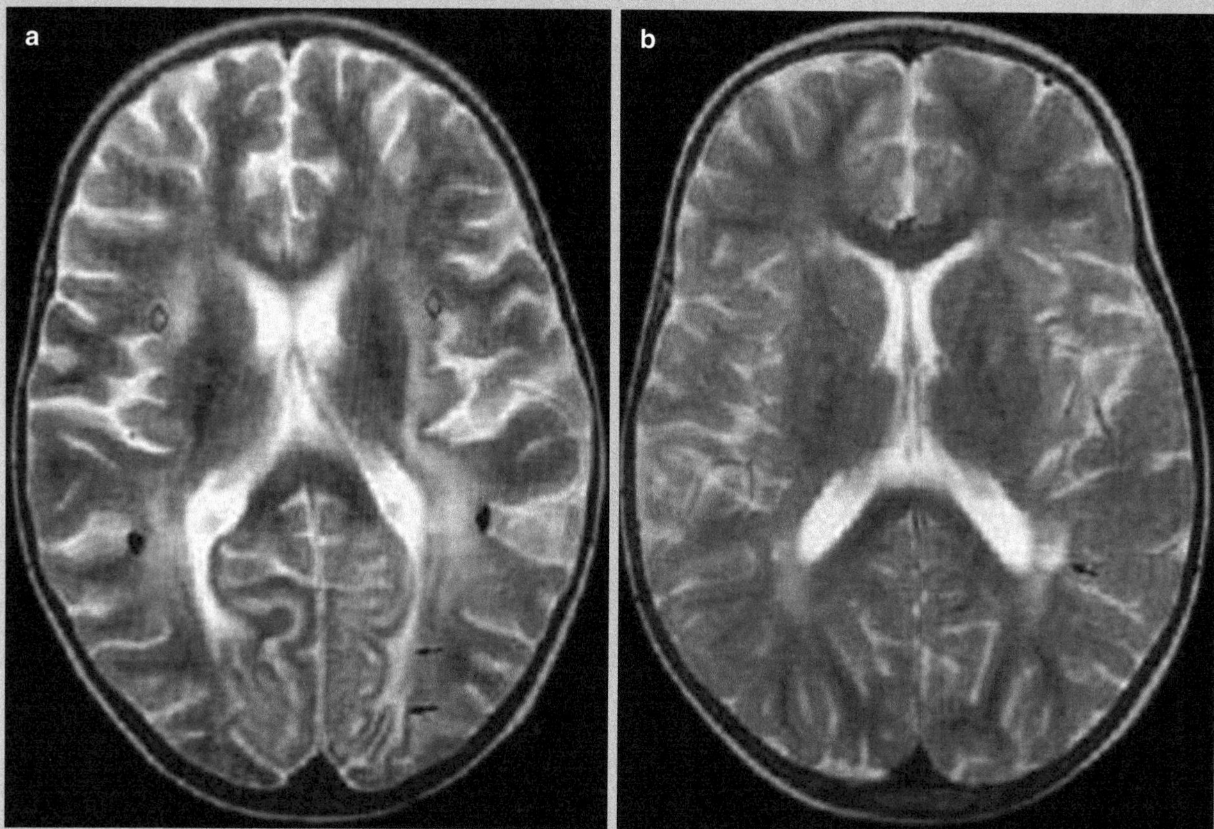

Fig. 17.5 Hemolytic uremic syndrome. (**a**) One week after hospitalization, T2WI demonstrates high signals at the white matter of the left occipital lobe (indicated by *arrows*), the bilateral periventricular white matter, and the bilateral capsula externa. (**b**) Reexamination after 10 months by T2WI demonstrates high signals at the left paraventricular white matter and shrinkage of the lesions (indicated by *arrows*) (Reproduced with permission from Signorini E, et al. *Pediatr Nephrol*, 2000, 14 (10-11): 990)

17.8 Diagnostic Basis

17.8.1 Diagnosis of Other Infectious Diarrhea

The definitive diagnosis of other infectious diarrhea should be based on the following evidence.

17.8.1.1 Epidemiological Data

Epidemiological data include the season and region of the occurrence, case history of eating or drinking contaminated food or water, history of group occurrence, history of contact to animals, and history of contact to contaminated water.

17.8.1.2 Clinical Data

1. The patients experience frequent bowel movements for above three times per day, with abnormal appearance of the stool. It can be loose, watery, mucous, bloody purulent, or bloody. The patients may also experience nausea, vomiting, abdominal pain, fever, poor appetite, and general upset. In some severe cases, the patient also sustains dehydration, acidosis, electrolyte disturbance, and shock. The conditions may also be life threatening.
2. Diarrhea caused by O_1 and O_{139} serogroups of *Vibrio cholerae*, *Shigella*, *Entamoeba histolytica*, *Salmonella typhosa*, and *Salmonella paratyphi* A, B, and C has been excluded.

17.8.1.3 Laboratory Test

The laboratory tests include routine laboratory tests, serological test, etiological examination, and immunologic assay. The definitive diagnosis depends on successful culture and isolation of the pathogen in stool specimens and examinations with favorable specificity.

17.8.2 Diagnosis of Other Infectious Diarrhea-Related Complications

17.8.2.1 Rotavirus Encephalitis

The cases of other infectious diarrhea complicated by rotavirus encephalitis experience obvious neurological abnormalities. MR imaging demonstrates long T1 and long T2 signals at the splenium of corpus callosum, which facilitates the diagnosis.

17.8.2.2 Guillain-Barre Syndrome

Case History

Most of the patients have a history of nonspecific viral infection or vaccination.

Clinical Manifestation

The clinical manifestation is characterized by symmetrical delayed paralysis of limbs, abnormal sensation of limbs, voluntary neurological symptoms, as well as occasional symptoms of cranial nerve palsy and respiratory muscles palsy.

Cerebrospinal Fluid Examination

The cerebrospinal fluid examination demonstrates increased protein content and normal cell counts.

Electrophysiological Examination

The examination demonstrates F waves or delayed/absent H reflex, slowed NCV, and prolonged distal latency.

MR Imaging

MR imaging demonstrates thickened and enhanced cauda equina and spinal nerves, with frog sign in typical cases.

17.8.2.3 Reye Syndrome

Case History

The child patients experience a history of prodromic viral infection before the onset. After that, the patients experience acute progressive cerebral symptoms such as convulsion and disturbance of consciousness, but no neurological focal lesions.

Liver Function Test

The patients show liver dysfunction, with elevated ALT and AST, prolonged prothrombin time, increased blood ammonia, and decreased blood glucose.

Cerebrospinal Fluid Examination

The cerebrospinal fluid has increased pressure, with decreased glucose as well as normal cell counts and protein quantification.

Liver Biopsy

Liver biopsy demonstrates typical histological changes.

Head CT Scanning or MR Imaging

Head CT scanning or MR imaging mainly demonstrates cerebral edema, which provides evidence for the early diagnosis.

17.8.2.4 Pneumonia

Clinical Manifestation

The patients with infectious diarrhea clinically experience pulmonary infection.

Radiological Examination

Both X-ray and CT scanning demonstrate patches of shadows and consolidation at the lung, which are the basis for definitive diagnosis.

17.8.2.5 Intussusception

Infant cases with paroxysmal crying and screaming, vomiting, and jam-like bloody stool, and sausage-like mass palpable at the abdomen can be definitively diagnosed with intussusceptions. The atypical clinical manifestations, in combination to the acoustic shadows of concentric ring sign or target ring sign by ultrasound or in combination to the typical sleeve sign and sausage sign by CT scanning, can define the diagnosis.

17.8.2.6 Hemolytic Uremic Syndrome

Based on the triad of microvascular hemolytic anemia, acute renal insufficiency, and thrombocytopenia, the diagnosis of HUB can be defined. MR imaging demonstrates lesions at the basal ganglia, indicating involvement of the central nervous system by HIUS.

17.9 Differential Diagnosis

17.9.1 Bacillary Dysentery

The patients with bacillary dysentery typically experience fever, abdominal pain, diarrhea, mucous or bloody purulent stool, and tenesmus. The abdominal pain is commonly found at the lower abdomen or the left lower quadrant of the abdomen. Stool microscopy demonstrates relatively large quantities of leukocytes, erythrocytes, and macrophages. By stool bacterial culture, the finding of *Shigella* can define the diagnosis.

17.9.2 Other Thrombotic Microangiopathy

After diarrhea, HUS can be generally distinguished from other thrombotic microangiopathy. Almost all patients with HUS of *E. coli* O_{157}:H_7 infection experience prodromic diarrhea, with normal or slightly increased fibrous protein concentration and prolonged blood coagulation time. In addition, *E. coli* O_{157}:H_7 infection-related HUS has repeated occurrence.

References

Fukuada S, Kishi K, Yasuda K, et al. Rotavirus-associated encephalopathy with a reversible splenial lesion. Pediatr Neurol. 2009;40(2):131–3.

Johnsen SD, Bird CR. The thalamus and midbrain in Reye syndrome. Pediatr Neurol. 2006;34(5):405–7.

Koehl B, Boyer O, Biebuyck-Gougé N, et al. Neurological involvement in a child with atypical hemolytic uremic syndrome. Pediatr Nephrol. 2010;25(12):2539–42.

Kubota T, Suzuki T, Kitase Y, et al. Chronological diffusion-weighted imaging changes and mutism in the course of rotavirus-associated acute cerebellitis/cerebellopathy concurrent with encephalitis/encephalopathy. Brain Dev. 2011;3(1):21–7.

Shiihara T, Watanabe M, Honma A, et al. Rotavirus associated acute encephalitis/encephalopathy and concurrent cerebellitis: report of two cases. Brain Dev. 2007;29(10):670–3.

Suggested Reading

Awasthi S, Agarwal GG, Mishra V, et al. Four-country surveillance of intestinal intussusception and diarrhoea in children. Paediatr Child Health. 2009;45(3):82–6.

Donnerstag F, Ding X, Pape L, et al. Patterns in early diffusion-weighted MRI in children with haemolytic uraemic syndrome and CNS involvement. Eur Radiol. 2012;22(3):506–13.

Jang YY, Lee KH. Transient splenial lesion of the corpus callosum in a case of benign convulsion associated with rotaviral gastroenteritis. Korean J Pediatr. 2010;53(9):859–62.

Mao LY, Wang X, Fei GQ, et al. Reye Syndrome: clinical manifestations and radiological demonstrations. Chin J Comput Med Radiol. 2009;15(6):580–1.

Nathanson S, Kwon T, Elmaleh M, et al. Acute neurological involvement in diarrhea-associated hemolytic uremic syndrome. Clin J Am Soc Nephrol. 2010;5(7):1218–28.

Nie QH. Infectious diarrhea. Beijing: People's Medical Publishing House; 2011.

Park NH, Park SI, Park CS, et al. Ultrasonographic findings of small bowel intussusception, focusing on differentiation from ileocolic intussusception. Br J Radiol. 2007;80(958):798–802.

Steinborn M, Leiz S, Rüdisser K, et al. CT and MRI in haemolytic uraemic syndrome with central nervous system involvement: distribution of lesions and prognostic value of imaging findings. Pediatr Radiol. 2004;34(10):805–10.

Yikilmaz A, Doganay S, Gumus H, et al. Magnetic resonance imaging of childhood Guillain–Barre syndrome. Childs Nerv Syst. 2010;26(8):1103–8.

Zhang LX, Zhou XZ. Modern studies of infectious diseases. Beijing: People's Military Medical Press; 2010.

Pertussis

18

Yinglin Guo, Lili Liu, and Bailu Liu

Pertussis (whooping cough) is an acute respiratory infectious disease caused by *Bordetella pertussis*. It is clinically characterized by paroxysmal spasmodic cough, a crow-like inspiration sound, and increased peripheral lymphocytes. It has a long course of disease, which may last for as long as 2–3 months without treatment. Its occurrence is more commonly found in children, and there has been a recent increase of its incidence rate in adults.

18.1 Etiology

Bordetella pertussis is a short bacillus with its two ends densely stained, in a length of 1–1.5 μm and a width of 0.3–0.5 μm. It is categorized into the species of Bordetella and is a Gram-negative aerobic bacillus with no buds and flagellum. However, it is enveloped by capsule and is incapable of moving. The appropriate temperature and pH value for its growth is 35–37 °C and 6.0–7.0, respectively, with poor resistance to external physical and chemical factors. It is sensitive to ultraviolet ray and disinfectants. Its initial isolation should be on the Bordet-Gengou medium containing glycerinum, potato, and fresh blood.

During its growth and replication, *Bordetella pertussis* can produce endotoxin, exotoxin, and antigenic bioactive substances, which institute the main cause underlying its pathogenesis. (1) Pertussis toxin (PT), the key virulent factor of the bacteria, is a bacterial toxin with typical A-B transribosylase. A is composed of virulent subunit, which plays a role in promoting an increase of lymphocytes, activating insulin-producing cells, aggregating growth of CHO cells, and activating allergic reactions caused by histamine. B is composed of S2–S5 to participate in surface receptor binding of eukaryotic cells and transmembrane transport of subunit S1. (2) Filamentous hemagglutinin (FHA), another key virulent factor, adheres to *Bordetella pertussis* and lives in epithelial cells of respiratory organs. Meanwhile, it has a favorable immunogenicity to stimulate the immune system to generate specific protective antibodies. (3) Pertactin (Prn) is the outer membrane protein of *Bordetella pertussis* and plays an important role during infection and adhesion of *Bordetella pertussis* to respiratory epithelia cells of host. And it also has a favorable immunogenicity. (4) Agglutinogen (AGG) is one of the pathogenic factors of *Bordetella pertussis*, which contributes to adhesion of pathogenic bacteria to respiratory epithelial cells of host. (5) Other factors of pathogenic bacteria include lipopolysaccharide, adenylate cyclase toxin, dermotoxin, and tracheal cytotoxin.

18.2 Epidemiology

18.2.1 The Source of Infection

Human beings are the only host of *Bordetella pertussis*. The patients, asymptomatic patients, and *Bordetella pertussis* carriers are all the sources of the infection. The infectivity lasts from the very beginning of its incubation period to 6 weeks after the onset, especially the first 2–3 weeks after the onset.

18.2.2 Route of Transmission

While coughing, talking, and sneezing, the pathogenic bacteria spread along with droplets. Infection occurs after susceptible person inhales the droplets with the bacteria. The indirect transmission is unlikely due to the weak surviving ability of the bacteria in external environment.

Y. Guo (✉)
Department of Radiology, Taiping People's Hospital, Daowai District, Harbin, Heilongjiang, China
e-mail: guoyinglinhmu@126.com

L. Liu • B. Liu
CT Department, The Second Affiliated Hospital, Harbin Medical University, Harbin, Heilongjiang, China

H. Li (ed.), *Radiology of Infectious Diseases: Volume 2*, DOI 10.1007/978-94-017-9876-1_18

18.2.3 Susceptible Population

People are generally susceptible to pertussis, especially children aged under 5 years. Due to the shortage of protective antibodies of mothers to transfer to fetus, its incidence rate is higher in infants under the age of 6 months, including neonates. With the bacteria inoculation for over 12 years, the incidence rate can be up to 50 %. At the same time, the occurrence of pertussis tends to be found in young adults and adults. In the 1950s, PerV was manufactured for widespread vaccination; the incidence rate of pertussis has decreased to the lowest level since then. However, in the recent 20 years, its occurrence is slowly but stably increasing.

Lifelong immunity cannot be acquired after its infection and the protective antibodies against pertussis are IgA and IgG. IgA can inhibit the adhesion of the bacteria to surface of epithelial cells, while IgG has long-term protective effect.

18.2.4 Epidemic Features

Pertussis is commonly found in frigid zone and temperate zone, which occurs all year round, but more commonly occurs in winters and springs. Its prevalence is generally sporadic, with local epidemic in institutions such as kindergarten and child-care centers as well as in areas with poor living conditions.

18.3 Pathogenesis and Pathological Changes

18.3.1 Pathogenesis

The pathogenesis of pertussis has not been fully elucidated. After invading the respiratory tract of susceptible person, *Bordetella pertussis* firstly attaches to cilia of epithelial cells in the throat, trachea, bronchus, and bronchiole and then reproduces in the cilia and secretes various toxic substances. These toxic substances paralyze the cilia to cause degenerative necrosis of epithelial cells and systemic reactions. Thereby, the discharge of thick secretions caused by respiratory tract inflammation is impaired. The detained secretions continuously stimulate peripheral nerves of respiratory tract to cause spasmodic cough via coughing center until discharge of the secretions.

Because of the long-term stimulation of cough, persistent excitation lesions occur in the coughing center. Other stimulation such as pharyngeal examination and food intake can also reflexively cause episodes of spasmodic cough. In the cases with incomplete discharge of secretions, the respiratory tract may be blocked in different degrees to cause pulmonary infections, pulmonary atelectasis, emphysema, and bronchiectasia. In the cases with incessant spasmodic cough, brain hypoxia, hyperemia, and edema occur, which can be complicated by pertussis encephalopathy.

18.3.2 Pathological Changes

Though *Bordetella pertussis* mainly damages the mucosa of bronchus and bronchiole, the lesions can also be found in the nasopharynx, throat, and trachea. The main changes include mucosal hyperemia and infiltration of monocyte and neutrophil granulocyte at the base of mucosal epithelial cells with necrocytosis. Granulocytes and lymphocytes aggregate around the bronchus and alveolus to cause interstitial inflammation. The lymph nodes beside the trachea and bronchus are commonly enlarged. Obstruction of the bronchus by secretions can cause pulmonary atelectasis and bronchiectasia. In the cases with pertussis complicated by encephalopathy, hyperemia, edema, spots of hemorrhage, cortical atrophy, nerve cell degeneration, and hydrocephalus can be found by microscopy or naked eye observation.

18.4 Clinical Symptoms and Signs

The incubation period generally last for 2–21 days, commonly 7–14 days. The typical clinical course of pertussis can be divided into three stages in unvaccinated children and infants: prodromal stage, spasmodic cough stage, and convalescence stage.

18.4.1 Prodromal Stage

Generally, this stage begins at the onset and persists for 7–10 days until the occurrence of paroxysmal spasmodic cough. During this stage, the symptoms include low-grade fever, sneezing, lacrimation, and cough, presenting difficulty for its differentiation from other bacterial respiratory infections. At the onset, the cough is single acoustic dry cough. After the body temperature returns to normal after 3–4 days, cough begins to aggravate, which is especially severe at nights. Due to a lack of characteristic symptoms during this stage, it can be misdiagnosed or miss diagnosed.

18.4.2 Spasmodic Cough Stage

During this stage, obvious paroxysmal spasmodic cough occurs, generally lasting for 2–6 weeks or longer. The spasmodic cough is characterized by continual brief coughs with following deep and prolonged inhalation. A large quantity of air passes through the narrow glottis to produce a crow-like sound, with following continual brief cough till coughing up a large quantity of thick sputum, commonly with accompanying vomiting. Spasmodic cough is more frequent at nights, commonly with accompanying flushing face and cyanotic lips, lingual valgus, anxious expression, carotid artery expansion, and curved body. Feeding, crying, catching a cold, and receiving pharyngeal examination can induce spasmodic cough. During the interval of spasmodic cough, the children patients commonly have a normal life. In the cases with no complications, the body temperature is normal. Due to the accompanying vomiting to spasmodic cough, which can be induced by feeding, therefore, decreased body weight is common in children patients.

During spasmodic cough, the capillary pressure may increase to cause hemorrhage under the bulbar conjunctiva or nasal bleeding. Due to lingual valgus, the friction between glossodesmus and lower incisor may cause glossodesmus laceration. Due to the small glottises of children, it can be completely closed due to spasm of vocal cord. In addition to blockage by thick secretions, suffocation may occur that may further develop into asphyxial seizures with serious cyanosis. It commonly occurs at nights. Without emergency rescuing, death occurs due to asphyxia.

In adults and elder children, the symptoms are atypical, with manifestations of dry cough with no paroxysmal spasm and no obvious increases of leukocytes and lymphocytes. Therefore, pertussis in adults and elder children tends to be misdiagnosed as bronchitis or upper respiratory infection.

18.4.3 Convalescence Stage

During this stage, both frequency and severity of spasmodic cough decrease and terminally the spasmodic cough is absent. Such a course lasts for 2–3 weeks. In the cases with complications of pneumonia and pulmonary atelectasis, this stage may last as long as several weeks or even several months.

18.5 Pertussis-Related Complications

18.5.1 Respiratory Complications

18.5.1.1 Bronchopneumonia

Bronchopneumonia is the most common severe complication that is caused by secondary infection. It may occur in any stage of the disease but mostly occurs in the spasmodic cough stage. In the cases with bronchopneumonia, paroxysmal spasmodic cough may be temporarily absent, but symptoms of sudden fever, shallow and rapid respiration, as well as cyanosis can be found. By tests and examinations, pulmonary fine moist rales can be found, with an increase of peripheral WBC count that is predominantly an increase of neutrophil granulocyte.

18.5.1.2 Pulmonary Atelectasis

Pulmonary atelectasis is caused by partially obstructed bronchus or bronchioles by thick secretions, which is common in the middle and lower lung lobes. Its occurrence is related to insufficient drainage of secretions in the middle and lower lung lobes.

18.5.1.3 Emphysema and Cutaneous Emphysema

Spasm and blockage by secretions can cause emphysema. With the increase of alveolar pressure, alveolar rupture occurs to cause pulmonary interstitial emphysema which further develops into cervical subcutaneous emphysema via the tracheal fascia. Pulmonary interstitial emphysema may also develop into mediastinal emphysema via pulmonary hilum and pneumothorax via visceral pleura.

18.5.2 Complications of the Central Nervous System

As the most serious complication, pertussis encephalopathy commonly occurs in the spasmodic cough stage, with an incidence rate of 2–3 %. The mechanism underlying its occurrence is cerebral angiospasm caused by serious spasmodic coughs, which further leads to cerebral hypoxia and hemorrhage. The clinical manifestations include convulsion or repeated convulsions, high fever, and coma. In serious cases, the life is threatened. After its occurrence, the sequelae can be found, including epilepsy and mental retardation.

18.5.3 Other Complications

Increased capillary pressure can cause subconjunctival hemorrhage and nasal bleeding. Persistent severe spasmodic cough causes increased intra-abdominal pressure, which further leads to umbilical herniation and inguinal herniation. There are also reports about the complication of rib fracture.

18.6 Diagnostic Examinations

18.6.1 Laboratory Tests

18.6.1.1 Routine Blood Test

During the spasmodic cough stage, peripheral WBC count obviously increases that reaches as high as $(20–50)\times 10^9$/L that is predominantly an increase of lymphocytes, accounting for above 60 % of the count. In the cases with secondary infection, neutrophil granulocyte count increases.

18.6.1.2 Bacteriology Test

Bacterial culture has a high specificity. In the early stage of the disease, nasopharyngeal swab for culture has a high positive rate. The earlier culture has a higher positive rate. The culture during the prodromal stage has a positive rate of about 90 %, which gradually decreases thereafter to 50 % at the 4th week.

18.6.1.3 Serologic Test

Double serum samples are collected during the acute stage and the convalescence stage. By hemagglutination inhibition test or complement fixation test, specific antibody can be detected. Such a method is mainly applied for retrospective diagnosis or facilitating diagnosis for atypical cases. ELISA can be applied to detect specific IgM antibody of pertussis, which provides basis for the early diagnosis. Such a method has a positive rate of 70 % and is more significant for the cases with negative bacterial culture.

18.6.1.4 Molecular Biological Assay

Specific nucleic acid segment of bacteria can be detected in nasopharyngeal secretions by PCR, with a specificity of 97 % and a sensitivity of 94 %. Such a detecting procedure is especially important for cases with atypical symptoms, with a history of antibiotics use in the early stage of the disease and with a history of vaccination.

18.6.2 Diagnostic Imaging

When patients are attacked by the complications of respiratory system and central nervous system, it is appropriate to use X-rays, CT, and MRI to assess. In general, X-ray is the commonest way to test complications of respiratory system in chest. With no abnormality found by X-ray yet suspected thoracic disease in chest, doctors can use CT to make a definite diagnosis. With the encephalopathy accompanying with anoxia, hyperemia, and edema in brain, the first choice should be MRI examination.

18.7 Imaging Demonstrations

18.7.1 Respiratory System

18.7.1.1 Chest X-Ray

Chest X-ray may demonstrate no abnormalities or only thickened blurry pulmonary markings. When the conditions progress further, chest X-ray demonstrates network and small patches of blurry shadows with uneven density at both hili as well as in both the middle and lower lungs. Densely distributing lesions may fuse into large flakes of shadows. In the cases with inflammatory infiltration in the interstitium surrounding the hilum, the density of hilar shadow increases, with poorly defined contour and structures. Due to the partially obstructed bronchiole, accompanying emphysema occurs, characterized by localized increase of permeability or increased transparency of both lungs, enlarged thoracic cavity, widened intercostal space, as well as lower and flat diaphragm. In the cases with pulmonary atelectasis, there are triangular or ribbonlike dense shadows with its sharp end pointing to the hilus. In the cases with pulmonary edema, there are patches or butterfly-winglike shadows with low density in the middle and inner zone of both lungs that are symmetrical distributed with the hilus as its center. In the cases with bronchiectasia, there are cystoid or column-like dilation of the bronchus. In the cases with serious spasmodic cough, alveolar rupture may occur to develop into pneumothorax characterized by absence of pulmonary markings in the outer zone of the lung field. In the cases with a small quantity of pneumothorax, the pneumothoracic area is linear or stripe-like with no pulmonary markings. The compressed lung edge can be well defined and is more clearly defined during exhalation.

18.7.1.2 CT Scanning

By HRCT, early stage of pneumonia and mild cases can be demonstrated as thickened vascular bundle in bronchus of both lungs, with irregular changes and accompanying ground-glass opacities. These findings indicate inflammatory infiltration in the interstitium surrounding the bronchus and intra-alveolar inflammatory infiltration and a small quantity of exudates (Fig. 18.1). The serious cases have accompanying lobular consolidation, with demonstrations of scattering small flakes or triangular-like parenchyma shadows or diffusive flakes of shadows with poorly defined boundaries. The shadows may also fuse into large flake of parenchyma shadow. In the cases with emphysema, there is round-like transparent area in the small flakes of parenchyma shadows, with different sizes and ranges. CT scanning can demonstrate occurrence of a small quantity of pneumothorax, with demonstrations of transparent areas in the exterior zone of the lung with no pulmonary markings, its medial arch-shaped visceral pleura being in fine linear shadow with soft tissue density, and different degrees of compression of the lung tissues.

Case Study 1

A boy aged 6 weeks, with a body weight of 3.1 kg, T 35.8 °C, BP 70/42 mmHg, and WBC 7.2×10^9/L.

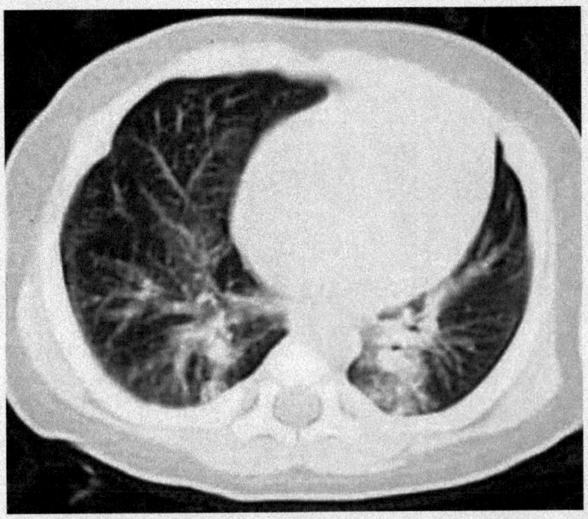

Fig. 18.1 Pertussis complicated by pneumonia. CT scanning demonstrates thickened vascular bundle of bronchus of both lungs, with poorly defined boundaries and flakes of ground-glass opacities and patches of shadows (Reprint with permission from Abe and Watanabe *Pediatr Emerg Care*, 2003, 19(4): 262)

18.7.2 Central Nervous System

The encephalopathies complicating pertussis include encephaledema and cerebral hypoxia that commonly involve the nuclei in basal ganglia.

18.7.2.1 CT Scanning

Encephaledema and cerebral hypoxia commonly occur in basal ganglia, which is demonstrated as symmetric low-density shadows or scattering low-density shadows with poorly defined boundaries. There are also demonstrations of blurry interface between gray and white matter and absence of some sulci. Brain parenchymal hemorrhage is demonstrated as spots, patches, and round shadows with high density in the brain parenchyma, which are possibly surrounded by low-density edema zone in different widths. Subarachnoid hemorrhage can be demonstrated as the absence sulci and cistern as well as increased density in cast-like appearance.

18.7.2.2 MR Imaging

Acute encephaledema and cerebral hypoxia commonly occur in the basal ganglia, which are demonstrated by symmetric long T1 long T2 signals. Otherwise, they can be demonstrated as multifocal or diffusive flakes of long T1 long T2 signals. By DWI, cytotoxic cerebral edema is demonstrated as high signal with obviously decreased ADC value, and interstitial cerebral edema is demonstrated as no high signals and slightly or moderately increased ADC value. In cases with acute hematoma, MR imaging demonstrates equal signal by T1WI and slightly decreased signal by T2WI. In cases with subacute and chronic hematoma, MR imaging demonstrates high signals by both T1WI and T2WI (Fig. 18.2).

Case Study 2
A boy aged 6 years, he had a history of vaccination against DPT. By physical examination, T was 36.3 °C and WBC 12×10^9/L.

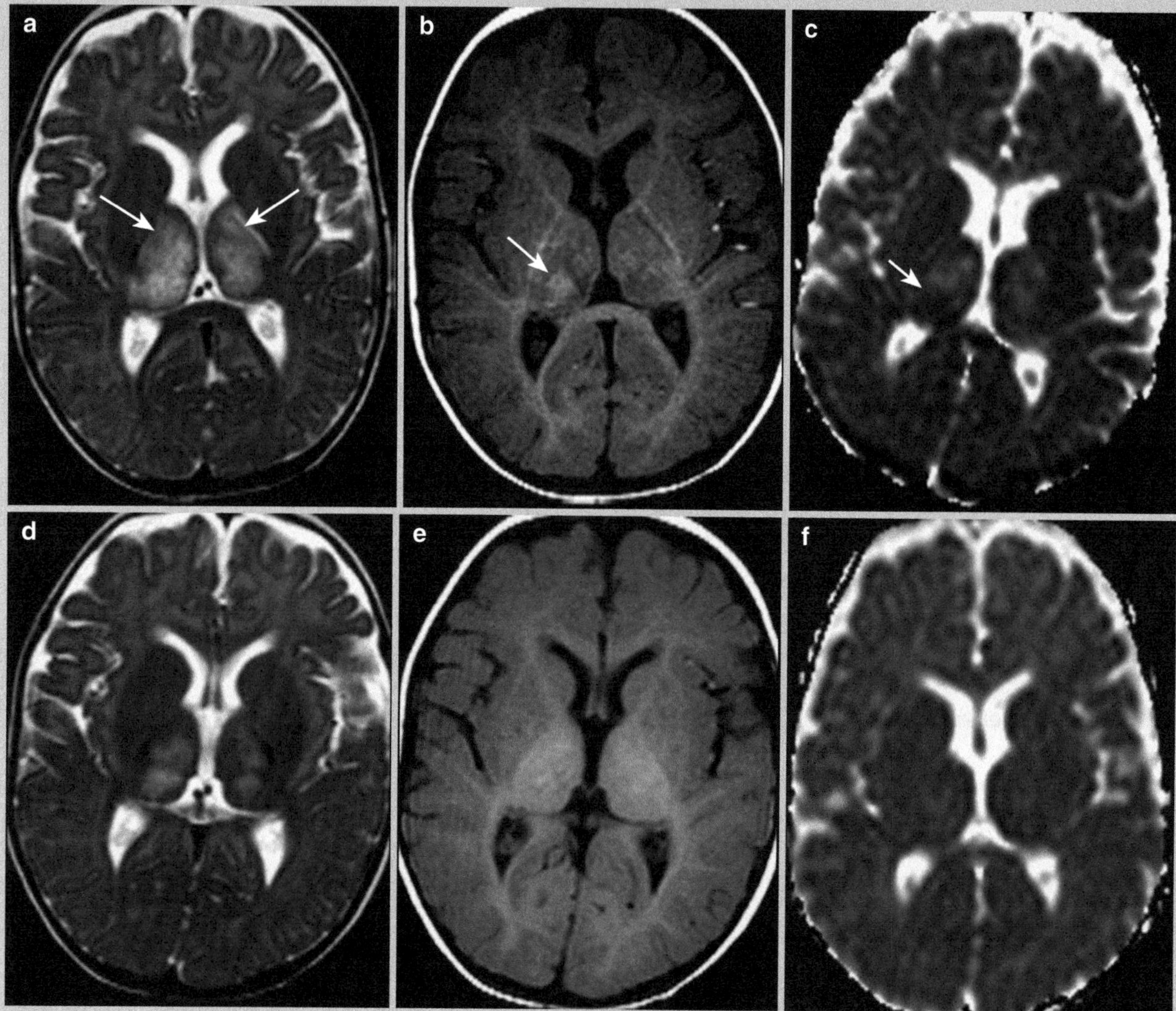

Fig. 18.2 Pertussis complicated by encephalopathy. (**a**) At day 3 after admission, MR imaging demonstrates symmetrical increased signal in bilateral basal ganglia and posterior limb of internal capsule by T2WI (*pointed by arrows*). (**b**) T1WI demonstrates high signal in the right thalamus, indicating cerebral hemorrhage (*pointed by arrow*). (**c**) Increased ADC value in bilateral thalamus and internal capsule, decreased ADC value in the high-signal area of the right thalamus by T1WI, indicating cerebral hemorrhage or cytotoxic cerebral edema (*pointed by arrow*). (**d**) Reexamination after 1 week, T2WI demonstrates decreased signal and range of the lesions in the bilateral thalamus. (**e**) T1WI demonstrates no increase of signal intensity of the lesions in the right thalamus. (**f**) Absence of the area with increased ADC value in the right thalamus (Reprint with permission from Aydin H, et al. *Pediatr Radiol*, 2010, 40(7): 1281)

18.7.3 Fracture

Fracture rarely occurs in the cases of pertussis. In the cases with pertussis complicated by fracture, X-ray and CT scanning demonstrate continual broken bone, with favorable demonstration of the location and quantity of fracture as well as displacement of fracture.

Case Study 3
A boy aged 11 years complained of sudden right chest pain for 3 h. He was diagnosed with pertussis 6 weeks ago.

For case detail and figures, please refer to Prasad and Baur, *J Paediatr Child Health*, 2001, 7(1): 91.

18.8 Diagnostic Basis

18.8.1 Diagnosis of Pertussis

18.8.1.1 Epidemiological Data

To patients with cough, especially children, the local prevalence of pertussis should be asked. A history of contact and a history of vaccination should be collected into the case history. This information facilitates the diagnosis of pertussis.

18.8.1.2 Clinical Manifestation

The typical symptoms include spasmodic cough and crow-like inhalation sound. After the body temperature returns to normal, cough tends to aggravate, especially at nights. But no other obvious lung signs can be found. In such cases, pertussis should be suspected.

18.8.1.3 Laboratory Examinations

By laboratory tests, increases of peripheral blood cell count and lymphocytes count are found. By bacteriological or molecular biological examination, positive finding is obtained. Based on these findings, the diagnosis of pertussis can be made.

18.8.2 Diagnosis of Pertussis-Related Complications

18.8.2.1 Respiratory Complication

Bronchopneumonia

In the children cases of pertussis complicated by bronchopneumonia, paroxysmal spasmodic cough is terminated, with fever and moist rales of the lungs. By laboratory test, peripheral WBC count increases that is predominantly an increase of neutrophil granulocyte. Diagnostic imaging demonstrates thickened and blurry pulmonary markings, network, and small patches of blurry shadows in both the hili and middle and lower lungs. In the serious cases, lobular consolidation can be found or fusion of small shadows into large flakes of consolidation shadow.

Pulmonary Atelectasis

X-ray and CT scanning demonstrate triangular or ribbonlike dense shadows, with its sharp end pointing to the hilus.

Pulmonary Emphysema and Subcutaneous Emphysema

Emphysema is demonstrated as focalized increase of permeability or increased transparency of both lung fields, widened intercostal space, and low and flat diaphragm. Subcutaneous emphysema is demonstrated as gas density shadow at the area of lesion.

18.8.2.2 Complications of the Central Nervous System

Children with pertussis have clinical manifestations of consciousness disturbance, high fever, and coma, with imaging demonstration of encephaledema and cerebral hypoxia. In combination to laboratory findings, the diagnosis of pertussis complicated by encephalopathy can be defined.

18.8.2.3 Rib Fracture

For children with pertussis, with no history of trauma, who have sudden severe chest pain, and with imaging demonstrations of continual fracture by CT scanning and X-ray, the diagnosis of pertussis complicated by fracture can be defined.

18.9 Differential Diagnosis

18.9.1 Acute Bronchitis and Pneumonia

The cases of bronchitis induced by influenza virus, adenovirus, respiratory syncytial virus, and parainfluenza virus have severe cough and spasmodic cough shortly after the onset, but with no crow-like inhalation sound after cough and with no aggravation at nights. By auscultation, scattering dry and moist rales can be heard with no fixed location that decreased or absent after cough. After treated, symptoms may be relieved or absent within a short period of time. X-ray and CT scanning demonstrate increased pulmonary markings or scattering small flakes of shadows in the middle and lower lungs.

18.9.2 Hilar Tuberculosis

Enlarged hilar lymph nodes may compress the trachea and bronchus or invade the bronchial wall to cause spasmodic cough, but with no crow-like inhalation sound and aggravation at nights. Such cases commonly have a history of tuberculosis. Based on the toxic symptoms, tuberculin test finding, as well as chest X-ray and CT scanning demonstrations, the diagnosis can be defined. CT scanning can favorably demonstrate enlarged hilar lymph nodes and mediastinal lymph nodes, with well-defined morphology, size, boundaries, and densities. Meanwhile, CT scanning can demonstrate early the primary foci and foci of caseous necrosis.

18.9.3 Pertussis Syndrome

The infection of *Bordetella parapertussis* and adenovirus I/II/III/V can cause symptoms resembling to pertussis. However, the toxic symptoms are generally more serious than pertussis. The cough and wheezing are more obvious than pertussis, with no obvious increase of lymphocyte. Chest X-ray demonstrates rough cardiac edge, namely, dense and irregular linear or jagged shadows surrounding the cardiac edge. Its differentiation from pertussis should be based on bacterial culture, virus isolation, and serological examination.

18.9.4 Pulmonary Atelectasis, Emphysema, and Bronchiectasia Caused by Other Factors

CT scanning demonstrates pulmonary atelectasis caused by bronchial lesions, extrapulmonary compression, and intrapulmonary scar contraction. CT scanning also facilitates identifying various types of emphysema. Bronchiectasia is caused by bronchial infection or traction of intrapulmonary lesions. CT scanning demonstrates the cause of bronchiectasis, such as pulmonary tuberculosis and chronic pulmonary interstitial fibrosis.

References

Abe Y, Watanabe T. Pertussis pneumonia complicated by a hyponatremic seizure. Pediatr Emerg Care. 2003;19(4):262–4.

Aydin H, Ozgul E, Agildere AM. Acute necrotizing encephalopathy secondary to diphtheria, tetanus toxoid and whole-cell pertussis vaccination: diffusion-weighted imaging and proton MR spectroscopy findings. Pediatr Radiol. 2010;40(7):1281–4.

Prasad S, Baur LA. Fracture of the first rib as a consequence of pertussis infection. J Paediatr Child Health. 2001;7(1):91–3.

Suggested Reading

Greenberg DP, von König CH, Heininger U. Health burden of pertussis in infants and children. Pediatr Infect Dis J. 2005;24(5):S39–43.

Ma YL. Studies of infectious diseases. Shanghai: Shanghai Science and Technology Press; 2011.

Yang YH, Su XL. Retrospective analysis of clinical data on pediatric pertussis. Guangzhou Med Pharm. 2011;42(1):39–40.

Zhang L, Zhang SM. Recent progresses in understanding epidemiology of pertussis. China Vaccines Immunol. 2008;14(6):559–64.

19 Plague

Ruili Li, Hong Jun Li, and Dan Wu

Plague, also known as Black Death, is a natural focal disease caused by *Yersinia pestis*. It prevails in wild rodents, with rats as its important source of infection. Its pathogen is commonly carried by rat fleas to infect humans, which causes bubonic plague after its invasion of human skin and pneumonic plague after its invasion via the respiratory tract. Plague, one of the most serious infectious diseases threatening human life, has strong infectivity and a high mortality rate. In the Prevention and Control Act of Infectious Diseases in China, it has been listed as the first infectious disease in class A. Three pandemics of plague occurred, with the first event occurring in the sixth century which spread from Mediterranean into Europe and nearly 100 million deaths reported. The second pandemic occurred in the fourteenth century, with the disease prevailing in Europe, Asia, and African. The third pandemic occurred in the eighteenth century, with the disease prevailing in 32 countries. The pandemic in the fourteenth century involved China. *Yersinia pestis* can be manufactured into bioterrorism weapon to threaten the world peace. Therefore, the prevention and control of plague is very important.

19.1 Etiology

Yersinia pestis, briefly known as plague bacillus, is categorized into *Yersinia* sp. and the family *Enterobacteriaceae*. By Meilan or Giemsa staining of the newly isolated strain, the bacteria are gram-negative oval-shaped short bacilli with their two ends being bluntly round and bipolarly thick. It is 1–1.5 μm in length and 0.5–0.7 μm in width, with no flagella, inability of moving, no spore forming, and capsules in the body of animals and during early cultures. It is facultative aerobic, which grows well but slowly in normal medium, while shows polymorphism at old culture medium and at suppurative plague foci. The optimal temperature for its culture is 28–30 °C, and the optimal pH value for its culture is 6.9–7.1. The thallus contains endotoxin and can produce murine toxin and some antigen components with pathogenic effects. The specific antigenic components of the bacteria include:

1. Fraction I antigen (FI) that can be further divided into two types, polysaccharide proteins (F-I) and proteins (F-IB). FI has strong antigenicity, high specificity, and leukocytic phagocytosis. It can be detected by agglutination, complement fixation, and indirect hemagglutination tests, which can be applied for the serological diagnosis of this disease. And its antibodies play protective roles.
2. The virulence V/W antigen on the cell surface where the V antigen is a protein to induce the production of the protective antibodies, while the W antigen is a lipoprotein that cannot induce protective effects. The V/W antigen conjugate is a thallus surface antigen, which plays role in promoting formation of capsules and inhibiting phagocytosis. In addition, it plays a role in the cells to protect growth and reproduction of the bacteria, functioning as the virulence factor of the bacteria and being related to the bacterial invasive capacity.
3. T antigen, namely, murine toxin. It exists within the cells and can cause local necrosis and toxemia, with favorable antigenicity.

After the infection of humans and animals, antitoxin antibodies can be produced. *Yersinia pestis* can produce two types of toxins, murine toxin or exotoxin (toxic protein) that has strong toxicity to mice and rats and endotoxin (lipopolysaccharide) that has stronger toxicity than other

R. Li • D. Wu
Department of Radiology, Beijing You'an Hospital, Capital Medical University, Beijing, China

H.J. Li (✉)
Beijing You'an Hospital, Capital Medical University, Beijing, China
e-mail: lihongjun00113@126.com

H. Li (ed.), *Radiology of Infectious Diseases: Volume 2*, DOI 10.1007/978-94-017-9876-1_19

gram-negative bacterial endotoxins and can cause fever, disseminated intravascular coagulation, hemolysis within tissues and organs, toxic shock, and local and systemic Schwarzman reaction. The endotoxin (lipopolysaccharide) is the lethal toxic substance of these pathogenic bacteria. *Yersinia pestis* can survive for a long period of time at low temperature and in organisms. For instances, it can survive for 10–20 days in purulent sputum, for weeks or months in dead bodies, and for over 1 month in flea feces. It is sensitive to light, heat, dryness, and common disinfectants.

19.2 Epidemiology

19.2.1 The Source of Infection

Plague is a typical natural focal disease that prevails in humans after its prevalence in rats and other rodents, especially marmots. The source of infection in humans is mainly ground squirrels and sewer rats. Other animals like cats, sheep, rabbits, camels, wolves, and foxes may also be the sources of infection.

Various types of patients with plague are also the source of infection. Due to the spread of pneumonic plague via droplets and large quantity of pathogenic bacteria in the sputum of patients with pneumonic plague, the patients with plague are important sources of infection. Attention should be paid on the carriers (including healthy carriers and convalescent carriers) as source of infection. The blood of early septicemic plague is infectious. Patients with bubonic plague are also the source of infection after the abscesses rupture or their blood is sucked by fleas. The three types of plague can develop into each other.

19.2.2 Route of Transmission

The transmission vector of plague from animal to human is mainly rat fleas, indicating the bacteria's route transmission from rats to fleas and then to humans. Before the prevalence of plague in humans, there is commonly prevalence of plague in rats, generally spreading from field mice to house mice. When fleas parasitizing on rats with plague suck the bacteria-infected blood, the bacteria multiply in the flea's stomach in a large quantity and form bacterial embolus blocking its forestomach. When the flea sucks human blood, blood flow is blocked by the bacterial embolus and flows back into the human body along with the bacteria, thus causing the infection. The bacteria also exist in flea feces, which may gain their access into the human body via skin scratch. A recent study has demonstrated another possible route of transmission, via ticks as the spreading medium.

19.2.2.1 Transmission via the Skin

Due to contact to bacteria containing sputum and pus from the patients, bacteria containing in the skin, blood, and flesh of the infected animals or feces of infected fleas, the bacteria can gain their access into the human body via skin wounds to cause the infection.

19.2.2.2 Transmission via the Digestive Tract

Humans can be infected by intake of meat of infected animals, with the digestive tract as the route of transmission.

19.2.2.3 Transmission via the Respiratory Tract

The bacteria in the sputum from patients infected with pneumonic plague can be transmitted from person to person via droplets, causing epidemic in humans. Generally, bubonic plague does not spread from person to his/her surrounding persons.

19.2.3 Population Susceptibility

Populations are generally susceptible to plague and the susceptibility has no gender and age differences. Plague may be asymptomatic and vaccination reduces the susceptibility. Individuals with a history of vaccination can be asymptomatically infected via close contacts with the patients. By throat culture, *Yersinia pestis* can be detected. And persistent immunity can be acquired after the infection. Slight cases of plague can be cured, but with insufficient immunity acquired after the infection.

19.2.4 Epidemiological Features

19.2.4.1 The Natural Foci of Plague

There are many natural foci of plague in the world, with persistent existence of rats plague. In Asia, Africa, and America, the naturally occurring rats plague is the most common. In China, the natural occurrence of rats plague is mainly in Yunnan province and Qingzang plateau.

19.2.4.2 Prevalence

Plague commonly spreads from the epidemic focus into its surrounding areas along with transportations to cause exogenous plague. Therefore, epidemics and even pandemics are resulted.

19.2.4.3 Seasonal Occurrence

The seasonal occurrence is related to hunting and reproduction of rat fleas. Human plague commonly occurs from June to September, and excessive rainfall is the most possible cause of the spreading of plague. Pneumonic plague commonly prevails after October.

19.3 Pathogenesis and Pathological Changes

19.3.1 Pathogenesis

After *Yersinia pestis* gains its access into the human body via the skin, it is firstly engulfed by the capsule and V/W antigen phagocytes for local replication. After that, under the effects of hyaluronic acid and soluble cellulose, the bacteria rapidly enter the local lymph nodes via the lymphatic vessels for replication which causes serious hemorrhagic necrotizing inflammation and primary lymph node inflammation (bubonic plague). After replication in a large quantity, the bacteria and the toxins in the lymph nodes enter the bloodstream causing systemic infection, sepsis, and serious toxic symptoms, with possible involvement of the spleen, liver, lungs, and central nervous system. When the bacteria spread to the lungs, secondary pneumonic plague occurs. After the bacteria are directly inhaled into the respiratory tract, they firstly replicate in the local lymphoid tissues and then spread to the lungs to cause primary pneumonic plague. On the basis of primary pneumonic plague, the bacteria enter bloodstream and cause septicemia, which is known as secondary septicemic plague. In extremely rare cases of serious infection, the bacteria infect the blood and replicate thus causing primary septicemic plague, which has an extremely high mortality rate.

19.3.2 Pathological Changes

The basic lesions are vascular and lymphatic endothelial cell injury, acute hemorrhagic and necrotic lesions. Regional lymph nodes have hemorrhagic inflammation and coagulation necrosis. The swollen lymph nodes commonly fuse with their surrounding tissues to form large or small masses, which are in dark red or grayish yellow. Extensive hemorrhage occurs in the spleen and bone marrow. Bleeding spots can be found on the skin mucosa, and hemorrhagic effusion can be found in the serous cavity. Hemorrhagic inflammation occurs in the heart, liver, and kidneys. The cases of pneumonia plague are demonstrated with bronchial or lobar pneumonia and hemorrhagic serous exudates in the bronchi and alveoli as well as necrotic nodules caused by scattered bacterial embolism.

19.4 Clinical Symptoms and Signs

The incubation period of plague is generally 2–5 days, with the incubation period of bubonic or septicemic plague being 2–7 days and primary pneumonic plague being as short as 1–3 days or even several hours. Individuals with a history of vaccination may experience longer incubation period, which lasts for 12 days. Plague has four clinical types, bubonic, pulmonary, septicemic, and slight. Except the clinical slight type, the early systemic toxic symptoms of other clinical types are almost the same, but with respective characteristic manifestations.

19.4.1 Bubonic Plague

It is the most common type of plague, accounting for 85–90 % of the plague cases, which commonly occurs in the early stage of an epidemic. In addition to fever and systemic toxic symptoms, it is characterized by acute lymphadenitis. Because the lower limbs are more highly possible to be bitten by fleas, inguinal lymphadenitis is more common, accounting for nearly 70 % of the bubonic plague cases, followed by subaxillary, cervical, and submaxillary lymphadenitis. Lymphadenitis is commonly unilateral, possibly with concurrent involvement of several parts. At the onset, the regional lymph nodes show swelling and pain. At days 2–3, the conditions rapidly deteriorate, with redness, swelling, heat, pain, and fusion of swollen lymph nodes with their surrounding tissues into masses with severe tenderness. The patient at this time is in a forced position. At days 4–5, the swollen lymph nodes are purulent and rupture and the conditions of the patient are generally relieved. In some cases, the conditions may develop into septicemia, severe toxemia, and heart failure or even pneumonic plague and thereafter death.

19.4.2 Pneumonic Plague

This type is the most serious clinical type, with an extremely high mortality rate. Pneumonic plague can be primary or secondary to bubonic plague, which is common at the epidemic peak. With acute and sudden onset as well as rapid development, it is characterized by, in addition to high fever and severe toxic symptoms, severe chest pain and cough with phlegm that first with mucous and then bubbly bloody sputum or bright-red bloody sputum in 24–36 h after onset. There are also shortness of breath that rapidly develops into dyspnea and cyanosis, a small quantity of scattered moist rales at the lungs, and pleural rales. Chest X-ray demonstrates signs of bronchitis, with less pulmonary signs that are inconsistent with the severe systemic symptoms. With no timely appropriate rescuing, the patients may die of heart failure, bleeding, and shock within 2–3 days. Before death occurs, the patients show systemic skin cyanosis purplish black in color; therefore, the disease is also known as Black Death.

19.4.3 Septicemic Plague

It is also known as fulminant plague, the most dangerous type. It can be primary or secondary. Primary septicemic plague develops rapidly due to the compromised immunity of the patients, large quantity of the bacteria, and their strong toxicity. The patients may experience sudden high fever or normal body temperature, unconsciousness, delirium, or coma. There are commonly no swollen lymph nodes but mucocutaneous bleeding, nasal bleeding, vomiting, bloody stools, hematuria, DIC, and heart failure. Death commonly occurs within 24 h after onset, and the patients rarely survive for more than 3 days. The mortality rate is as high as 100 %.

19.4.4 Slight Plague

Slight plague is also known as small plague, with slight fever and mild systemic symptoms. The patients are commonly able to work as usual but experience local lymphadenectasis with mild tenderness, occasional suppuration, and no bleeding. The blood culture may be positive. And the cases are more common at early and terminal stages of epidemics or in individuals with a history of vaccination.

19.4.5 Other Rarely Occurring Types of Plague

19.4.5.1 Cutaneous Type

After the invasion of the bacteria into local skin to cause painful red spots, these red spots develop into blisters within several hours to form pustules that may be mixed with blood. Otherwise, furuncles or carbuncles are developed, with black crusts covering on their surface, surrounding dark-red infiltrations, and hardened ulceration at the base, which appears like cutaneous anthrax. Occasionally, generalized pustules can be found, which appear like smallpox and are also known as smallpox-like plague.

19.4.5.2 Meningoencephalitic Type

It commonly occurs secondary to bubonic type or other types of plague, with obvious symptoms of meningeal irritation. The cerebrospinal fluid is purulent, with detection of *Yersinia pestis* by smears or culture.

19.4.5.3 Ocular Type

The bacteria invade the conjunctiva to cause conjunctival congestion, swelling, and pain, with consequent occurrence of purulent conjunctivitis.

19.4.5.4 Enteritic Type

In addition to the systemic toxic symptoms, the patients experience diarrhea with mucous and blood in stool, vomiting, abdominal pain, and tenesmus. The pathogenic bacteria can be detected from the feces.

19.4.5.5 Throat Type

The pathogenic bacteria invade the oral cavity to cause acute pharyngitis and tonsillitis, possibly with accompanying cervical lymphadenectasis. This type can also be asymptomatic, with detection of the pathogenic bacteria by culture of pharyngeal secretion. Such asymptomatic cases are common in individuals with a history of vaccination.

19.5 Plague-Related Complications

19.5.1 Sepsis

After the bacteria enter the bloodstream, they grow and replicate to produce toxins with consequent occurrence of systemic serious infection. Clinically, it is characterized by fever, severe toxemia, skin rashes and petechiae, hepatosplenomegaly, and increased WBC count. The slight cases only have general symptoms of infection, while the serious cases may have septic shock, DIC, and multiple organ failure.

19.6 Diagnostic Examinations

19.6.1 Routine Blood Test

WBC count increases significantly, which can be up to 30×10^9/L. Neutrophils also increase significantly. Mild-to-moderate anemia can also be detected.

19.6.2 Bacteriological Examinations

The results are important to define the diagnosis. The fluid harvested from puncture of the lymph nodes, pus, sputum, blood, and cerebrospinal fluid can be prepared for smear, microscopy, culture, and animal inoculation.

19.6.2.1 Bacterial Culture

Based on different conditions of the patients, the tissues from the liver or spleen tissues of animals or the fluid harvested from puncture of lymph nodes, pus, sputum, blood, and cerebrospinal fluid of patients can be collected. The following cultures on blood agar plate or broth medium can be performed to isolate the pathogenic bacteria. Further identification of the bacteria should be based on biochemical reaction, phage lysis test, or serological test.

19.6.2.2 Animal Inoculation

The aforementioned materials should be firstly harvested with following preparation into emulsion in saline solution. The emulsion is then subcutaneously or intraperitoneally injected into guinea pigs or mice. Death occurs within 24–72 h and the guinea pig or mouse is dissected for bacteriological examination.

19.6.3 Serological Tests

19.6.3.1 Indirect Hemagglutination Assay (PHA)

Using FI antigen of *Yersinia pestis*, the blood FI antibody is detected. The positive result can be detected in 5–7 days after the infection, which reaches its peak in 2–4 weeks. Thereafter, it gradually decreases, which may last for as long as 4 years. The assay is commonly applied for retrospective diagnosis and epidemiological investigation.

19.6.3.2 Enzyme-Linked Immunosorbent Assay (ELISA)

It is more sensitive to the blood FI antibody than PHA. Anti-plague IgG can also be used to detect FI antigen. The detected titer being above 1:400 is defined positive. The erosive animal specimens 30 days after its death can be treated with formaldehyde for the assay, with the titer not affected.

19.6.3.3 Radioimmunoprecipitation Test (RIP)

This test can detect the small quantity of F1 antibody from individuals who had a history of plague 28–32 years ago. Therefore, it can be applied for retrospective diagnosis and immunological studies.

19.6.3.4 Fluorescent Antibody Method (FA)

By using fluorescein-labeled specific antiserum, the specimens from suspected cases can be examined, which can define the diagnosis rapidly and accurately.

19.6.4 Molecular Biological Examination

The molecular biological examinations include DNA probes and polymerase chain reaction (PCR). Both are widely applied in recent years, with rapid, sensitive, and specific detecting results.

19.6.5 Diagnostic Imaging

Chest X-ray and CT scanning are conventional radiological examinations for pneumonic plague.

19.7 Imaging Demonstrations

Case Study 1

Animal experiment of pneumonic plague (Fig. 19.1).

(Note: The case and figures are cited from Layton RC, et al. *Plos Negl Trop Dis*, 2011a, 5(2): e959.)

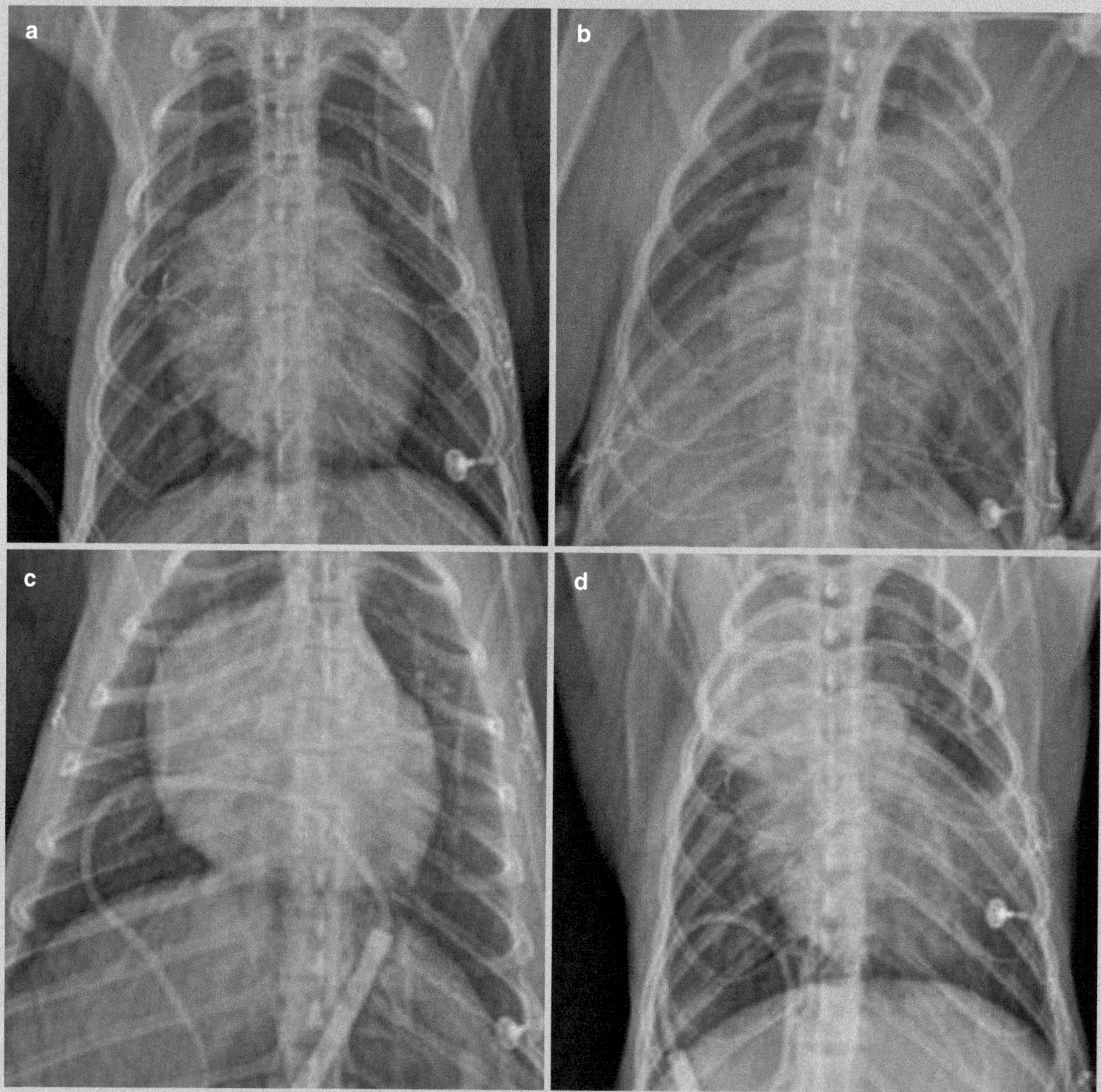

Fig. 19.1 Pneumonic plague. (**a**) Chest X-ray demonstrates clear pulmonary markings in both lungs in nontreatment group of African green monkeys before their infection of *Yersinia pestis*; (**b**) chest X-ray demonstrates flakes of high-density shadows in the left lung field and in the right lower lung at day 5 after infection of *Yersinia pestis*; (**c**) chest X-ray demonstrates clear pulmonary markings in both lungs in the treatment group of African green monkeys before their infection of *Yersinia pestis*; (**d**) with medication of lenofloxacin immediately after the onset of symptoms, chest X-ray demonstrates flakes of high-density shadows at day 5 after the infection only in the left lower lung and in the right upper lung field, which have smaller range than that in nontreatment group

Chest X-ray demonstrations of pneumonic plague include hemorrhagic necrotizing inflammation with pulmonary segment as the center, which may involve multiple pulmonary lobes or segments. The manifestations are mass-like lesions that may fuse into flakes and even white lung change (Fig. 19.2). After 2 weeks of treatment, the symptoms improve significantly, but the absorption of pulmonary shadows is slow, especially in the cases with respiratory failure.

(For case detail and figures, please refer to Layton RC, et al. *Plos Negl Trop Dis*, 2011, 5(2): e959.).

Case Study 2

Animal experiment of pneumonic plague.

(Note: L for left. Reproduced with permission from Layton et al. RC, et al. *J Med Primatol*, 2011b, 40(1): 6.)

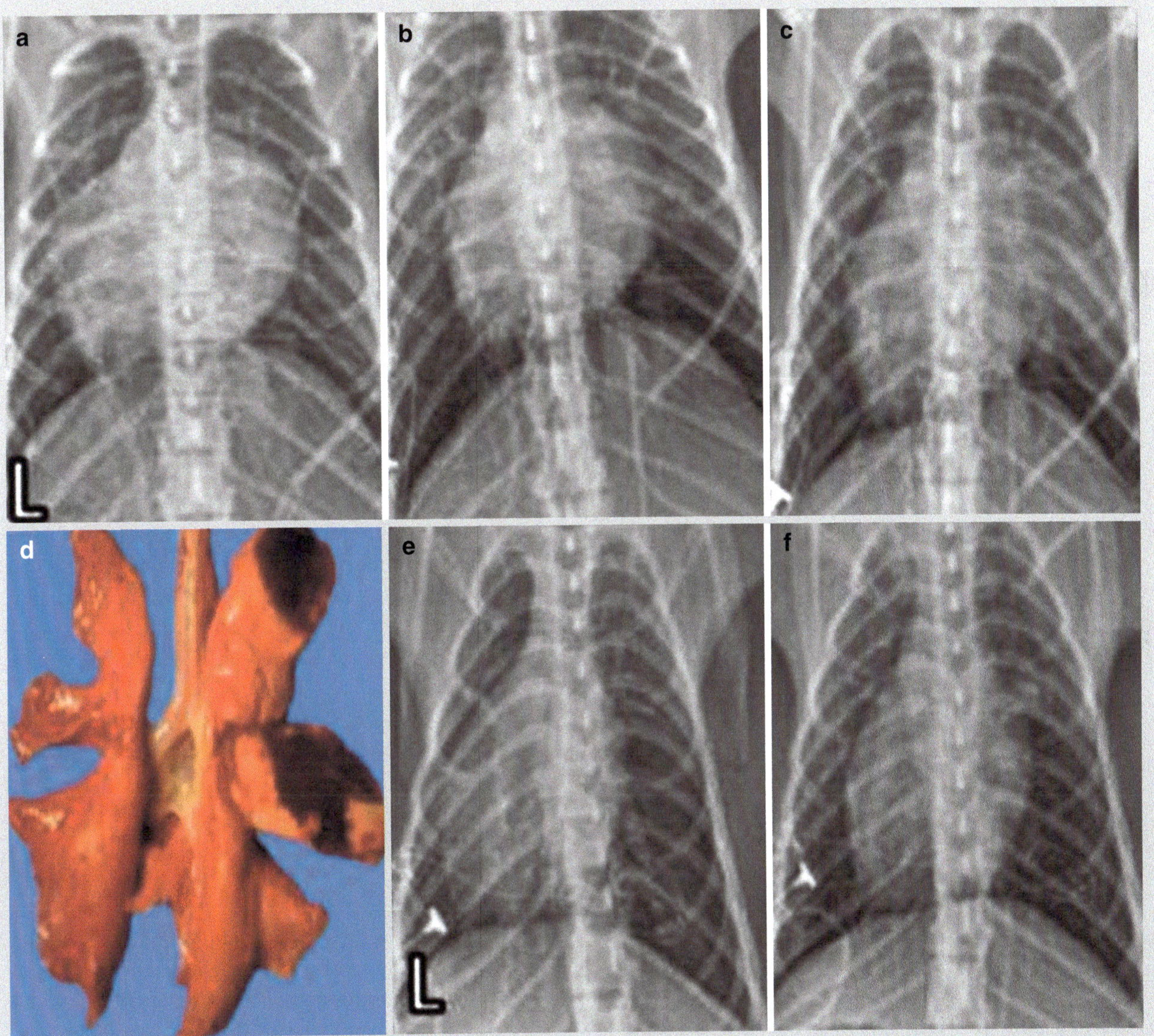

Fig. 19.2 Pneumonic plague. (**a**) Chest X-ray demonstrates clear pulmonary markings in both lungs in African green monkeys (X775) before their infection of *Yersinia pestis*; (**b**) chest X-ray demonstrates pale flakes of shadows in the right middle lung lobe at day 3 after the infection; (**c**) chest X-ray demonstrates flakes of high-density shadows in the right middle lung lobe and pale shadows in the right upper lung lobe 4 days later; (**d**) autopsy of the gross specimens after euthanasia demonstrates flakes of necrotic areas in the right middle and upper lung lobes; (**e**) chest X-ray demonstrates clear pulmonary markings in both lungs in African green monkeys (X784) before their infection of *Yersinia pestis*; (**f**) chest X-ray demonstrates pale flakes of shadows in the right middle lung lobe at day 3 after the infection; (**g**) chest X-ray demonstrates flakes of pale shadows and high-density shadows in the middle lobes of both lungs and in the left lower lung lobe; (**h**) autopsy of the gross specimens after euthanasia demonstrates spots and flakes of necrotic necroses areas in the upper lobes and lower lobes of both lungs

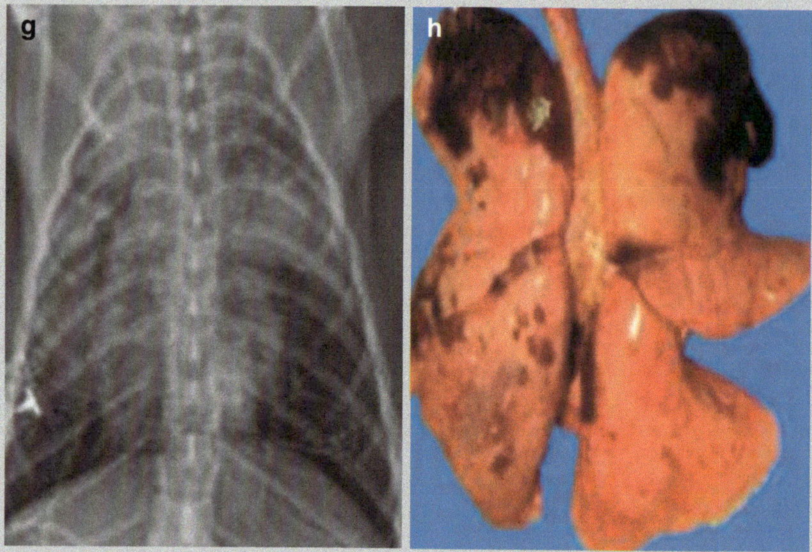

Fig. 19.2 (continued)

Case Study 3
A male patient aged 53 years complained of high fever with chills and a body temperature of 40 °C, cough with frothy bloody sputum, chest pain, obvious dyspnea, and mild headache. Reverse indirect agglutination test of sputum specimen at day 2 after the onset demonstrated *Yersinia*-specific F1 antigen positive, moist rales in both lungs, phlegm rales in the left lung, lower breath sounds in the right lung, and dullness on percussion.

For case detail and figures, please refer to DaWa WJ, et al. *Chinese Journal of Tuberculosis and Respiratory Disease*, 2011, 34(6): 404. (In Chinese)

Case Study 4
A female patient aged 40 years complained of high fever, cough with light yellowish foam-like sputum in small quantity and with blood streaks, chest pain, and breathing difficulty. Her SpO_2 was 80 %, with coarse breathing sounds in both lungs and moist rales in the left middle lung. Reverse indirect agglutination test of sputum specimen demonstrated *Yersinia*-specific F1 antigen positive.

For case detail and figures, please refer to DaWa WJ, et al. *Chinese Journal of Tuberculosis and Respiratory Disease*, 2011, 34(6): 404. (In Chinese)

Case Study 5
A male patient aged 37 years complained of fever with a body temperature of 39.8 °C, chest pain, slight breathing difficulty, and cough with yellowish thick sputum that is difficult to be coughed up with no blood in it. Extensive moist rales and a little phlegm rales can be heard in the left lung. Reverse indirect agglutination test of sputum specimen demonstrated *Yersinia*-specific F1 antigen positive.

For case detail and figures, please refer to DaWa WJ, et al. *Chinese Journal of Tuberculosis and Respiratory Disease*, 2011, 34(6): 404. (In Chinese)

Case Study 6
A male patient aged 20 years complained of fever with a body temperature of 39 °C, slight cough, expectoration with blood streaks, and occasional chest pain. A few moist rales can be heard in the right middle lung. And his conditions are relatively slight. Reverse indirect agglutination test of sputum specimen demonstrated *Yersinia*-specific F1 antigen positive.

For case detail and figures, please refer to DaWa WJ, et al. *Chinese Journal of Tuberculosis and Respiratory Disease*, 2011, 34(6): 404. (In Chinese)

Case Study 7

A male patient aged 38 years complained of fever and body temperature of 37.5 °C, cough with frothy bloody sputum, chest pain, obvious dyspnea, fatigue, myalgia, and nausea with vomiting. Reverse indirect agglutination test of sputum specimen at day 3 after the onset demonstrated *Yersinia-specific* F1 antigen positive, phlegm rales in the right lung, and lower breath sounds in the left lung (Fig. 19.3).

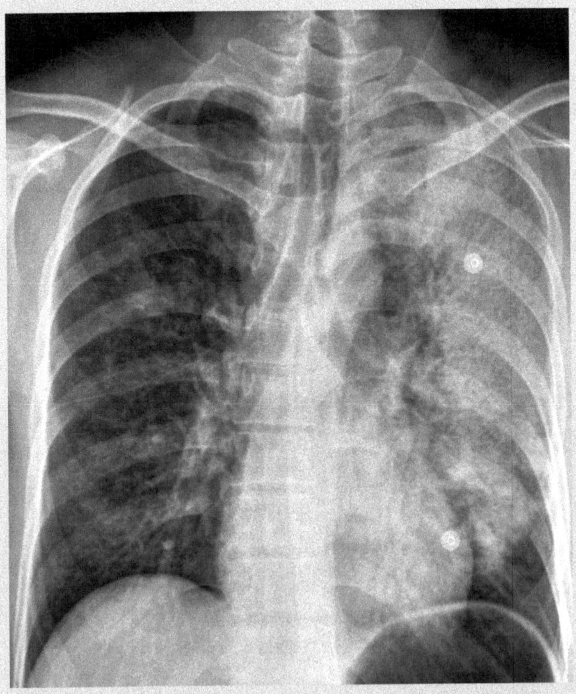

Fig. 19.3 Pneumonic plague. At day 2 of the illness course, chest X-ray demonstrates spotted and flocculent shadows in the right upper lung field and large flakes of shadows in the left lung field

Case Study 8

A male patient aged 50 years with a body temperature of 38.5 °C and obnubilation and had the fidgets and hemorrhage spots in the skin. Bilateral anisocoria, left 2 mm, right 3 mm, light reflex slow. His SpO_2 cannot be measured, with coarse breathing sounds in both lungs and some moist rales. Reverse indirect agglutination test of sputum specimen at day 3 after the onset demonstrated *Yersinia*-specific F1 antigen positive (Fig. 19.4).

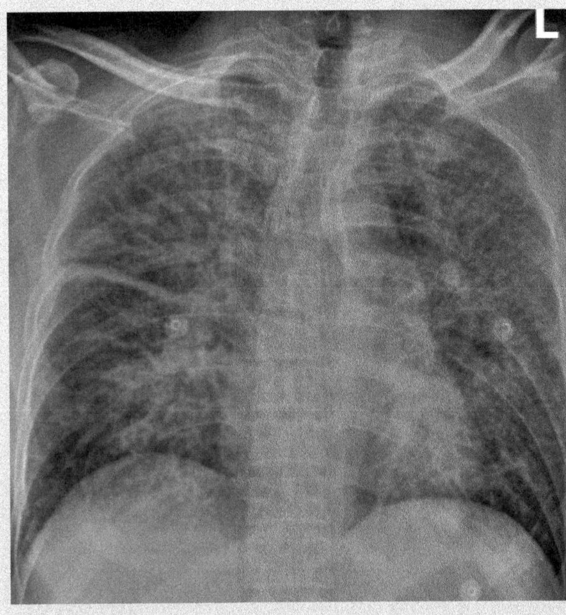

Fig. 19.4 Pneumonic plague. (**a**) At day 2 of the illness course, chest X-ray demonstrates increase of pulmonary markings in both lungs and little flakes of shadows in the both lower lung fields, especially around the hila; ribbon thickened along the interlobar pleura

19.8 Diagnostic Basis

Early diagnosis, especially the timely identification of the first case, is critically important for the prevention and control of plague. In epidemic areas, the cases in early stage of epidemics or atypical sporadic cases should be paid special attention. Based on the epidemiological data and typical clinical manifestations, the diagnosis can be generally made. Slight cases should be distinguished from acute lymphadenitis, tsutsugamushi disease, leptospirosis, and tularemia. The suspected cases should receive bacteriological or serological examinations, with serological test being based on at least four times increase of the titer by double sera test. Successful detection of *Yersinia pestis* is the most important evidence to define the diagnosis.

19.8.1 Epidemiological Data

The patients may have lived in an area that ever had prevalence of plague in rats or the patients visited an epidemic area of plague 10 days prior to the onset. Otherwise, the patients may have a history of contact to animals or patients with plague.

19.8.2 Clinical Manifestation

The clinical manifestations include sudden onset, high fever, severe systemic toxic symptoms and early tendencies of failure and bleeding, lymphadenectasis, pulmonary involvement, or sepsis.

19.8.3 Laboratory Tests

19.8.3.1 Routine Tests

Routine Blood Test

The total WBC count commonly increases to 20–30 × 10^9/L. Lymphocyte count increases in the early stage, followed by an increase of neutrophil count and decrease of RBC, hemoglobin, and platelet counts.

Routine Urine Test

The amounts of urine reduce, with proteinuria and hematuria.

Routine Stool Test

The patients with enteritic type of plague have bloody stool or with mucous and blood which is always positive by bacterial culture.

19.8.3.2 Bacteriological Examinations

The fluid by puncture of the lymph nodes, pus, sputum, blood, and cerebrospinal fluid should be collected for bacteriological examinations.

Smear

The aforementioned specimens can be prepared for smear or imprints, and the following gram staining can detect short bacillus with both G^- ends thickly stained. About 50–80 % of the cases are positive.

Bacterial Culture

The aforementioned specimens are inoculated in the ordinary agar or broth culture medium for bacterial culture. The positive rate of early bubonic plague by blood culture is 70 % and that of late bubonic plague by blood culture is about 90 %. The positive rate can reach 100 % during sepsis.

Animal Inoculation

The above specimens are first prepared into emulsion with saline solution. The emulsion is then subcutaneously or intraperitoneally injected into guinea pigs or mice. Death occurs within 24–72 h and the organs can be harvested for bacteriological examination.

Phage Lysis Test

Plague phage is added into the detected bacteria that are not defined. The following fission and bacteriolysis can be observed.

19.8.3.3 Serological Test

By indirect hemagglutination, F1 antigen can be used to detect the F1 antibody in sera of patients or infected animals. F1 antibody persists for 1–4 years and therefore is commonly applied for epidemiological investigation and retrospective diagnosis.

By fluorescein antibody staining, the fluorescein-labeled specific antiserum is used to detect suspected specimen. It has high specificity and sensitivity.

Other enzyme-linked immunosorbent assay or radioimmunoprecipitation test can be applied to detect the Fl antibody. Both have a high sensitivity that is widely applied for large-scale epidemiological investigation.

19.8.4 Radiological Examinations

Chest X-rays of pneumonic plague demonstrate hemorrhagic necrotic inflammation with the pulmonary segment as the center. Multiple pulmonary lobes or segments may be involved. The manifestations include mass-like lesions that may fuse together to form flake and even white lung sign. After 2 weeks of treatment, the symptoms improve significantly, but the absorption of pulmonary shadows is slow, especially in the cases with respiratory failure.

19.9 Differential Diagnosis

19.9.1 Bubonic Plague

19.9.1.1 Acute Lymphadenitis

The patients with acute lymphadenitis commonly have obvious trauma, lymphangitis, and slight systemic symptoms.

19.9.1.2 Lymphatic Filariasis (Swollen Lymph Nodes Filariasis)

In the acute stage of the disease, lymphadenitis and lymphangitis often concur, which can be self-healed after several days. The systemic symptoms are mild. In the evening, microfilariae can be found through blood film examination. Ultrasound or CT scanning can demonstrate enlarged lymph nodes, based on which the differentiation is still difficult.

19.9.1.3 Tularemia

It is caused by infection of tularemia pathogens, with mild systemic symptom. The swollen glands are well defined, mobile, and painless with normal skin color. There is no forced posture with favorable prognosis.

19.9.2 Septicemic Plague

It should be differentiated from septicemia of other causes, leptospirosis, epidemic hemorrhagic fever, epidemic cerebrospinal meningitis, and hemorrhagic fever with renal syndrome. The pathogens or antibodies should be timely identified. And the differentiation should be based on epidemiological data, symptoms, and signs.

19.9.3 Pneumonic Plague

It should be differentiated from pneumonia of other causes, such as lobar pneumonia, severe acute respiratory distress syndrome, pulmonary hemorrhagic leptospirosis, *Chlamydia* and *Mycoplasma* pneumonia, and pulmonary anthrax. Based on the clinical manifestations and pathogenic detection of the sputum, the differential diagnosis can be made. Key points for differentiation based on the radiological findings are the following.

19.9.3.1 Lobar Pneumonia

Chest X-ray demonstrates flakes of dense shadows with not very high density that are evenly distributed and visible air bronchogram. CT scanning demonstrates evenly high-density shadows with poorly defined boundaries and visible air bronchogram in the lesions.

19.9.3.2 Severe Acute Respiratory Distress Syndrome

There are diffuse infiltrative shadows in both lungs.

19.9.3.3 Pulmonary Hemorrhagic Leptospirosis

Chest X-ray demonstrates varying lesions in different clinical stages of the disease. The demonstrations include thickened pulmonary markings, miliary and nodular opacities, and patches and flakes of fused shadows along with the progress of the conditions.

19.9.4 Mycoplasma Pneumonia

Chest X-ray in the early stage of the disease demonstrates increased and thickened pulmonary markings with poorly defined boundaries and reticular shadows, corresponding to the stage of acute interstitial inflammation. The lesions further develop into alveolar infiltration, demonstrated as patches of dense shadows that are segmentally distributed in the lower lungs. The shadows are fan-shaped dense shadow from the hilus radiating to the lung field, with poorly defined boundaries.

References

DaWa WJ, Pan WJ, Gu XY, et al. Primary pneumonic plague: report of 5 cases. Chin J Tuberc Respir Dis. 2011;34(6):404–8.

Layton RC, Mega W, Mc Donald JD, et al. Levofloxacin cures experimental pneumonic plague in African green monkeys. PLoS Negl Trop Dis. 2011a;5(2):e959.

Layton RC, Brasel T, Gigliotti A, et al. Primary pneumonic plague in the African Green monkey as a model for treatment efficacy evaluation. J Med Primatol. 2011b;40(1):6–17.

Suggested Reading

Clark EA, Walker N, Ford DC, et al. Molecular recognition of chymotrypsin by the serine protease inhibitor ecotin from Yersinia pestis. J Biol Chem. 2011;286(27):24015–22.

Cornelius CA, Quenee LE, Overheim KA, et al. Immunization with recombinant V10 Protects cynomolgus macaques from lethal pneumonic plague. Infect Immun. 2008;76(12):5588–97.

Dutt AK, Akhtar R, Mcveigh M. Surat plague of 1994 re-examined[J]. Southeast Asian J Trop Med Public Health. 2006;37(4):755–60.

Gamble C, Jacobsen KO, Leffel E, et al. Use of a low-concentration heparin solution to extend the life of central venous catheters in African green monkeys (Chlorocebus aethiops). J Am Assoc Lab Anim Sci. 2007;46(3):58–60.

Hinnebusch BJ, Erickson DL. Yersinia pestis biofilm in the flea vector and its role in the transmission of plague. Curr Top Microbiol Immunol. 2008;322:229–48.

Li LJ. Studies of infectious diseases. Beijing: Higher Education Press; 2011.

Rossi CA, Ulrich M, Norris S, et al. Identification of a surrogate marker for infection in the African green monkey model of inhalation anthrax. Infect Immun. 2008;76(12):5790–801.

Smiley ST. Current challenges in the development of vaccines for pneumonic plague. Expert Rev Vaccines. 2008;7(2):209–21.

Sun YC, Koumoutsi A, Darby C. The response regulator PhoP negatively regulator yersinia pseudotuberculosis and yersinia pestis biofilm. FEMS Microbiol Lett. 2009;290(1):85–90.

Van Andel R, Sherwood R, Gennings C, et al. Clinical and pathologic features of cynomolgus macaques (Macaca fascicularis) infected with aerosolized Yersinia pestis. Comp Med. 2008;58(1):68–75.

Psittacosis

20

Haifeng Mi, Hongjun Li, and Jianan Yu

Psittacosis, also known as ornithosis, is an acute infectious disease caused by *Chlamydia psittaci* (Cps) and commonly prevails in poultry and other species of bird. Humans infected by *Chlamydia psittaci* may suffer from unapparent subclinical infection, with symptoms ranging from mild flulike illness to severe SARS. As a typical animal-based infectious disease, psittacosis rarely has pulmonary signs but a long illness course, despite its clinical manifestation characterized by severe pulmonary lesions. Repeated onsets of psittacosis may lead to chronic diseases.

20.1 Etiology

Initially isolated from parrots, *Chlamydia psittaci* (Cps) is the pathogen of psittacosis. With a diameter of 150–200 nm, the elementary body is ring-shaped and characterized by a narrow protoplasmic margin around the nucleoplasm, a non-glycogen inclusion body and iodine staining negative. Cps develops well in several cell culture systems, among which HeLa cells, Vero cells, and L cells as well as McCoy cells are commonly used. The Cps can also develop in the yolk sac of the chicken embryo. The number of susceptible animals is relatively large, and the laboratory rats are usually used in the animal inoculation. As Cps and *Chlamydia trachomatis* share the same antigen, both of them cannot be distinguished by the complement fixation test (CFT). With a weak resistance to the surroundings, Cps can be easily killed by the general chemical disinfectants. It can be inactivated in 48 h at 37 °C, in 10 min at 60 °C, in 24 h with 0.1 % formaldehyde or 0.5 % phenol, and in 30 min with diethyl ether or with ultraviolet radiation. It is resistant to low temperature and can remain infectious for several years if it is kept at –70 °C.

H. Mi • H. Li • J. Yu (✉)
Department of Radiology, Beijing You'an Hospital, Capital Medical University, Beijing, China
e-mail: lihongjun00113@126.com

20.2 Epidemiology

20.2.1 Source of Infection

Birds which are infected by psittacosis or serve as the pathogen carriers are considered as the source of infection. Currently, more than 140 types of birds are known to contract or carry the pathogen which is mostly found in secretions and feathers. Infections in birds are unapparent and the signs are characteristic. Although most of the infected birds show no or mild symptoms, the pathogens can be excreted for several months. A patient can also become a minor source of infection if he/she excretes pathogens in sputum.

20.2.2 Route of Transmission

Psittacosis can be transmitted via the respiratory tract. Besides being directly transmitted to humans via droplet, the bacteria can be indirectly transmitted by inhaling an aerosol of infected birds' feces via the respiratory tract. However, according to the reports, few patients experience the onsets without the contact history of birds. Psittacosis is rarely transmitted via direct person-to-person contact.

20.2.3 Susceptible Population

Populations are generally susceptible and the occurrence has no significant gender difference. It is an epidemic disease all year round. The infection rate is closely related to the frequency of bird contact: parrot and poultry raisers easily contract the disease. Although certain immunity can be acquired after the infection is cured, it is not strong enough to prevent the repeated onsets and the following infection.

H. Li (ed.), *Radiology of Infectious Diseases: Volume 2*, DOI 10.1007/978-94-017-9876-1_20

20.2.4 Epidemic Features

Psittacosis affects many areas around the world. Although severe outbreaks have occurred, few cases have been reported in recent years. Ritter reported the case of human psittacosis in Switzerland in 1879. In the early 1960s, psittacosis was proved to exist in China. The disease usually spread sporadically, while outbreaks and epidemics occur on a small scale sometimes. As people who are often exposed to poultry and birds have a higher infection rate, psittacosis is considered as an occupational disease for poultry workers.

20.3 Pathogenesis and Pathological Changes

20.3.1 Pathogenesis

The pathogenesis of psittacosis is still not clear. After being inhaled by humans via the respiratory tract, Cps enters the blood circulation, then attacks the mononuclear macrophage system, and proliferates inside. After the above process, Cps invades the lung and other organs via blood. Thus, human psittacosis may be a respiratory tract infection (RTI) or a general infection mainly with respiratory symptoms. The pulmonary lesions often occur in the hilum of the lung and then spread around, resulting in the lobular pneumonia and interstitial pneumonia. Via microscopic examination, infiltration of the mononuclear lymphocytes can be discovered in the alveolar wall and interstitial tissue; deciduous epithelial cells, fibrous protein, lymphocytes, and few neutrophils can be found in the pulmonary alveoli; the inclusion bodies and pathogens can be seen in the cytoplasm of the macrophage in the exudation of pulmonary alveoli. SARS and lobular pneumonia often occur. In severe cases, necrosis of lung tissue may occur accompanying pleurisy. Beside the lung, relative lesions can be found in other involved organs such as the liver, spleen, kidney, meninges, cardiac muscles, and endocardium.

20.4 Clinical Symptoms and Signs

The incubation period generally lasts for 7–40 days, with symptoms ranging from mild to severe. Documents and reports show that the shorter the incubation period, the more severe the symptoms. Mild cases can lead to flulike illness or even no apparent symptoms, while severe cases can result in death. Although SARS is considered as the major manifestation, there is no specific clinical manifestation of psittacosis. Manifestations can be divided into the following types based on the clinical symptoms.

20.4.1 Pneumonia

20.4.1.1 Fever and Flulike Symptoms

The onset is acute, with body temperature up to 40 °C in 1–2 days, chills, general upset, headache, muscular soreness, and obvious muscle shapes in the neck and back. In some cases, patients may suffer from conjunctivitis, epistaxis, and rash. The high body temperature may gradually decline in 1–2 weeks. The fever course is 3–4 weeks, while it may last for several months in some cases.

20.4.1.2 Pneumonia

Pneumonia often occurs after the 1st week of onset, accompanying worsening coughs, which are mostly dry coughs with a small amount of phlegm or bloody sputum, choking sensation in chest, and chest pain. In severe cases, patients may suffer from dyspnea, cyanosis, tachycardia, delirium, and even coma. The physical signs of the lung are often milder than the symptoms. At the beginning stage of the onset or in mild cases, patients have no apparent physical signs or only suffer from moist rales in the lung and pharyngeal hyperemia. As the disease develops, signs of lung consolidation and moist rales occur, accompanying pleural friction rub and pleural effusion in few cases.

20.4.1.3 Other Symptoms

Digestive symptoms such as anorexia, nausea and vomiting, abdominal pain, and diarrhea may occur. The liver and spleen may be enlarged accompanying the occurrence of jaundice. The onset of myocarditis, endocarditis, and pericarditis may be triggered, with circulatory failure and pulmonary edema in the severe cases. Psychiatric symptoms such as headache, insomnia, slow response, and nervousness may occur, with sleepiness, delirium, mental disorientation, and unconsciousness in severe cases. The disease can result in serious conditions and adverse outcomes.

The above symptoms are lack of the specificity. The manifestations of pneumonia as well as the enlargement of the spleen play the most important role in the diagnosis of psittacosis.

20.4.2 Typhoid Sepsis and Blood Poisoning

The symptoms include high fever and headache, accompanying relative bradycardia and enlargement of the spleen. Complications such as myocarditis, endocarditis, and meningitis easily occur. In severe cases, the coma and renal failure may lead to patients' death.

The illness course is long, with a fever course lasting for 3–4 weeks or even several months. The recurrence rate may reach 20 %.

20.5 Psittacosis Related Complications

The complications of psittacosis seldom occur. In severe cases, the cardiovascular system and nervous system can be negatively affected. Cardiac complications include myocarditis, endocarditis, and pericarditis. Cps may attack the aortic valves and mitral valves as well. The disease may lead to artery embolization and have a negative effect on the liver, kidney, skin, and other organs.

20.6 Diagnostic Examinations

20.6.1 Laboratory Tests

20.6.1.1 Routine Tests

At the acute stage, the WBC count is normal or slightly lower, with a normal or slightly accelerating ESR. Transient proteinuria can be discovered via the uronoscopy.

20.6.1.2 Etiological Tests

Etiological tests serve as the diagnostic basis of psittacosis. In clinical cases, blood, sputum, and throat swab are taken at the acute stage to detect Cps.

20.6.1.3 Serological Tests

Serological tests are often used in the diagnosis of psittacosis.

Microimmunofluorescence Test

The test is applied to detect the IgM-specific and IgG-specific antibodies. The positive result of IgM can be found in the early stage of the diagnosis. The positive rate reaches 80–95 %. It is reported that the microimmunofluorescence test is more sensitive than CFT.

CFT or Hemagglutination Inhibition (HI)

A diagnosis is needed if the paired serum titers increased at a four-time speed during the detection of specific antibodies.

20.6.2 Diagnostic Imaging

20.6.2.1 X-Ray Radiology and CT Scanning

X-ray radiology and CT scanning are commonly applied for the diagnosis as well as the differential diagnosis of the psittacosis pneumonia.

20.6.2.2 CT Scanning and MR Imaging

MR imaging is commonly applied for the diagnosis of the neurological complications caused by psittacosis.

20.7 Imaging Demonstrations

Pneumonia is the major manifestation when psittacosis invades the lung. The imaging demonstrations have certain characteristics and are similar to other types of pneumonia but are lack of specific manifestations.

20.7.1 X-Ray Radiology

The X-ray demonstration is abnormal in 80–95 % of cases. It may demonstrate the patches of infiltration shadows in the pulmonary segment or the lung lobe and the fan-shaped shadows distributed from the pulmonary segment in the radial pattern as well as the wedge-shaped shadows under the pleura. Most shadows are found in the inferior lobe with an inhomogeneous density, accompanying the signs of diffuse panbronchiolitis and interstitial pneumonia. Corn-shaped nodules and obvious consolidation can be found in some cases (Fig. 20.1) and even cover the whole pulmonary lobe of severe patients.

Case Study 1

A male patient, aged 35 years, was admitted to hospital on the sixth day of the continued high fever, with chills, muscular soreness, general upset, and mental confusion. Pleurisy occurred in the left thorax 9 months before being admitted to hospital, accompanying no fever. The X-ray demonstrates the pneumonia in the inferior lobe of the left lung with pleural effusion. Two days after being admitted to hospital, pain occurred under the sternum, accompanying dry coughs. The patient had a contact history of cockatiel and rabbit fur. He was diagnosed as having psittacosis via serological tests, with the *paired serum titers of 1:8–1:32.*

For case detail and figures, please refer to Mcphee SJ, et al. *West J Med*, 1987, 146(1): 91.

Case Study 2

A man aged 12 years, with pain occurring in the left upper quadrant. He once suffered from gastric ulcer. The pain transferred from the left upper quadrant to the axilla, chest, and back, accompanying the respiratory failure, bilateral pneumonia, and pleurisy. In the microimmunofluorescence test, the results of the specific-antibody titers were as follows: IgG 1:16, IgM 1:32. He had no contact history of parrots.

For case detail and figures, please refer to Homma T, et al. *J Med Microbiol*, 2011, 60 (4): 547.

Case Study 3
A female patient, aged 69 years, was admitted to hospital due to dyspnea, accompanying general upset, fever, intense coughs, and diarrhea. The patient once worked in the poultry processing room and had a contact history of infected parrots. The biopsy demonstrated the extensive bronchopneumonia in the left lung and the small lesions of the diffuse pneumonia in the inferior lobe of the right lung. In the microimmunofluorescence test, the results of the serum specimen were as follows: IgM 1:16, IgG 1:512. The clinical diagnosis was psittacosis pneumonia.

For case detail and figures, please refer to Petrovay and Balla *J Med Microbiol*, 2008, 57(10): 1296.

Case Study 4
A female patient aged 69 years, with a high fever for 2 weeks, dry coughs, and dyspnea. The manifestations include respiratory failure, hypoxia and apparent symptoms of poisoning, accompanying the failure of several organs. The oxygen saturation is 26 %. In the microimmunofluorescence test, the results were as follows: IgG 1:256, IgA 1:32. The clinical diagnosis was psittacosis pneumonia.

For case detail and figures, please refer to Petrovay and Balla *J Med Microbiol*, 2008, 57(10): 1296.

Case Study 5
A female patient, aging 35 years, was admitted to hospital due to a high body temperature of 38 °C accompanying general upset, chills, fever, dizziness, anorexia, and nausea. She had the positive results of the infectious mononucleosis, with a slight increase in AST and ALT. She was diagnosed as having the virus hepatitis. After she took the aspirin, the fever was not reduced. Dry coughs and dyspnea as well as moist rales occurred as the disease developed. She had a contact history of parrots. In the microimmunofluorescence test, the results were as follows: IgG 1:128, IgM 1:128. The clinical diagnosis was psittacosis pneumonia.

For case detail and figures, please refer to Mcphee SJ, et al. *West J Med*, 1987, 146(1): 91.

Case Study 6
A female patient, aging 57 years, was admitted to hospital due to a high fever and chills for 5 days. Other symptoms included mild dry coughs, nausea, vomiting, trance, and tachycardia. She had the contact history of two infected parrots, one of which contracted the respiratory system disease. In the microimmunofluorescence test, the antibody titers increased. The clinical diagnosis was psittacosis pneumonia.

For case detail and figures, please refer to Convelli HD, et al. *West J Med*, 1980, 132(3): 245.

20.7.2 CT Scanning

Via the CT scanning, shadows in the shape of ground glass can be found. The CT scanning can also demonstrate the thickened markings and obscurity of the involved bronchus and blood vessels. Small lesions in the lung can be discovered via the CT scanning, which is helpful to the early diagnosis of the disease. Shadows in the shape of ground glass surround the nodule lesions of the consolidation in the lung, with a density lower than that of the consolidation nodules and accompanying halo-shaped signs. The air bronchography can be seen in the lung field outside the areas of lesions and consolidation. A small amount of pleural effusion can be discovered via the CT scanning.

Case Study 7
A male patient aged 30 years, with a high fever for 5 days, accompanying general upset and collapse and diffuse hernia pain in the stomach. He had the contact history of parakeets. In the microimmunofluorescence test, the results of the specific-antibody titers were 1:64. The clinical diagnosis was psittacosis pneumonia.

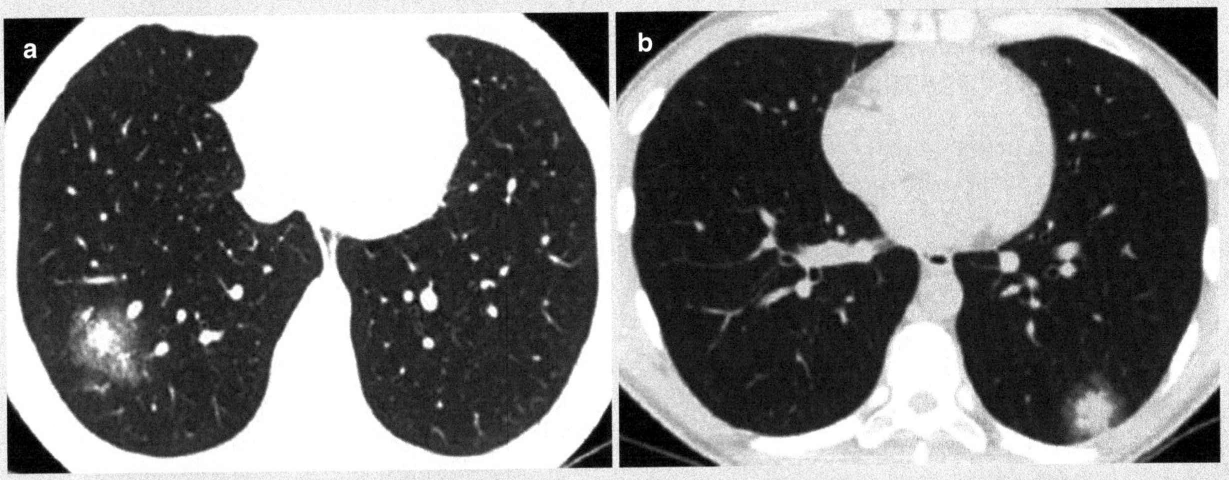

Fig. 20.1 Psittacosis pneumonia. (**a**, **b**) HRCT demonstrates two high-density shadows of nodules in the posterior segment outside the inferior lobe, with the shadows in the shape of ground glass surrounded around the nodule lesions. The signs are halo-shaped, with clearly defined boundaries (Reproduced with permission from Hochhegger B, et al. *J Thrac Imaging*, 2009, 24(2): 136.)

Case Study 8
A male patient, aging 76 years, served as a businessman in the parrots sales. He was admitted to hospital due to general upset and fever, with no cough or sputum. His wife, aging 77 years, was admitted to hospital due to a high fever, with no cough and sputum as well. In the microimmunofluorescence test, their results of the specific-antibody titers increased. The clinical diagnosis was psittacosis pneumonia.

For case detail and figures, please refer to Saito T, et al. *J Chin Microbiol*, 2005, 43(6): 3011.

Case Study 9
A female patient aged 76 years, with a fever for 1 week, anorexia, dry coughs, tachycardia, and dysentery. She had a contact history of parakeet. In the physical examination, moist rales can be heard in the superior lobe of the left lung, the middle field of the right lung, and the posterior lobe of the right lung. CFT showed that the antibody titters increased. The clinical diagnosis was psittacosis pneumonia.

For case detail and figures, please refer to Ito I, et al. *Intern Med*, 2002, 41(7): 580.

20.8 Basis for the Diagnosis

20.8.1 Epidemiological Materials

The contact histories of infected birds serve as the epidemiological data.

20.8.2 Clinical Manifestations

The clinical manifestations include high fever, severe headache, muscular soreness, relative bradycardia, enlargement of the spleen, and symptoms of systemic sera. In addition, patients may suffer from the pneumonia with severe symptoms. Cyanosis, tachycardia, delirium, and coma may occur in the severe cases.

20.8.3 Laboratory Diagnosis

Pathogens can be detected in the etiological examination. The disease can also be diagnosed via the CFT of serum, with the single serum titer exceeding 1:64 and paired serum titers increasing at a four-time speed. Pathogens of birds should be detected in patients' bodies.

20.8.4 Imaging Diagnosis

The X-ray and CT demonstrate the patch-shaped, cloud-shaped, nodule-shaped, and corn-shaped shadows in the lung field, expanding from the hilum of the lung in a fan-shaped or wedge-shaped pattern. The infiltration is commonly found in the inferior lobes of the bilateral lungs. Lesions are often found in the lobule, often accompanying the symptoms of diffuse panbronchiolitis and interstitial pneumonia. The lobar inflammation may occur as well, with an obvious demonstration of the chest X-ray and few pulmonary signs.

20.9 Differential Diagnosis

The clinical manifestation of psittacosis is lack of specificity. Psittacosis should be differentiated from other types of pneumonia caused by other pathogens, such as the *Legionella* pneumonia, *Mycoplasma* pneumonia, and SARS.

20.9.1 *Legionella* Pneumonia

The clinical manifestations include fever, profuse sweating, coughs, white phlegm, dyspnea, and relative bradycardia. The WBC count may increase in the laboratory test. As the WBC count of the psittacosis carriers is usually normal, psittacosis can be easily differentiated from *Legionella* pneumonia and other bacterial pneumonia. The chest X-ray demonstrates the leaf-shaped, cotton-shaped, and cloud-shaped shadows. Lesions can spread either diffusely or focally, accompanying swellings. If the patient tests positive for the *Legionella* via the special stain of the lung tissues in the biopsy, he/she may contract *Legionella* pneumonia.

20.9.2 *Mycoplasma* Pneumonia

Characterized by the intensive coughs, the *Mycoplasma* pneumonia often occurs in autumn and winter. The frequency and severity of coughs may increase in 1–2 days after the onset, accompanying the fever, headache, and general upset. Muscular soreness and gastrointestinal symptoms are seldom seen in the cases of *Mycoplasma* pneumonia. *Mycoplasma* pneumonia is mainly characterized by the apparent imaging manifestations as well as few positive physical signs in the lung. The X-ray demonstration is characterized by the interstitial changes, with the thickened and straight markings expanding from the hilum of the lung in the fan-shaped pattern. The X-ray also demonstrates the cloudy patches of the infiltration shadows with a low density and unclearly defined boundaries. The lesions are usually distributed segmentally on a small scale.

20.9.3 Virus Pneumonia

With the flulike symptoms, the psittacosis may sometimes be misdiagnosed as the virus pneumonia. Virus pneumonia is mostly caused by the influenza virus. With an acute onset, the variable symptoms of the virus pneumonia include fever, asthma, accelerating respiratory rate, and coughs with a small amount of sputum. The physical signs of the lung are inapparent. The X-ray may demonstrate the net-shaped shadows in the lung, accompanying the thickened and obscure markings. In severe cases, the diffuse nodule-shaped shadows with homogeneous density can be found in the middle and inferior field of the lung. The consolidation is seldom seen.

20.9.4 SARS

SARS is a respiratory infection cause by the SARS *Coronavirus*, sharing similar symptoms with psittacosis. The clinical symptoms including the high fever, dry coughs, small amount of sputum, headache, muscular soreness, and anorexia can be found in both diseases. In severe cases, patients may suffer from the respiratory distress. The demonstration of the chest X-ray may be normal at the early stage, while in some cases, the thickened and disorderly markings as well as the patch-shaped and cloud-shaped shadows can be found in the lung. The lesions may be discovered in both the unilateral and bilateral field of the lung. The typical changes are characterized by the shadows in the shape of the ground glass as well as the pulmonary consolidation (the air bronchus sign).

References

Covelli HD, Husky DL, Dolphin RE. Psittacosis: clinical presentation and therapeutic observations. West J Med. 1980;132(3):242–5.

Hochhegger B, Marchiori E, Irion KL, et al. Psittacosis presenting as a halo sign on high-resolution computed tomography. J Thorac Imaging. 2009;24(2):136–7.

Homma T, Yamaguchi T, Komatsu N, et al. A case of acute psittacosis with severe abdominal pain. J Med Microbiol. 2011;60(4):547–9.

Ito I, Ishida T, Mishima M, et al. Familial cases of psittacosis possible person-to-person transmission. Intern Med. 2002;41(7):580–3.

McPhee SJ, Erb B, Harrington W. Psittacosis. West J Med. 1987; 146(1):91–6.

Petrovay F, Balla E. Two fatal cases of psittacosis caused by Chlamydophila psittaci. J Med Microbiol. 2008;57(10):1296–8.

Saito T, Ohnishi J, Mori Y, et al. Infection by chlamydophilia avium in an elderly couple working in a Pet shop. J Clin Microbiol. 2005; 43(6):3011–3.

Suggested Reading

Kay RS. Psittacosis in Egypt: a case study. J Travel Med. 1997;4(1):48–9.

Ma YL. Studies of infectious diseases. Shanghai: Shanghai Science and Technology Press; 2011.

Matsushima H, Takayanagi N, Ubukata M, et al. A case of fulminant psittacosis with rhabdomyolysis. Nihon Kokyuki Gakkai Zasshi. 2002;40(7):612–6.

McGuigan CC, McIntyre PG, Templeton K. Psittacosis outbreak in Tayside, Scotland, December 2011 to February 2012. Euro Surveill. 2012;17(22):1–3.

Suwa T, Ando S, Hashimoto N, et al. Pathology of experimental chlamydiosis in chicks. Nihon Juigaku Zasshi. 1990;52(2):275–83.

Tanaka H, Nakahara K, Mimoto H, et al. A case of fulminant psittacosis showing Chlamydia in TBLB specimens. Nihon Kyobu Shikkan Gakkai Zasshi. 1991;29(1):118–23.

Zhang Q, Tang GJ, Wang SL, et al. Imaging manifestations of psittacosis pneumonia. Chin J Radiol. 2005;39(11):1134–7.

Pulmonary Tuberculosis

21

Yuxin Shi, Weiren Zhang, Min Yuan, and Xinhua Zhou

Pulmonary tuberculosis is a chronic infectious disease caused by invasion of *Mycobacterium tuberculosis hominis* or *Mycobacterium tuberculosis bovis* to the lungs. Accounting for about 90 % of human tuberculosis, pulmonary tuberculosis is the most common type. The *Mycobacterium tuberculosis* (MTB) at the intrapulmonary lesions can spread along bronchi within the lungs and even pass through the pleura to cause tuberculous pleuritis. Otherwise, MTB disseminates along with blood and lymph flows to cause both intrapulmonary and extrapulmonary tuberculosis.

21.1 Etiology

MTB is categorized into the genus of *Mycobacterium*, the family of *Mycobacteriaceae* and the order of *Actinomycetales*. It is an obligate aerobe that grows slowly. On solid medium, its generation time is 18–20 h, requiring 8 days to 8 weeks for culture. On most of the culture medium, the bacterial colony is rough. MTB is also known as acid-fast bacillus characterized by acid-fast and acid-fast alcohol decolorization. It has quite strong resistance to both physical and chemical factors. For instances, MTB in sputum can be killed by boiling for 5 min, and the MTB in dry sputum can survive for several weeks in darkness. However, MTB has quite weak resistance to ultraviolet radiation. It can be killed under sunshine for 2–7 h or in 75 % ethanol for 5 min or at a temperature of 60 °C for 10–30 min or at a temperature of above 80 °C for 5 min. The optimal way for sterilizing is to autoclave (120 °C) for 30 min. The *M. tuberculosis* complex includes various types of *Mycobacterium*, which share common properties and high genome homology. However, the main pathogenic type to humans is *M. tuberculosis*, *M. bovis*, and *M. africanum*.

21.2 Epidemiology

21.2.1 Source of Infection

The main sources of infection are patients with sputum smear positive or sputum culture positive. The patients with sputum smear positive for pulmonary tuberculosis have the strongest infectivity.

21.2.2 Route of Transmission

MTB spreads via the respiratory tract. When the patients with active pulmonary TB cough, sneeze, or speak aloud, droplet with singular MTB as the core suspends in the air to infect other people. In addition, MTB excreted by coughs dries and adheres to dust to form MTB carrying dust, which can also infect individuals. MTB rarely spreads via the gastrointestinal tract, urogenital system, and skin.

21.2.3 Susceptible Population

Populations are generally susceptible to pulmonary TB. Diabetes, HIV/AIDS, silicosis, neoplasm, organ transplantation, and long-term use of immunosuppressant or adrenal cortical hormone can be complicated by tuberculosis. The sociological high-risk factors of tuberculosis include poverty, poor living conditions, and malnutrition.

Y. Shi (✉) • M. Yuan
Department of Radiology, City Public Health & Clinical Center, Fudan University, Shanghai, China
e-mail: Shiyx828288@163.com

W. Zhang
Department of Radiology, Provincial Institution for Infectious Diseases Prevention and Control, Harbin, Heilongjiang, China

X. Zhou
Department of Radiology, Affiliated Luhe Hospital, Capital Medical University, Beijing, China

H. Li (ed.), *Radiology of Infectious Diseases: Volume 2*, DOI 10.1007/978-94-017-9876-1_21

21.2.4 Epidemiological Features

Recently, due to increasing mobility of populations as well as the increasing incidences of drug-resistant tuberculosis and HIV/AIDS complicated by tuberculosis, the occurrence of tuberculosis has been increasing worldwide. Based on data released by WHO in 2000, 2 billion people have a history of MTB infection, with 8 million new cases of tuberculosis each year and 3 million cases of death. China is one of the 22 countries with serious prevalence of tuberculosis and meanwhile is one of the 27 countries with serious prevalence of multidrug-resistant tuberculosis. Currently, about 1.3 million new cases of tuberculosis are reported each year in China, accounting for 14.3 % of the total new cases in the world and ranking the second worldwide.

21.3 Pathogenesis and Pathological Changes

21.3.1 Pathogenesis

21.3.1.1 Pathogenicity and Virulence of MTB

The virulence of MTB is possibly related to its components. For instances, repeated injection of small doses of lipoid cord factors (6,6 double mycolic acidic trehalose) into the abdominal cavity of mice can cause obvious toxic effects. Other lipoids, like sulfolipid, can strengthen the toxicity of cord factors and suppress the fusion of lysosome with phagosome to promote the growth and proliferation of MTB in macrophages. Phospholipid can stimulate the multiplication of monocytes, epithelioid cellularization, and formation of the Langerhans cells. Waxiness D is the complex of mycolic acid arabinose Yutian galactan and mucopeptide, which contributes to the formation of liquefaction, necrosis, dissolution, and cavities of tubercular caseous lesions. In addition to the above lipid components, coexistence of polysaccharide with other substances shows bioactivities, which is an important component of complete antigen and plays an adjuvant role in inducing chemical taxis response of neutrophils. The bacterial protein of MTB is a complete antigen, stimulating responses to tuberculin.

21.3.1.2 Biological Process of MTB Infection and Its Onset

Dannenberg et al. divided the process of MTB infection and its onset into initial stage, T-cell response stage, symbiotic stage, and extracellular multiplication and dissemination stage. The MTB invading the respiratory tract is engulfed by alveolar macrophage, where they survive and replicate themselves with the following spread to adjacent nonactivated alveolar macrophage to cause initial lesions of infection. The initial growth of MTB in alveolar macrophage causes tubercular lesions with central solid caseous necrosis to restrict its further multiplication. During the T-cell response stage, The T-cell-mediated immunity (CMI) and delay type hypersensitivity (DTH) are induced, which play a crucial role in the occurrence, development, and prognosis of TB. In only rare cases, primary tuberculosis occurs during the T-cell response stage. In most cases, MTB is symbiotic with its host. Enwrapped by fibers, the core of caseous necrosis is the place where MTB persistently survives, and an environment with low oxygen, low pH value, and inhibitory fatty acid is unfavorable for its multiplication. However, the immunosuppression of the host is favorable for its multiplication, with reactivated MTB to multiply themselves. Finally, a large quantity of MTB is released from the liquefied caseous lesions to disseminate.

21.3.1.3 Immune Responses of the Human Body to MTB Infection

The immune responses of the human body to MTB infection include two types: CMI and DTH, both of which are mediated by T cells.

21.3.2 Pathological Changes

21.3.2.1 Basic Pathological Changes of Tuberculosis

Human immunity and hypersensitivity as well as the quantity and virulence of the invading MTB are closely related to the quality, range, pathological basis, and developing speed of the lesions.

Exudative Lesion

The exudative lesions are demonstrated with congestion, edema, and infiltration of leukocytes. In the early exudative lesions, there are neutrophils, which are gradually replaced by macrophages and lymphocytes. The engulfed MTB can be detected inside the macrophages. The exudative lesions are usually observed at the early stage of the inflammation or during deterioration of the lesions. In addition, it can be detected in patients with serous tuberculosis. When the conditions improve, the exudative lesions can be completely absorbed.

Proliferative Lesion

After macrophage engulfs and digests the invading MTB, the phospholipid of MTB enlarges the macrophage to a flat shape resembling to epithelial cell, which is known as epithelioid cell. The epithelioid cell is the major component of proliferative lesions, showing certain specificity for the diagnosis of tuberculosis. Infiltration of the epithelioid cells, Langerhans cells, and lymphocytes forms the typical epithelioid granuloma node, which is the characteristic lesion of tuberculosis. The formation of such node is a development process of phagocytosis by macrophages to kill MTB, confine the lesion, and prevent its dissemination. Most invading MTBs are killed during the formation of phagocytosing and killing the *M. tuberculosis*, which localizes the lesion and prevents the *M.*

tuberculosis from spreading. Most *M. tuberculosis* is killed in during the formation of the epithelioid granuloma node. Therefore, by acid-fast staining, MTB is commonly not detectable in the node. The pathological changes with predominant proliferative lesions occur mostly in patients with infection of MTB of a small quantity or in patients with strong CMI.

Degenerative Lesion (Caseous Necrosis)

Degenerative lesions occur commonly based on exudative or proliferative lesions. In the patients with compromised immunity or strong allergic responses, or in the patients infected by a large quantity of MTB, the MTBs in exudative lesions successfully fight against the macrophages for multiplication in a large quantity. Consequently, the cells are turbid and swollen to show fatty degeneration, with dissolution, fragmentation, and finally necrosis. The apoptotic inflammatory cells release a proteolytic enzyme to dissolve the tissue, inducing coagulative necrosis. Due to a large quantity of adipose, the degenerative lesion is grayish yellow by naked eye observation, with loose and crisp texture resembling to dry cheese, which is therefore known as caseous necrosis. Under a microscope, an area of coagulated red-stained unstructured necrotic tissue can be observed. The caseous necrosis is subject to liquefaction and cavities, which can be disseminated along the bronchus. Most caseous lesions can be cured after calcification.

The above three types of lesions can concurrently exist in the same one pulmonary lesion, with one predominating. For instances, at the center of exudative lesion and multiplicative lesion, a small quantity of caseous necrosis can be found; in the pulmonary lesion with caseous necrosis predominating, different degrees of exudation and epithelioid granuloma node can be observed.

21.3.2.2 The Prognosis of the Lesions

The prognosis of the lesions of tuberculosis mainly includes absorption, fibrosis, calcification, dissemination, and deterioration. When the immunity is strong and (or) antituberculosis therapy is used, the lesions can be gradually cured. Exudative lesion can be absorbed via phagocytosis of mononuclear phagocytic system, even leaving no scar. The healing of lesions is commonly accompanied by proliferation of fibrous tissue to form stripe- or cord-like scar. Caseous lesion can also be healed after dehydration, contraction, calcium salt deposition, and calcification of the lesions. The deterioration of tuberculosis is manifested as expansion and dissemination of the lesions. After the initial infection of MTB, the bacteria can be engulfed by macrophages, which reach the hilar lymph nodes along with lymph flow. A small quantity of MTB can gain their access into the blood flow to disseminate all over the body, but with no obvious clinical symptoms (asymptomatic septicemia). In the cases with invasion of vascular vessel by necrotic lesion, the MTB can induce systemic miliary tuberculosis along with blood flow, with the lungs, meninges, bone, kidney, and other organs involved. And the bacteria can also spread to other organs along with lymph flow. After pulmonary tubercular caseous necrosis is liquefied, the bacteria can spread along the bronchus to form new lesions in other parts of the lung. After sputum containing a large quantity of MTB is swollen into the gastrointestinal tract, intestinal tuberculosis and peritoneal tuberculosis may occur. In addition, direct dissemination of pulmonary TB into the pleura is possible, with consequent occurrence of tubercular pleuritis.

21.4 Clinical Symptoms and Signs

According to the Health Industry Standards of P.R. China issued in 2001, tuberculosis is categorized into five types: primary tuberculosis, hematogenous disseminated pulmonary tuberculosis, secondary pulmonary tuberculosis, tubercular pleuritis, and other extrapulmonary tuberculosis.

21.4.1 Clinical Symptom

21.4.1.1 Systemic Symptom

The patients with pulmonary tuberculosis often experience some symptoms of tubercular toxic symptom, which is commonly irregular low-grade fever after noons with a body temperature of 37.4–38 °C that persists for several weeks. In the cases of acute hematogenous disseminated pulmonary tuberculosis, caseous pneumonia with cavitation or complicated by pulmonary infection, the patients may experience high fever and night sweats. Other systemic symptoms include fatigue, poor appetite, emaciation, insomnia, menstrual disorder, and even amenorrhea.

21.4.1.2 Cough

Cough is always the chief complaint by the patients in their first clinic visit. The cases with cough for at least 3 weeks with bloody sputum should be highly suspected as pulmonary tuberculosis. The patients with pulmonary tuberculosis mainly complain of dry cough. In the cases complicated by bronchial tuberculosis, the patients often experience severe irritated cough. In the cases complicated by compressed trachea and bronchus by mediastinal or hilar lymphatic tuberculosis, the patients may experience spasmodic cough.

21.4.1.3 Expectoration

Expectoration is rare in patients with pulmonary tuberculosis. The sputum is usually white thick. The patients with pulmonary TB complicated by infection or bronchiectasis often expectorate yellowish thick phlegm. In the cases with caseous liquefaction and necrosis, the patients may also expectorate yellowish thick sputum and even expel necrotic tissue.

21.4.1.4 Chest Pain

Chest pain is not a specific manifestation of pulmonary tuberculosis. The lesion close to the pleura may adhere to the pleura to cause dull pain or stabbing pain, which has insignificant relationship with respiration. Pulmonary tuberculosis complicated by tubercular pleuritis can cause severe chest pain, which is related to respiration.

21.4.1.5 Dyspnea

Generally, the patients in the early stage of pulmonary TB rarely experience dyspnea. Only in the cases of pulmonary tuberculosis complicated by a large quantity of pleural effusion or pneumothorax, the patients may experience dyspnea. Bronchial tuberculosis causes narrowing of the trachea or large bronchus, with consequent manifestation of dyspnea. Otherwise, mediastinal, hilar, and paratracheal lymphatic tuberculosis may compress the trachea or bronchus to cause dyspnea. In the cases of advanced pulmonary TB, extensive lesions at both lungs can cause respiratory failure or right cardiac insufficiency, which may also induce dyspnea.

21.4.1.6 Tubercular Allergy

Pulmonary tuberculosis can cause systemic allergy. Its clinical manifestations resemble to rheumatic fever, mainly including erythema nodosum, multiple arthralgia, behcet disease, and follicular keratoconjunctivitis. The allergy is more common in young female patients, which is nonresponsive to nonsteroidal anti-infective drugs but can be effectively treated by antituberculosis therapy.

In general, pulmonary tuberculosis commonly has no specific clinical manifestations. Some patients are even asymptomatic, with the diagnosis defined by routine physical examinations. In the cases with accompanying immunosuppression, the clinical manifestations are atypical, with implicit onset and clinical course. Otherwise, the patients experience acute onset with severe clinical symptoms which are unveiled by primary disease and are subject to misdiagnosis.

21.4.2 Signs

The pulmonary signs are related to the location, quality, range, and severity of the lesions. In the cases with mild conditions, the pulmonary signs are not obvious, with no specificity. In the cases with extensive pulmonary lesions, corresponding physical signs can be detected. In the cases with obvious cavities or complicated by bronchiectasis, fine moist rales can be heard by auscultation. In the cases with large areas of caseous pneumonia, signs of pulmonary consolidation are detectable, such as strengthened vocal fremitus, flatness or dullness by percussion, and bronchial breathing sound by auscultation. In the cases with huge cavity, hyperresonance or tympany can be heard by percussion and amphoric breathing sound by auscultation. In the cases of bronchial tuberculosis, localized wheezing can be heard. In the cases with extensive fibrosis at both lungs, the affected side of the thorax is subject to collapse, with narrowed intercostal space and shift of bronchus. The other parts may be subject to corresponding signs due to compensatory emphysema, such as hyperresonance by percussion or decreased breathing sound by auscultation.

21.5 Pulmonary Tuberculosis-Related Complications

21.5.1 Hemoptysis

When necrotic lesion of tuberculosis involves the pulmonary capillary wall, the patients expectorate bloody phlegm. In the cases with the major vessel involved, hemoptysis in different quantities occurs. In the cases with ruptured aneurysm in the cavity or ruptured bronchial artery, massive hemoptysis occurs possibly to cause death. Tubercular bronchiectasis induced by healing and fibrosis of lung tissue can cause repeated and long-term hemoptysis or bloody sputum after pulmonary TB is cured.

21.5.2 Spontaneous Pneumothorax

Pulmonary TB is a common cause of pneumothorax. A variety of lesions in the cases of pulmonary TB can cause pneumothorax, such as penetration of subpleural lesion or cavity into the thoracic cavity, emphysema, or ruptured lung bullae induced by fibrosis or scarring of tubercular lesions. The lesions of miliary tuberculosis may affect the pulmonary interstitium to cause interstitial emphysemic lung bullae rupture. The penetration of the lesion or cavity into the thoracic cavity often causes increased exudative fluid in the thoracic cavity, inducing pneumoserothorax or pyopneumothorax.

21.5.3 Bronchiectasis

The lesions of pulmonary TB damage the bronchial wall and tissue surrounding the bronchus to cause bronchiectasis. Otherwise, bronchial tuberculosis itself causes bronchial deformation and dilation, which is known as tubercular bronchiectasis, which may be accompanied by hemoptysis.

21.5.4 Secondary Lung Infection

Cavities (especially fibrous cavities), pleural thickening, airway obstruction caused by bronchiectasis, atelectasis, and bronchial tuberculosis are the pathological basis for secondary lung infection or other secondary bacterial infections to bronchial tuberculosis. The pathogenic bacteria are mostly Gram-negative bacilli, with infection of mixed pathogenic bacteria being more commonly found.

21.5.5 Cardiac and Pulmonary Failures

Cardiac and pulmonary failures are serious complications of pulmonary TB. When pulmonary TB is ineffectively treated, the conditions develop into chronic to destroy lung tissue, resulting in emphysema and pulmonary bulla. These conditions further affect the pulmonary functions and lead to chronic respiratory failure. Pneumothorax and complicating infections can cause acute respiratory failure. Long-term hypoxia and traction of the vascular wall by intrapulmonary fibrous tissue induce pulmonary arterial hypertension, which may further develop into cardiopulmonary disease and right heart failure.

21.6 Diagnostic Examinations

21.6.1 Laboratory Test

21.6.1.1 Common Test

The common tests are nonspecific. The peripheral blood WBC count is commonly within normal range, possibly with decreased hemoglobin (HGB). At the acute progressive stage, the WBC count can be detected with an increase. In the cases of severe infection, hemogram resembling to leukemia can be detected, with rapid blood sedimentation rate and elevated CRP.

21.6.1.2 Etiological Test

Smear Test

Various excretions and secretions such as sputum, urine, pleural effusion, and feces as well as suctions of lymph node puncture can be prepared into smear for examination. The finding of acid-fast bacilli facilitates the diagnosis, but with a low positive rate.

Isolation of Pathogenic Bacteria

The separation of pathogenic bacteria for culture has a higher detection rate than the smear test. Meanwhile, it can be applied to exclude the possibility of non-tuberculosis mycobacteria infection, which is a standard test for diagnosis. By using rapid radioactive culture, the drug sensitivity and the bacterial serotype identification can be tested, which increases the primary separation rate by 10 % compared to the modified routine Lowenstein-Jensen culture. The time needed for the detection is also shortened. In addition, the BacT/Alert 3D system can be used to detect tuberculosis mycobacteria and drug sensitivity, with even shorter time required. Direct microscopy requires no costly equipment but is simple and rapid with high sensitivity and specificity, which are, respectively, 97.5 % and 94.4 %.

Detection of Specific Nucleic Acid

Nucleic acid probe, PCP, and DRA blotting hybridization can be applied to detect DNA of MTB. The gene chip technology is also applied in identifying MTB, testing drug resistance, and analyzing genes of MTB.

21.6.1.3 Serological Test

Along with the further studies into molecular biology and immunology of *Mycobacterium*, ELISA, ELI-SPOT stratification assay, indirect immunofluorescence (IIF), and Western blotting have been applied in clinical practice to detect the relevant antibody in serum, sputum, and pleural effusion. Serological test is an auxiliary test for the rapid diagnosis of pulmonary TB but still with poor specificity.

21.6.1.4 Tuberculin Skin Test

Currently the commonly applied tuberculin skin test in clinical practice is the purified protein derivative (PPD) of BCG. PPD 5 IU is percutaneously injected at the forearm, with the following observation of the callosity after 72 h at the injection site. A callosity with a diameter being 5–9 mm is defined as weak positive, while 10–19 mm is defined as positive, both of which indicate MTB infection. Strong positive finding in adults, namely, callosity with a diameter no less than 20 mm or smaller than 20 mm but with blisters or necrosis, indicates active tuberculosis.

21.6.1.5 Endoscopic Examination

Endoscopic examinations include fiber bronchoscope and thoracoscopy, and fibro-colonoscopy provide etiological and pathological diagnoses for certain types of tuberculosis.

21.6.1.6 Biopsy

As for patients with tuberculosis but no bacterial excretion or tuberculosis with no communication with external environment, such as tuberculosis of the lymph node, bone, joint, liver, and spleen, biopsy can be applied for etiological and pathological diagnosis.

21.6.2 Diagnostic Imaging

Routine chest X-ray is a radiological examination of choice for suspected cases of pulmonary TB. In most cases, in combination to clinical case history and sputum examination, the diagnosis can be defined. CT scanning can be ordered as a supplementary examination. It can demonstrate acute miliary tuberculosis earlier, tuberculosis lesions at hidden positions, mediastinal and hilar lymphadenectasis, and density changes within lesions. Therefore, CT scanning has an important value for differential diagnosis of some types of tuberculosis, such as tuberculoma.

21.7 Imaging Demonstrations

21.7.1 Imaging Demonstrations of Pulmonary Tuberculosis

21.7.1.1 Primary Pulmonary TB

Primary Syndrome

Typical primary syndrome is characterized by primary lesions and interconnecting lesions of lymphangitis and enlarged hilar lymphadenitis to form a dumbbell-like appearance. However, such a radiological sign is rarely found. In some patients, the primary lesion is large to cover the lesions of lymphangitis and lymphadenitis. Local pleural thickening has a corresponding radiological sign.

X-Ray

The primary lesion is mostly singular, with cloudy or round-like shadow with increased density. Otherwise, the primary lesion is demonstrated as flakes or large flakes of shadows with increased density at the pulmonary segment or lobe, with a size of 0.5–2 cm and poorly defined boundary. The lesions are often located at the posterior segment of the upper lung lobe or the dorsal segment of the lower lung lobe near the pleura.

The lesion of lymphangitis can be found from the primary lesion to the enlarged lymph node, characterized by one or several blurry cord-like shadows with increased density.

Hilar and/or mediastinal lymphadenectasis is radiologically demonstrated as mass-like shadow that protrudes out of the normal tissue contour.

CT Scanning

The primary lesion is demonstrated as lobular shadow and acinar nodular shadow with poorly defined boundary by CT scanning. CT scanning can well define the primary lesion, draining lymphangitis, and swollen hilar lymph node (Figs. 21.1 and 21.2). CT scanning can also well define lobar or segmental atelectasis caused by compression of the bronchus by swollen lymph nodes and the pleural changes in the vicinity of the primary lesion.

Case Study 1

A male patient aged 16 years was diagnosed with primary pulmonary tuberculosis (primary syndrome).

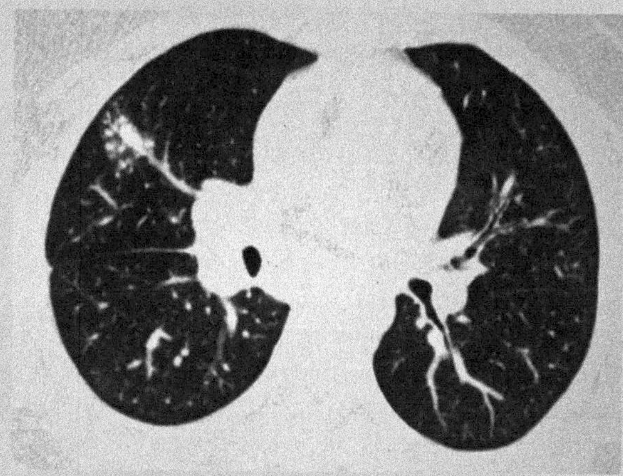

Fig. 21.1 Primary syndrome. CT scanning demonstrates a small quantity of spot-like shadows at the lateral segment of the right middle lobe with fusion of some spot-like shadows, enlarged right hilum that is caused by right hilar lymphadenectasis, and unobstructed adjacent bronchus

Cast Study 2

A female patient aged 20 years was diagnosed with primary pulmonary tuberculosis (primary syndrome).

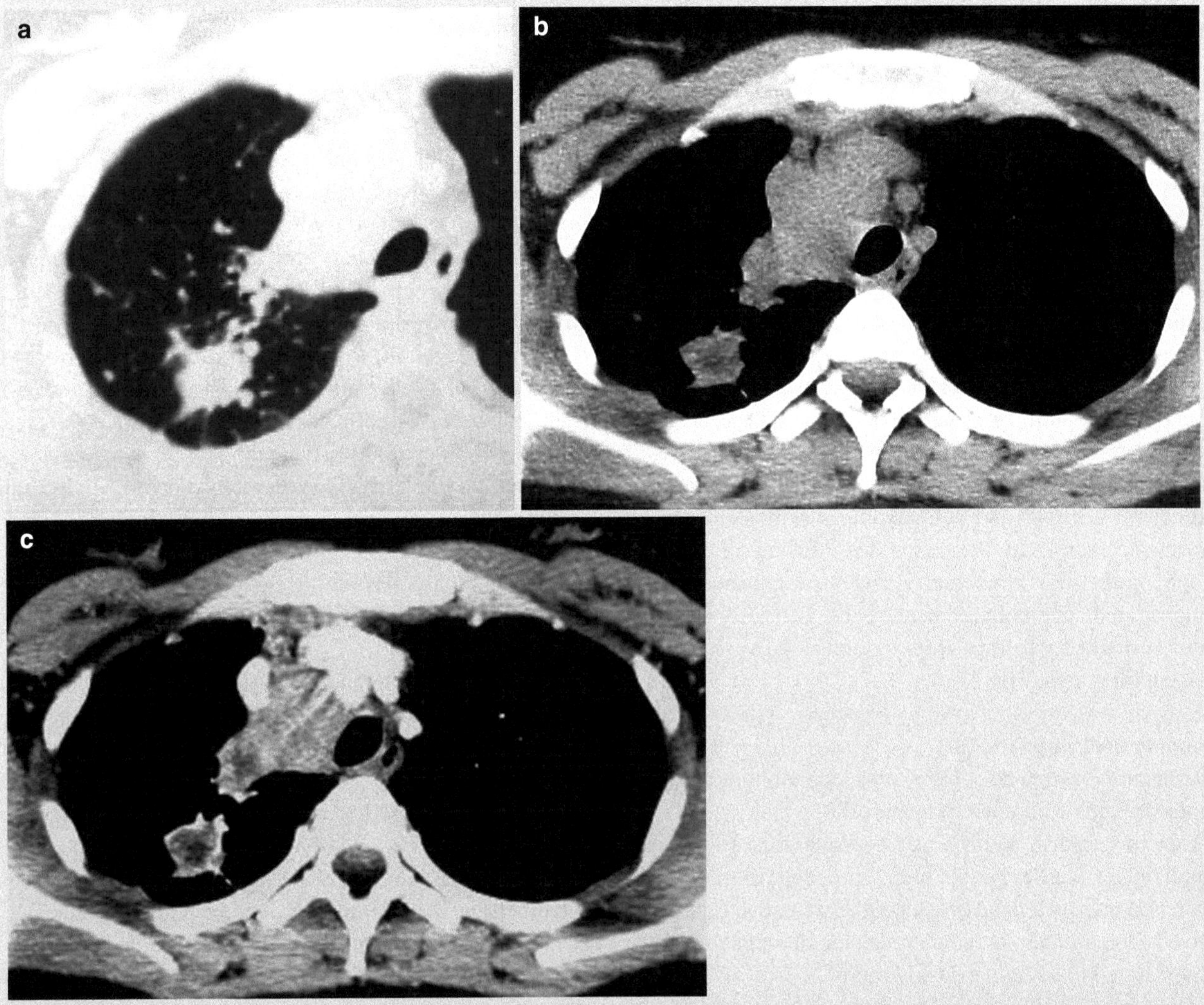

Fig. 21.2 Primary syndrome. (**a**) CT scanning demonstrates irregular nodular shadows at the apical segment of the right upper lobe, surrounding spot- and cord-like shadows, and flakes of shadows near mediastinum that connect to the mediastinum. (**b**) CT scanning demonstrates uneven density of the nodules at the right upper lobe, low-density area in the parenchyma, lymphadenectasis at the 2R area of the mediastinum, poorly defined surrounding adipose space, and connection of some adipose spaces with intrapulmonary lesions. (**c**) Contrast scanning demonstrates marginal enhancement of the nodules at the right upper lung, central low-density area with no enhancement, and uneven enhancement of mediastinal lymph nodes

Intrathoracic Lymphatic TB

Due to rapid absorption of primary lesion in the lung but relatively slow absorption of hilar and mediastinal lymphatic lesion, primary tuberculosis is only demonstrated as enlarged hilar and/or mediastinal lymph nodes, which is known as intrathoracic lymphatic tuberculosis. Hilar lymphatic tuberculosis can be further divided into the following two types: inflammatory lymphatic tuberculosis, with enlarged lymph node and surrounding inflammatory infiltration, and mass lymphatic tuberculosis, with absorption of inflammatory lesion surrounding the lymph node and well-defined boundary of the lymph node.

Hilar Lymphatic TB

Mass Lymphatic Tuberculosis

The lesion of mass type is commonly located at the right hilum, specifically superior margin of the right hilum and the angular area of the right hilum around the right inferior pulmonary artery. The lesion at the left hilar area is commonly located at the superior and exterior margin of the left pulmonary arterial arch and around the left inferior pulmonary artery.

The fully exposed lymph node is nodular, round, or oval in shape with well-defined intact boundary. The partially exposed lymph node is half arch in shape protruding towards the lung field due to its partial overlapping with the hilar vascular vessels. The fusion of large lymph nodes is demonstrated like a mass, with its exterior margin lobulated like plum petals. Plain CT scanning demonstrates some adipose spaces between the lymph nodes, based on which the mass can be distinguished to be formed by fused nodules.

The density of the lesion is homogeneous or heterogeneous (caseous necrosis and liquefaction within lymph lodes). Even calcification can be found.

Contrast CT scanning demonstrates less enlarged lymph nodes with slightly even enhancement and most enlarged lymph nodes with ring-shaped enhancement (peripheral granulation of the lymph node is demonstrated as a ring-shaped or marginal enhancement by contrast scanning, and central necrosis and liquefaction is demonstrated with no enhancement). In the cases with fusion of multiple lymph nodes into large mass, separated enhancement is demonstrated. The enhancement degree of enlarged lymph nodes is markedly distinct from that of blood vessels in the adjacent hilar area (Fig. 21.3).

Inflammatory Lymphatic TB

Inflammatory lymphatic TB shares common radiological demonstrations with mass lymphatic TB.

Due to caseous necrosis and capsular rupture of some lymph nodes, these lymph nodes are demonstrated with rough and poorly defined margin. Otherwise, due to the exudative lesion around the lymph node, the marginal density is demonstrated to be lightened and blurry.

The major vascular branches at the hilar area are mostly demonstrated with smooth blood flow, well-defined and smooth vascular lining, and occasional enlarged lymph nodes. In the cases with the adjacent bronchus involved or with concurrent adjacent bronchial TB, the involved bronchial segment is subject to thickened bronchial wall and narrowed bronchial lumen.

Mediastinal Lymphadenectasis

The lesion is commonly located at the paratracheal area and tracheobronchial region, especially the right lung.

For the cases with well-defined lymph node, pathological examination indicates intact capsule encapsulating the swollen lymph node. X-ray demonstrates the swollen lymph node in a half arch shape protruding towards the lung field, with wavelike mediastinum. Plain CT scanning demonstrates round- or oval-shaped lymph node with surrounding adipose space, especially prevascular space. There are also swollen lymph nodes anterior to the right trachea and posterior to the vena cava, at the left aortic-pulmonary window and in the right azygoesophageal recess. For the cases with unclearly defined lymph node, its surrounding adipose spaces are partially absent and partially present. The pathological examination indicates caseous necrosis of the lymph node and its penetration out of its capsule. For the cases with fusion of multiple lymph nodes into irregular mass, the mass is commonly located between the major vascular vessels in the mediastinum.

By plain CT scanning, the density of most lymph nodes is homogeneous, and the density of rare lymph nodes is uneven due to caseous necrosis and liquefaction. In some cases, the lymph nodes are demonstrated with internal or marginal calcification. Contrast CT scanning demonstrates homogeneous enhancement of the small lymph nodes, peripheral irregular wall enhancement of large lymph nodes, ring-shaped enhancement of the thin wall, and separated enhancement. By pathology, the enhanced area is indicated to be tubercular granulation tissue with abundant blood flow, and the area with no enhancement is indicated to be mostly caseous necrosis. The separated enhancement is pathologically indicated to be the fusion of multiple lymph nodes containing lesions of caseous necrosis (Figs. 21.4 and 21.5).

Case Study 3

A male patient aged 16 years was diagnosed with intrathoracic lymphatic TB.

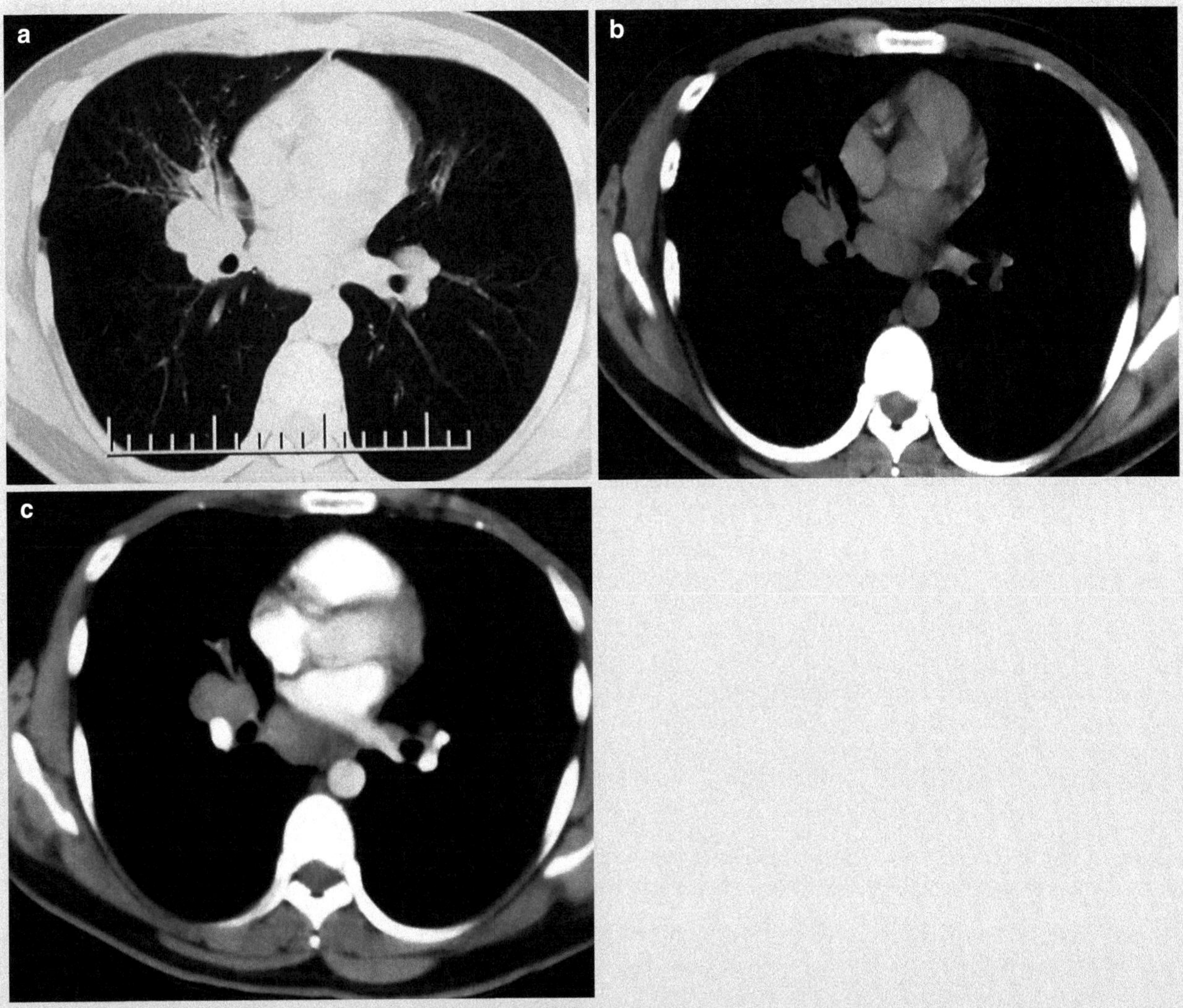

Fig. 21.3 (**a**, **b**) Plain CT scanning demonstrates swollen lymph nodes at the right lower lung hilum with nodular shadows and unobstructed right middle bronchus. (**c**) Contrast CT scanning demonstrates homogeneous enhancement of the hilar major vascular vessels that obviously distinct from its adjacent nodular shadows of lymph nodes. Obstructive pneumonia is demonstrated at the right middle lung lobe

Case Study 4

A male patient aged 21 years was diagnosed with intrathoracic lymphatic TB.

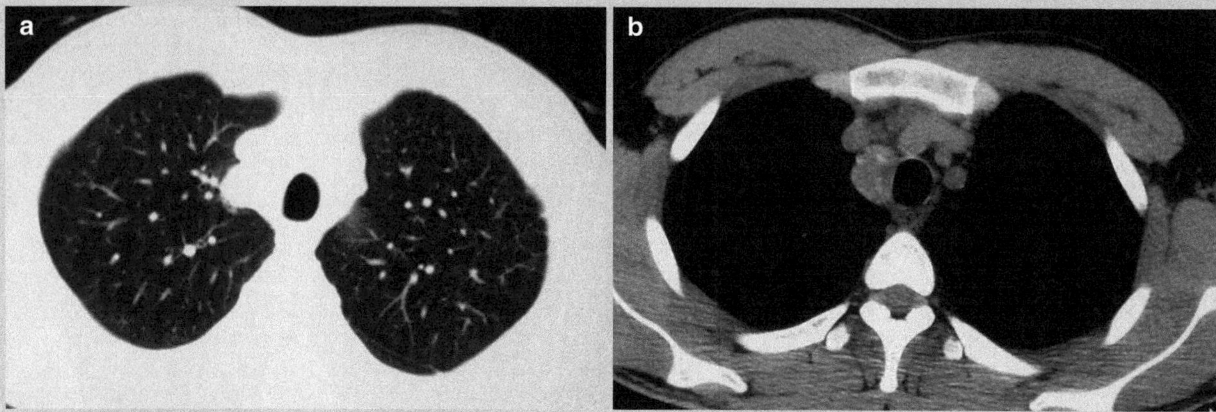

Fig. 21.4 Mediastinal lymphatic TB. (**a**) CT scanning demonstrates paratracheal nodular shadow at the right upper mediastinum, which is in arch shape protruding towards the lung field. (**b**) The nodules are in bean shape, with marginal or internal spots of calcification

Case Study 5

A female patient aged 23 years was diagnosed with mediastinal lymphatic TB.

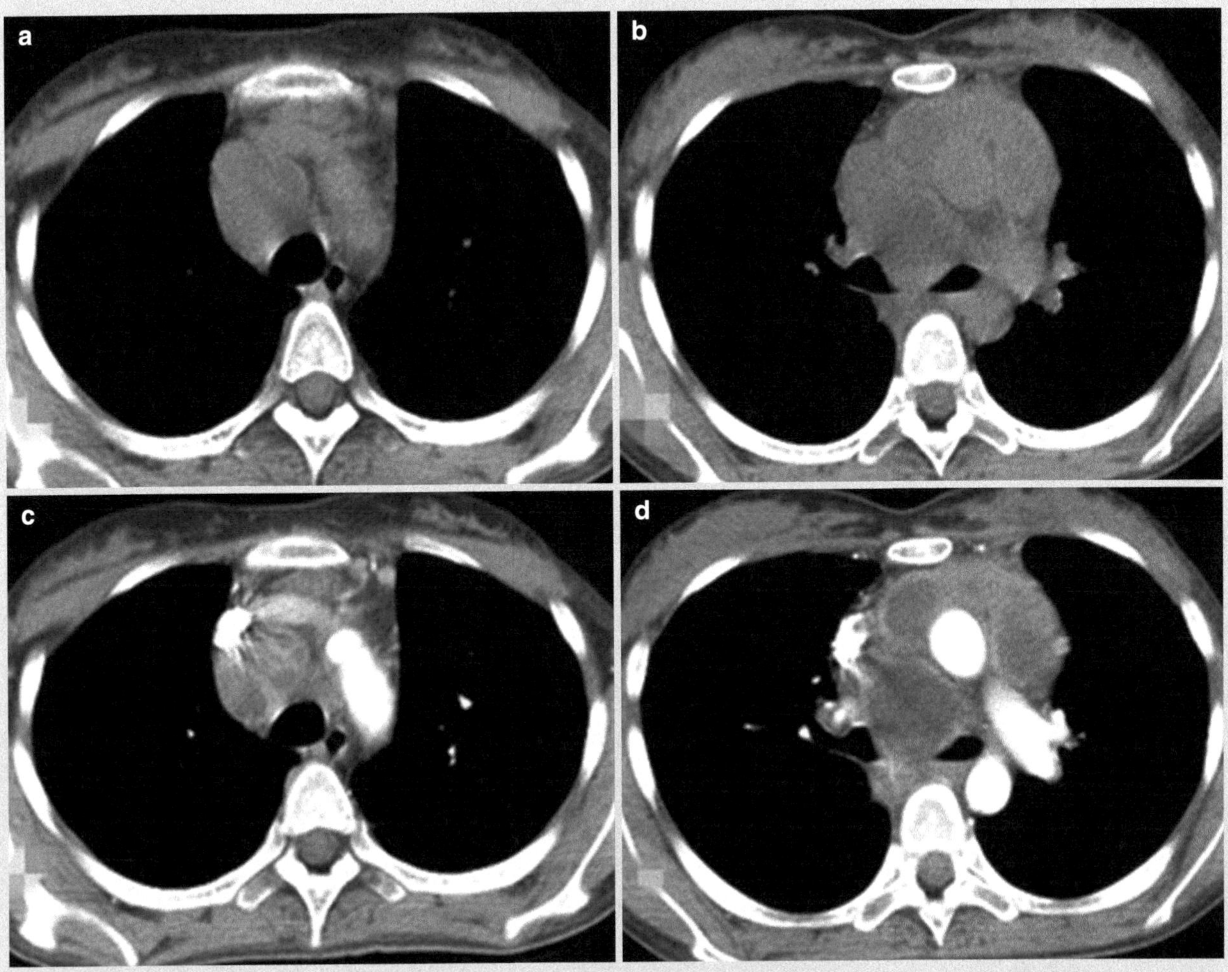

Fig. 21.5 Mediastinal lymphatic TB. (**a**, **b**) Plain CT scanning demonstrates swollen lymph nodes at the 3R and 4R areas of the mediastinum, absent adipose space between some of the lymph nodes and vascular vessels, and uneven density. (**c**, **d**) Contrast scanning demonstrates heterogeneous enhancement of the lymph nodes, with ring-shaped or separated enhancement

By plain MR imaging, the mediastinal lymph nodes are demonstrated as equal T1 and equal T2 signals, with internal patches of slightly long T1 slightly and long T2 signals. By contrast MR imaging, the mediastinal lymph nodes are demonstrated as nodular, ring-shaped, separated, or uneven enhancement. The demonstrations of no central enhancement, peripheral enhancement, and ring-shaped enhancement are characteristic, with high diagnostic value.

21.7.1.2 Hematogenous Pulmonary TB

Acute Hematogenous Pulmonary TB

It is caused by invasion of a large quantity of MTB into the blood flow for once or several times within a short period of time. It is more common in children and during the stage of primary pulmonary TB.

X-Ray

X-ray demonstrates extensively and evenly distributed miliary sized nodular shadows with increased density. It is characterized by even distribution, even size, and even density, which is known as the three-evens sign. Due to a large quantity of lesions with dense distribution, both lungs are demonstrated with ground-glass opacity. The miliary shadows have a diameter of 1–2 mm and a round or oval shape, with well-defined boundary. In the cases with exudative lesions, the miliary shadows are demonstrated with poorly defined boundary. At the early stage, X-ray only demonstrates enhanced lung markings. After about 2 weeks, typical miliary nodules can be demonstrated. In the advanced stage, the miliary increased density shadows tend to fuse together.

CT Scanning

Pulmonary interstitial miliary nodules are demonstrated with diffusely distributed military shadows at the interstitium of both lungs. The nodules have a diameter of 1–3 mm with even distribution and even density. Most nodules are well defined and rarely with poorly defined boundary. In the cases with no immediate treatment, the nodules may enlarge to a diameter of about 5 mm. The nodules are morphologically irregular and may fuse into focalized consolidation lesion.

Miliary nodules may be complicated by confined ground-glass opacity, with light density and blurry boundary.

Interlobular septal thickening and intralobular reticular shadows are caused by congestion and edema of alveolar septa during the acute stage, which often coexists with ground-glass opacity. Most patients experience their absence after treatment. In some rare patients, they develop into irreversible reticular fibrosis.

Clustering thin wall cyst shadows can be demonstrated at the progressive stage of the conditions in rare patients, which are reversible.

In the patients with acute hematogenous pulmonary TB but receiving delayed or inappropriate therapy, the conditions progress. The caseous substances formed by TB lesions may involve the alveolar cavity and disseminate along the bronchus. The nodular shadows in both lungs can be demonstrated with random and confined distribution of centrilobular branch shadow and the tree bud sign that may be well defined or poorly defined (Figs. 21.6 and 21.7).

Case Study 6

A female patient aged 14 years was diagnosed with acute hematogenous pulmonary TB.

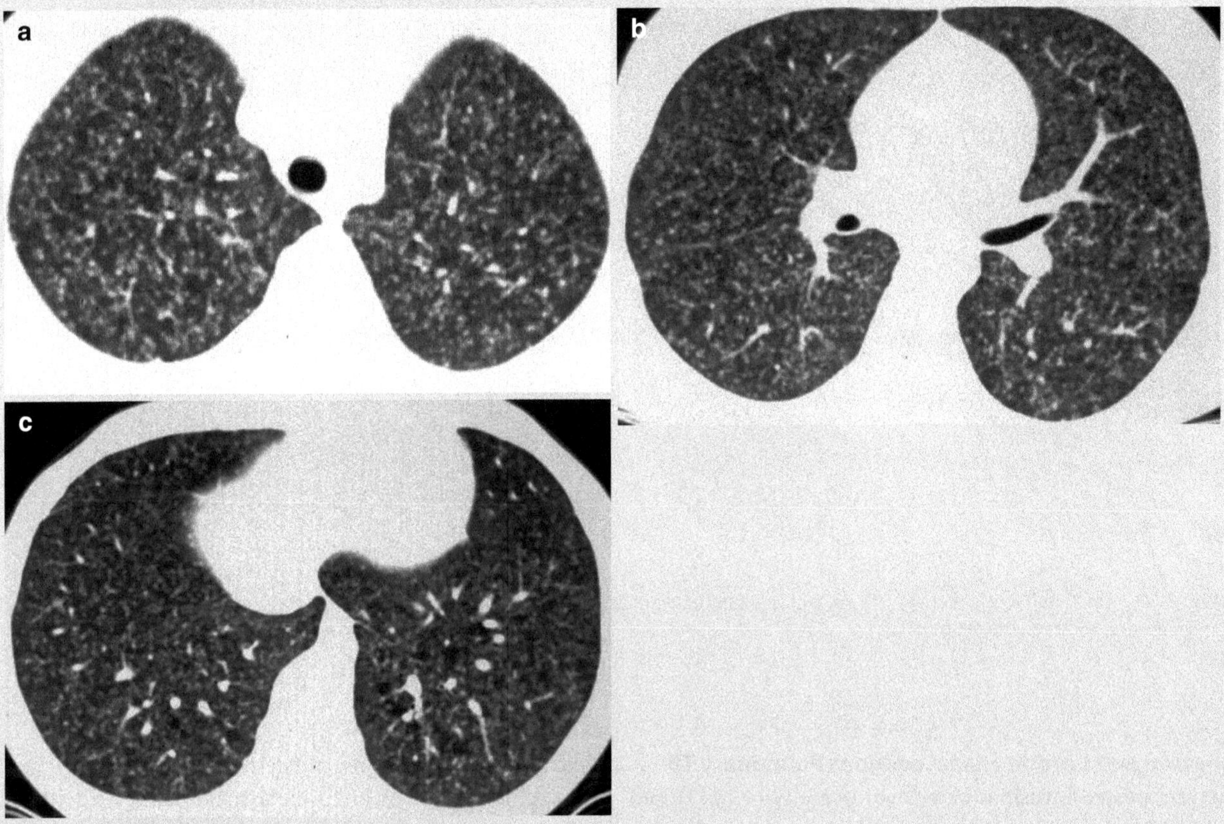

Fig. 21.6 Acute hematogenous pulmonary TB. (**a–c**) CT scanning demonstrates diffuse miliary shadows at both lungs, with even size, even density and even distribution

Case Study 7

A female patient aged 25 years was diagnosed with acute miliary pulmonary TB. During the recent 10 days, the patients experience fever and cough after abortion, with difficulty expectorating. The fever occurs commonly after noons, with a body temperature fluctuating around 37.8 °C, and the cough is paroxysmal.

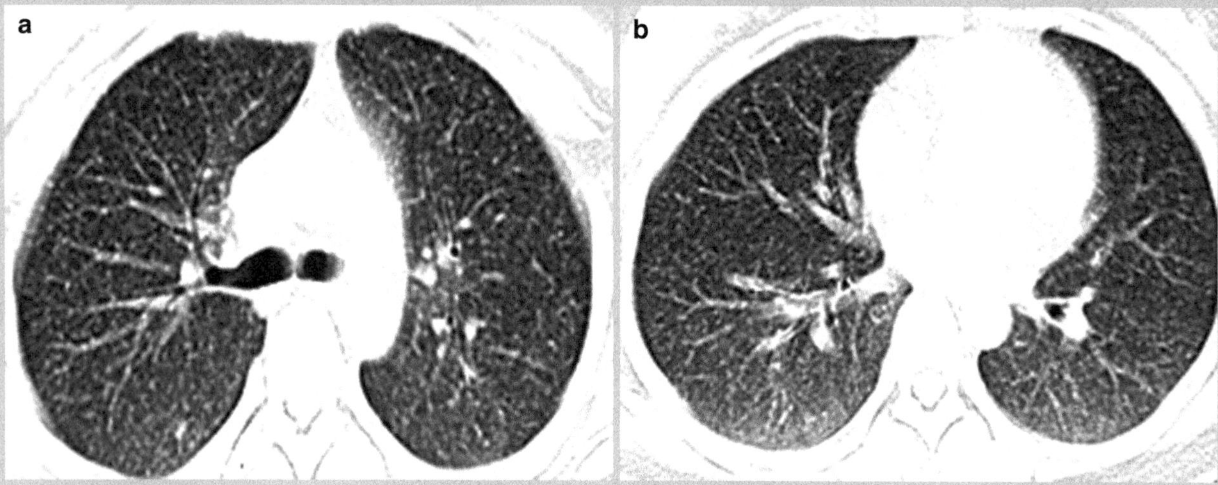

Fig. 21.7 Acute miliary pulmonary TB. (**a**, **b**) CT scanning demonstrates diffuse miliary nodular shadows at both lungs with even size, even density, and even distribution

Subacute and Chronic Hematogenous Pulmonary TB

Due to repeated invasions of a small quantity of MTB into the blood flow during a long period of time, subacute or chronic hematogenous pulmonary TB occurs. The source of their dissemination is commonly infected veins after urogenital TB or osteoarticular TB.

X-Ray

X-ray demonstrates three-unevens sign. The size of lesions ranges from miliary to 1 cm in diameter. The density of exudative or proliferative lesions is light, while the density of calcification is dense, with blurry or sharp boundary. The lesions are unevenly distributed at the upper and middle lung fields. The old hard nodular calcifications are mostly distributed at the lung apex and subclavicular area, while the new exudative and proliferative lesions are mostly distributed at the lower lungs.

CT Scanning

CT scanning demonstrates unevenly distributed lesions that are more commonly distributed at the middle and upper lungs, the lesions with different sizes due to fusion of miliary nodules, and the lesions with uneven density due to inner calcification. These findings are known as the three-unevens sign. Compensatory emphysema can be demonstrated between lesions or at the lower lungs (Fig. 21.8).

Case Study 8

A male patient aged 24 years was diagnosed with subacute hematogenous pulmonary TB.

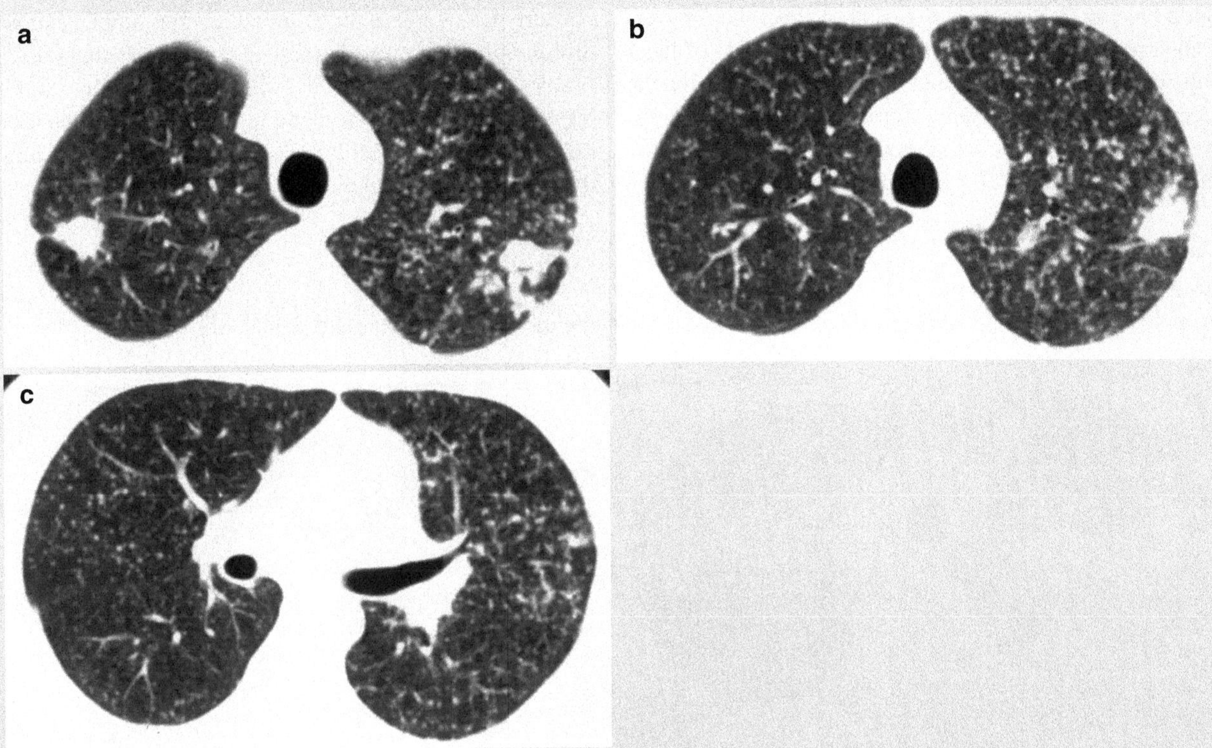

Fig. 21.8 Subacute hematogenous pulmonary TB. (**a–c**) CT scanning demonstrates diffuse miliary nodules at both lungs, with different size and density. Some miliary nodules fuse together at the upper lobe of both lungs

Secondary Pulmonary TB

Secondary pulmonary TB is a major type of pulmonary TB, and it is the most common type of pulmonary TB.

Infiltrative Pulmonary TB

CT Scanning

CT scanning sometimes demonstrates traces of primary infection of tuberculosis. The calcification in the intrapulmonary primary lesions is demonstrated in spots of and nodular lesions with high density. Peripheral inflammation can be demonstrated around the old lesions, with central high density and peripheral patches and small flakes of light blurry shadows. Hilar and mediastinal lymph nodes are demonstrated with calcification.

The lesions of secondary infection of MTB are commonly located at the apical posterior segment of the upper lung lobe and dorsal segment of the lower lung lobe. Multiple lesions can be found within one pulmonary segment or lobe or within unilateral or bilateral lung fields. The exudative lesions are demonstrated as cloud-like shadow with patches, small flakes, or flakes of shadows with increased density. The density of lesions is even or uneven with blurry boundary. The patches of shadows may fuse into flakes of shadows. The proliferative lesions are demonstrated as spots, small nodules, and patches of shadows with increased density and well-defined boundary. The proliferative lesions rarely fuse together. Caseous necrosis can be found at the lesions to induce low-density or semitransparent cavity, which is demonstrated as a transparent area with different sizes and shapes. Infiltrative TB at different stages can be demonstrated with no wall cavity, thin wall cavity, caseous thick wall cavity, tension cavity, and purified cavity. Around the cavity, spots of small nodular shadows are demonstrated, which are technically known as satellite lesions. Bronchial lesions are commonly found at the unilateral or bilateral middle and lower lung fields disseminated from cavity. The calcifications are demonstrated as high-density spots of linear or patches of shadows with well-defined boundary but in regular or irregular shape. At the middle and advanced stages of infiltrative TB, calcification is commonly demonstrated in the lesions. The finding of calcifications in the lesion or at the margin of lesion greatly facilitates the qualitative diagnosis. Meanwhile the finding of calcification indicates that the conditions are tending to stabilize or be improved. The fibrous lesions are demonstrated as cords like or stellate-like shadows with high density and rough boundary. Within a short period of time, the progress and absorption of the lesions are slower than those of lobar pneumonia, lobular pneumonia, mycoplasma pneumonia, and common viral pneumonia. Accompanying pleural effusion occurs. In the cases complicated by hematogenous disseminated pulmonary TB, in addition to intrapulmonary infiltrative lesions, there are also demonstrations of acute or subacute and chronic hematogenous disseminated pulmonary TB (Figs. 21.9, 21.10, 21.11, and 21.12).

Infiltrative pulmonary TB is demonstrated with common concurrence of at least two types of lesions among exudates, proliferation, caseous necrosis, cavity, calcification, and fibrosis. Radiologically, it is characterized by multiple lesions, multiple densities, and multiple shapes. The typical radiological sign of infiltrative pulmonary TB is lesions at the apical posterior segment of both upper lung lobes.

Case Study 9

A male patient aged 20 years was diagnosed with secondary pulmonary TB (infiltrative pulmonary TB).

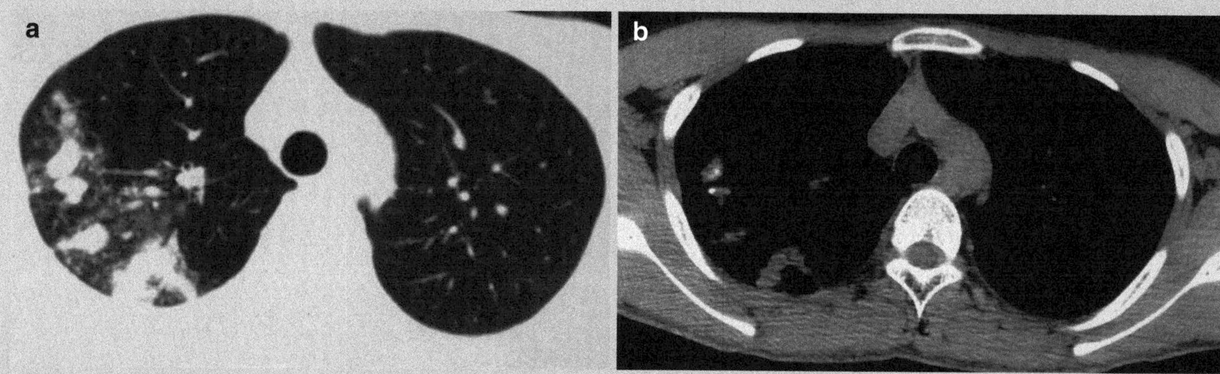

Fig. 21.9 Infiltrative pulmonary TB. (**a**, **b**) CT scanning demonstrates spots of small nodular and small patches of shadows at the right upper lung lobe and calcification in the lesions at the apical segment of the right upper lung lobe

Case Study 10

A male patient aged 25 years was diagnosed with secondary pulmonary TB (infiltrative pulmonary TB).

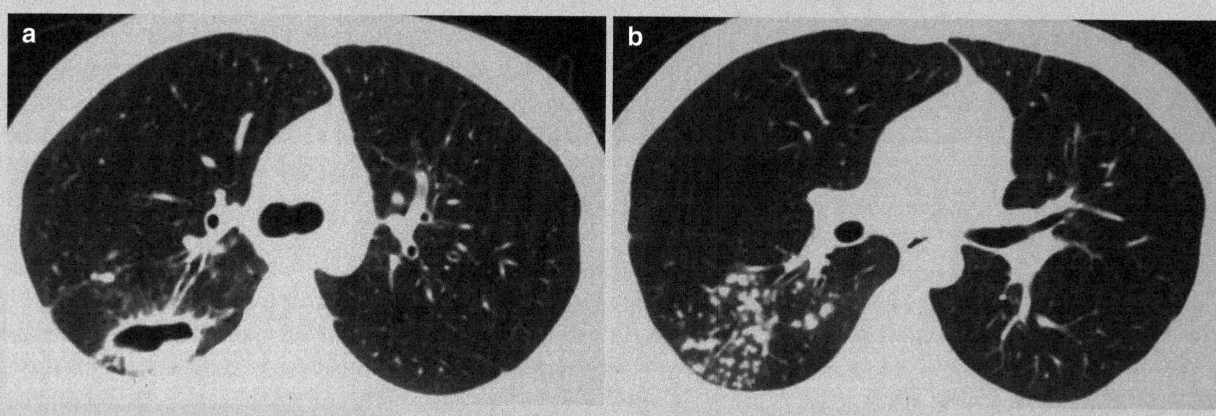

Fig. 21.10 Infiltrative pulmonary TB. (**a**, **b**) CT scanning demonstrates a transparent area at the posterior segment of the right upper lung lobe, double rail-like draining bronchi between the transparent area and the hilum, spot-like satellite lesions around the transparent area, and spots of bronchial lesions at the right lower lung lobe

Case Study 11

A female patient aged 77 years complained of cough for over 4 months, with rare phlegm, fatigue, chest distress, and shortness of breath. By sputum smear, acid-fast bacillus is positive.

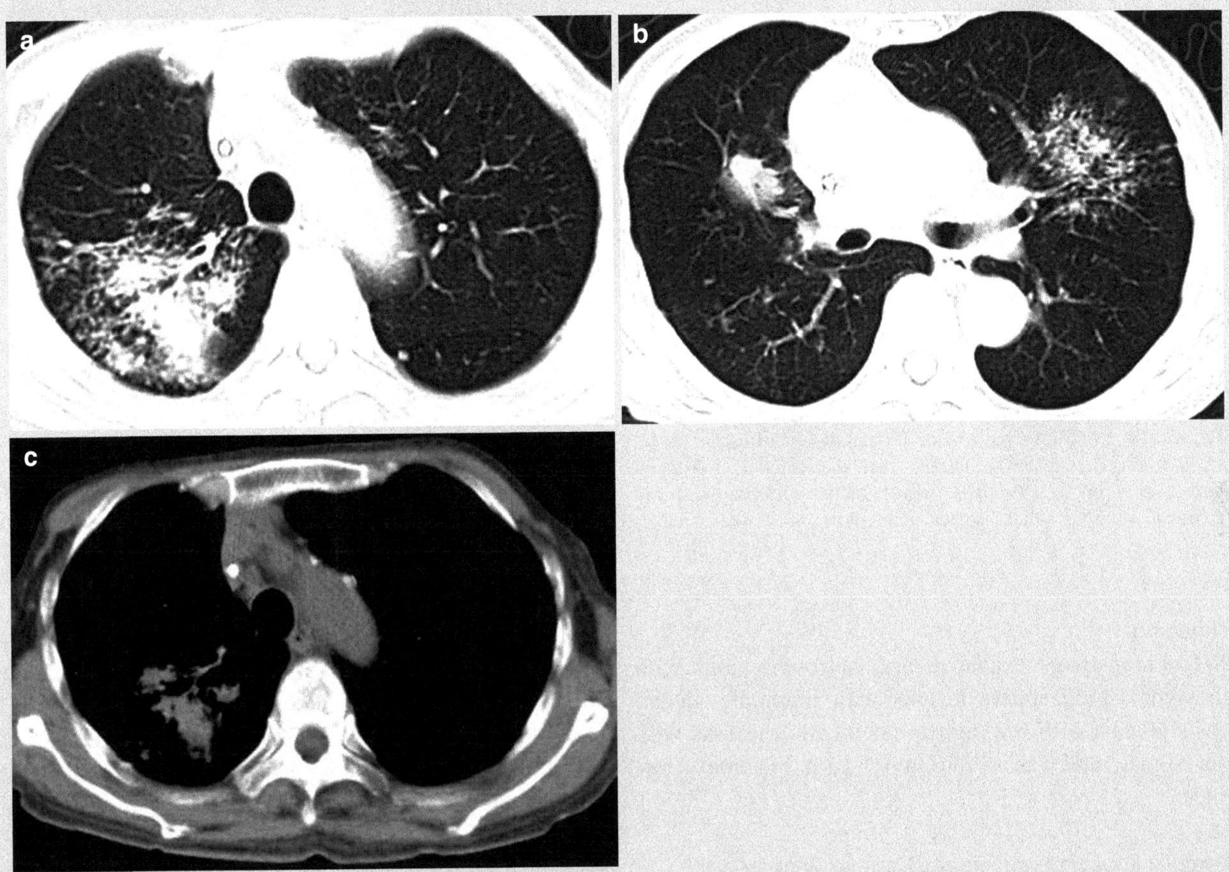

Fig. 21.11 Infiltrative pulmonary TB. (**a**–**c**) CT scanning demonstrates flakes and nodular blurry shadows at both lungs, dilation of local bronchial lumen, thickening of local bronchial wall, and calcification of some lymph nodes

Case Study 12

A female patient aged 43 years. By sputum smear, acid-fast bacillus is positive.

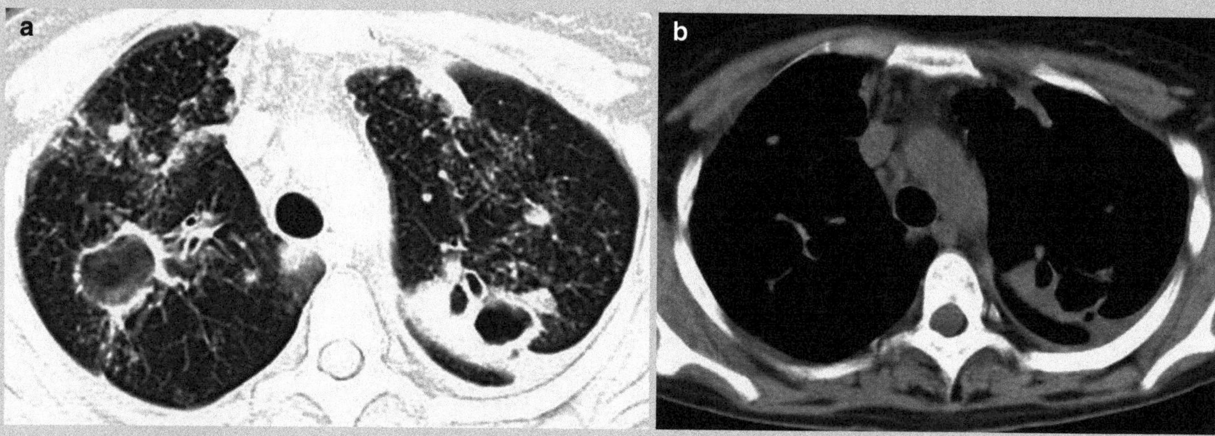

Fig. 21.12 Infiltrative pulmonary TB and pleural effusion. (**a**, **b**). CT scanning demonstrates multiple thick wall cavities in different sizes at both upper lung lobes, uneven thickness of the thick wall cavities, multiple small patches and cotton wool like shadows around the lesions, observable tree bud sign, and scattering multiple nodular or cord-like shadows in both lungs. There are also enlarged mediastinal lymph nodes and bilateral pleural effusion in small quantities

MR Imaging

T2WI demonstrates exudative and caseous lesions with high signal, proliferative lesions with moderate signal, fibrosis lesions with low signal, calcification lesions with lower signal, and gas in the cavity with extremely low signal.

Tubercular Lobar Pneumonia and Caseous Pneumonia

Tubercular Lobar Pneumonia

Tubercular lobar pneumonia is an uncommon type of secondary pulmonary TB, which is also known as bronchial pneumonia TB.

By CT scanning, the lesions are commonly located at the upper lung lobe, especially the apical posterior segment. The lesions are commonly demonstrated as large flakes of shadows occupying a whole segment, lobe, or even a lung field. The central area is demonstrated with a large area of consolidation, with light and poorly defined boundary. These demonstrations resemble to those of lobar pneumonia. The large flakes of consolidation are demonstrated with inner air bronchus sign. In some cases, the air bronchus is demonstrated with column-like or bead string-like dilation. The cloud-like shadows are demonstrated with spots of and small nodular high-density lesions. The small nodular shadows are demonstrated at the margin of flakes of shadows, with some marginal lesions being blurry and some others well defined. By radiological examinations, a large flake of lesions is surrounded by many small lesions, which scatter unevenly. Such findings facilitate its differential diagnosis from lobar pneumonia. In the large flake of consolidation or at the marginal flake of consolidation, there are slightly low-density semitransparent areas or small transparent areas, indicating the occurrence of small caseous necrosis and dissolution. The disease progresses rapidly, with infiltration of the lesions, occurrence of surrounding inflammation, and fusion of the lesions. At the affected lung field or contralateral lung field, scattering polymorphic spots of small nodular or patches of TB lesions greatly facilitate its diagnosis (Fig. 21.13).

Case Study 13

A male patient aged 36 years was diagnosed with secondary pulmonary TB (tubercular lobar pneumonia).

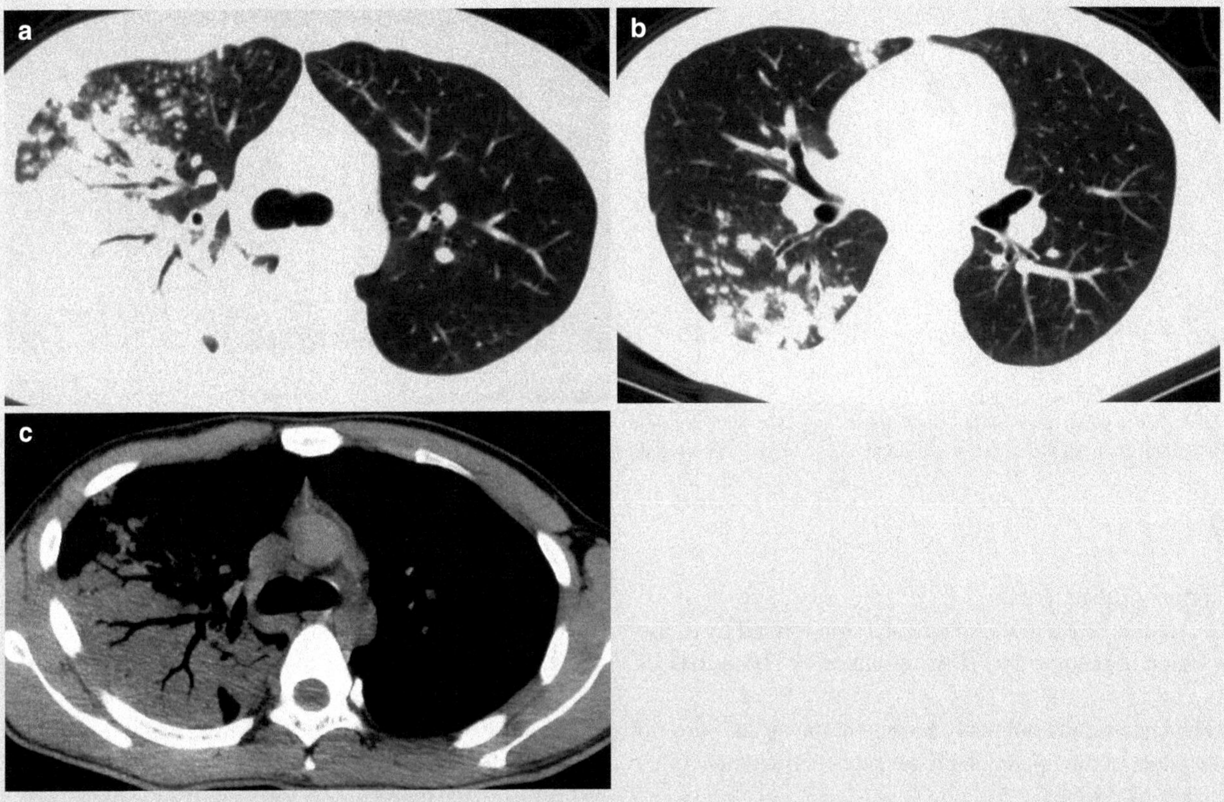

Fig. 21.13 Tubercular lobar pneumonia. (**a–c**) CT scanning demonstrates a large flake of consolidation at the right upper lung lobe with inner air bronchus sign. The margin of lesions is demonstrated to be poorly defined with small patches and spots of shadows. The middle and lower lobes of right lung are demonstrated with small patches and spots of shadows

Caseous Pneumonia

Caseous pneumonia is the acutest and severest type of secondary pulmonary TB. Some cases of caseous pneumonia are developed from caseous necrosis of exudative lesions due to tubercular lobar pneumonia.

1. X-ray and CT scanning

Caseous lobar pneumonia is demonstrated with large flakes of cloud-like shadows, which gradually develop into a large flake of consolidation shadow with moderate density. The lesion is commonly located at the upper lung lobe, occupying a whole segment, lobe, or even lung field, with poorly defined boundary. The lesion has uneven density, with extensive multiple worm-bitten-like low-density semitransparent area or transparent area in different sizes at the large flake of consolidation shadow. The cavities are morphologically varied, with irregular, unsmooth, and poorly defined cavity wall. Such a sign is more clearly demonstrated by HRCT. Without timely and effective treatment to control its development, the conditions continue to deteriorate with further expansion of multiple worm-bitten-like cavities in different sizes and their fusion. Consequently, large area of the lung is destructed by formation of huge cavity (Fig. 21.14). Bronchial lesions caused by dissemination can be demonstrated at the homolateral or contralateral lung field. Caseous lobular pneumonia is demonstrated with multiple scattering small flakes, small nodules, and spots of shadows at the unilateral or bilateral upper and middle parts of the lung. The small flakes of shadows may fuse into a large flake. In the flakes of, small flakes of and nodular lesions, irregular lesions of caseous necrosis and dissolution can be found in different sizes to show low-density semi-transparent or transparent area. Such a sign is of great significance for the diagnosis. At the middle and advanced stages, the lung tissue is subject to extensive and severe damage to cause shrinkage of the lung lobe and thickening of the adjacent pleura.

2. MR imaging

The demonstrations of secondary pulmonary TB based on caseous lesions by MR imaging morphologically resemble to those by CT scanning. The lesions of caseous necrosis are demonstrated with moderate or slightly low T1WI signal and heterogeneous high T2WI signal. In the cases with peripheral fiber or granulation tissue, enhancement can be demonstrated, while the caseous necrotic tissue is demonstrated with no enhancement. In the cases with accompanying large calcification, no signaling shadow can be demonstrated.

Case Study 14

A female patient aged 30 years was diagnosed with secondary pulmonary TB (caseous pneumonia).

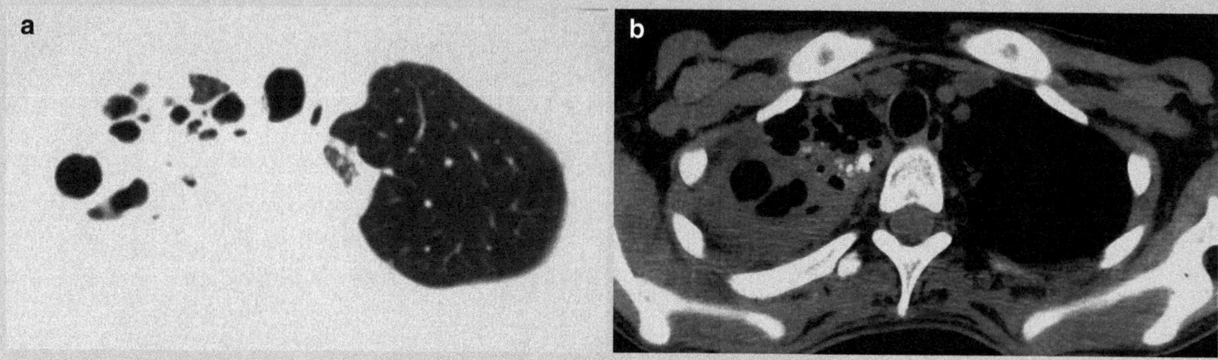

Fig. 21.14 Caseous pneumonia. (**a**) CT scanning demonstrates large flakes of shadows at the right upper lung lobe with multiple irregular transparent areas in different sizes in the lesions and cord-like shadows at the left upper lung lobe. (**b**) Spots of calcification are demonstrated in the lesion

Pulmonary Tuberculoma

Tuberculoma refers to the spherical lesion formed by a caseous lesion of pulmonary TB encapsulated by fibrous tissues.

1. The lesions are commonly located at the apical posterior segment of the upper lung lobe and dorsal segment of the lower lung lobe.
2. The lesion is mostly singular, but in rare cases, the lesions are multiple.
3. The lesions are round or oval in shape, those with a diameter being less than 2 cm are referred to as fibrous caseous lesion, and those with a diameter being larger than 2 cm are referred to as tuberculoma.
4. The contour of lesion is clear and regular, rarely with incisura and lobulation.
5. The density of the lesion may be homogeneous or with inner semitransparent area due to dissolution. The dissolution area is commonly located near the hilum in the spheric shadow. Cavity can also be demonstrated.
6. At the lung field near the spherical shadow, scattering proliferative or fibrous lesions are commonly found in spots of small nodular and cord-like shadows, namely, the satellite lesions.
7. Between the tuberculoma and hilum of the lung, cord-like shadows are demonstrated, which are residual draining bronchi after formation of the tuberculoma derived from the cavity.
8. Calcification can be found within or at the margin of tuberculoma. The typical demonstration is laminar ring-shaped calcification shadow or scattering spots of calcification.
9. Contrast CT scanning demonstrates linear enhancement of the tuberculoma capsule and no or slight central enhancement (Figs. 21.15, 21.16, and 21.17).

Case Study 15

A male patient aged 39 years was diagnosed with secondary pulmonary TB (pulmonary tuberculoma).

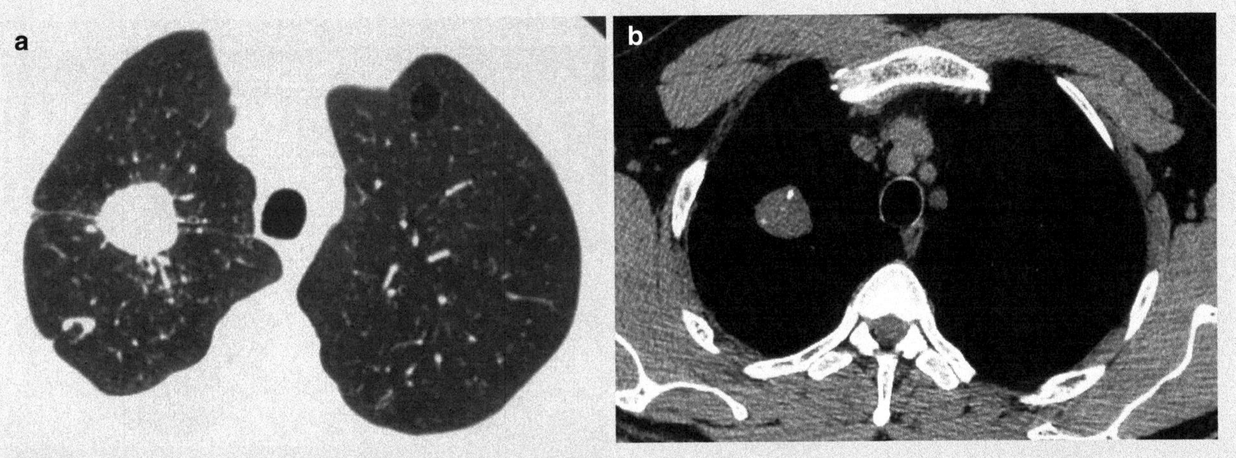

Fig. 21.15 Pulmonary tuberculoma. (**a**) CT scanning demonstrates round-like nodular shadow at the apical segment of the right upper lung lobe, with a well-defined and smooth boundary, multiple linear shadows in different lengths radiating from the nodule outwards, and spots of satellite lesion around the lesion. (**b**) Spots of calcifications can be demonstrated in the lesion

Case Study 16

A female patient aged 43 years experienced cough and hemoptysis for several months. By sputum smear, acid-fast bacillus is positive.

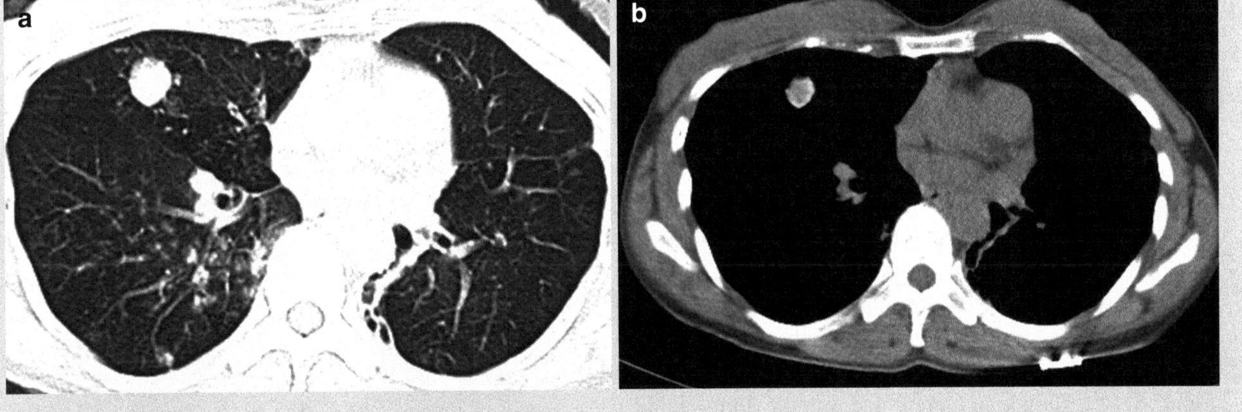

Fig. 21.16 Pulmonary tuberculoma, infiltrative pulmonary TB. (**a**, **b**) CT scanning demonstrates spherical lesion at the right middle lung lobe, with marginal irregular calcification and well-defined boundary. The lesion is demonstrated with surrounding satellite lesions. And multiple nodules are demonstrated at the right lower lung

Case Study 17

A male patient aged 35 years experienced cough for over 20 days, with no known causes. He coughed up rare sputum that was white and foamy, with no blood and odor. By sputum smear, acid-fast bacillus is positive.

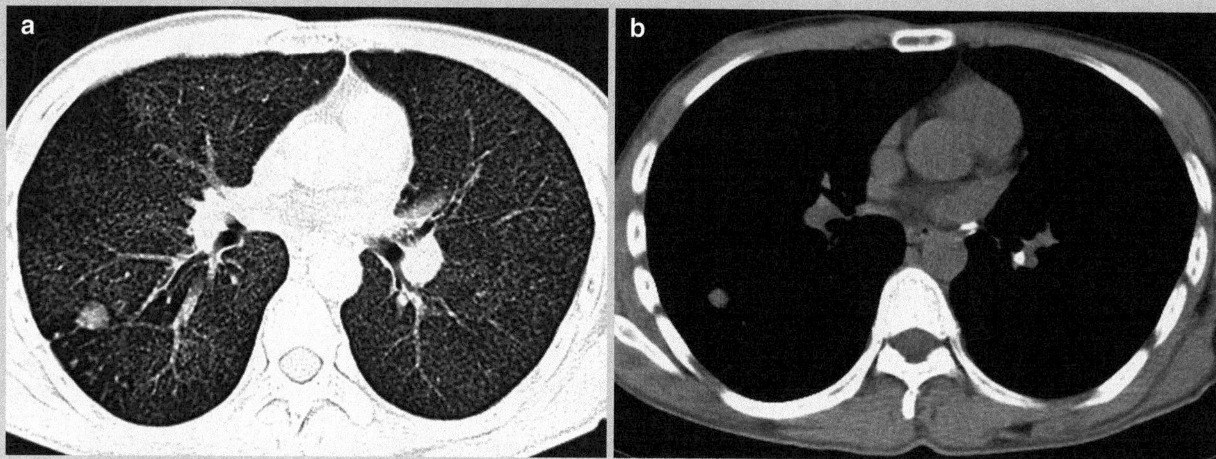

Fig. 21.17 Pulmonary tuberculoma and acute hematogenous pulmonary TB. (**a**, **b**) CT scanning demonstrates spherical lesion at the right lower lung lobe near pleura with poor defined boundary and surrounding satellite lesions. There are diffuse miliary TB lesions at both lungs and calcified lymph nodes at the mediastinum and left hilum

Chronic Fibro-Cavity Pulmonary TB

Tuberculosis has a long illness course, with alternated deterioration and alleviation. Local or most of the lung tissue is subject to severe damage, with concurrent extensive proliferation and repair of fiber tissue around the lesion, namely, the occurrence of fibro-cavity.

1. Irregular fibro-cavities are located at the apical posterior segment of the upper lung lobe or the dorsal segment of the lower lung lobe, namely, the supraclavicular or subclavicular region. Extensive cord-like shadows are demonstrated to surround the lesion. Local lung volume shrinks, commonly leading to elevated hilum at the affected lung. The lung markings are demonstrated like willow. And the trachea and mediastinum are demonstrated to shift to the affected lung.
2. Both old and new tuberculosis lesions are commonly found at the unilateral upper and middle lung fields, namely, concurrence of various lesions including exudative lesions, proliferative lesions, caseous lesions, cavities, fibrous lesions, and calcification.
3. Bronchial lesions due to dissemination are commonly found at the middle and lower lung fields of the affected lung as well as at the contralateral lung field.
4. The unaffected lung field is subject to compensatory emphysema. CT scanning demonstrates bullae of the lung, which is demonstrated as thin wall bullae within or at the margin of the lung.
5. The pleura of the affected lung is subject to long-term invasion, thickening, and adhesion to cause narrowing of local intercostal space and collapse of thorax. Meanwhile, due to shrinkage of the upper lung volume as well as traction by pleural thickening and adhesion, the arches of the superior mediastinum and trachea shift towards the affected lung.
6. CT scanning, especially HRCT, is superior to X-ray in detecting secondary bronchiectasis. The demonstrations are commonly multiple thin wall small bubbles with a honeycomb-like sign (Figs. 21.18, 21.19, and 21.20).

Case Study 18

A male patient aged 44 years was diagnosed with secondary pulmonary TB (chronic fibro-cavity pulmonary TB).

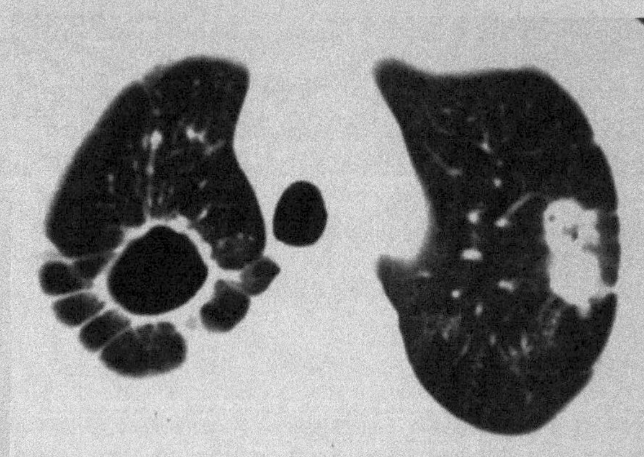

Fig. 21.18 Chronic fibro-cavity pulmonary TB. CT scanning demonstrates transparent area at the posterior segment of the right upper lung lobe, smooth and regular lining of the cavity, multiple cord-like shadows at the exterior margin of the cavity that radiate from the cavity wall outwards, and connection of most cord-like shadows with adjacent pleura. Around the transparent area, spots of shadows scatter. Spots and patches of shadows are demonstrated at the apical posterior segment of the left upper lung lobe

Case Study 19

A male patient aged 44 years experienced cough. By sputum smear, acid-fast bacillus is positive.

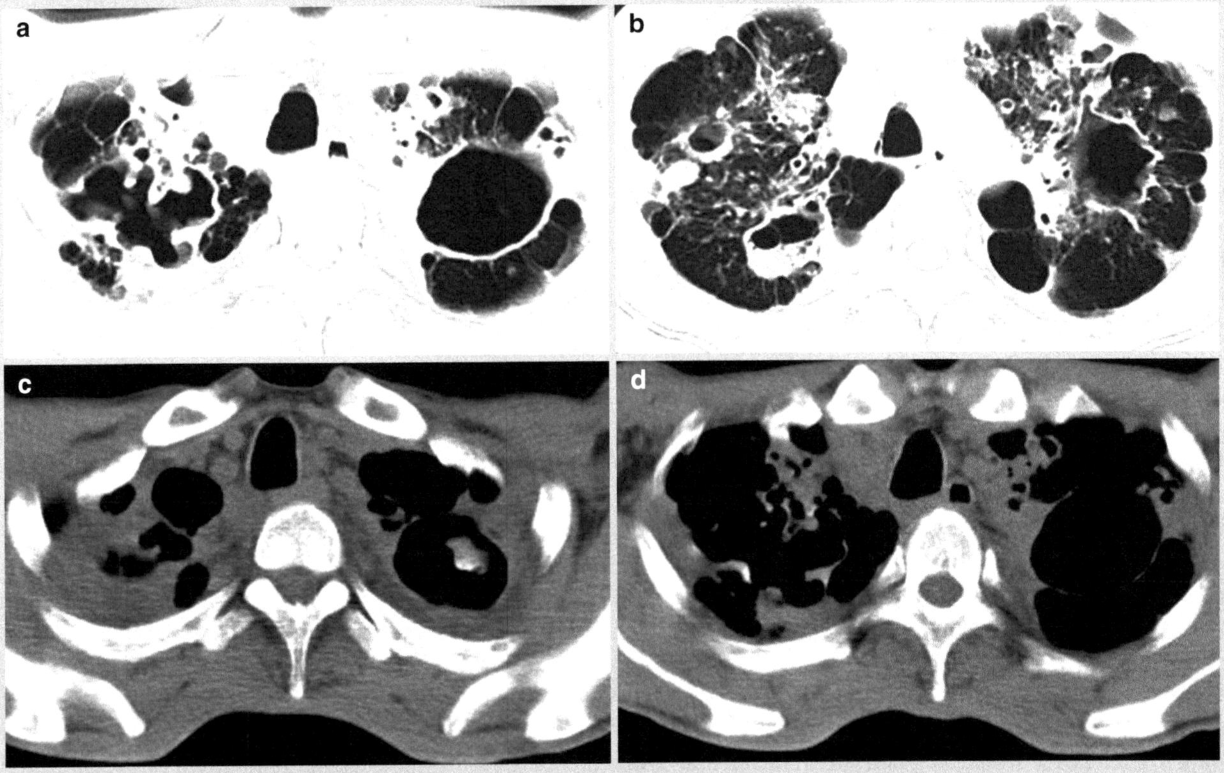

Fig. 21.19 Chronic fibro-cavity pulmonary TB. (**a**–**d**) CT scanning demonstrates multiple thick wall cavities at the upper lobe of both lungs, accompanying bronchial lesions due to dissemination, and pleural thickening

Case Study 20

A male patient aged 59 years. By sputum smear, acid-fast bacillus is positive.

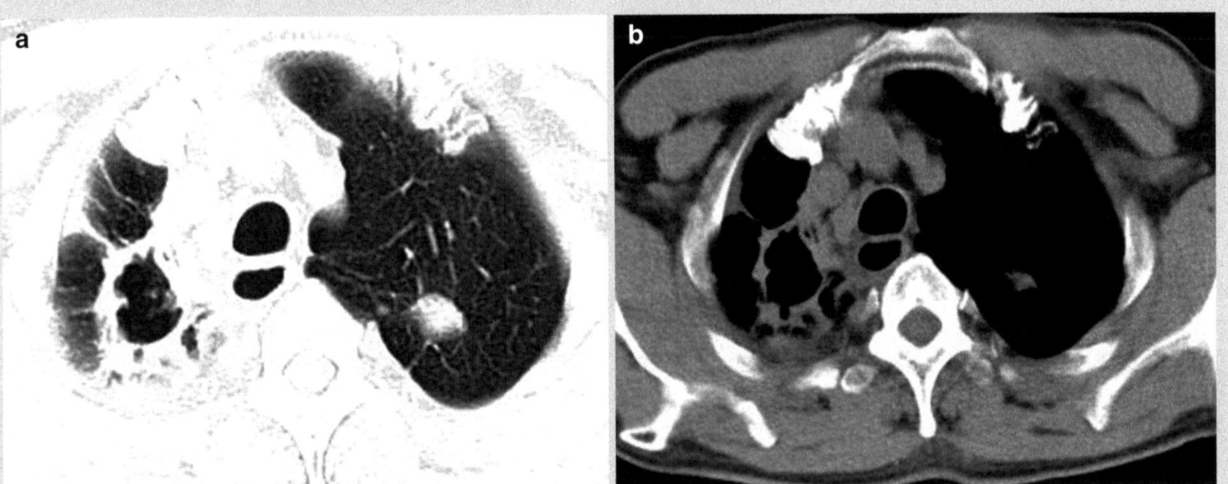

Fig. 21.20 Chronic fibro-cavity pulmonary TB. (**a**, **b**) CT scanning demonstrates singular thick wall cavity at the right upper lung lobe and surrounding cord-like shadows

Tuberculous Pleuritis

Tuberculous pleuritis is a pleural inflammation caused by access of MTB and its metabolites into the pleural cavity. Clinically, it is categorized into dry pleuritic and exudative pleuritis.

Dry Pleuritis

Due to rare protein exudates, X-ray demonstrates dry pleuritis with no abnormalities. When local pleura develops thickening and adhesion, local decrease of transparency can be demonstrated, with a dome-shaped shadow at the diaphragm. CT scanning is more sensitive to pleural thickening. In addition, CT scanning can demonstrate slight protrusion of the pleura towards the lung field due to a small quantity of areas with liquid density, with poorly defined boundary (Figs. 21.21 and 21.22). MR imaging demonstrates linear moderate or low T1WI signal shadow and slightly high or high T2WI signal shadow.

Exudative Pleuritis

Based on the quantity, location, and state of pleural effusion, exudative pleuritis can be categorized into free pleural effusion type and localized pleural effusion type.

Free Pleural Effusion

Free pleural effusion refers to pleural effusion that is not confined or restricted within a certain part of the pleural cavity, whose distribution can change along with change of body posture and is consistent to the distribution of liquid gravity. Based on the volume of pleural effusion, it can be further divided into three types: small quantity, moderate quantity, and large quantity.

Concerning the small quantity type, in the cases with pleural effusion exceeding 250–300 ml, X-ray at the standing posture demonstrates blunt and shallow costophrenic angle at the affected side as well as the normal shape and contour of the diaphragm. CT scanning demonstrates arch shape and narrow strip of liquid density shadow at the medial posterior thoracic wall that is parallel to thoracic wall. The shadow has smooth and regular margin (Figs. 21.23 and 21.24).

Concerning the moderate quantity type, the superior borderline of effusion is commonly above the anterior plane of the 4th rib, but below the anterior plane of the 2nd rib. Ultrasound demonstrates a triangular no echo area of the costrophrenic angle or no echo area due to a small quantity of effusion superior to the liver top. X-ray at standing posture demonstrates the superior borderline of effusion as arch shape shadow with higher exterior and lower interior, which has upper light density and lower dense and even density, and completely absent contour of the diaphragm. CT scanning demonstrates crescent liquid density shadow at the medial posterior thoracic wall, with even density and regular margin. The local lung tissue is slightly compressed.

Concerning the large quantity type, the superior borderline of effusion surpasses the anterior plane of the 2nd rib. The affected lung field has dense and even shadow, with widened intercostal space and lowered diaphragm. The mediastinum shifts towards the unaffected side. In some cases, only the transparent lung apex of the affected thoracic cavity can be found. CT scanning demonstrates the thoracic cavity being occupied by liquid density shadow and the lung being compressed with soft tissue shadows at the hilum.

Localized Pleural Effusion

Encapsulated pleural effusion refers to effusion limited in a certain part of the pleural cavity due to adhesions of visceral and parietal pleura. By ultrasound, the no echo area is limited at a certain part of the pleural cavity with semicircular or irregular shape. In most cases, the no echo area is close to the thoracic wall with wide base, and does not change along with change of body posture. By X-ray radiology, the encapsulated pleural effusion is commonly located at the medial posterior thoracic wall at the lower thoracic cavity. X-ray at tangential position demonstrates semicircular or D-shaped liquid density shadow protruding from the thoracic wall to the lung field, with well-defined and smooth boundary. And the angulation of its superior and inferior margins with the thoracic wall is obtuse. By CT scanning, the encapsulated pleural effusion at the lateral thoracic cavity is demonstrated as a convex-shaped liquid density shadow protruding from the thoracic wall to the lung field, which has broad basement and closely adheres to the thoracic wall. Its angulation with the thoracic wall is commonly obtuse, and its margin is smooth. The adjacent pleura is commonly subject to thickening to form a pleural tail sign. Local lung tissue may be subject to compression (Fig. 21.25).

Interlobar effusion refers to effusion confined to the horizontal fissure and oblique fissure. By X-ray, the cases with oblique fissure effusion are demonstrated with effusion confined at the upper or lower oblique fissure. Based on the demonstrations by anterior-posterior X-ray, the diagnosis can be hardly defined, while the demonstrations by lateral X-ray can facilitate to define the diagnosis. Lateral X-ray demonstrates the typical spindle-shaped shadow at the interlobar fissure, with even density and well-defined boundary. After free pleural effusion gains its access into the interlobar fissure, the effusion is commonly confined at the lower part of the oblique fissure, with triangular increased density shadow with the sharp top pointing upwards to the hilum. By CT scanning, the interlobar area with less vascular vessels is demonstrated with flakes or strips of high-density shadow, sometimes with spindle or sphere shape. In the cases with a large quantity of effusion, mass-like shadow is demonstrated, with the thickened interlobar pleura at its both ends. The lesion is located at the interlobar fissure with liquid density, based on which the diagnosis can be defined. By MR imaging, the morphology and signal of effusion can be demonstrated from multiple perspectives.

Infrapulmonary effusion refers to effusion within the pleural cavity between the diaphragm and the base of the lung. It is more commonly found at the right lung. And its radiological demonstrations change along with change of body posture. By X-ray at standing posture, the diaphragmatic surface at the affected lung is demonstrated with elevation, with outward shift of the highest point of the diaphragmatic dome to the exterior 1/3 part of the diaphragm. X-ray at supine posture demonstrates generally increased density of the affected lung field due to perfusion of liquid into the unilateral thoracic cavity and normal position of the diaphragmatic muscle.

Case Study 21

A male patient aged 41 years was diagnosed with tuberculous pleural thickening.

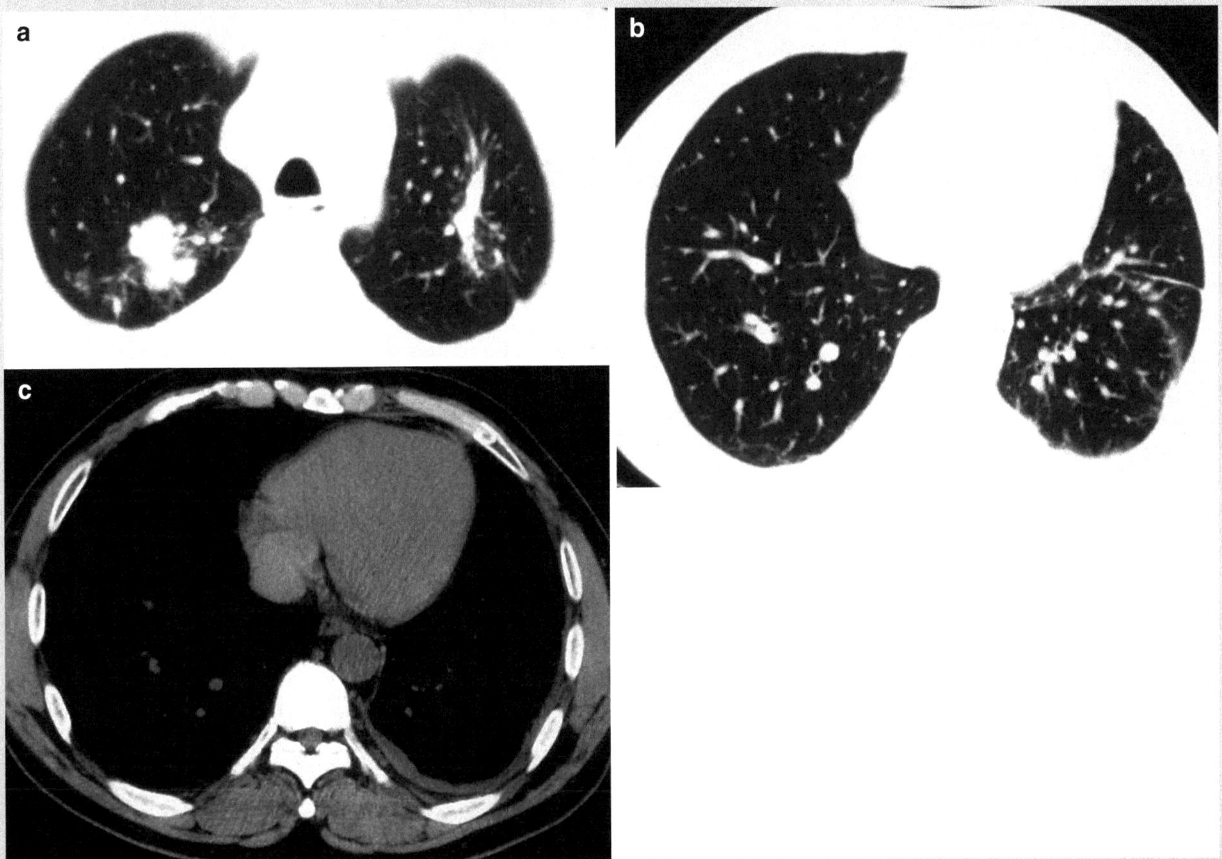

Fig. 21.21 Infiltrative pulmonary tuberculosis and dry pleuritis. (**a**) CT scanning demonstrates spots and patches of shadows at the posterior segment of the right upper lung lobe. (**b**) CT scanning demonstrates cord-like shadow at the apical posterior segment of the left upper lung lobe. (**c**) Arc-shaped cord-like shadow with soft tissue density is demonstrated at the posterior inferior part of the left pleura, with well-defined and smooth pleural surface

Case Study 22

A male patient aged 43 years was diagnosed with pleural tuberculoma, pleural thickening, and calcification.

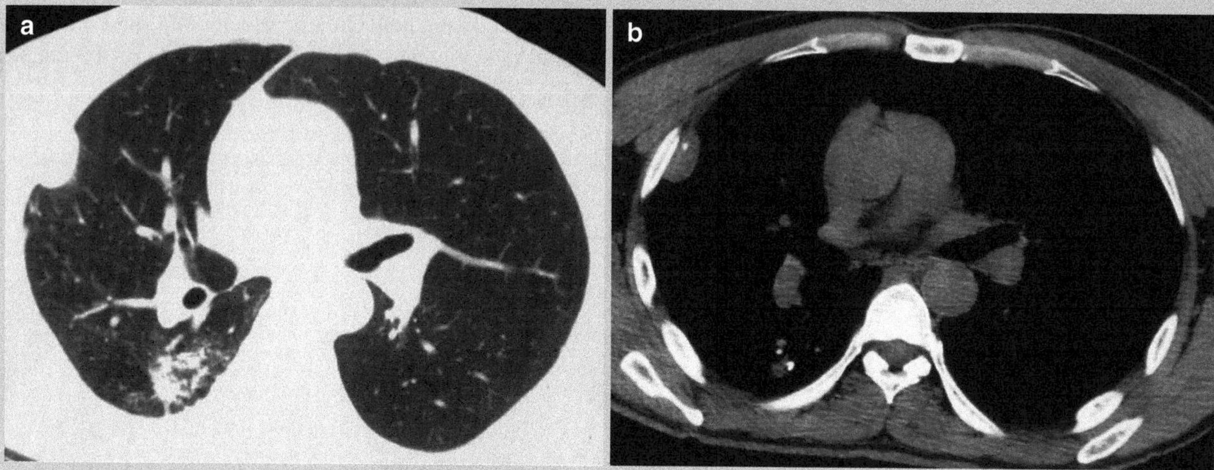

Fig. 21.22 Pleural tuberculoma, pleural thickening, and calcification. (**a**, **b**) CT scanning demonstrates patches of shadows at the dorsal segment of the left lower lung lobe, with calcification in the lesion. D-shaped shadow with soft tissue density is demonstrated exterior and anterior to the adjacent right pleura, with well-defined and smooth pleural surface and internal spots of calcification

Case Study 23

A male patient aged 22 years was diagnosed with tuberculous pleural effusion.

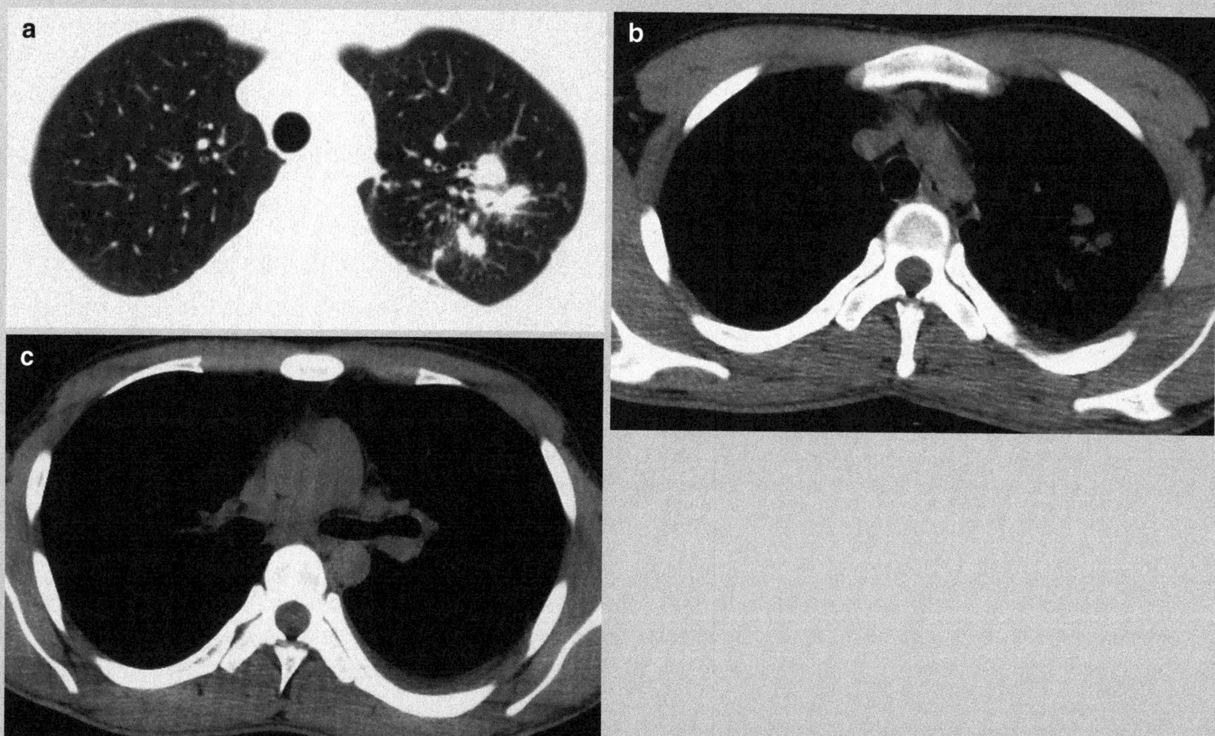

Fig. 21.23 Tuberculous exudative pleuritis (free pleural effusion). (**a**–**c**) CT scanning demonstrates spots and patches of shadows at the apical posterior segment of the left upper lung lobe and crescent-shaped liquid density shadow at the left thoracic cavity

Case Study 24

A male patient aged 61 years experienced fever and cough. By sputum smear, acid-fast bacillus is positive.

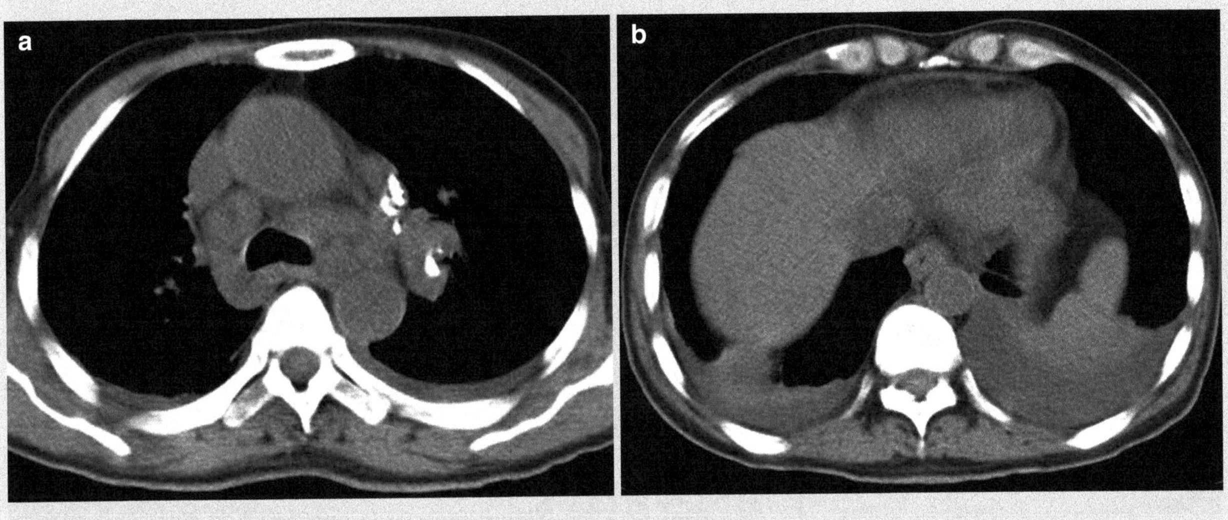

Fig. 21.24 Tuberculous exudative pleuritis (free pleural effusion). (**a**, **b**) CT scanning demonstrates small quantities of pleural effusion at bilateral thoracic cavity and enlarged mediastinal lymph nodes

Case Study 25

A male patient aged 66 years experienced fever and cough. By sputum smear, acid-fast bacillus is positive.

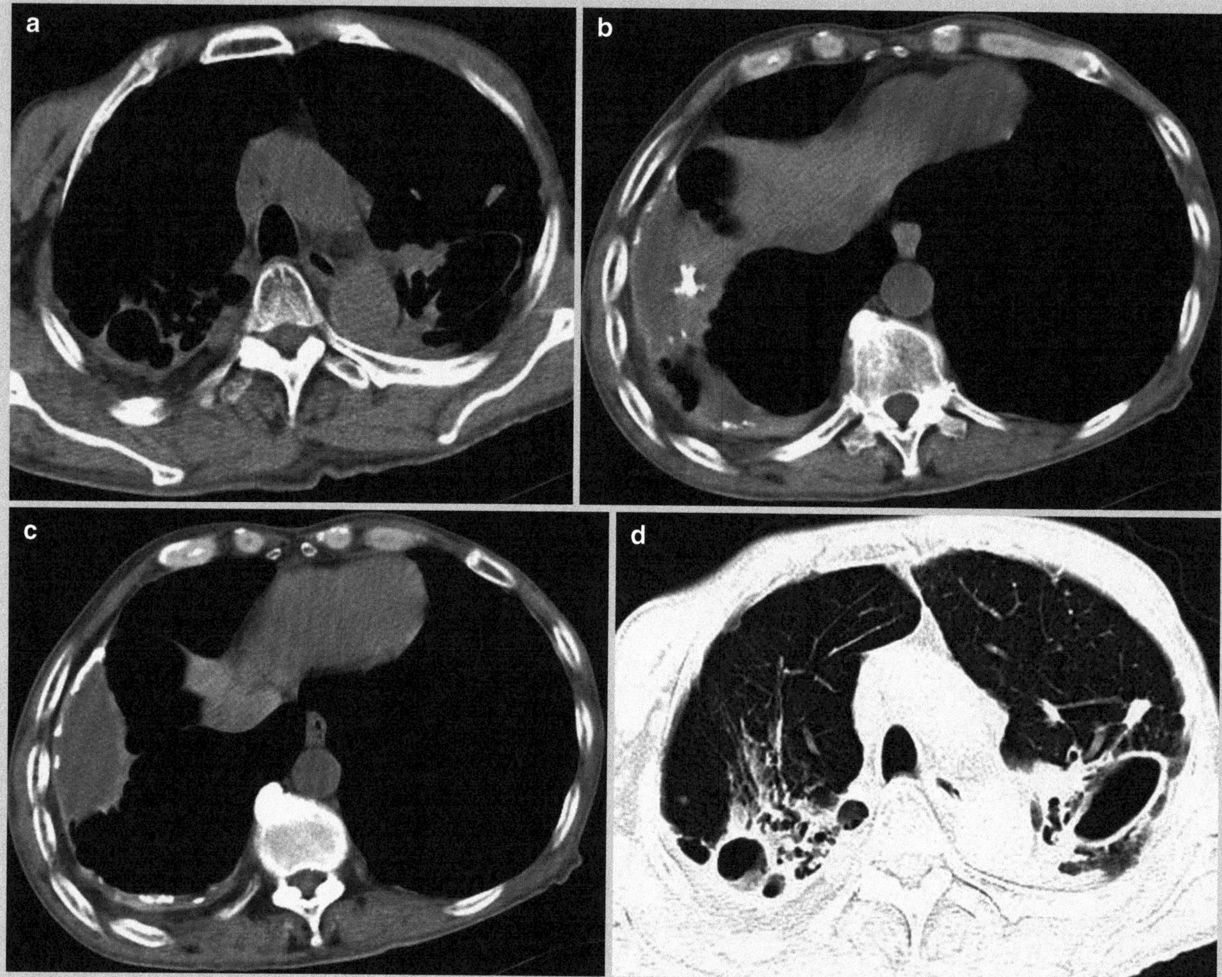

Fig. 21.25 Tuberculous exudative pleuritis (encapsulated pleural effusion), pleural thickening, calcification, and cavity. (**a–d**) CT scanning demonstrates encapsulated pleural effusion, pleural thickening, calcification, and multiple cavities at both lungs

Studies by PET/CT have demonstrated that an abnormal increased of ^{18}F-FDG uptake can be induced by pulmonary TB, tuberculous granuloma, chronic tuberculous lymphadenitis, tuberculous pleuritis (peritonitis), and bone tuberculosis. In addition, the uptake of ^{18}F-FDG varies in different pathological stages. The nodular lesion of pulmonary TB is demonstrated with hypermetabolism, even in the cases with obvious calcification at the lesion, which indicates active TB with chronic inflammation. Pathologically, the chronic inflammations include infiltration of inflammatory cells, proliferation of macrophages, and formation of granuloma. The non-demonstrated lesions by ^{18}F-FDG PET are caseous and old fibrosis and calcification, which are present in the cases with inactive tuberculosis. For such cases, following up observations is necessary. In the cases with hilum and mediastinal lymph nodes involved, hypermetabolism is demonstrated by ^{18}F-FDG, indicating tuberculous lymphadenitis and proliferative lesion (Figs. 21.26, 21.27, 21.28, and 21.29). PET/CT facilitates in assessing the extrapulmonary active tuberculosis, while ^{18}F-FDG PET can also be applied to assess the therapeutic efficacy against TB. Soussan M et al. divided FDG PET/CT examination for tuberculosis into two types, one is for lung TB and the other for lymphatic TB. The relationship between the two types and the immunity of the patients has been studied. They found that the lesions confined within the lungs with slight hypermetabolism can be defined as lung TB, indicating normal immune functions and the effective immune responses. In the patients with compromised immunity, the lesions caused by MTB cannot be confined within the lungs, and the lymph nodes are involved, with or without involvement of the bone, liver, and spleen. An obvious hypermetabolism demonstrated by FDG indicates lymphatic TB.

By ^{18}F-FDG PET examination, attention should be paid to the differential diagnosis of active tuberculous nodule and lung cancer, for both of which exhibit hypermetabolism. The lesion with signs of lobulation, speculation, vacuole sign, air bronchus, or pleural depression sign supports the diagnosis of lung cancer. In combination to ^{18}F-FLT, the differential diagnosis of benign pulmonary nodule and malignancy can be accurately made. However, well-differentiated lung cancers can also be demonstrated as no or low uptake of ^{18}F-FDG.

Case Study 26

A female patient aged 45 years experienced coughing up bloody sputum for 4 months. And the conditions showed no response to anti-infective therapy. By PPD test 2 months ago, strongly positive was indicated, and the patient received anti-TB therapy. The reexamination after treatment for 2 months, the lesions are demonstrated to be thick and dense at the right upper lung lobe by CT scanning. Following PET/CT examination was ordered. Pathological diagnosis after surgery was pulmonary TB.

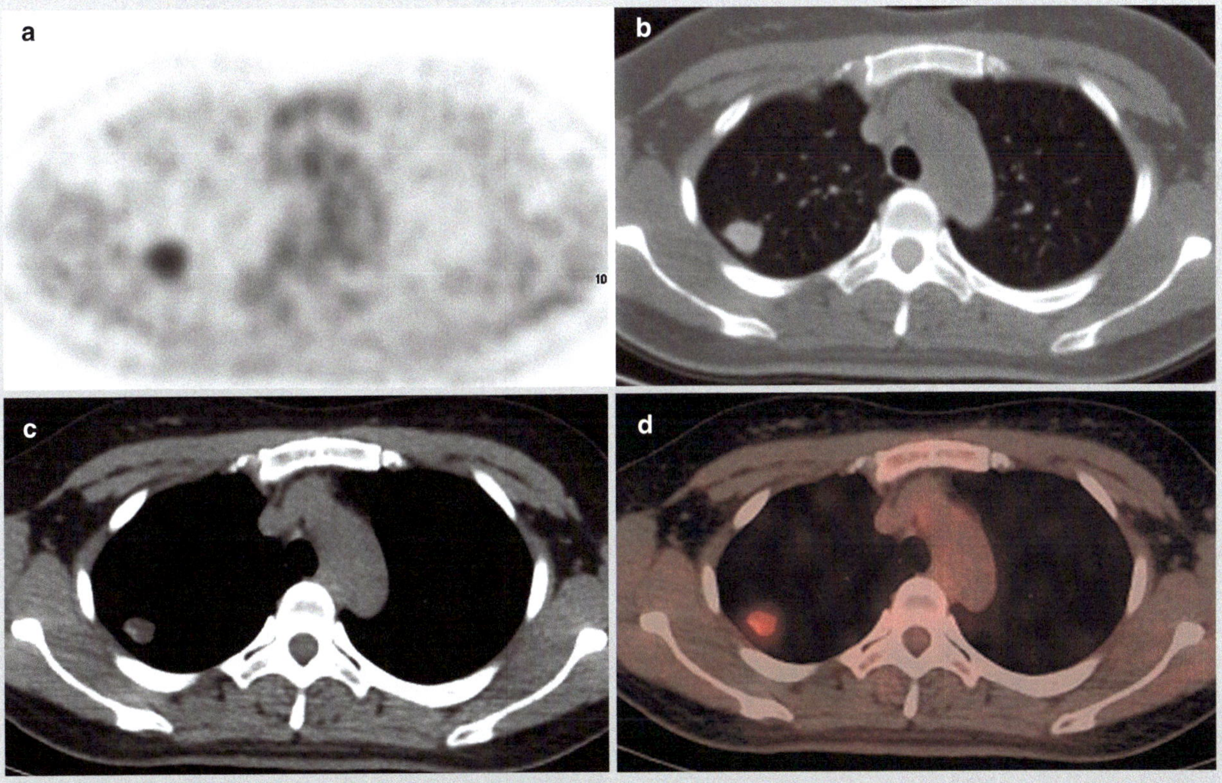

Fig. 21.26 Tuberculoma. (**a**) PET demonstrates increased radioactive uptake by nodules at the right upper lung lobe, with SUV max 2.9. (**b**, **c**) CT scanning demonstrates a nodule in size of 1.7 cm × 1.3 cm at the posterior segment of the right upper lung lobe. The nodule is shallowly lobulated with smooth and regular margin and internal spots of calcification. (**d**) PET/CT demonstrations of the lesion

Case Study 27

A male patient aged 46 years experienced fever and right abdominal pain for over 1 month. The patient reported fever and right abdominal pain more than 1 month ago with no known causes. The fever occurred after noons with a body temperature of 38–40 °C and night sweating. After receiving anti-infective therapy, he showed no improvement. By PPD test, strongly positive and the conditions were obviously improved after anti-TB treatment. The clinical diagnosis was tuberculosis.

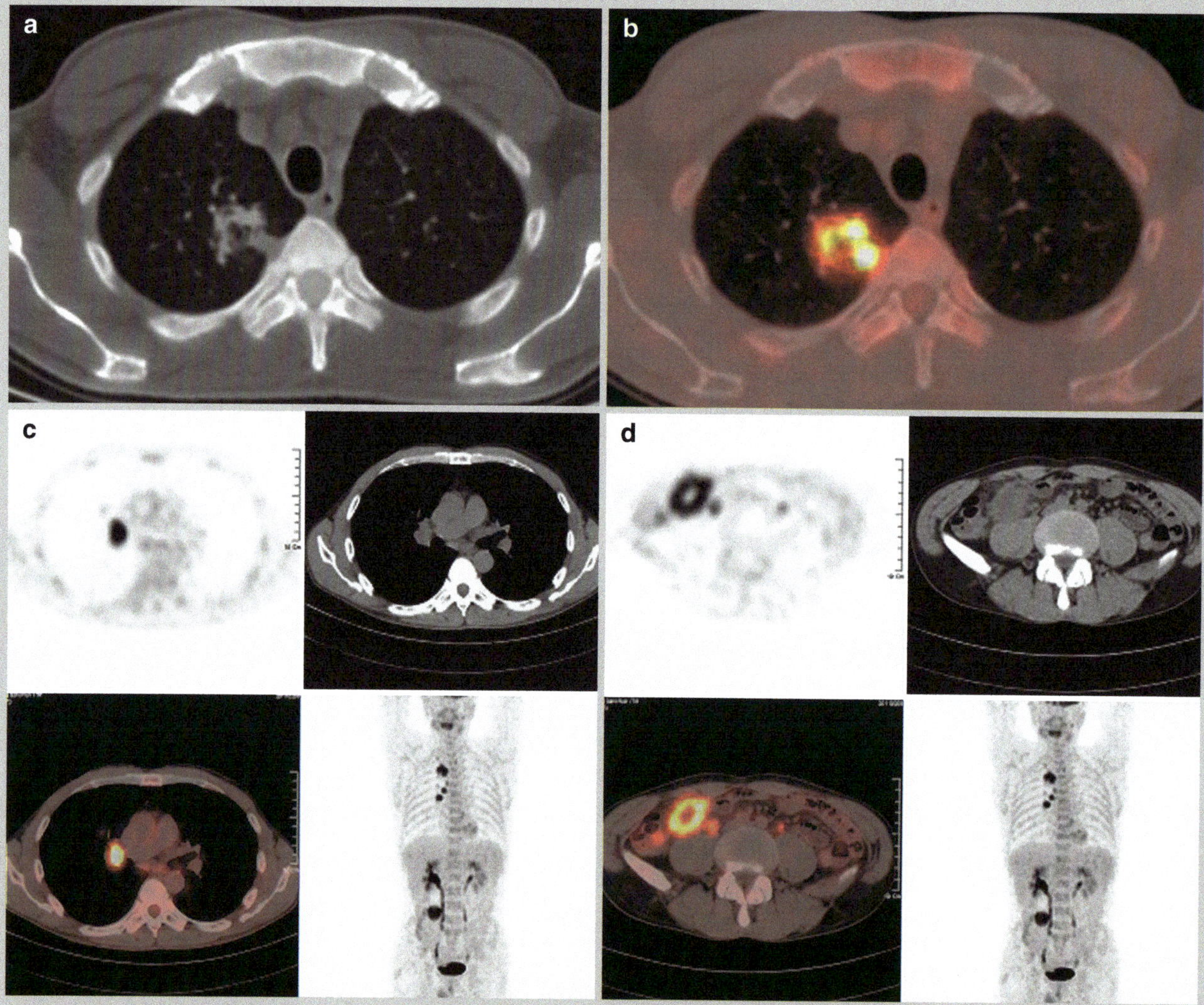

Fig. 21.27 Pulmonary TB and abdominal TB. (**a**) CT scanning demonstrates irregular spots of shadows comprising a nodular lesion at the apical posterior segment of the right upper lung lobe, with lower density at the center. (**b**) PET/CT demonstrates increased HDG metabolism around the lesion, with SUVmax11.2 and defective metabolism of the central low-density area. (**c**) It is demonstrated with enlarged hilar lymph nodes at the right lung, with high FDG metabolism and SUVmax12.8. (**d**) The abdominal cavity is demonstrated with a mass in size of 4.7 × 3.2 cm, which shows irregular ring-like abnormal increase of the radioactive uptake, with SUVmax9.8, which shows an increase to SUVmax12.4 after 1 h. The central low-density area is demonstrated as caseous change with no metabolism

Case Study 28

A male patient aged 64 years experienced cough with bloody sputum for over 1 year. He had a medical history of pulmonary TB 2 years ago and received anti-TB therapy. After oral medication for 14 months, the symptoms showed no improvement. He reported no recent subjective upset.

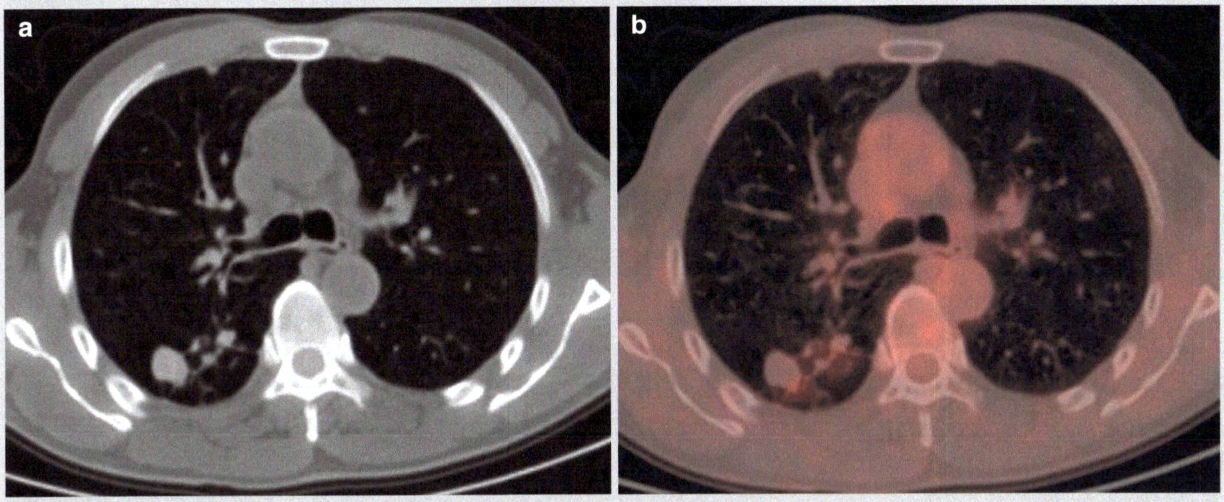

Fig. 21.28 Pulmonary TB. (**a**) CT scanning demonstrates spots of nodular and cord-like TB lesions at the posterior segment of the right upper lung lobe, with well-defined boundary. (**b**) The lesion is demonstrated with no significant increase of the radioactive uptake, with SUVmax1.6

Case Study 29

A male patient aged 71 years was detected with lesions by a routine physical examination.

(Note: the cases of 26–29 and the corresponding figures were provided by Xia GL at the Affiliated Tumor Hospital, Nantong University, Nantong, Jiangsu, China)

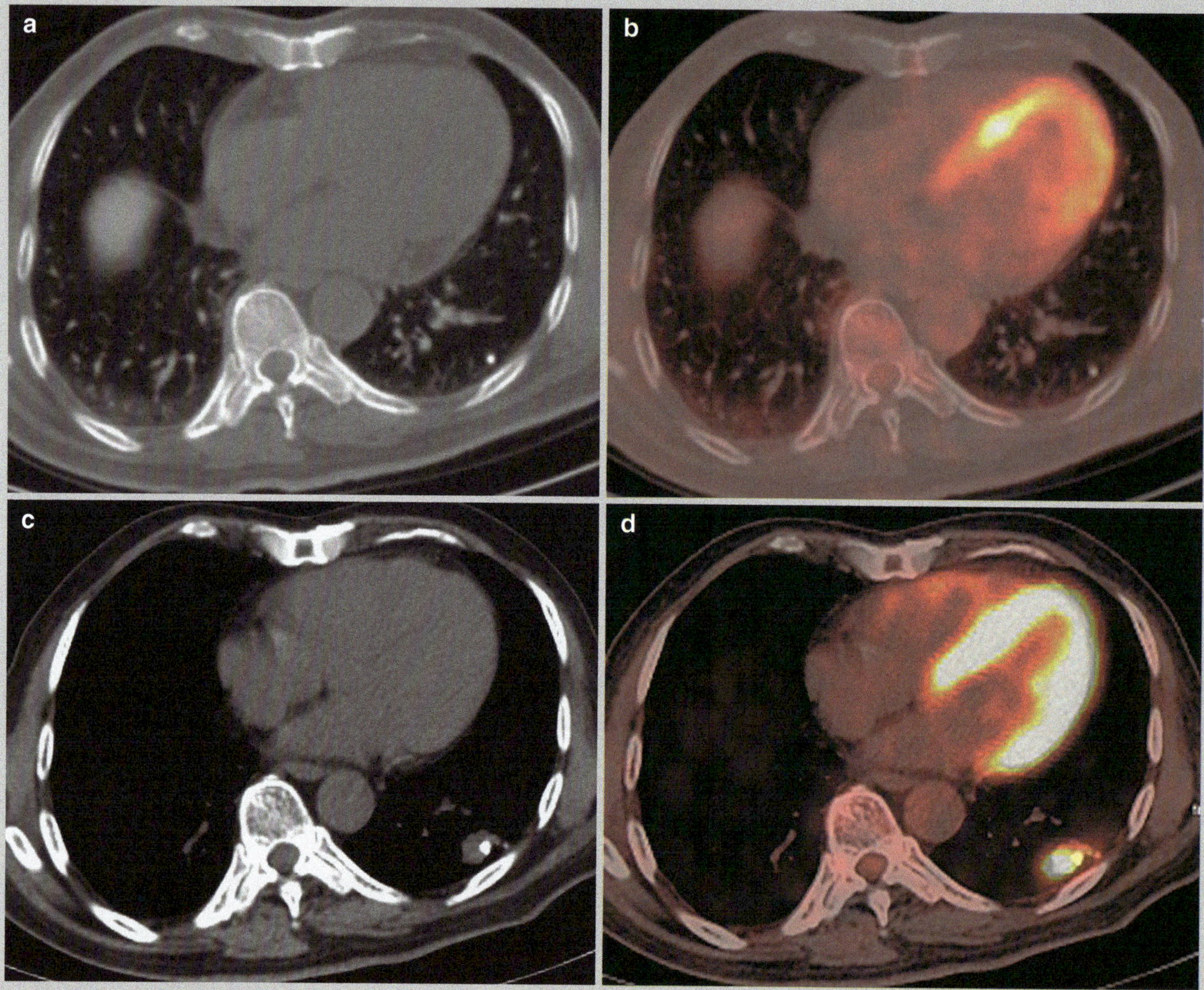

Fig. 21.29 Tuberculoma. (**a**, **b**) During a routine physical examination 18 months ago, CT scanning demonstrates spots of calcifications at the posterior basilar segment of the left lower lung lobe. PET/CT demonstrates no metabolism at the lesion. (**c**, **d**) By a recent reexamination, CT scanning demonstrates that calcification is surrounded by soft tissue density shadows with smooth and regular margin. PET/CT demonstrates increased metabolism of the soft tissue density shadows with SUVmax11.0, which is suspected to be lung cancer. Pathology after surgery indicates tuberculosis

21.7.2 Extrapulmonary Tuberculosis

21.7.2.1 Tuberculous Meningoencephalitis

Tuberculous meningoencephalitis is a disease caused by the invasion of MTB along with blood flow or directly into the subarachnoid space to involve the pia mater and arachnoid membranes and further involvements of the cranial nerves, brain parenchyma, cerebrovascular vessels, and spinal cord.

CT Scanning

CT scanning demonstrates increased meninx density, which is commonly found at the suprasellar cistern, ambient cistern, and lateral cerebral fissure. Extensive thickening and increased density are demonstrated at the contours of the cistern and sulcus as well as the meninx. By contrast scanning, obvious enhancement can be demonstrated.

CT scanning also demonstrates miliary lesions at the brain parenchyma. The fine miliary nodular shadows with equal density are extensively distributed at the cerebral cortex or brain tissue. By contrast scanning, enhancement can be demonstrated.

By CT scanning, ring shape, disk like, mass like and spots of shadows are demonstrated, which are characteristic signs of cerebral tuberculoma. Contrast scanning demonstrates ring-shaped enhancement with central low density and peripheral high density. The surrounding edema is comparatively mild, with slight space-occupying effect.

Ventricular dilation and hydrocephalus can also be demonstrated by CT scanning. Due to various degrees of obstruction at different locations of the passage for cerebrospinal fluid flow, the ventricle is subject to different degrees of dilation. In the cases with slight dilation, the anterior horn of the lateral ventricle is blunt. In the cases with moderate dilation, the lateral ventricle undergoes slight dilation. In the cases with severe dilation, the lateral ventricle undergoes obvious expansion, with compression of the adjacent brain parenchyma. Ventricular dilation and effusion are also commonly demonstrated at the 3rd ventricle.

Cerebral edema is another important sign by CT scanning. The flakes of shadows are demonstrated with low density and poorly defined boundary. The lesion is commonly located around the cerebral TB lesions or around the dilated ventricle due to hydrocephalus. By contrast scanning, the area with hydrocephalus is demonstrated with no enhancement.

Cerebral infarction is demonstrated to be singular or multiple and the lesion is in low density. Due to different sizes of the lesions, the shape of the lesions varies, which are commonly located at the area supplied by the middle cerebral artery. By contrast scanning, the lesion of cerebral infarction is demonstrated with no enhancement.

Cord-like or nodular shadows are also demonstrated by CT scanning. Cord-like shadows are demonstration of tuberculous arteritis, with increased density, and can be enhanced by contrast scanning. Nodular shadows are formed by small tuberculous proliferative lesions, with increased density, and can be enhanced by contrast scanning.

Calcification demonstrated by CT scanning is possibly located at the nodules of cerebral tuberculoma, cistern, and meninges.

MR Imaging

MR imaging can demonstrate early or small lesions and can demonstrate early tuberculous meningitis with abnormal signal shadows at the basal cistern, cerebral convex meninges, and sylvian cistern, with relative high T1WI signal and high T2WI signal. After the injection of Gd-DTAP, T1WI demonstrates meningeal enhancement at the basal cistern and diffuse meningeal enhancement (Figs. 21.30 and 21.31).

Brain tuberculoma is demonstrated by T1WI with equal signal to the gray matter and by T2WI with mostly uneven low signal or slightly high signal. Edema around brain tuberculoma is mild with high T2WI signal. After the injection of Gd-DTAP, the lesion of brain tuberculoma is demonstrated with nodular enhancement or ring-shaped enhancement (Fig. 21.32).

Case Study 30

A boy aged 13 years was diagnosed with tuberculous meningitis. In June 2012, he experienced repeated severe headache, non-ejective vomiting of gastric content, and intermittent attacks of fever with the highest body temperature of 39 °C. By laboratory tests, examination of the cerebrospinal fluid following lumbar puncture showed positive protein and WBC 300×10^6/L. The clinical diagnosis was tuberculous meningitis, and the patient was given anti-TB treatment. The symptoms such as headache and vomiting then were improved, and the body temperature returned to normal, but still with intermittent dizziness and poor appetite.

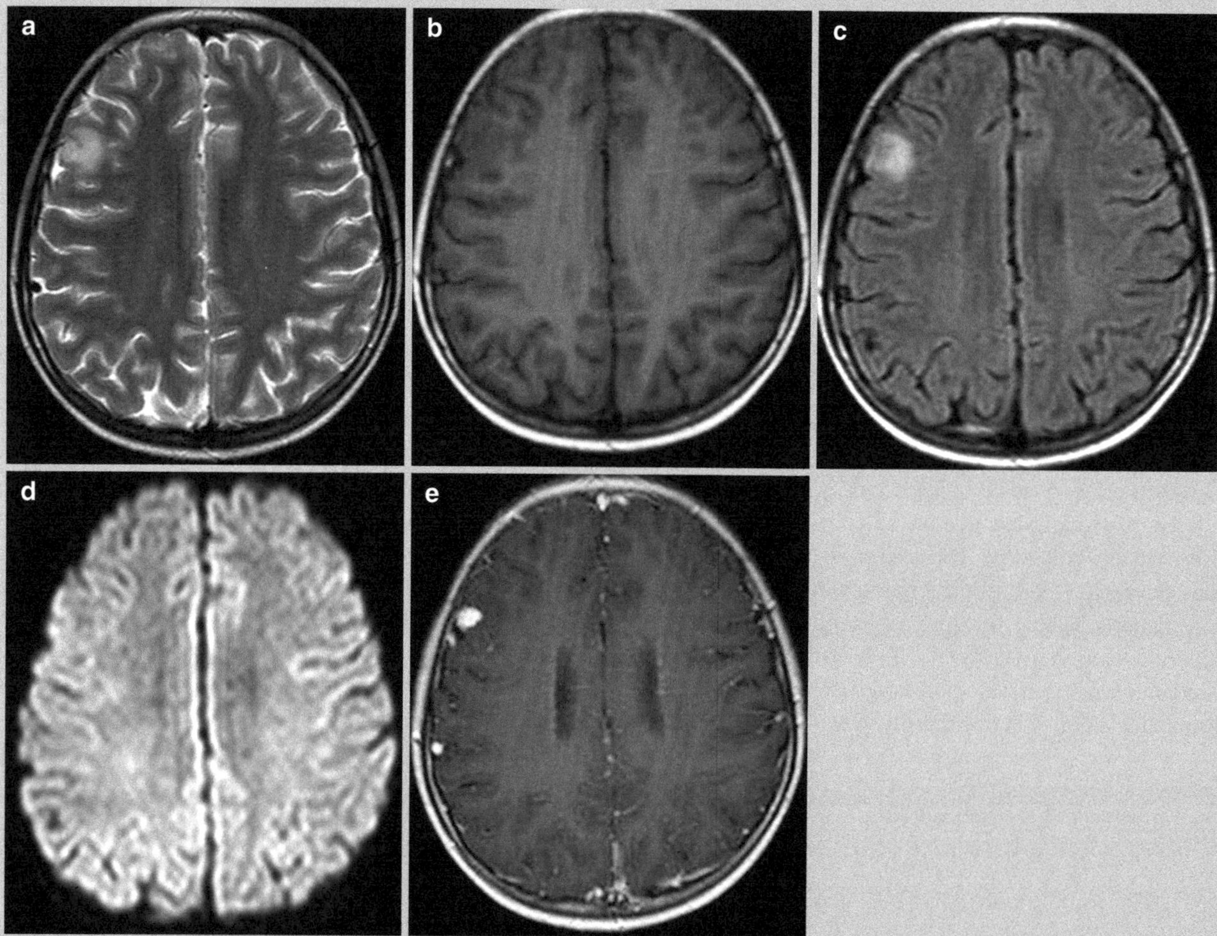

Fig. 21.30 Tuberculous meningitis. (**a**–**e**) MR imaging demonstrates multiple nodular abnormal signal shadows at both brain hemispheres, with low T1WI signal and high T2WI signal. The water suppression sequence demonstrates high signal, and DWI slightly low signal. The lesions are poorly defined with obvious surrounding edema. By contrast imaging, the lesions are demonstrated with nodular enhancement

Case Study 31

A female patient aged 23 years was diagnosed with tuberculous meningitis. In February 2011, she experienced sudden nausea, frequent vomiting of gastric content with no known causes. She also developed aversion to cold, fever, and headache, but no chills. Her highest temperature reached 38.3 °C. After oral intake of the analgesic-antipyretic drug with no prescription, her headache did not improve, but gradually worsened. The high body temperature can return to normal, but with repeated occurrence. On March 7, the patient experienced severe and unbearable headache. By lumbar puncture and following examination, the WBC count increases, indicating infection of the central nervous system.

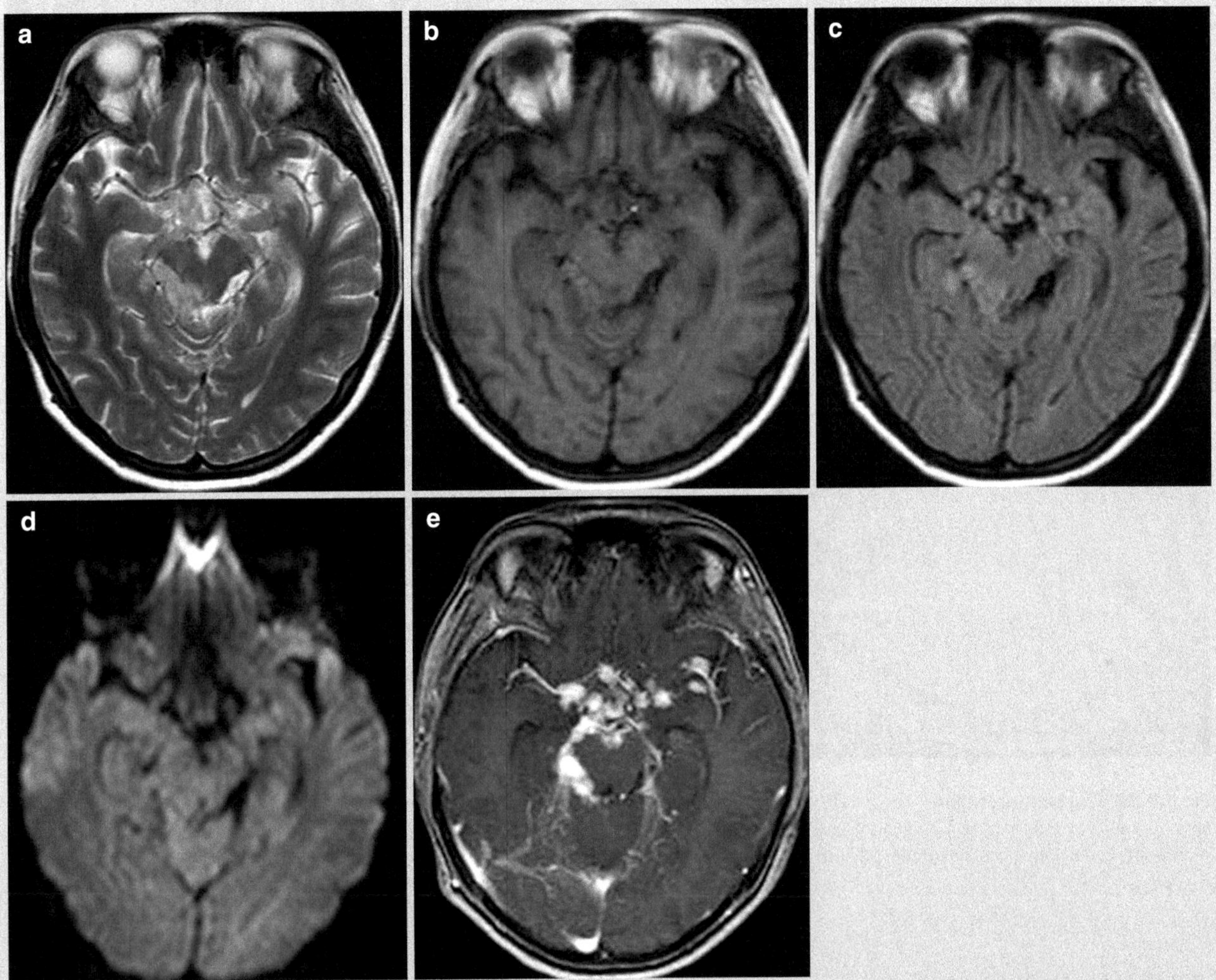

Fig. 21.31 Tuberculous meningitis. (**a**–**e**) MR imaging demonstrates obvious thickening of meninges at the suprasellar cistern and quadrigeminal cistern, with low T1WI signal and high T2WI signal. The water suppression sequence demonstrates high signal, while DWI slightly high signal. Contrast imaging demonstrates nodular enhancement

Case Study 32

A male patient aged 21 years was diagnosed with cerebral tuberculosis.

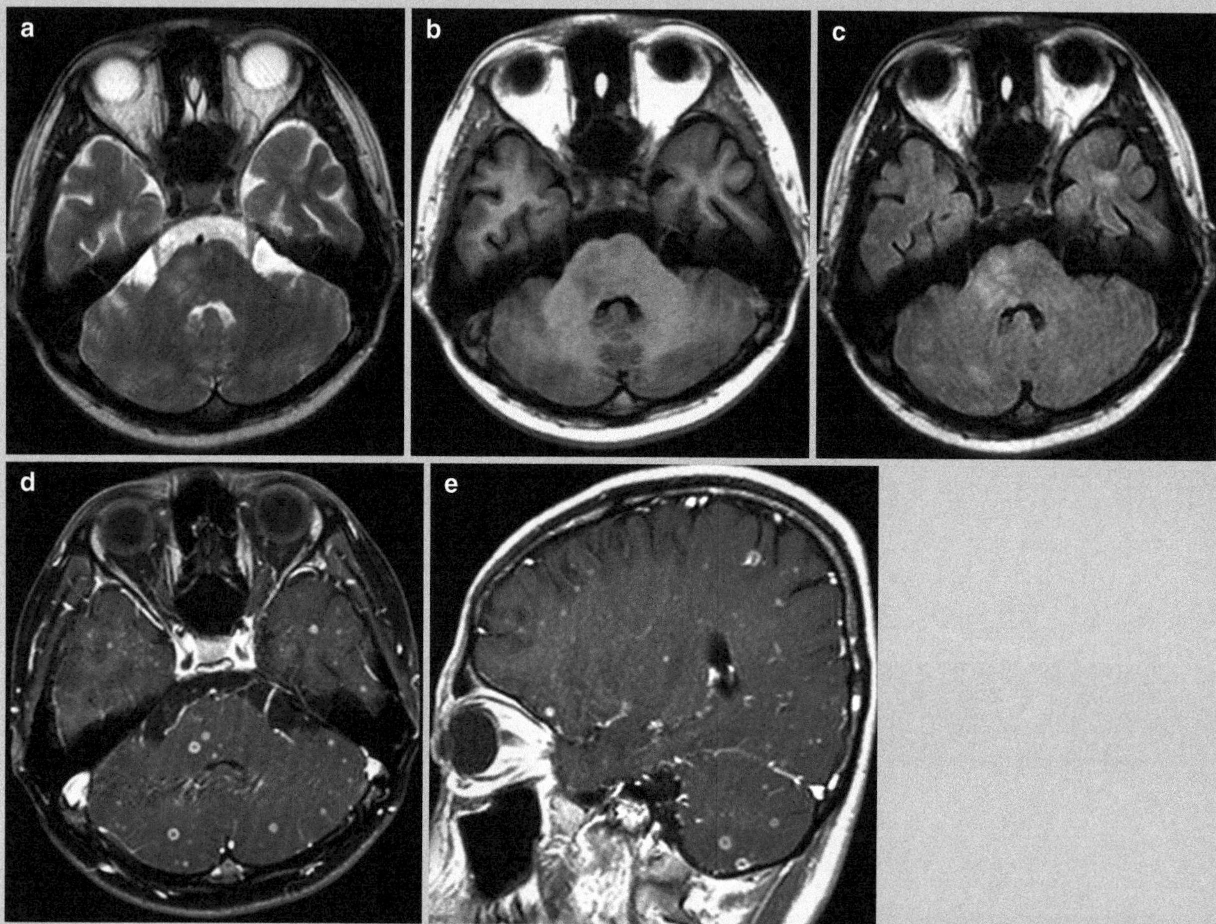

Fig. 21.32 Cerebral tuberculosis. (**a–c**) MR imaging demonstrates slightly long T1 slightly long T2 signal of patches of shadows at the brainstem, cerebellum, and left temporal lobe, with poorly defined boundary. (**d, e**) Contrast imaging demonstrates multiple military, nodular enhancement of the lesions at the brainstem, cerebellum, and bilateral brain hemispheres and ring-shaped enhancement of some lesions

21.7.2.2 Hepatic Tuberculosis

Ultrasound

Different pathological types of hepatic TB granuloma are demonstrated with different ultrasound findings. The lesions based on liquefaction, necrosis, and sparse pus are demonstrated with no echo but internal fine light spots. The lesions based on caseous necrosis is demonstrated with low echo, with internal even echo and well-defined boundary. The lesions of fibrous proliferation and calcification are demonstrated as an irregular strong echo.

CT Scanning

For the cases with miliary hepatic TB, CT scanning demonstrates enlarged liver and multiple miliary lesions with low density in the liver.

For the cases with nodular hepatic TB, CT scanning demonstrates uneven density in the nodular shadow, commonly with fine spots and spots of calcification. By contrast scanning and marginal enhancement can be demonstrated.

MR Imaging

MR imaging demonstrates hepatic TB lesion with low T1WI signal and equal or high T2WI signal.

Case Study 33

A female patient aged 46 years was diagnosed with hepatic TB (Fig. 21.33).

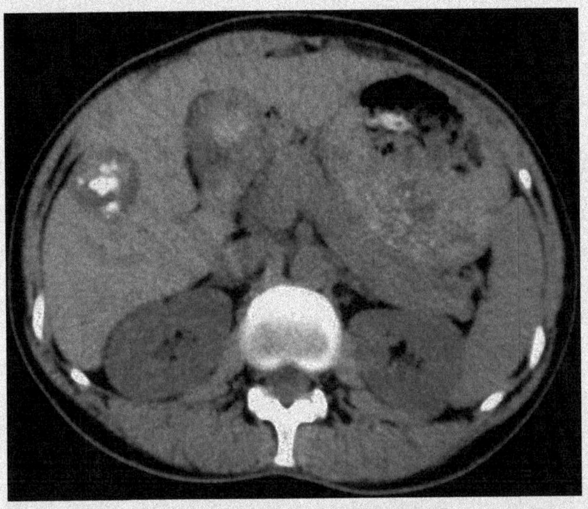

Fig. 21.33 Hepatic TB. CT scanning demonstrates round-like shadow at the right liver lobe with mixed density, internal low-density shadow, and scattering spots of calcification. The margins of the lesions are mostly well-defined and regular

21.7.2.3 Splenic Tuberculosis

Ultrasound

Nodular splenic TB is demonstrated by ultrasound as weak echo nodule with well-defined boundary and regular shape. The internal echo is uneven, with less blood flow signal. The demonstrations of abscess splenic TB by ultrasound resemble to those of non-tuberculous splenic abscess, with space-occupying effect of cystic consolidation in the spleen. There are commonly fibrous proliferation and calcification, with irregular strong echo.

CT Scanning

CT scanning commonly demonstrates splenomegaly. For the cases with nodular splenic TB, CT scanning demonstrates low or equal density nodular shadows with poorly defined boundary. By contrast scanning, the lesions are demonstrated with no enhancement and ring-shaped enhancement of rare lesions. For the cases of abscess splenic TB, CT scanning demonstrates singular or multiple round-like low-density shadows in the spleen. Contrast scanning demonstrates marginal enhancement. The spleen is also demonstrated with spots or small nodular lesions of calcification.

MR Imaging

Nodular splenic TB is commonly demonstrated as mostly equal or low T2WI signal. Abscess splenic TB is demonstrated as equal or low T1WI signal and high T2WI signal or centrally irregular high surrounded by low signal by T2WI.

21.7.2.4 Intestinal Tuberculosis

Barium Meal Radiology

Barium meal radiology or barium enema examination is important for the diagnosis of intestinal tuberculosis. For the cases complicated by intestinal obstruction, barium enema examination is appropriate to avoid aggravated intestinal obstruction by barium meal.

The Ulcerative Type

At the early stage, due to the stimulation by inflammation and ulceration to the involved intestinal segment, obvious irritation sign as barium passes through is demonstrated. The manifestations include accelerated emptying of barium, with no or a small quantity residue of barium, while favorable filling state of proximal and distal lesion, just like a skip of barium over an intestinal segment, which is known as skip sign. The mucosa at the lesion is subject to irregular thickening and derangement, while the intestinal wall is demonstrated with spots and serration-like niche. In the advanced stage of the lesion, due to shrinkage of fibrous tissue, fibrous proliferation, and thickened intestinal wall, the intestinal lumen is subject to stenosis, deformation, as well as dilation and stasis of the proximal part. In addition, ileocecal TB can induce confined peritonitis to cause adhesion of the peritoneum to its surrounding intestine.

The Proliferative Type

This type is mainly manifested as irregular deformation and stenosis of the intestinal lumen, with accompanying rough and deranged mucosa, multiple small polypoid, or space-occupying filling defect. But niche and irritation sign are rare. In the cases of simplex proliferative TB, the irritation sign is not obvious. But if accompanied by ulceration, the irritation sign may be observable. Due to submucosal and subserosal proliferation of fibrous tissue, the intestinal wall is thickened to cause intestinal stenosis. In severe cases, partial intestinal obstruction occurs, with dilation of the proximal ileum. When the ileocecal valve is invaded, it is subject to proliferation and thickening, with depression at the inner wall of cecum to affect the emptying of small intestines. When the cecum and ascending colon are involved, the intestinal lumen is subject to narrowing and shortening. The mucosal folds are subject to derangement and proliferation, mostly with polypoid filling defect, which should be differentiated from intestinal cancer. In the cases with ileum and ileocecal valve involved, the diagnosis should be suspected as tuberculosis. If accompanied by lumen adhesion, the intestinal lumen is disorderly arranged and accumulated, and the loops can hardly be separated, with tenderness. In the cases with ascites, the flexure intervals are widened with a floating-like appearance. The flexure can also be compressed to the middle abdomen by ascites, commonly with no intestinal flexure in the pelvic cavity.

CT Scanning

CT scanning demonstrates the involved intestinal segment with obvious thickening of the intestinal wall. Contrast scanning demonstrates obvious enhancement of the involved intestinal segment with stratification. In the cases complicated by abdominal lymphatic TB, the swollen lymph nodes are demonstrated with ring-shaped enhancement. Intestinal TB can involve surrounding tissues of the intestinal canal to cause tuberculous inflammation or tuberculous granulation tissue and caseous necrosis. By plain scanning, the surrounding adipose is demonstrated to be turbid with increased density. If accompanied by caseous necrosis, the density is uneven, with obvious peripheral enhancement and no or slight enhancement of caseous necrosis. The mesenteric lymph nodes are enlarged and calcified. The ring-shaped enhancement of lesions around the affected intestinal canal and the enlarged and calcified mesenteric lymph nodes are important and characteristic signs for the diagnosis of abdominal TB.

Case Study 34

A male patient aged 30 years was confirmatively diagnosed with HIV infection 2 months ago. After intake of Zongzi (glutinous rice dumpling), he experienced intermittent abdominal pain and accompanying abdominal distention, nausea, and vomiting. He also reported terminated anal discharge of gas and stool. Abdominal plain scanning suggested intestinal obstruction. Pathology after an exploratory laparotomy demonstrated the diagnosis of abdominal lymphatic TB and mesenteric necrosis (Fig. 21.34).

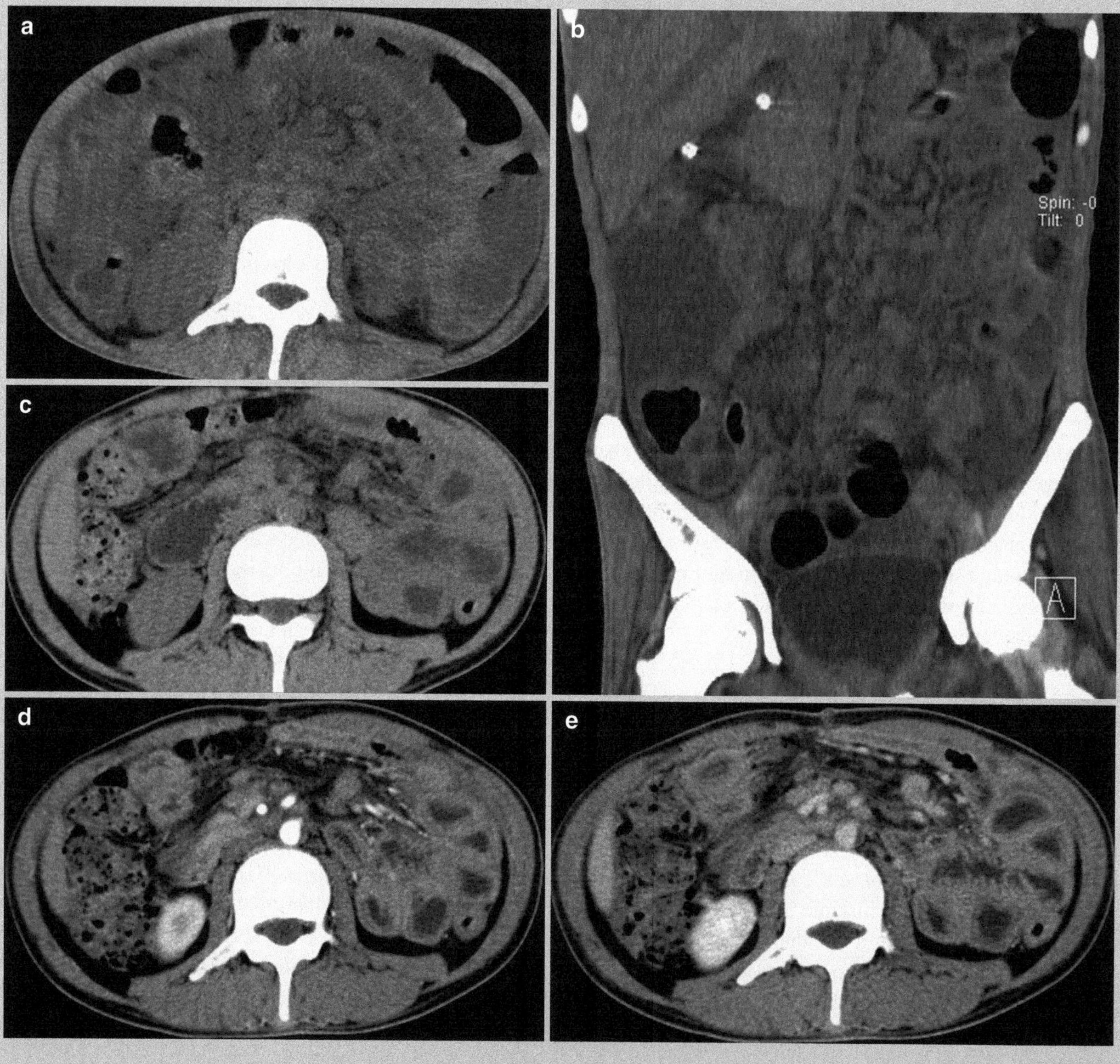

Fig. 21.34 Intestinal TB. (**a**, **b**) Plain CT scanning demonstrates thickened intestinal wall with edema, multiple enlarged lymph nodes at the mesenteric root and retroperitoneum, and abdominal effusion. (**c**–**e**) By reexamination after exploratory laparotomy and following treatment for 2 months, CT scanning demonstrates absent ascites, enlarged lymph nodes at the abdominal cavity, and retroperitoneum. By contrast scanning, the lesions are demonstrated with ring-shaped enhancement

21.7.2.5 Kidney TB

Ultrasound

In the cases of kidney TB with cold abscess or caseous necrosis at the renal parenchyma, ultrasound demonstrates the renal parenchyma with low echo area or liquid dark area with poorly defined boundary. In the cases with fibrosis or calcification, ultrasound demonstrates bright light spots, masses, or strips. In the cases with calcification, posterior acoustic shadow can be demonstrated.

CT Scanning

At the early stage of kidney TB, CT scanning demonstrates no abnormalities. But at the advanced stage, CT scanning is superior to intravenous urography in demonstrating the lesions, with protrusion of local kidney contour outwards or enlarged kidney. Thinning and atrophy of mainly renal cortex can also be demonstrated due to stenosis of renal arteries induced by fibrosis of renal TB. The renal parenchyma is demonstrated with multiple round or oval liquid-like density shadows with different sizes and poorly defined boundaries. The renal parenchyma is also demonstrated with spots, small nodules, or egg shell-like calcification. The renal pelvis wall is demonstrated to be thickened, partially with linear or arch-like calcification shadow. The ipsilateral urethral wall is demonstrated to be thickened (Fig. 21.35). The renal pelvis and urethral wall of the affected kidney are subject to dilation and effusion. Contrast CT scanning demonstrates no obvious enhancement of the early lesions at the early stage, and based on which it should be differentiated from neoplasms. Meanwhile, the function of the affected kidney can be assessed.

Intravenous Pyelography (IVP)

The typical demonstration by IVP is destructed renal calices. The renal calices are subject to irregular worm-bitten-like margin, narrowed cervix with irregular margin, and deformation. The renal parenchyma is subject to cavities with different sizes and shapes. The pelvis margin is destructed and deformed. The pelvis and urethra of the affected kidney are subject to effusion. Meanwhile, based on the rate and degree of imaging, the function of the affected kidney can be assessed.

Case Study 35

A male patient aged 53 years was diagnosed with right kidney TB.

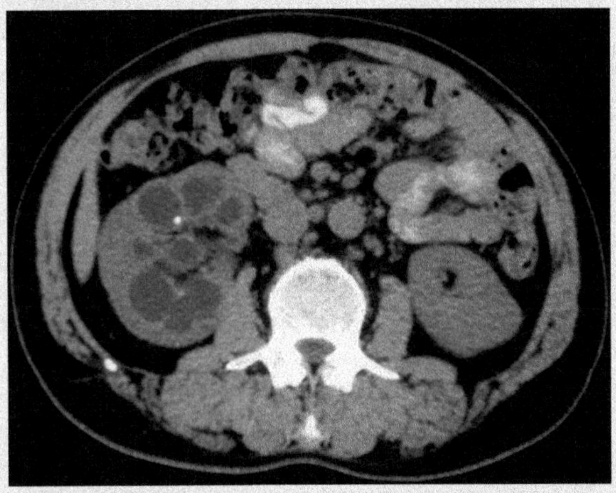

Fig. 21.35 Kidney TB. CT scanning demonstrates enlarged right kidney, and wavelike local kidney margin. There are also multiple oval shape liquid density shadows with different sizes and poorly defined boundaries at the right renal parenchyma, with marginal calcification at one shadow

MR Imaging

By T1WI, the corticomedullary interface is absent, with low-density lesions of different sizes at the kidney. The renal sinus shifts or is absent. By T2WI, the lesions are demonstrated with high signal.

21.7.2.6 Spinal TB

Ultrasound

By ultrasound, cold abscess is demonstrated as unilateral or bilateral paravertebral even or uneven low echo areas under the anterior longitudinal ligament with different sizes. In the abscess cavity or on the abscess wall, there are spots and patches of strong echoes, which are caused by calcification of abscess or fragments of sequestra.

CT Scanning

1. Bone destruction

   In the cases of spinal TB, bone destruction is common at the vertebra but rare destruction of vertebral appendix. The lesions are morphologically irregular, with worm-bitten-like margin. In some bone destruction areas, small fragments of sequestra can be observed.

2. Narrowed intervertebral space

   The bone destruction at the upper or lower margin of the vertebral body leads to flattening of the affected vertebra, which further causes destruction of adjacent intervertebral disks. By 3-dimensional reconstruction, the lesions of adjacent two vertebral TB induce narrowing of the intervertebral space between the two vertebrae.

3. Paravertebral soft tissue mass

   Around the affected vertebra, soft tissue swelling can be observed. In the swollen soft tissue, there are liquid-like low-density areas with poorly defined boundary and commonly accompanying spots and patches of calcification.

4. Involvement of the spinal canal

   After bone destruction of the vertebra and appendix, the caseous lesions, fragments of sequestra, and granulation tissues penetrate into the adjacent spinal canal to cause secondary spinal canal stenosis (Fig. 21.36).

MR Imaging

Spinal TB is demonstrated as low T1WI signal and often mixed high T2WI signal. MR imaging can demonstrate the location and range of paravertebral soft tissue abnormality and cold abscess. Paravertebral soft tissue shadow is commonly demonstrated as low T1WI signal and mixed high T2WI signal, and some are demonstrated as homogeneous high signal. MR imaging can demonstrate the degree and range of spinal involvement as well as spinal ischemia and degeneration (Fig. 21.37).

Case Study 36

A female patient aged 46 years was diagnosed with thoracic spinal TB.

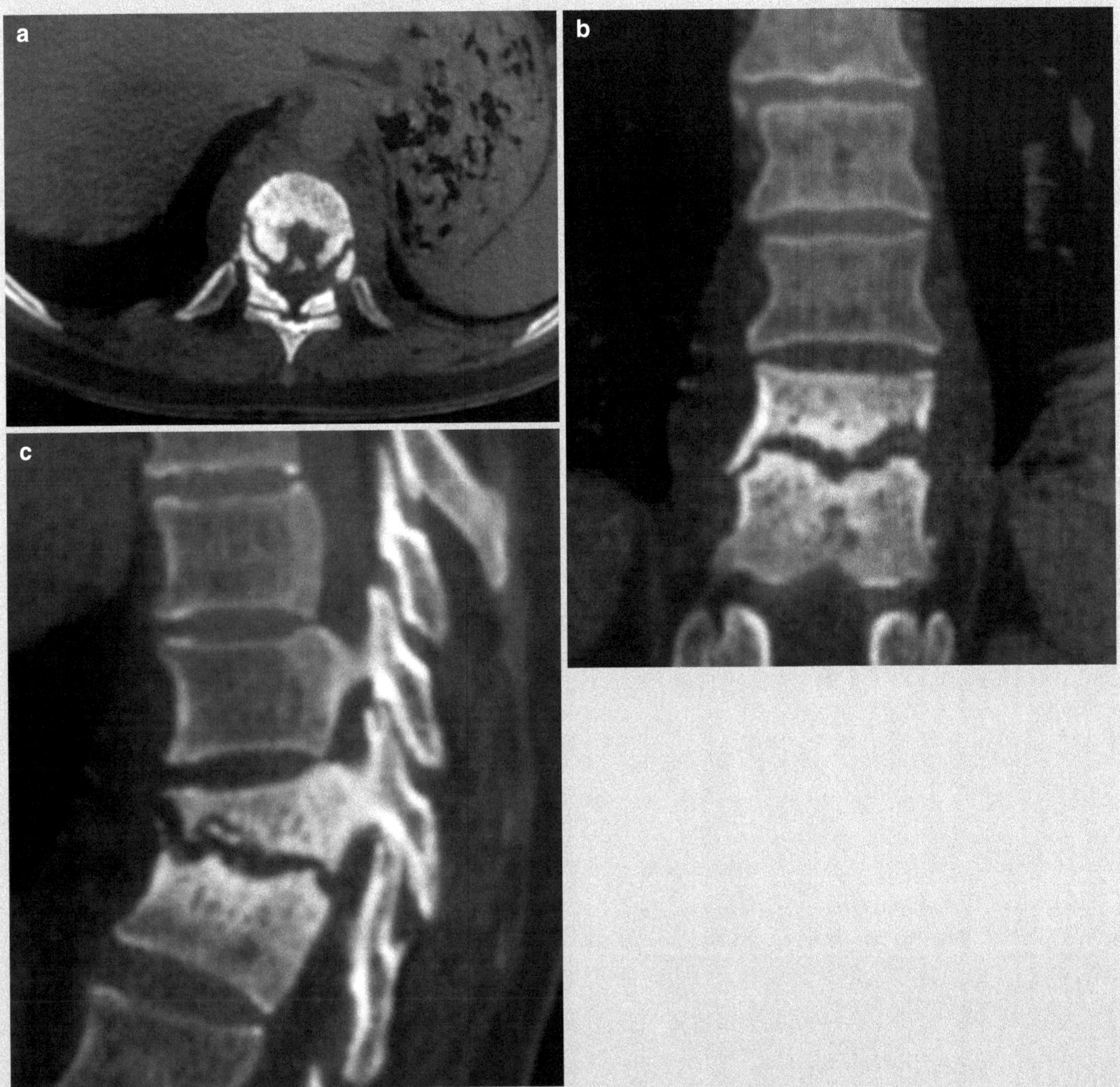

Fig. 21.36 Thoracic spinal TB. (**a–c**) CT scanning demonstrates bone destruction of adjacent two thoracic vertebrae with worm-bitten-like margin. At the superior vertebra, small sequestra shadow is observable. The intervertebral space between the two affected vertebrae is narrowed. The spine is subject to slight kyphosis with the two vertebrae as the center. In the paravertebral soft tissue, spindle-shaped abscess shadow can be observed

Case Study 37

A female patient aged 25 years experienced repeated pain at the lower back and the back 3 months ago. The symptoms aggravated several weeks later, with slight impaired movement and numbness of the lower limbs. Chest CT scanning demonstrated abnormal density at the lung and bone destruction at the T9 vertebra, with paravertebral abscess. The diagnosis was then suspected to be tuberculosis. PPD skin test was positive.

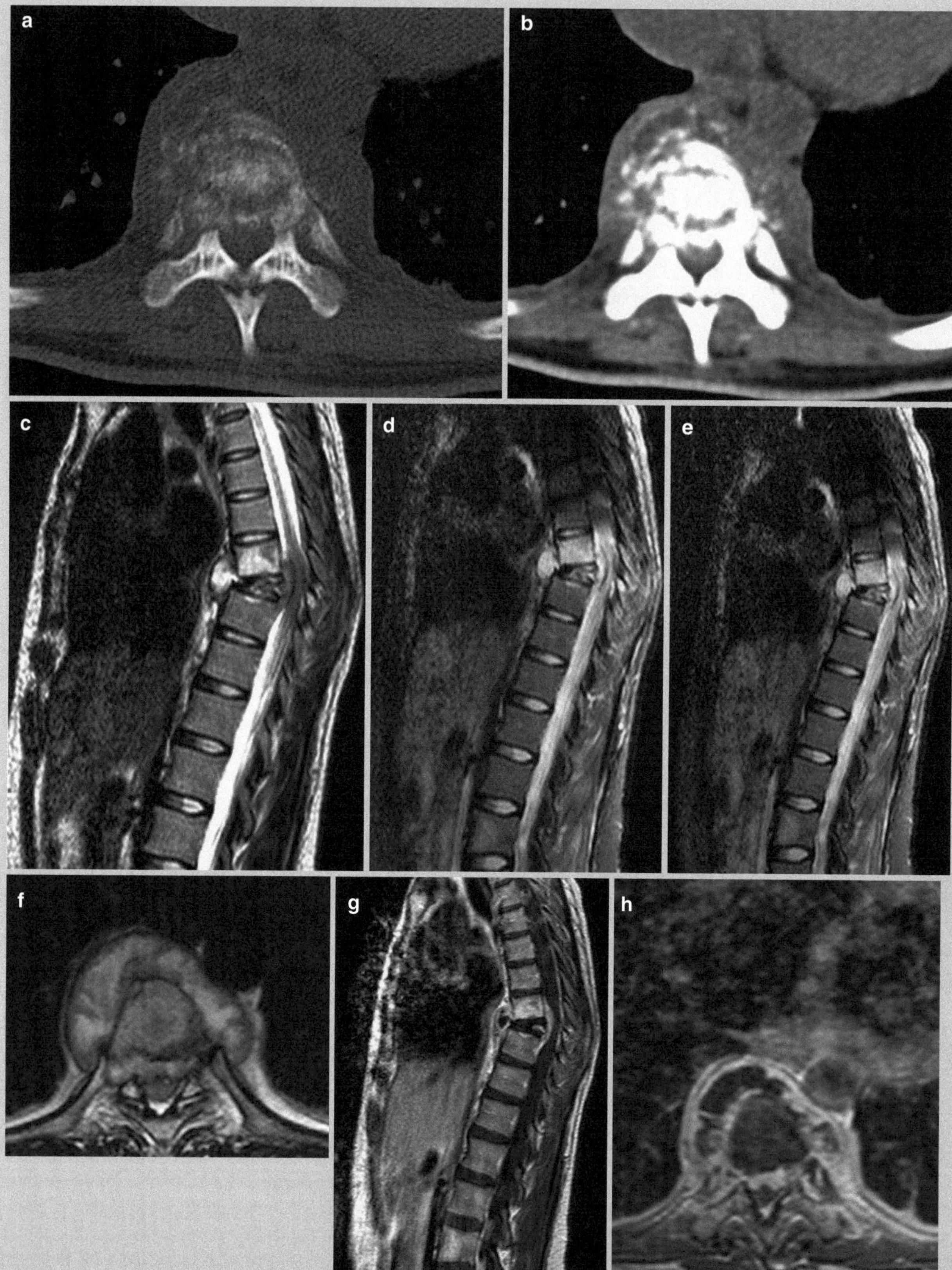

Fig. 21.37 Thoracic spinal TB. (**a**, **b**) CT scanning demonstrates obvious bone destruction at the vertebral body, paravertebral abscess, and stenosis of the vertebral canal. (**c–h**) MR imaging demonstrates obvious compression and bone destruction at T9, with decreased T1WI signal of the vertebral body and increased T2WI signal, with wedge shape change. Local angular deformity penetrates into the vertebral canal, with thin spinal cord at the corresponding level. The adjacent intervertebral discs are demonstrated with decreased T2WI signal and thick homogeneous ringlike signals at paravertebral area of T9, with internal long T1 and long T2 signal. Contrast imaging by Gd-DTPA demonstrates ring-shaped enhancement. T8 and L3 are demonstrated with flakes of high T2WI signal, with enhancement by contrast imaging

21.8 Diagnostic Basis

The diagnosis of pulmonary TB requires comprehensive analysis of epidemiological data, clinical manifestations, laboratory findings, and radiological demonstrations. The diagnoses are mainly based on findings by X-ray, CT scanning, and sputum examination for pathogenic bacteria. Positive finding by sputum smear for acid-fast bacillus or sputum MTB culture, tuberculous granuloma by biopsy of lung tissue, and tubercles or caseous necrosis are the gold criteria for the diagnosis of pulmonary TB.

21.8.1 Diagnosis of Pulmonary TB

21.8.1.1 Primary Pulmonary TB

It is more common in children and adolescents.

The patients experience mild TB toxic symptoms, such as erythema nodosum as well as joint swelling and pain.

The respiratory signs are rare. The children patients often experience hepatomegaly, splenomegaly, and rarely cervical superficial lymphadenectasis.

Fibro-bronchoscopy demonstrates bronchial stenosis, chronic inflammation of bronchial mucosa, and lympho-bronchial fistula.

PPD skin test is commonly positive.

Sputum smear for acid-fast bacillus is positive, or gastric fluid examination for acid-fast bacillus is significant to define the diagnosis.

Radiological examinations demonstrate bipolar dumbbell sign or hilar lymphadenectasis and hilar inflammatory infiltration.

21.8.1.2 Hematogenous Disseminated Pulmonary TB

Prior to onset, the patients may experience conditions to compromise immunity, such as acute infectious disease, alcoholism and catching a cold, fatigue, delivery, and use of large doses of immunosuppressants. Otherwise, they are high-risk population before the onset.

The onset is acute and sudden, with high fever, night sweating, weakness, and dyspnea. The patients may also experience hepatosplenomegaly, cerebral meningeal irritation sign, and sometimes choroidal tubercle at the ocular fundus.

By laboratory tests, blood erythrocyte sedimentation rate is accelerated, with change of WBC count. PPD skin test is positive (negative cannot be excluded). Anti-TB antibody is positive. Sputum smear for acid-fast bacillus is positive.

By radiological examinations, typical miliary nodular shadows are demonstrated at both lungs, with three-evens sign or three-unevens sign.

Various biopsies facilitate to define the diagnosis.

21.8.1.3 Secondary Pulmonary TB

The clinical manifestations include repeated or prolonged cough with sputum, low-grade fever, night sweating, emaciation, and poor appetite for over 2 weeks. Regular anti-infective therapy is ineffective. High-risk population of TB should be attended more carefully.

By physical examination, no obvious positive sign can be found.

By laboratory test, the blood WBC count is commonly normal, possibly with anemia and rapid ESR. CRP obviously increases and PPD skin test is positive. Sputum smear for acid-fast bacillus is positive, and/or sputum MTB culture is positive. Biopsy of lung tissue can define the diagnosis of TB. BALF smear for acid-fast bacillus is positive. The finding of TB lesions by bronchial or lung tissue biopsy can define the diagnosis. DNA detection of MTB, serum anti-TB antibody test, and effective trial anti-TB therapy facilitate the diagnosis of TB.

X-ray and CT scanning demonstrate cloud-like, nodular patches of lesions with mixed existence, especially the accompanying cavities and its satellite lesions. These lesions fail to be absorbed after short-term anti-infective treatment.

21.8.2 Diagnosis of Extrapulmonary TB

21.8.2.1 Tuberculous Pleuritis

Tuberculous Dry Pleuritis

Based on the case history, the patients with clinical manifestations of low-grade fever or moderate fever, dry cough, severe stabbing chest pain, and local pleural friction can be diagnosed with tuberculous dry pleuritis. X-ray and CT scanning demonstrate pleural thickening with poorly defined boundary. MR imaging demonstrates linear moderate or low T1WI signal shadow and slightly high or high T2WI signal.

Tuberculous Exudative Pleuritis

The patients commonly have a past history of TB and clinically experience moderate fever, early chest pain with following alleviation, and dyspnea.

Radiological examinations demonstrate pleural effusion.

By diagnostic thoracic puncture for routine examination of pleural effusion, biochemical examination and bacterial culture are necessary examinations to define the diagnosis. In such ways, about 75 % of cases with pleural effusion can be etiologically diagnosed.

21.8.2.2 Tuberculous Meningoencephalitis

The patients commonly have a past history of TB and an unobvious onset with TB toxic symptoms, including intracranial hypertension, meningeal irritation sign, cerebral nerve impairment, and consciousness disturbance.

By laboratory tests, the cerebrospinal fluid is demonstrated with abnormalities, including cell count increase that is mainly lymphocytes, increased protein level, decreased glucose and chloride levels, and detected MTB.

CT scanning and MR imaging demonstrate meningeal thickening that is mainly at the cranial base, obvious enhancement of the choroid and/or tuberculoma at the cerebral parenchyma, and tuberculous granuloma.

21.8.2.3 Hepatic TB

The patients experience hepatic pain and upset, TB toxic symptoms, extrahepatic TB, and a past history of TB.

Laboratory findings support the diagnosis of TB, such as PCR, TB-Ab, and PPD skin test.

Radiological demonstrations are varied. Localized hepatic TB is commonly located at the marginal liver, with singular or multiple low-density lesions and accompanying fine spots or spots of calcification. In the abdominal cavity, calcified swollen lymph nodes are demonstrated, with ring-shaped enhancement of the lesions by contrast radiological examination.

The diagnosis of hepatic TB can be defined based on liver tissue biopsy.

21.8.2.4 Splenic TB

The patients usually have extrasplenic TB lesion or a past history of TB, with TB toxic symptoms and signs.

By laboratory tests, the findings include anemia, rapid ESR, as well as increased neutrophils and lymphocytes.

By radiological examinations, the spleen is enlarged, with multiple round lesions in the spleen but no enhancement or slight marginal enhancement.

Puncture of lymph node for biopsy, laparoscopy, or spleen puncture for biopsy demonstrates infection of MTB. By serous cavity fluid examination, MTB is detected.

Experimental anti-TB therapy is effective to alleviate the symptoms.

21.8.2.5 Intestinal TB

The patients are commonly young and middle age adults with extrenteral TB, especially open pulmonary TB with accompanying gastrointestinal symptoms.

The patients experience fever, night sweating, abdominal pain, diarrhea, and constipation. In addition, the patients may also experience right lower abdominal tenderness, mass, and intestinal obstruction with no known causes.

Barium meal radiology demonstrates irritation sign, barium filling defect, intestinal canal stenosis, as well as intestinal canal shortening and deformation.

21.8.2.6 Kidney TB

The diagnosis of kidney TB is mainly based on detected MTB in urine specimen and the corresponding radiological demonstrations. The commonly applied radiological examinations include urography and CT scanning, which can demonstrate the range, severity, and stage of the lesions. Especially, urography can demonstrate early renal calices lesion. But CT scanning can sensitively detect the lesions with calcification. Both facilitate to define the diagnosis.

21.8.2.7 Spinal TB

The symptoms of spinal TB are unobvious, with long illness course. It refers to osteolytic destruction of at least two vertebrae with narrowed or absent intervertebral space and spinal kyphosis. Paravertebral abscess and soft tissue calcification are characteristic X-ray demonstrations of spinal TB. CT scanning can define the unobvious bone destruction as well as the position and range of paravertebral abscess. MR imaging can detect early vertebral TB lesions, which fail to be demonstrated by X-ray and CT scanning. It is superior to CT scanning in demonstrating soft tissue changes and invasions into the spinal canal.

21.8.3 Pulmonary TB-Related Complications

21.8.3.1 Hemoptysis

The patients commonly have a history of pulmonary TB and recent history of hemoptysis.

CT scanning demonstrates pulmonary tuberculosis and patches of ground-glass shadows. Reexamination of CT scanning demonstrates obvious absorption or complete absorption of the lesions.

21.8.3.2 Spontaneous Pneumothorax

X-ray and CT scanning demonstrations provide main evidence to define the diagnosis. The typical demonstrations include increased transparency of the lesion, absent lung markings, and fine linear soft tissue density shadow. In combination to the symptoms, signs, and etiological factors, the diagnosis can be defined.

21.8.3.3 Tuberculous Bronchiectasis

The patients commonly have a history of pulmonary TB. After appropriate anti-TB treatment, the conditions are stable, with the following occurrence of hemoptysis and expectoration. In addition, bubble sound at the fixed location is commonly heard.

X-ray demonstrates cord-like patches and curled hairlike shadows. CT scanning demonstrates larger diameter of bronchus than its accompanying bronchial artery.

21.9 Differential Diagnosis

21.9.1 Lobar Pneumonia

Tuberculous lobar pneumonia and caseous pneumonia are radiologically demonstrated as lobar or segmental exudative consolidation shadows at the lungs. Both commonly occur at the upper lung lobe. Tuberculous exudative lesion is commonly concurrent with proliferative lesion and caseous lesion.

Lobar pneumonia is radiologically demonstrated as lobar or segmental exudative consolidation shadows. Its occurrence is commonly at each lung lobe, with basically even density of flakes of shadows. In the cases with the flakes of shadows involving adjacent interlobar fissure, interlobar pleural septum can be sharply demonstrated. With the interlobar pleura as the separation, the affected side is demonstrated with consolidation shadow, while the contralateral side of the interlobar fissure is the unaffected lung.

21.9.2 Bronchial Pneumonia, Mycoplasma Pneumonia, and Allergic Pneumonia

Exudative lesion of pulmonary TB is radiologically demonstrated as spots and patches of shadows with poorly defined boundary. In the cases of primary pulmonary TB, the primary lesions are commonly small, commonly concurrent with cord-like shadow of lymphangitis between the lesion and the hilum as well as the hilar and mediastinal lymphadenectasis. Infiltrative lesion of pulmonary TB is commonly located at the apical posterior segment of the upper lung lobe and dorsal segment of the lower lung lobe. The lesion is commonly complicated by proliferative lesion, caseous lesion, cavity, calcification, and fibrosis. Radiologically, the demonstrations are characterized by multiple lesions, multiple densities, and multiple shapes. By short-term observation, the lesions show no obvious change.

Bronchial pneumonia commonly occurs at the middle and medial parts of the middle and lower lung fields at both lungs. The lesions are demonstrated as small flakes or patches of shadows distributed along the bronchi. The density of the lesion is almost the same, which is light with poorly defined boundary. The multiple adjacent small lesions may fuse. And by short-term observation, the lesions show rapid change.

Mycoplasma pneumonia commonly occurs at the low lung lobe. The characteristic demonstration is patches and flakes of shadow extending from the hilum to the peripheral lung field. The density of the shadow is almost the same, which is light with poorly defined boundary and internal courses of lung markings. For about 2 weeks, the lesions can be obviously or completely absorbed.

The lesions of allergic pneumonia are commonly multiple, which are distributed at multiple lobes or segments along the bronchus mostly at the middle and lower lung fields. The lesions are demonstrated as patches or flakes of shadow with equal light density, poorly defined boundary, and internal lung markings. The characteristic demonstration is the rapid change of migrating lesions, namely, the primary lesions are absorbed within several days and new lesions are then present at other lung fields.

21.9.3 Interstitial Pneumonia

Radiologically, acute hematogenous disseminated pulmonary TB and subacute/chronic hematogenous disseminated pulmonary TB share some commonalities. The lesions disseminate from the hilum to the middle and lower lung fields, mostly bilaterally symmetric at both lungs. The densely distributed lesions at both lung fields cover the lung markings to show decreased lung markings. The lesions of acute hematogenous disseminated pulmonary TB are demonstrated as miliary and small spots of shadows with even density, even size, and even distribution. The lesions of subacute/chronic hematogenous disseminated pulmonary TB are demonstrated as spots of small nodular and patches of shadows and cavities at the upper lung field due to the fusion of small lesions, which are morphologically varied. However, the lesions at the middle lung field are mostly demonstrated as miliary and small nodular shadows, with almost even distribution. The lesions at the upper lung field are mostly old, while the lesions at the middle lung field are mostly new.

The lesions of interstitial pneumonia are commonly located at the middle and lower lung fields, rarely involving the apex of the lung. The lesions may be distributed at unilateral lung or bilateral lung fields with strips of and cord-like shadows or grid-like shadow with well-defined boundary. The lesions are mostly distributed along the lung markings. The strips and grid-like shadows are commonly accompanied by miliary and small spots of shadows with well-defined boundary. Sometimes, at the lateral part of the middle lung field, honeycomb-like transparent shadow and ground-glass shadow are demonstrated. The key point for its differentiation from hematogenous disseminated pulmonary TB is the enhanced lung markings at the affected lung field.

21.9.4 Pulmonary Abscess and Bronchiectasis

Cavities caused by pulmonary TB are commonly located at the apical posterior segment of the upper lung lobe and dorsal segment of the lower lung lobe, with smooth lining and no liquid in them. Calcification can be commonly demonstrated at the wall of cavity, with consolidation shadow at their external wall. The lesions can also be transparent area formed by proliferative lesion and fibrosis with unsmooth and irregular margin. There are cords like high-density shadow radiating from the cavity wall. Cord-like or double rail-like draining bronchi are commonly found between the cavity and hilum. Around the cavity, spots of satellite lesions are demonstrated. At the ipsilateral or contralateral upper lung field, spots and patches of polymorphic TB lesions are mostly found with different densities. At ipsilateral or contralateral middle and lower lung field, spots and patches of bronchial disseminated lesions are commonly found. Cavity induced by TB lesion mostly remains stable for a long period of time.

At the early stage, pulmonary abscess is demonstrated as a large flake of exudative consolidation shadow, which is commonly found at each lung lobe. The shadow may be found at different lobes or segments with poorly defined boundary. At the shadow, a confined central low-density area can be demonstrated with poorly defined boundary. The lesion further develops to show a characteristic sign of acute pulmonary abscess, namely, a large flake of exudative consolidation shadow with deep gas fluid level and poorly defined boundary of the consolidation shadow. In combination to the clinical acute onset with symptoms of high fever, chills, purulent sputum with unpleasant odor or purulent bloody sputum, as well as laboratory findings of increased WBC count and neutrophil count, the diagnosis can be defined. Treatment for a short period of time, the lesions can be demonstrated with improvement and absorption.

The abscess type of bronchiectasis commonly occurs at the lower lung lobe. The lesions are demonstrated as multiple round or oval thin wall transparent areas of different sizes. Most of the abscess wall has even thickness, with clear and smooth inner and outer abscess wall. Gas or gas fluid level is demonstrated within the abscess. The lesions are commonly accompanied by bronchiectasis and other pathological changes such as thickening of the bronchial wall and widened bronchial lumen. When dilated bronchus is filled with mucus, column shape or bead string-like liquid density shadow can be demonstrated to be accompanied by adjacent vascular vessels with a larger diameter than the vascular vessels. In combination to its long illness course and repeated occurrence of respiratory infection, the diagnosis can be defined.

21.9.5 Peripheral Lung Carcinoma and Lung Hamartoma

Tuberculoma commonly occurs at the apical posterior segment of the upper lung lobe and the dorsal segment of the lower lung lobe. The lesion is commonly singular with round or oval shape and clear regular margin. The density of the lesion is mostly uneven. The finding of spots or egg shell-like calcification at the internal or marginal tuberculoma facilitates the diagnosis. Tuberculoma composed of cavities is demonstrated with transparent area in the nodular shadow. In some cases, cord-like or double rail-like draining bronchus can be demonstrated between the tuberculoma and hilum. Around the lesion of tuberculoma, spots of satellite lesions are commonly demonstrated. At the ipsilateral or contralateral lung field of tuberculoma, spots, patches, and cord-like lesions are demonstrated with various shapes and densities. Contrast CT scanning demonstrates no or slight enhancement of tuberculoma. The lesion of tuberculoma may be stable, with no change for a long period of time.

Peripheral lung carcinoma may occur at any lung lobe, with more common occurrence at the anterior segment of the upper lobe. The lesion is commonly singular with round-, oval-, or potato-like shape, demonstrated as nodular or mass-like shadow. The lesion has soft tissue density, mostly even and sometimes vacuole sign. In most cases, the lesion is well defined, with lobulation sign and spicule sign. In the nodule, calcification rarely occurs, sometimes with vascular bundle sign between mass-like shadow and hilum. Contrast CT scanning demonstrates mostly obvious enhancement of the nodular shadow of lung carcinoma. The nodular shadow of the peripheral lung carcinoma commonly enlarges during 1–3 months. Clinical symptoms include cough up bloody sputum, with no fever.

Lung hamartoma commonly occurs adjacent to the pleura, mostly singular with round or oval shape. In the nodular shadow, calcification can be observed. The characteristic sign of lung hamartoma is popcorn-like calcification, while its typical manifestation is the concurrent soft tissue density, calcification density, and adipose density within one nodular shadow. Its margin is clear and smooth, with no spicule sign or obvious lobulation sign. By long-term observation, lung hamartoma has no obvious change, and most patients experience no clinical symptoms.

Suggested Reading

Boehme CC, Nabeta P, Hillemann D, et al. Rapid molecular detection of tuberculosis and rifampin resistance. N Engl J Med. 2010; 363(11):1005–15.

Boehme CC, Nicol MP, Nabeta P, et al. Feasibility, diagnostic accuracy, and effectiveness of decentralised use of the Xpert MTB/RIF test for diagnosis of tuberculosis and multidrug resistance: a multicentre implementation study. Lancet. 2011;377(9776):1495–505.

Li L, Li HJ. HIV/AIDS complicated by pulmonary tuberculosis: radiological demonstrations by PET/CT. Pract Radiol. 2011;21(10): 1043–5.

Mazurek GH, Jereb J, Vernon A, et al. Updated guidelines for using Interferon Gamma Release Assays to detect Mycobacterium tuberculosis infection-United States, 2010. MMWR Recomm Rep. 2010;59(RR-5):1–25.

Soussan M, Brillet PY, Mekinian A, et al. Patterns of pulmonary tuberculosis on FDG-PET/CT. Eur J Radiol. 2012;81(10):2872–6.

Steingart KR, Flores LL, Dendukuri N, et al. Commercial serological tests for the diagnosis of active pulmonary and extrapulmonary tuberculosis: an updated systematic review and meta-analysis. PLoS Med. 2011;8(8), e1001062.

Tang SJ, Gao W, Xiao HP, et al. Clinical tuberculosis. Beijing: People's Medical Publishing House; 2011.

Tuon FF, Higashino HR, Lopes MI, et al. Adenosine deaminase and tuberculous meningitis–a systematic review with meta-analysis. Scand J Infect Dis. 2010;42(3):198–207.

van Zyl-Smit RN, Binder A, Meldau R, et al. Comparison of quantitative techniques including Xpert MTB/RIF to evaluate mycobacterial burden. PLoS One. 2011;6(12), e28815.

Yang GD, Lu PX, Xiao Y, et al. Radiological demonstrations of singular tuberculoma by 18F-FDG PET/CT. Pract Radiol. 2011;21(9): 934–7.

Scarlet Fever

22

Li Li, Qun Lao, and Haiyan Zhao

Scarlet fever is an acute respiratory infectious disease caused by group A β-hemolytic streptococcus. Its clinical symptoms include fever, angina, general diffusive red skin rashes, and the obvious desquamation after deflorescence of the red skin rash. After infection of scarlet fever, complications of allergic cardiopathies, nephropathies, and arthropathies are occasionally found.

22.1 Etiology

Group A β-hemolytic streptococcus, also known as Streptococcus pyogenes, is Gram-positive with a diameter of 0.5–2.0 μm. After its isolation from tissues of the human body, it commonly has capsule but no flagella and spore. The bacteria are most likely to grow in the culture medium containing blood, producing complete hemolysis or β-hemolysis. Based on the different polysaccharide antigens in the cell walls of the bacteria, streptococcus can be categorized into 19 groups, namely, from group A to group U excluding groups I and J. Group A is the pathogen of scarlet fever. Group A β-hemolytic streptococcus has four surface antigens: M, R, T, and S. The disease-related surface antigen is protein M, which is the component of the bacterium and has immunotoxic effect on neutrophils and platelets. In addition, protein M and the bacterial capsule bear resistance to phagocytosis. Lipoteichoic acid has a high affinity with the biological membrane, contributing to the streptococcal adhesion to human epithelial cells.

The pathogenicity of group A β-hemolytic streptococcus stems from the bacteria themselves and the produced toxins and proteases. The produced toxins by the bacteria include (1) pyrogenic exotoxin: it is also known as erythrogenic toxin, including four different types of pyrogenic exotoxin with different antigenicities that is nominated as A, B, C, and D. Their antibodies, having no cross protection, can cause fever and skin rashes of scarlet fever. In addition, these antibodies can inhibit the activities of phagocytic system and the T cells and trigger Shwartzman reaction (endotoxin hemorrhagic necrosis). (2) streptolysin: streptolysin, including O streptolysin and S streptolysin, is capable of lysing the erythrocytes, killing leukocytes and platelets, and impairing the heart. The proteases produced by group A β-hemolytic streptococcus include (1) streptokinase (fibrinolysin) that dissolves the blood clot and prevents the clotting of plasma; (2) hyaluronidase (diffusion factor) that dissolves the hyaluronic acid between tissues and thus facilitates the bacterial diffusion within the tissues; (3) streptodornase, also known as DNase, that cracks DNA with high viscosity and destructs the host tissues and cells; (4) nicotinamide adenine dinucleotide phosphate enzyme that impairs the tissues and cells containing nicotinamide adenine dinucleotide phosphate; (5) serum opacity factor, a α-lipoprotein lipase, that turbids horse serum, inhibits the specific and non-specific immune responses produced in organisms, and facilitates bacterial infection and spread.

Group A β-hemolytic streptococcus has a weak resistance to hotness and dryness. Generally, it can be inactivated after heated at a temperature of 56 °C for 30 min. However, it can survive for several weeks in phlegm and pus.

22.2 Epidemiology

22.2.1 Sources of Infection

The common sources of infection include patients with scarlet fever and persons carrying the pathogenic bacteria.

L. Li (✉) • H. Zhao
Department of Radiology, Beijing You'an Hospital, Capital Medical University, Beijing, China
e-mail: sycrbyxx@126.com

Q. Lao
Department of Radiology, The City Children's Hospital, Hangzhou, Zhejiang, China

H. Li (ed.), *Radiology of Infectious Diseases: Volume 2*, DOI 10.1007/978-94-017-9876-1_22

Patients in the period from the 24 h before the onset to the peak phase of scarlet fever have the strongest infectivity. And patient with angina caused by group A β-hemolytic streptococcus angina is the most significant source of infection because such patients have large quantities of bacterial discharge and tend to be ignored for isolation and detection.

22.2.2 Route of Transmission

Scarlet fever is commonly transmitted via droplets. Occasionally, it can be transmitted indirectly via contaminated appliances, books, and drinks. In some cases, the bacteria can invade skin wound or maternal birth canal to cause surgical scarlet fever or obstetric scarlet fever.

22.2.3 Susceptible Population

Populations are generally susceptible. After infection, the antibacterial and antiviral immunity is produced in organisms. The antibacterial immunity originates from the antibody against protein M, and such immunity has type specificity, with protection against the invasion by the same type of streptococcus but no protection against the invasion by different types of streptococcus. Anti-erythrogenic toxin has a long-term immunity. However, due to the five different serotypes of erythrogenic toxin with no cross immunity, infection of group A β-hemolytic streptococcus producing another type of erythrogenic toxin causes scarlet fever once again.

22.2.4 Epidemiological Features

22.2.4.1 Season

Scarlet fever occurs all year round, with more common occurrence in winters and springs, indicating its correlationship with the dry climate.

22.2.4.2 Age

Scarlet fever occurs at any age but is more common during the ages of 1–15 years.

22.2.4.3 Region

Scarlet fever is more commonly found in temperate regions but rare in frigid and tropical regions. In China, its occurrence is more common in northern areas than in southern areas.

22.2.4.4 Progress of the Disease

The prevailing types of bacteria are different during different periods in different regions. Accordingly, the conditions of the disease tend to be mild, with more cases of slight manifestations but rarer cases of toxic manifestations. The death rate from scarlet fever is significantly decreasing.

22.3 Pathogenesis and Pathological Changes

After invasion of the pathogen into the human body, three types of pathological changes can be found.

22.3.1 Suppurative Changes

Assisted by LTA, group A β-hemolytic streptococcus adheres to the epithelial cells of the mucosa to invade the tissues, causing inflammation. They fight against phagocytosis via M protein and the bacterial capsule. With collaborative effects of streptokinase and hyaluronidase, the inflammation spreads to cause tissue necrosis.

22.3.2 Toxic Changes

After the toxins produced by the streptococcus gain their access into the blood flow, symptoms of systemic toxemia occur including fever, dizziness, headache, and other toxemic symptoms. The erythrogenic toxin causes congestion and edema of cutaneous blood vessels, along with epithelial cell proliferation and leukocyte infiltration that is the most obvious around hair follicles, to produce typical scarlet fever-like skin rashes. Finally, dead epidermis sheds off to form desquamation. The mucosa may also be congested, sometimes presenting as spot bleeding to form exanthem. In addition, mononuclear cells infiltration may be found around the interstitial blood vessels in the liver, spleen, and lymph nodes, with accompanying different degrees of congestion and fatty degeneration. Furthermore, watery degeneration, and in some serious cases even necrosis, may be found in the myocardium. Interstitial inflammation can be found in the kidney. And the central nervous system in the cases of toxic type may have changes of malnutrition.

22.3.3 Allergic Changes

Occasionally, patients may sustain allergic changes in the second or third week of the illness course, commonly as cardiac, renal, and joint synovial inflammations. The cause may be cross immune reaction between some types of group A β-hemolytic streptococcus and antigens of myocardium, glomerular basement membrane, and synovial capsule in infected patients. The allergic changes may also be caused by immune impairments due to sedimentation of antigen-antibody complex at the above-mentioned positions.

22.4 Clinical Symptoms and Signs

The incubation period of scarlet fever ranges from 1 to 7 days, commonly lasting 2–3 days.

22.4.1 Clinical Manifestations

Scarlet fever has a rapid onset, with common clinical manifestations of fever, angina, and skin rashes.

22.4.1.1 Fever

The fever is commonly persistent, with a body temperature of about 39 °C and accompanying toxic symptoms such as headache, stomach upset, and poor appetite. The changes of body temperature and its duration are consistent with the severity changes of skin rashes. The fever commonly persists for 1 week.

22.4.1.2 Angina

About 98 % of the cases with scarlet fever develop angina, with manifestations of sore throat, odynophagia, local congestion, and coverage of purulent exudates. Congestion or hemorrhagic mucosal rashes can be found at jaws whose occurrence may be prior to skin rashes.

22.4.1.3 Skin Rashes

Within 24 h after the onset of fever, skin rashes occur, which commonly begin on the chest and neck and behind the ears, followed by quick spread to the whole body. The typical skin rashes are evenly distributed papules with a size of needle tip that are diffusive and congestive. The color fades away when the rashes are pressed, with accompanying sense of itching. In some cases, skin rashes with a head of yellowish white pus can be found that are difficult to be squeezed to burst, which is referred to as miliary eruption. In some serious cases, hemorrhagic rashes occur. In the skin folds where the rashes are densely distributed or bleeding due to frictions is present, purplish lines of rashes may occur, which are known as linear eruption or Pastia lines. In some cases, only congestion occurs in the face with no skin rashes, and congestion around the mouth and nose is not obvious but is grayish white, which is known as circumoral pallor. At the jaws, there is also visible congestion or hemorrhagic mucosal rashes. The eruption of skin rash reaches its peak in 48 h, followed by fading away in the order of eruptions in 2–3 days. However, in some serious cases, the skin rashes may persist for about 1 week. After the skin rashes completely fade away in 2–3 days, desquamation begins, which is more obvious at the positions with more dense skin rashes. Desquamation is especially serious at the positions with miliary eruptions. Desquamation may be star-like flaky or otherwise sleeve-like on the palms, soles, toes, and fingers and chaff-like on the face and trunk. In recent years, the number of cases with slight symptoms is increasing, commonly with symptoms of low-grade fever, mild sore throat, scarce skin rashes that fade rapidly, and slight desquamation. However, further complications due to allergic reactions may occur.

Tongue papilla swelling may simultaneously occur with skin rashes. At the early stage, the surface of tongue may be covered by whitish coating and the reddish swollen papillae protrude out of the whitish coating, which is known as strawberry tongue. After 2–3 days, the whitish coating begins to shed off, with smooth surface of the tongue and protruding tongue papillae, which is known as bayberry tongue.

22.4.2 Types

Scarlet fever has varying clinical manifestations and different prognoses. Generally, it can be divided into the following five types.

22.4.2.1 Common Type

During its prevalence, more than 95 % of the cases belong to the common type. The clinical manifestations include fever, angina and characteristic red skin rashes, systemic toxic symptoms, and non-suppurative inflammations at submaxillary and cervical lymph nodes. The course of illness lasts for about 1 week.

22.4.2.2 Mild Type

During recent years, the mild type of cases is more common, characterized by low-grade fever, mild pharyngodynia, scare rashes that are only found on the trunk and rapidly fade, no obvious desquamation, and short course of illness. However, complications due to allergic reactions may occur.

22.4.2.3 Septic Type

Septic type of scarlet fever rarely occurs, which has clinical manifestations of severe suppurative inflammation of the pharynx with large quantity of exudates that may develop into suppurative pseudomembrane and local mucosal necrosis that develops into ulceration. The bacteria can spread into adjacent tissues to cause suppurative otitis media, sinusitis, mastoiditis, cervical lymphadenitis, and even inflammation of cervical soft tissues. In addition, septic scarlet fever may cause septicemia and migrating suppurative lesions.

22.4.2.4 Toxic Type

Toxic type of scarlet fever is rare, commonly with obvious toxic symptoms including high fever, headache, serious vomiting, and even unconsciousness. The clinical manifestations may also include toxic myocarditis, toxic hepatitis, and infective toxic shock. Angina is commonly not serious but skin rashes are obvious, possibly with bleeding. In the cases of shock, the skin rashes are dimly visible. The death rate from toxic type of scarlet fever is high.

22.4.2.5 Surgical/Obstetric Type

The pathogenic bacteria gain their access to the human body via wound or birth canal to cause the disease. Therefore, angina fails to occur in such type of cases. The skin rashes begin from the surrounding areas of wound and birth canal and spread all over the body. The toxic symptoms are mild, with favorable prognosis.

22.5 Scarlet Fever-Related Complications

22.5.1 Infective Complications

Infective complications are caused by direct invasion of the bacteria into the adjacent tissues. Such complications include otitis media, lymphadenitis, and bronchopneumonia.

22.5.2 Toxic Complications

Toxic complications are non-suppurative diseases caused by *Streptococcus*, such as toxic myocarditis and toxic nephritis. Such complications are generally transient, with favorable prognosis.

22.5.3 Allergic Reactive Complications

Such complications occur in the second and third week of the illness course, with an incidence of 3–20 %.

22.5.3.1 Acute Glomerular Inflammation

The occurrence of acute glomerular inflammation is related to the type of group A streptococcus. After the infections of types 1, 4, 12, 18, and 25, especially the infection of type 12, nephritis commonly occurs. Therefore, these types are also known as nephritic types.

22.5.3.2 Rheumatism

Generally, rheumatism is not related to the type of infected group A streptococcus, whose occurrence is commonly after 2–4 weeks during the illness course. The clinical manifestations commonly include migrating rheumatic arthritis with both major and minor joints involved. The involved joints may be red and swollen, with serous exudates from the articular cavity. Some patients may develop rheumatic myocarditis, endocarditis, and pericarditis. After the acute phase, even valve damages may occur. The occurrence of rheumatism is related to immune responses but not related to H antibody of M protein.

22.5.3.3 Poststreptococcal Reactive Arthritis (PSRA)

Poststreptococcal reactive arthritis (PSRA) has recently been recognized as a disease independent of rheumatic fever. Its clinical manifestations include arthritis with acute onset, whose occurrence is symmetric or asymmetric, persistent or repeated, and non-migratory. PSRA may involve any joints and the major joints of lower limbs, like the knee and ankle, are especially vulnerable. The therapies of salicylic acid and other nonsteroidal medications are ineffective or have a poor therapeutic efficacy.

22.6 Examination Options

22.6.1 Laboratory Tests

22.6.1.1 Routine Laboratory Tests

Routine Blood Test

WBC count reaches $(10–20) \times 10^9$/L or above. Neutrophil counts usually are above 75 %, with visible toxic particles in the cytoplasm.

Routine Urine Test

Small quantity of protein can be found in urine sample from patients, which is commonly transient. In the cases with complicating nephritis, the protein level increases, with findings of erythrocytes and leukocytes.

22.6.1.2 Serological Examination

Examination of pharyngeal swab smear by immunofluorescence can be performed for a rapid diagnosis.

22.6.1.3 Etiological Examination

By culture of pharyngeal swab or secretions from other lesions, the finding of hemolytic streptococcus can define the diagnosis.

22.6.2 Diagnostic Imaging

Diagnostic imaging is commonly applied for the diagnosis and differential diagnosis of scarlet fever-related complications, such as pulmonary infections.

22.7 Imaging Demonstrations

22.7.1 Bronchopneumonia

22.7.1.1 Chest X-Rays

Lesions are commonly found in the inner and middle parts of middle and inferior fields of both lungs, distributing along the bronchi, showing spots or flakes of shadows with increased density. These shadows are unclearly defined, which may fuse into flakes or large flakes of shadows (Figs. 22.1 and 22.2). In the cases of bronchial inflammatory blockages, chest X-ray may find triangular-shaped dense shadow of atelectasis and the finding of compensatory emphysema in the adjacent lung field. In the cases of inflammatory lesions with the pleura involved, the pleura can be found with congestion, edema, and exudation, with pleural effusion.

Case Study 1

A female aged 18 years was admitted to the hospital due to the complaint of cough for 7 days and fever for 1 day. At 7 days before her admission, she'd had paroxysmal cough with phlegm that cannot be expectorated, with no obvious known causes. In addition, no wheezing or shortness of breath occurred. The oral medication of azithromycin alleviated the cough. On the day of admission, she complained of skin rashes and fever. Her fever was irregular, with the highest body temperature of 39 °C, with no chill or convulsion. The oral medication of azithromycin failed to control her body temperature and she vomited two to three times.

On physical examination, the following were obtained: T 39 °C, P 130/min, and R 32/min. The general mucosa has no yellowish staining and bleeding spots, but little reddish macula on the neck, chest, and back can be found. The throat is red, with both tonsils swollen and exudates visible. The respiratory sound of both lungs is coarse, with unstable moist rales in the right lung. By laboratory tests, the following were obtained: serum CRP 69.2 mg/L, normal levels of IgM and IgG, and antistreptolysin O 25 UI/ml.

(The case and the figure are provided by Tang, YH at Ruijin Hospital, Shanghai, China)

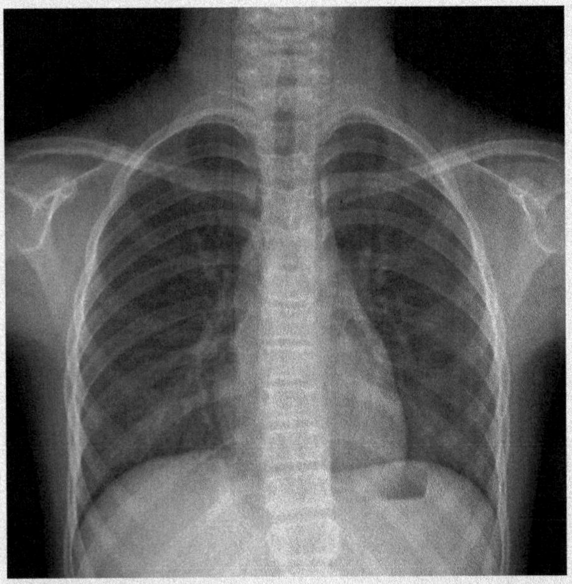

Fig. 22.1 Scarlet fever complicated by bronchopneumonia. The chest X-ray demonstrates thickened pulmonary markings in both lower lungs, with spot-shaped shadows that are more obvious in the right lower lung

Case Study 2

A girl patient has chief complaint of fever and rash for 1 day with accompanying chill.

On physical examination, her temperature is 37.7 °C (rectal temperature), with pharyngeal congestion. The tonsils are swollen at the degree of 1, raspberry tongue. Many reddish maculopapules can be found on the skin all over the body that slightly protrude out of the skin surface. The color of these maculopapules fades away when pressed. The skin between maculopapules has obvious congestion. By auscultation, the respiratory sound is coarse in both lungs, with rare moist rales in the left lower lung. By laboratory tests, routine blood test found WBC 13.76 × 109/L, N 0.823, L 0.097, RBC 4.87 × 1,012/L, PLT 290 × 109/L, and CRP 14 mg/L; pharyngeal swab found viridans streptococci (++), streptococci positive, Neisseria (++), and no detected fungus.

(The case and the figure are provided by Lao, Q at the City Children's Hospital, Hangzhou, China)

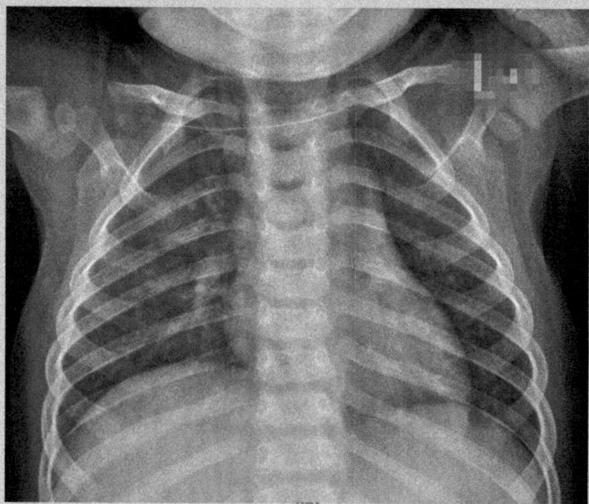

Fig. 22.2 Scarlet fever complicated by bronchopneumonia. The chest X-ray demonstrates increased blurry pulmonary markings of both lungs and scattered small patches of shadows in the inner zone of the middle and upper lung fields in the right lung

22.7.1.2 CT Scanning

CT scanning demonstrates thickened bronchovascular bundle. The lesions are diffused patches of shadows, with unclearly defined boundaries. Otherwise, they are scattered small flakes of parenchymal shadows or fused large flakes of shadows. Surrounding the small flakes of parenchymal shadows, obstructive emphysema or pulmonary atelectasis is commonly found. The adjacent lung field of obstructive atelectasis may have demonstrations of compensatory emphysema. In addition, CT scanning can detect small quantity of pleural effusion that tends to be missed by chest X-rays.

22.7.2 Reactive Arthritis After Streptococcal Infection

X-ray demonstrates cystic absorption and slight osteohyperplasia in the joints of the ankle, knee, hip, and sacroilium, with asymmetric narrowing of the articular space.

22.8 Basis for Diagnosis

22.8.1 Scarlet Fever

The clinical diagnosis of scarlet fever can be defined based on a history of contacting patients with scarlet fever or angina; clinical characteristic manifestations of typical skin rashes and desquamation, strawberry tongue, Pastia lines, and circumoral pallor; and laboratory findings of obviously increased level of peripheral blood routine test indicators. The definitive diagnosis can be made based on detected group A streptococci by pharyngeal swab or pus culture.

22.8.2 Scarlet Fever-Related Complications

22.8.2.1 Bronchopneumonia

Children with scarlet fever have signs and symptoms of respiratory infection.

Diagnostic imaging demonstrates lesions in the inner and middle zones of both lower lungs that distribute along bronchi. The lesions are demonstrated as multiple scattering patches, with obstructive emphysema or lobular atelectasis.

22.8.2.2 Reactive Arthritis After Streptococcal Infection

Typical arthritis has the following features: (1) Arthritis with an acute onset is usually non-migratory, asymmetric, or symmetric, with involvement of any joint; (2) typical arthritis is persistent or recurrent; and (3) therapies of salicylic and other nonsteroidal medication are ineffective or have a poor therapeutic efficacy.

The evidence of group A streptococcus infection before the occurrence of articular symptoms is found.

The findings fail to meet the Jones diagnostic criteria for rheumatic fever.

The diagnostic imaging demonstrates cystic absorption and slight osteohyperplasia of extremities and sacroiliac joint, with asymmetric narrowing of the articular space.

22.9 Differential Diagnosis

22.9.1 Scarlet Fever

22.9.1.1 Differentiation of Scarlet Fever from Other Diseases with Skin Rashes

Measles

Patients with measles have obvious catarrhal symptoms of the upper respiratory tract. The skin rashes occur at the fourth day, with different sizes and shapes, and are especially more common in the face. The rashes are dark reddish maculopapules, with normal skin between the rashes.

Rubella

Measles-like rashes occur at the first day of the disease onset. On the following day, the rashes increase on the trunk and some may fuse into flakes, just like the appearance in the cases of scarlet fever. However, the cases of rubella commonly have no manifestations of diffusive skin flushing, which is commonly found in the cases of scarlet fever. At this time, the rashes on the extremities are still measles-like, and the rashes on the face are in the same quantity as those on the body. The rashes fade away at day 3 after the onset of rubella, with no desquamation. There are also no pharyngeal inflammations but commonly enlarged retroauricular lymph nodes.

Drug Rashes

Patients commonly have a history of medication. In some cases, the rashes have diverse manifestations, with some scarlet fever-like rashes and some other urticaria-like rashes. The skin rashes are unevenly distributed and the sequence of eruption is not the same as those in the cases of scarlet fever from bottom up and from the trunk to the extremities. There are also no bayberry-like tongue and commonly no symptoms of angina. In some cases, medication by patients with angina may also cause drug rashes.

Staphylococcus aureus Infection

Some staphylococcus aureus can produce erythrogenic toxin, which may also cause scarlet fever-like rashes. Their differentiation is commonly based on bacterial culture.

22.9.1.2 Differentiation of Scarlet Fever from Other Diseases with Angina

Before the eruption of skin rashes, angina of scarlet fever cannot be distinguished from the common acute angina. Angina in patients with diphtheria is more slight than that in patients with scarlet fever, with more tough pseudomembrane that is difficult to be wiped away. The purulent secretions in the pharynx of patients with scarlet fever can be wiped away easily. However, scarlet fever and diphtheria may concur, and the bacterial examination is facilitative to the diagnosis.

22.9.2 Differential Diagnosis of Scarlet Fever-Related Complications

22.9.2.1 Bronchopneumonia

Simplex Pulmonary Eosinophilia

The disease has slight systematic symptoms or no symptoms but occasional findings of pulmonary lesions by physical examinations for health management. Its demonstrations by diagnostic imaging are similar to those of bronchopneumonia, including multiple small flakes of infiltration shadows in unilateral or bilateral lungs with even density and unclearly defined boundaries and fading of the lesions in 6–12 days. Being different from bronchopneumonia, cases of scarlet fever show transient or migrating pulmonary shadows, concurrent absorption of one lesion and occurrence of new lesion within short period of time, and accompanying characteristic peripheral eosinophilia. Increased eosinophil count in blood, sputum, and bronchial alveolar lavage fluid as well as increased serum IgE and IgM levels above normal range can facilitate the differential diagnosis.

Mycoplasma Pneumonia

In the early stage of mycoplasma pneumonia, pulmonary interstitial inflammation occurs, with following patches of parenchymal shadows in the air cavity resembling bronchopneumonia. The progression of mycoplasma pneumonia may resemble lobar pneumonia.

22.9.2.2 Reactive Arthritis After Streptococcal Infection

Rheumatic Fever

The clinical symptoms of rheumatic fever include migrating joint swelling and/or pain that may recover in two weeks. Rheumatic fever has favorable therapeutic response to the medication of nonsteroidal drugs. And X-ray demonstrates slight osteohyperplasia.

Reactive Arthritis

The clinical symptoms include persistent asymmetric joint swelling and/or pain. And X-ray demonstrates cystic absorption, osteohyperplasia, asymmetric narrowing of articular space, and other changes in sacroiliac joint as well as osteohyperplasia, slight narrowing of articular space, or blurry and destructed bone surface in joints of extremities.

Suggested Reading

Li N. (translator from English into Chinese). Oxford studies of infectious diseases. Beijing: People's Health Publishing House; 2011.

Li LJ. Studies of infectious diseases. Beijing: Higher Education Press; 2011.

Liang YM, Yang YH. Correlationship between Group A β-hemolytic streptococcus and scarlet fever. J Microbiol. 2009;29(4):89–92.

Liu G. Group A streptococcus induced acute pharyngotonsillitis and scarlet fever. J Clin Pediatr. 2006;24(6):447–8.

Zhang ZY, Zhang YQ. Differential diagnosis of scarlet fever complicated by arthritis and rheumatoid arthritis. General Pract Commun China. 2010;12(18):80.

Syphilis

23

Haifeng Mi, Yunfang Li, and Hongjun Li

Syphilis is a chronic and systemic sexually transmitted disease (STD) caused by *Treponema pallidum* (TP). It mainly spreads via sexual contact, blood, and vertical transmission. The disease has extremely complex clinical manifestations, involving nearly all organs in the human body. During its early stage, syphilis invades the genitals and the skin, while during the late stage, the cardiovascular system, nerve, skeleton, eyes, and other organs. Syphilis can be transmitted to fetus via placenta of infected mother, which is hazardous to human health.

23.1 Etiology

In 1905, Schaudinn and Hoffmann discovered *Treponema pallidum* (TP) in the primary lesion of a patient with syphilis. TP is also known as treponema pallor, which is categorized into the genus of *Treponemas*, the family of treponemas, the order of spirochete. The thallus of TP is slim with its length ranging from 5 to 20 μm (a mean length of 6–10 μm) and its transverse diameter being about 0.15 μm. The thallus has an even arrangement of 6–12 spirals and is invisible to the naked eyes. And only its refractivity can be observed by dark-field microscopy. TP is active, with moving patterns of spinning, crawling, and flexing. At the anterior part of TP, there are 4–6 flagella like fine fiber bundles, with curling endings. Without any impact from external factors, the spirals are regular in shape, with slow and regular motion. The commonly applied dyes fail to stain them, but the bacteria can be observed by dark-field microscopy or phase contrast microscopy. TP, an anaerobic microorganism, can survive and reproduce for a long period of time in the human body. And they can hardly survive in vitro, which can be rapidly killed by boiling, dryness, sunshine, soap water, and common disinfectants. However, it is cold tolerant, being capable of surviving 48 hours at 0 °C refrigerator, 3 days at 4 °C, and even being infectious at −78 °C for several years.

23.2 Epidemiology

23.2.1 Source of Infection

Patient with syphilis is the only source of infection, and TP can be found in their skin lesions, blood, seminal fluid, and breast milk. Caries callosa in the cases of primary syphilis and syphiloderm in the cases of secondary syphilis contain large quantities of TP.

23.2.2 Route of Transmission

23.2.2.1 Sexual Contact

Sexual contact is the major route of transmission, accounting for about 95 % of all syphilis cases. It spreads via tiny injuries of skin and mucosa. The untreated patients are the most infectious during the initial 1–2 years after the infection, and their infectivity is decreasing along with the development of the disease. The patients with an illness course of above 4 years hardly transmit the disease by sexual contact.

23.2.2.2 Vertical Transmission

Infected pregnant woman can transmit the disease to her fetus via placenta to cause intrauterine fetus infection. It mostly occurs after 4 months of gestation, leading to fetus syphilis, abortion, premature birth, and stillbirth. It is

H. Mi • Y. Li • H. Li (✉)
Department of Radiology Beijing You'an Hospital, Capital Medical University, Beijing, China
e-mail: lihongjun00113@126.com

H. Li (ed.), *Radiology of Infectious Diseases: Volume 2*, DOI 10.1007/978-94-017-9876-1_23

generally believed that pregnant women with a shorter course of syphilis are at a higher risk of transmitting the disease to the fetus. Their infectivity is decreasing along with the development of syphilis. However, woman with syphilis for 2 years can still transmit the disease to her fetus via placenta.

23.2.2.3 Other Routes

TP can also spread via indirect contact. Occasionally, patients are infected via kissing, shaking hands, breast feeding, or contacts to secretions of the patients, contaminated clothes, or contaminated utensils by the patients with syphilis.

23.2.3 Susceptible Population

The high-risk populations of infecting syphilis include prostitutes, male homosexuals, and drug abusers. And male homosexuals have especially high risk of infection. Currently, an increasingly large population is infected with syphilis, with common occurrence in sexual workers, peasant workers, and senior citizens. Syphilis is the most commonly found in the age group of 20–50 years, who have active sexual behaviors. In addition to no congenital immunity against syphilis in human being, this age group is generally susceptible to syphilis regardless of gender.

23.2.4 Epidemiological Features

Syphilis is an endemic sexually transmitted disease throughout the world. According to WHO, about 12 million new cases of syphilis are reported all over the world each year, with common occurrence in South Asia, Southeast Asia, and Africa. In Southeast Asia, the most new cases are reported each year, with its peak incidence age at 15–30 years and with no significant difference between males and females. In the early stage after the People's Republic of China was founded, syphilis was the major sexually transmitted disease, with more occurrence in residence areas of minorities than that in urban areas. With implementation of a series of control measures, sexually transmitted diseases were basically eradicated in China during the 1960s. However, after the 1980s, the incidence rate of syphilis has been increasing along with increasingly more international communications. By May 31, 2013, the yearly reported cases of syphilis was 189,559 in China, which increased by 0.7 % compared to the reported cases of the previous year (totally 188,321 cases). The geographic region with incidence of syphilis is increasingly large and the hazards caused by the disease are increasingly serious.

23.3 Pathogenesis and Pathological Changes

23.3.1 Pathogenesis

After TP gains its access into the human body via mucosa or skin defect, it invades the adjacent lymph nodes within several hours. After 2–3 days, it enters into the blood stream to spread throughout the body. After 2–3 weeks incubation period after its invasion into the human body, characteristic primary skin lesions form at the defected mucosa or skin, typically caries callosa. After that, antibodies are produced in the body. An experimental study on rabbits with syphilis has demonstrated that syphilis at the early stage is histologically characterized by mononuclear cell infiltration, with lymphocyte infiltration at day 6 after the infection. Meanwhile, TP can be found in the epithelial cell space of caries callosa and in the depressions or phagosomes of epithelial cells. Otherwise, TP can be found between the fibroblast plasma cells and the endothelial cells of tiny capillaries, in the lymphatic vessels, or in regional lymph nodes. Due to rapid elimination of TP from the lesions by immunity, most TPs are killed 24 days after the infection and the conditions develop into asymptomatic incubation period, namely, the primary incubation of syphilis.

23.3.2 Pathological Changes

23.3.2.1 Endarteritis Obliterans and Minor Perivascular Inflammation

Endarteritis obliterans refers to proliferation of endothelial cells and fibrocytes in arterioles, which leads to thickened vascular wall as well as stenosis and occlusion of vascular lumen. Minor perivascular inflammation refers to perivascular infiltrations of mononuclear cells, lymphocytes, and plasmocytes. And constant emergence of plasmocytes is one of the characteristic pathological changes in the cases of minor perivascular inflammation.

23.3.2.2 Syphilitic Gumma

Syphilitic gumma, also known as syphiloma, has grayish white lesions with different sizes. Under a microscope, the structure of lesion can be observed like tuberculous nodule, with central coagulative necrosis. Morphologically, the lesion resembles to caseous necrosis. But necrosis of the lesion is incomplete, with preservation of elastic fibers. By staining of the elastic fibers, the outline of original vascular walls in the lesion can be observed. In the granulation tissue around necrosis, there are abundant lymphocytes and plasmocytes but rare epithelioid cells and Langerhans cells. Endarteritis obliterans and periarteritis definitely occur. At the late stage of syphilitic gumma, the lesion can be absorbed, with following occurrence of fibrosis, and finally develops into deformed organs but rare occurrence of calcification. Syphilitic gumma may involve any organ in the human body, commonly skin, mucosa, liver, bone, and testis. Lesions of vasculitis can be found at any stage of syphilis, while syphilitic gumma commonly occurs in the cases of tertiary syphilis.

23.4 Clinical Symptoms and Signs

23.4.1 Acquired Syphilis

23.4.1.1 Primary Syphilis

The common manifestations include caries callosa and sclerotic lymphadenitis, usually with no systemic symptoms.

Caries Callosa

Caries callosa commonly occurs about 3 weeks after the infection, with 90 % of the cases at external genital organs. During the early stage, the lesion is a red bean-sized hard nodule, which develops necrosis at its surface to form painless ulcers with accompanying edema. By palpation, hardness of the lesion touches like cartilage, with serous secretion at the surface, which is known as caries callosa. It contains a large quantity of TP, with strong infectivity.

Sclerotic Lymphadenitis

Sclerotic lymphadenitis occurs 1–2 weeks after emergence of caries callosa, commonly with unilateral groin or adjacent lymph nodes involved. The lesion is a hard protrusion, with no redness, swelling, and ulceration at the surface and being painless. It usually disappears after several months. By puncture of the lymph node, a large quantity of TP can be detected.

23.4.1.2 Secondary Syphilis

In the cases with untreated or incompletely cured primary syphilis, TP disseminates throughout the body along with the blood flow and local lymph nodes to cause skin and mucosa lesions as well as systemic lesions, which is known as secondary syphilis. It commonly occurs 7–10 weeks after the infection, or 6–8 weeks after emergence of caries callosa.

Skin and Mucosa Lesion

In patients with secondary syphilis, 80–85 % of the cases develop skin and mucous lesion. The common manifestations include syphiloderm, condyloma, syphilitic alopecia, and mucosa lesion.

Bone and Joint Lesion

Invasion of TP into the skeletal system can cause periostitis, arthritis, osteitis, osteomyelitis, bursitis, or tenosynovitis. And the periostitis is the most common, with common involvement of long bone. For instance, syphilitic periostitis is commonly found at the tibia, with manifestations of slightly thickened periosteum, subjective persistent dull pain, obvious tenderness, slight conditions during daytime, and physical activities and aggravated conditions at nights. Arthritis commonly involves shoulder, elbow, knee, hip, ankle, and other joints, which is usually symmetric with manifestations of articular effusion, articular swelling, and tenderness. The symptoms are slight during daytime and serious at nights.

Ocular Lesion

Ocular lesion is the most common in the cases of secondary syphilis and its incidence rate is low. The lesion is commonly caused by iritis, iridocyclitis, choroiditis, and retinitis, with adverse effect on vision in different degrees.

Neurological Lesion

The neurological lesion is mainly caused by asymptomatic neurosyphilis, syphilitic meningitis, and cerebrovascular syphilis. Asymptomatic neurosyphilis is only manifested by abnormalities of cerebrospinal fluid, and syphilitic meningitis can cause symptoms of intracranial hypertension, cerebral nerve palsy, and others. Cerebrovascular syphilis is commonly concurrent with syphilitic meningitis, mainly invading the cerebral artery to cause thickened vascular wall and vascular stenosis, which further lead to insufficient blood supply to the brain.

Multiple Sclerotic Lymphadenitis

The incidence of multiple sclerotic lymphadenitis is 50–80 %, with manifestation of systemically enlarged painless lymph nodes.

Organ Syphilis

Organ syphilis rarely occurs, which may involve the liver, kidney, bile duct, and gastrointestinal tract to cause syphilitic hepatitis, syphilitic nephritis, pericholangitis, and gastrointestinal lesions.

23.4.1.3 Tertiary Syphilis

Tertiary syphilis is also known as advanced syphilis, with a history of above 2 years. About 40 % of untreated patients or patients incompletely cured with early syphilis may experience the development of the conditions into tertiary syphilis after 3–4 years.

Skin and Mucosa Lesion

The manifestations include nodular syphiloderm and syphilitic gumma.

Bone Syphilis

Bone syphilis has the most common manifestation of periostitis, which is characterized by affected limb pain, periosteal proliferation, thickened diaphysis, and saber-shaped tibia in the cases with involved tibia. In the cases with osteomyelitis, osteitis, and arthritis, pathological fracture, osteoperforation, and joint deformity can be found.

Ocular Syphilis

The manifestations resemble to those of secondary syphilis, including iritis, iridocyclitis, retinitis, optic neuritis, interstitial keratitis, and other ocular lesions.

Cardiovascular Syphilis

Its incidence rate is 10 %, which commonly occurs 10–30 years after the infection. The manifestations include simplex aortitis, incomplete closure of aortic valve, stenosis of coronary orifice, aortic aneurysm, and myocardial gumma.

Neurosyphilis

Its incidence rate is 10 %, which commonly occurs 3–20 years after the infection. Neurosyphilis can be classified into several types, and the commonly found types include asymptomatic neurosyphilis, meningeal syphilis, meningovascular syphilis, brain parenchymal syphilis, and gumma neurosyphilis.

23.4.2 Congenital Syphilis

Congenital syphilis is also known as placenta transmitted syphilis, which is caused by spreading of TP from mother to the blood flow of the fetus via placenta and the umbilical vein. It can be categorized into early congenital syphilis, advanced congenital syphilis, and latent congenital syphilis. Congenital syphilis is characterized by no occurrence of caries callosa. The early lesions of congenital syphilis are more serious than those of acquired syphilis. Compared to acquired syphilis, congenital syphilis has rarer involvement of the cardiovascular system but more common involvement of the skeleton and sensory organs. Congenital syphilis may affect the growth and development of the infant. Otherwise, physical signs of congenital syphilis permanently remain.

23.4.2.1 Early Congenital Syphilis

Early congenital syphilis commonly occurs in infants at the age of less than 2 years. Patients usually experience premature delivery, with retarded growth, malnutrition, elderly like appearance, weak and hoarse crying voice, and restlessness. The skin and mucosa lesions resemble to those in the cases of secondary acquired syphilis. Perioral and perianal rhagades commonly occur, with formation of radiating shaped scars after healed, which are characteristically early congenital syphilis. Bone syphilis is relatively common, with possible manifestations of chondritis, osteomyelitis, periostitis, and syphilitic dactylitis, which further cause syphilitic pseudoparalysis, such as limbs pain and limited limbs activities. In addition, the common manifestations also include syphilitic rhinitis, systemic lymphadenectasis, hepatosplenomegaly, and meningitis.

23.4.2.2 Advanced Congenital Syphilis

It commonly occurs at the age of above 2 years, generally at the age of 5–8 years. Various symptoms consecutively occur at the age of 13–14 years, mainly invading eyes, teeth, and nervous system but rarely invading the cardiovascular system. In the cases of skin and mucosa syphilis, syphilitic gumma is common, while in the cases of bone syphilis, periostitis is common, with possible occurrence of saber-shaped tibia and Clutton joint. Neurosyphilis is mainly characterized by cranial nerve lesions, especially auditory nerves and optic nerves. In some rare cases, juvenile paralytic dementia and juvenile tabes can be found. In addition, parenchymatous keratitis, Hutchinson teeth, and nerve deafness are integratively known as Hutchinson triad.

23.4.2.3 Latent Congenital Syphilis

Latent congenital syphilis may be asymptomatic. Otherwise, the early symptoms are untreated but disappear. However, both cases are serologically detected positive for syphilis.

23.4.3 Latent Syphilis

The cases with a history of syphilis, no symptoms or disappearance of symptoms, serologically positive for syphilis but no other positive findings, and normal findings in cerebrospinal fluid examination are defined as latent syphilis. Its occurrence is related to strong immunity of the human body or temporary suppression of TP due to therapies.

23.5 Syphilis-Related Complications

Syphilis-related complications are commonly found in the cases of tertiary syphilis, which involve multiple organs with variant clinical manifestations. The common complications include bone syphilis, cardiovascular syphilis, and neurosyphilis.

23.5.1 Bone Syphilis

Bone syphilis is caused by infection of TP by bones and joints. Based on the route of infection and time of onset, bone syphilis is categorized into congenital and acquired. Congenital bone syphilis occurs due to spread of TP from the blood flow of mother into fetus via the placenta, which is divided into early onset and late onset. The cases with syphilis occurring in infants aged under 2 years is referred to as early congenital bone syphilis, while the cases with syphilis occurring in children aged above 2 years are referred to as late congenital bone syphilis. Acquired bone syphilis occurs due to sexual contact, blood contact, or other ways of contact.

23.5.1.1 Early Congenital Bone Syphilis

It is mainly manifested as metaphysitis, periostitis, and osteomyelitis, among which metaphysitis is more common. And its clinical manifestations are various, including skin rashes, large bullous or large flakes of desquamation, systemic lymphadenectasis, bone changes, and hepatosplenomegaly, among which skin rash and bone changes are more common.

23.5.1.2 Late Congenital Bone Syphilis

Late congenital bone syphilis is caused by reactivation of potential lesion after invasion of TP into fetal bone. Generally, its onset occurs in children aged 4–15 years, which is clinically characterized by keratitis, deafness, saddle nose sign, and saber tibia sign. In addition, it also leads to swelling of joint, difficulty walking, even developmental disorder, and hypophrenia.

23.5.1.3 Acquired Bone Syphilis

Its onset is caused by invasion of TP, along with blood flow, to bones, which commonly occurs in patients suffering from secondary and tertiary syphilis. The main symptoms include obvious local stabbing pain and tenderness, which may aggravate during rests. The serological test for syphilis is positive. The manifestation is commonly periostitis. And osteitis and osteomyelitis are also possible manifestations.

23.5.1.4 Syphilitic Arthritis

Both congenital and acquired syphilis can lead to syphilitic arthritis. In the early stage, the disease firstly involves synovium of joint, with manifestations of joint swelling and effusion as well as widened joint space. When the disease further develops to involve articular cartilage and destruct the bone under articular cartilage, the articular space is narrowed, with blurry, discontinuous, and absence of bony articular surface. In the cases with the epiphysis involved, the lesions develop toward the diaphysis, with extensive osteoproliferation and bone destruction.

23.5.2 Neurosyphilis

Neurosyphilis is a systemic chronic infectious disease caused by invasion of TP into the central nervous system, accounting about 10 % of the syphilitic cases. It is more common in young and middle-aged male adults. Neurosyphilis can be found at any stage of syphilis infection. Inappropriate and insufficient treatment of early syphilis is an important factor contributing to the occurrence and development of neurosyphilis. The disease can mainly be categorized into the following types.

23.5.2.1 Asymptomatic Neurosyphilis

It refers to the cases with positive findings by laboratory cerebrospinal fluid examination, such as positive VDRL in the cerebrospinal fluid, but no symptoms and signs related to the nervous system.

23.5.2.2 Meningeal Syphilis

Meningeal syphilis usually onsets 2 months to 2 years after the infection, with main manifestations of syphilitic meningitis, which is clinically characterized by fever, headache, nausea, vomiting, psychiatric disorder, positive meningeal irritation sign, and manifestations of involved cranial nerve. And the commonly involved cranial nerves include the facial nerve and the vestibulocochlear nerve.

23.5.2.3 Meningovascular Syphilis

Its onset is usually 4–7 years after the infection, with typical manifestation of diffuse encephalitis complicated by focal lesions of the nervous system. Its early symptoms include changes of personalities, emotional change, changes of consciousness, and insomnia.

23.5.2.4 Brain Parenchymal Syphilis

Its onset is usually 4–7 years after the infection, which is more common in males, including paralytic dementia and myelophthisis. Paralytic dementia is manifested as diffuse parenchymal lesion of the cerebral cortex, with psychiatric and neurological changes. Myelophthisis is manifested as degeneration and atrophy of posterior root of spinal nerves and posterior column of spinal cords, with lightening pain of lower limbs, abnormal sensation, absent reflexes, and ataxia. The characteristic manifestations of brain parenchymal syphilis include absent lower tendon reflexes and deep sensory disturbance, which develop slowly but may have acute onset.

23.5.2.5 Gumma Neurosyphilis

Gumma neurosyphilis can be categorized into cerebral gumma and spinal gumma. Cerebral gumma neurosyphilis is manifested like brain tumor, brain abscess, or brain tuberculosis, while spinal gumma neurosyphilis is manifested as dural granuloma.

23.5.3 Cardiovascular Syphilis

Cardiovascular syphilis, one of the conditions that may cause death in the cases of advanced syphilis, is a cardiovascular disease caused by invasion of TP into the human body. Cardiovascular syphilis mostly derives from acquired syphilis, lasting for 10–25 years from the infection of TP to the onset of cardiovascular syphilis. In rare cases, symptoms of cardiovascular syphilis occur 1–2 years after the infection. Most patients with cardiovascular syphilis simultaneously experience neurosyphilis. Cardiovascular syphilis can be divided into the following five types, simplex syphilitic aortitis, syphilitic incomplete closure of aortic valve, syphilitic aortic aneurysm, syphilitic stenosis of coronary orifice, and syphilitic myocardial gumma.

23.5.4 Other Syphilis-Related Complications

In the advanced stage, TP can also invade multiple organs to cause various complications, including respiratory syphilis, gastrointestinal syphilis, hepatosplenic syphilis, urogenital syphilis, and endocrine glands syphilis. In addition, TP may also involve the eyes, ears, and lymph nodes to cause complications.

23.6 Diagnostic Examinations

23.6.1 Laboratory Tests

The laboratory tests for diagnosis of syphilis include pathogenic test, serological test, histopathological test, genetic diagnosis, and cerebrospinal fluid examination. Serological test and cerebrospinal fluid examination are commonly applied tests for diagnosis and assessment of syphilis.

23.6.1.1 Pathogenic Test

By dark-field microscopy, the finding of TP with typical morphology and characteristic motion is defined as positive, which is applied to define the diagnosis.

23.6.1.2 Serological Test

The serological test for diagnosis of syphilis can be divided into the following two types.

Serological Test for Non-TP Antigen

1. Venereal disease research laboratory test (VDRL): It can be quantitatively and qualitatively applied by using cardiolipin, lecithin, and cholesterin as the antigen.
2. Rapid plasma reagin test (RPR): It is an improved version of VDRL, with availability of results by naked eyes. It is one of the commonly used examinations across mainland China.
3. Unheated serum reagin test (USR): It is also an improved version of VDRL, with its sensitivity and specificity being close to those by VDRL.

Serological Test for TP Antigen

1. Fluorescent treponemal antibody absorption test (FTA-ABS): The test is the most sensitive examination for TP, but its technical operations are relatively challenging.
2. *Treponema pallidum* hemagglutination assay (TPHA): It is more applicable than FTA-ABS with favorable stability. However, it is less sensitive to primary syphilis than FTA-ABS.
3. *Treponema pallidum* particle assay (TPPA): Its sensitivity to syphilis is close to that by TPHA and is mainly applied to screen and define the suspected positive cases. TPPA is one of the commonly used laboratory tests to define TP infection. Meanwhile, it is also one of the examinations for definitive diagnosis of TP infection adopted by CDC of the United States.

Molecular Biological Detection

PCR is an important laboratory test for the diagnosis of syphilis and can be applied for various clinically collected specimens, with both high sensitivity and specificity. It can also be applied to define the genotype of TP. Currently, it is the most complicated examination for the diagnosis of TP infection.

Cerebrospinal Fluid Examination

Cerebrospinal fluid examination is applied for the diagnosis of neurosyphilis, whose indices include WBC count, protein, VDRL test, PCR detection, and colloidal gold test. VDRL test provides reliable evidence for the diagnosis of syphilis. In the cases with active neurosyphilis, the WBC count usually increases ($>5\times10^6$/L). Therefore, it is also a sensitive indicator for assessing therapeutic efficacy of the therapies against syphilis.

23.6.2 Diagnostic Imaging

23.6.2.1 X-Ray

X-ray examination of bones has relatively high sensitivity and specificity to congenital bone syphilis. Chest X-ray can also facilitate the diagnosis of cardiovascular syphilis.

23.6.3 Ultrasound

Ultrasound is a commonly used examination for cardiovascular syphilis.

23.6.3.1 CT scanning

CT is a commonly applied examination for the diagnosis of cardiovascular syphilis and neurosyphilis.

23.6.3.2 MR Imaging

MR imaging is commonly applied for understanding of the location, range, and severity of neurosyphilis.

23.7 Imaging Demonstrations

23.7.1 Bone Syphilis

23.7.1.1 Early-Onset Congenital Bone Syphilis

About 10 % of infant patients aged within 1 year show negative by serological test for syphilis. Therefore, radiological examination is important for the diagnosis of congenital bone syphilis. Early-onset congenital bone syphilis is the most commonly manifested as metaphysitis, followed by periostitis and osteomyelitis. It is characterized by multiple symmetric lesions, which is mainly metaphysitis with accompanying diffuse irregular osteoproliferation and bone destruction.

Syphilitic Metaphysitis

The lesions are multiple and symmetric, with common occurrence at the long bone of four limbs, such as femur and tibia. And the lesions are especially obvious at distal ulna and radius, proximal medial tibia, and proximal humerus. The early manifestations include widened area of prior calcification with marginal high density and serrated appearance as well as unevenly increased density. With the development of the lesions, the prior calcification area is coarse, with inferior transparent strips and dense lines to form sandwich sign. Along with granulation, unilateral bone destruction of metaphysis occurs to show bone defects, with clearly defined margin, which is known as cat-bite sign (Figs. 23.1, 23.2, and 23.3). The metaphysis at the bilateral superior medial tibia and the bilateral inferior medial femur shows symmetric bone destruction, which is surrounded by osteoproliferation with irregularly increased density. Such lesions are known as Wimberger sign, which has diagnostic value for early-onset congenital bone syphilis. After the lesions develop into the advanced stage, the prior calcification can be destructed, with partially or completely destructed metaphysis and different degrees of osteoproliferation. The lesions usually show no involvement in epiphysis, which is also characteristically early-onset congenital bone syphilis.

Syphilitic Periostitis

Periostitis, the most common condition in the cases of congenital bone syphilis, usually coexists with metaphysitis. The lesions are commonly found at radius, ulna, and femur. X-ray examination demonstrates linear, stratified, or shell-like thickening of periosteum at diaphysis, which parallels to diaphysis of long bone (Fig. 23.4). The lesions develop in a wide range and commonly involve the whole diaphysis and metaphysis. In some cases, periosteum is subject to obvious thickening to form sarcophagus sign. Some parts of thickened periosteum fuse into the diaphysis to show appearance of thickened diaphysis.

Syphilitic Osteomyelitis

It may occur at long bone, mostly resulted from expansion of metaphysitis toward diaphysis. The range with lesions is relatively large, and the lesions may involve more than half of the length of the diaphysis. The manifestations include local worm-eaten-like destruction of bone cortex, relatively wide osteoproliferation and sclerosis, thickened periosteum, and absence of bone marrow cavity, but no formation of sequestrum. Syphilitic osteomyelitis usually coexists with metaphysitis and periostitis. X-ray examination demonstrates transparent areas in the diaphysis with different sizes, which are actually bone destruction caused by syphilis.

23.7.1.2 Late-Onset Congenital Bone Syphilis

Its X-ray demonstrations resemble to those of early-onset congenital bone syphilis. However, late-onset congenital bone syphilis has obviously decreased range with lesions and obviously less serious conditions, with only diffuse changes of chronic periostitis. Periostitis is the most commonly found at the bilateral tibia, with stratified or lacelike proliferation of periosteum. The typical X-ray demonstrations include proliferation of convex periosteum at bilateral tibia and thickened diaphysis, which appears like a curved knife and is known as saber shin.

23.7.1.3 Acquired Bone Syphilis

The most common change of acquired bone syphilis is syphilitic osteomyelitis, which mainly involves diaphysis of long bone. The manifestations include periosteal proliferation in different degrees, which are common at tibia, skull, rib, and sternum. Periosteal proliferation at the anterior margin of bilateral tibia results in thickened bone cortex, appearing like a saber. Osteitis is manifested as diffuse osteoproliferation and osteosclerosis, thickened bone cortex, as well as thickened and deformed diaphysis with internal low-density areas, which are caused by bone destruction. Focal lesion of osteitis is syphilitic gumma, which is commonly found at bone cortex. The manifestations include defective bone cortex at certain part of bone, which is surrounded by osteoproliferation and osteosclerosis as well as periosteal proliferation.

Case Study 1

Syphilitic metaphysitis and syphilitic periostitis

For case detail and figures, please refer to Peng F et al. *Journal of Medical Radiology*, 2011, 21(6): 912 (In Chinese).

Case Study 2

A baby girl patient aged 20 days, with tenderness of the right lower limb for 2 days.

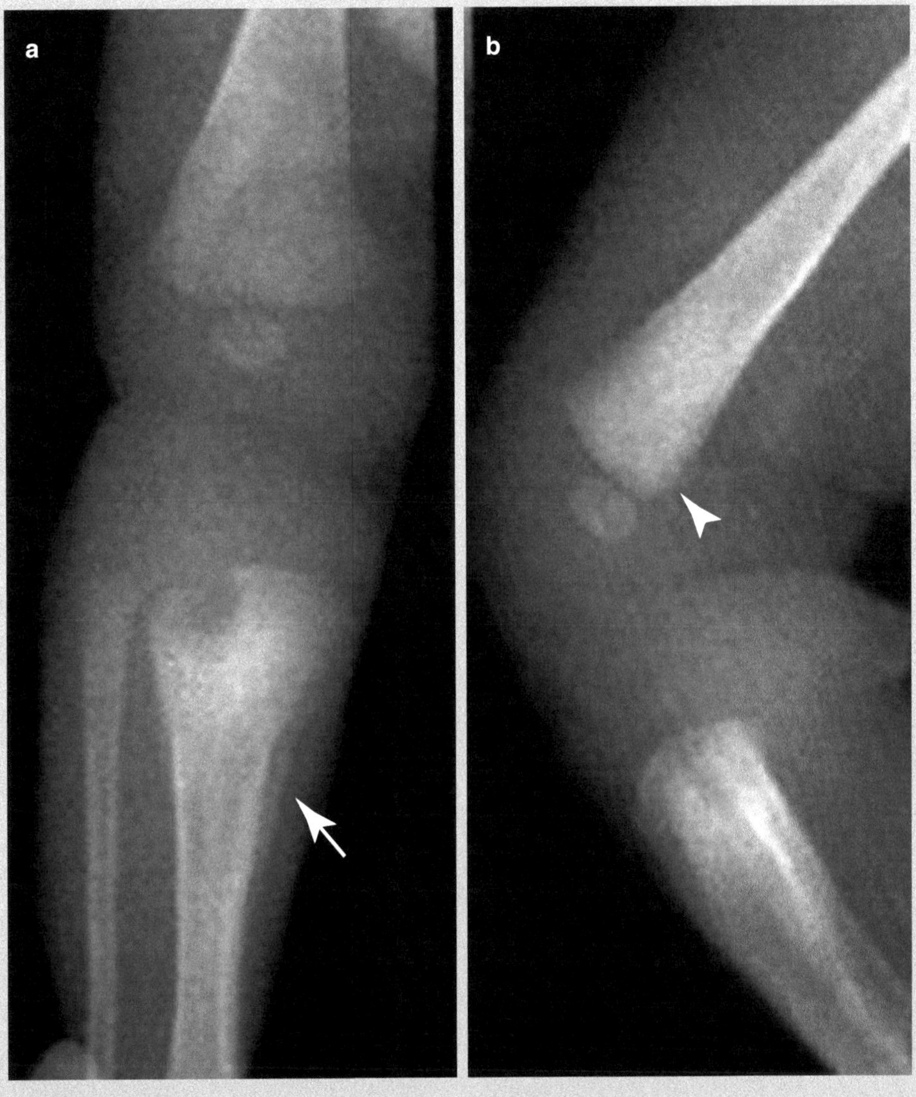

Fig. 23.1 Syphilitic osteomyelitis complicated by metaphysitis and periostitis. (**a**) Posterior-anterior and lateral X-rays demonstrate worm-eaten-like bone destruction at the left superior tibia, with surrounding high-density area and neighboring periosteal thickening (indicated by *arrow*). (**b**) Linear transparent area of bone destruction is demonstrated at the metaphysis of left distal femur (indicated by *arrowhead*)

Case Study 3

A baby boy patient aged 2 days, with RPR of 1:128.

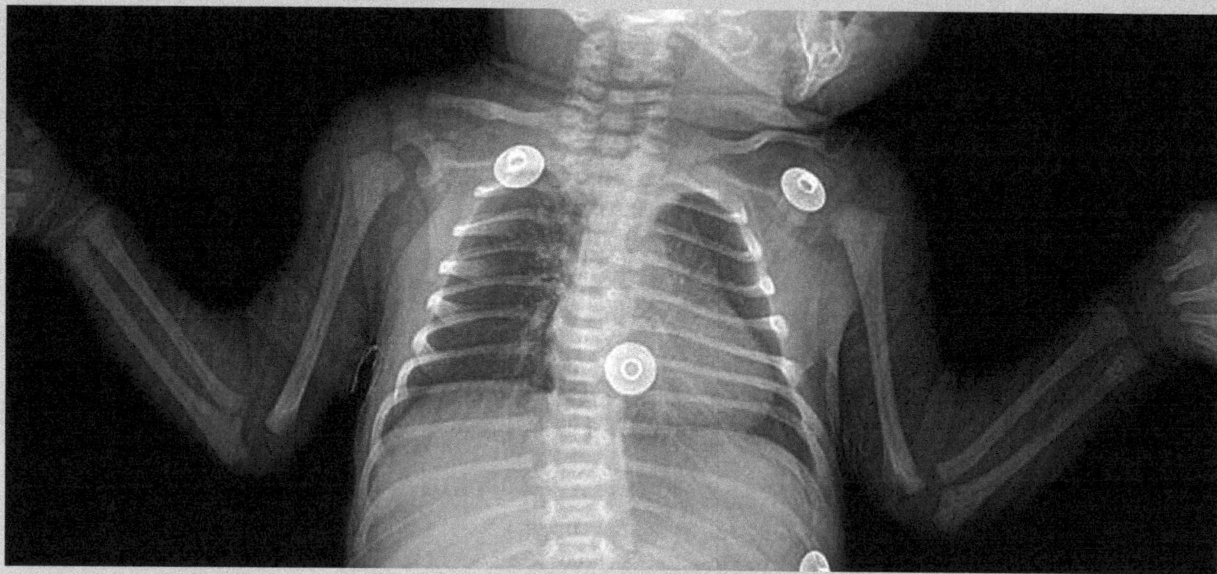

Fig. 23.2 Syphilitic metaphysitis. X-ray demonstrates round-like low-density bone lesion at the right inferior humerus

Case Study 4

A baby boy patient aged 2 months, with skin rashes for 1 month and fever and abdominal distension for 5 days.

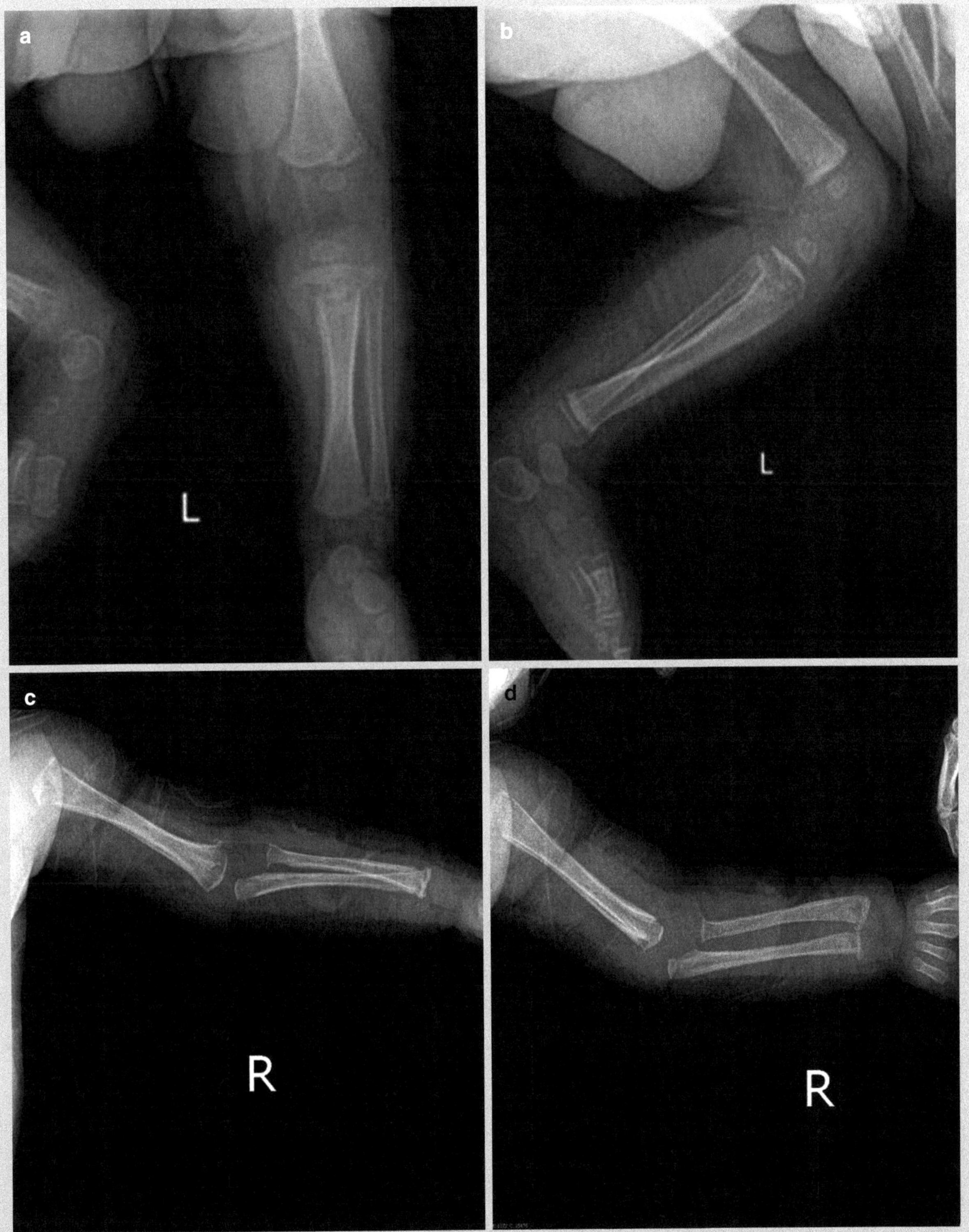

Fig. 23.3 Syphilitic metaphysitis. (**a**, **b**) Posterior-anterior and lateral X-rays demonstrate bone destruction at the proximal metaphysis of left tibia, widened space between metaphysic and swollen adjacent soft tissue; (**c**, **d**) Posterior-anterior and lateral X-rays demonstrate coarse bone cortex at the metaphysis of right radius and ulna

(The case study 2 and the case study 3 as well as the figures are provided by Zhang N et al. from the Department of Radiology, Chengdu Infectious Diseases Hospital, Sichuan, China)

Case Study 5
A baby boy patient aged 5 months, with abnormalities by serological test for above 3 months.

For case detail and figures, please refer to from Zhang GY et al. *Journal of Medical Research*, 2012, 41(2): 166 (In Chinese).

Case Study 6
A baby boy patient aged 10 weeks, with pain at bilateral upper limbs. He was suspected with greenstick fracture of the left humerus.

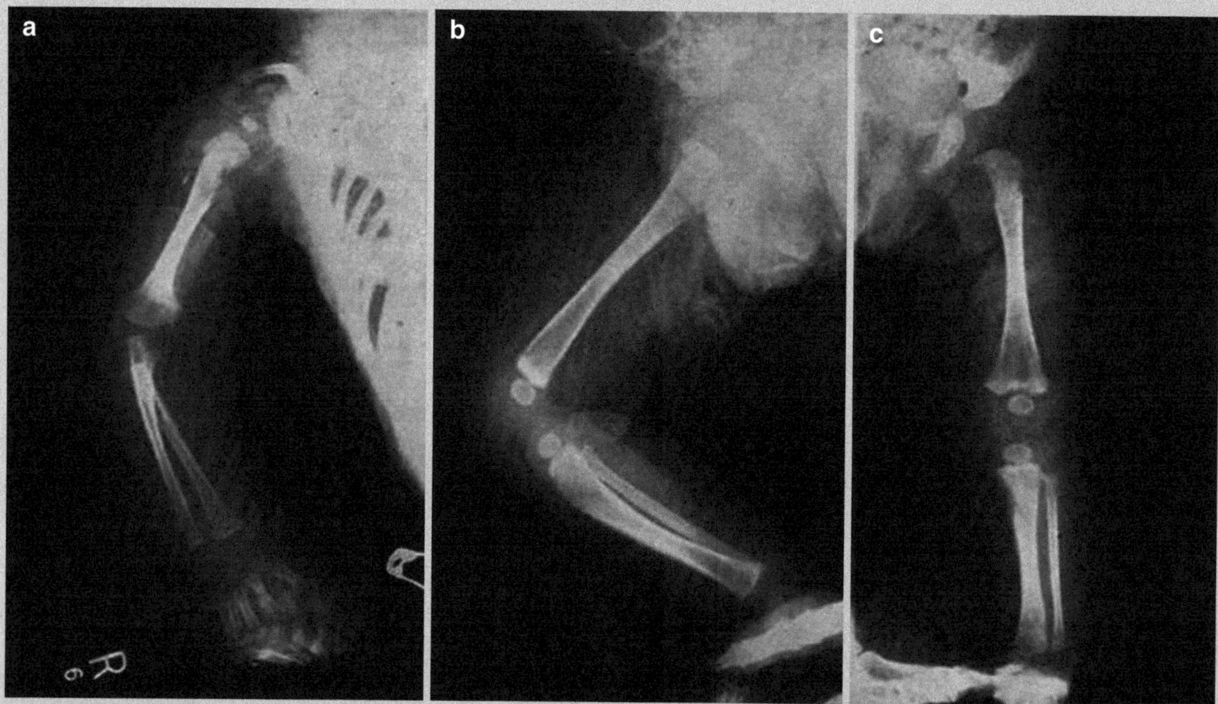

Fig. 23.4 Syphilitic metaphysitis and periostitis. (**a**) X-ray demonstrates parallel thickening of periosteum at the right radius and ulna and transparency shadow below the metaphysis. (**b**) Thickened prior calcification is demonstrated at the left femur. (**c**) Irregular decalcification is demonstrated at the left proximal tibia (Reprint with permission from Marks KL. *Br Med J*, 1954, 1 (4869): 1018)

23.7.2 Neurosyphilis

The radiological examinations for the diagnosis of neurosyphilis mainly include CT scanning and MR imaging. X-ray and ultrasound provide information with limited diagnostic value.

23.7.2.1 Asymptomatic Neurosyphilis

The radiological examinations usually demonstrate no abnormalities of the brain parenchyma.

23.7.2.2 Meningeal Syphilis

In its early stage, CT scanning demonstrates no abnormalities. But by contrast scanning, linear enhancement of meninges sometimes can be demonstrated. By MR imaging, the meninges and brain surface are demonstrated with diffuse linear long or equal T_1 signal and long T_2 signal. The meningeal lesions are generally more serious at the base of brain, which can be demonstrated with obvious enhancement by contrast imaging (Fig. 23.5). There are also demonstrations of swollen adjacent brain tissues, enlarged and widened cisterns and sulci, and increased signal strength of cerebrospinal fluid. Due to accumulated and increased inflammatory exudates at the base of brain, communicating hydrocephalus commonly occurs. The meningeal lesions can disseminate along the cranial nerves at the base of brain to invade the cranial nerves, with common involvement of VII and VIII cranial nerves. Syphilitic myelitis is demonstrated as long T_1 long T_2 signals of the involved spinal cords. By contrast imaging, uneven enhancement can be demonstrated (Figs. 23.6 and 23.7). Due to common involvement of the meninges, the condition is also known as syphilitic meningomyelitis, manifested as inflammatory thickening of dura matter and its adhesion with pia matter of arachnoid membrane. The condition may further develop to cause lesions at the supplying vascular vessels and the nerve roots of the spinal cords, leading to spinal cord degeneration.

23.7.2.3 Meningovascular Syphilis

Meningovascular syphilis is pathologically characterized by proliferation of arteriolar endothelial cells and fibrocytes, thickening of vascular walls, stenosis, and blockage of the vascular lumen. After formation of cerebral infarction, MR imaging demonstrates typical T_1WI low signal and T_2WI high signal. By contrast imaging, the lesions are demonstrated with patches and cortical gyrus-like enhancement. After occurrence of encephalomalacia, the signal is the same as that of the cerebrospinal fluid.

23.7.2.4 Brain Parenchymal Syphilis

Brain parenchymal syphilis includes paralytic dementia and myelophthisis. In the early stage of brain parenchymal syphilis, CT scanning demonstrates extensive low-density change, with accompanying edema. In the advanced stage of brain parenchyma syphilis, the cortex is subject to diffuse atrophy and expanded lateral ventricles, but no ischemia and inflammatory changes. T_1WI and T_2WI of MR imaging demonstrate atrophy of different degrees at bilateral frontal and temporal lobes that is more obvious at the anterior parts, bilaterally symmetric dilation of brain ventricles, and glial proliferation of subcortex and hippocampus (Fig. 23.8).

23.7.2.5 Gumma Neurosyphilis

Gumma neurosyphilis can be found at any part of brain tissues, mostly at the cerebral cortex and subcortex. The round-like lesions may be singular or multiple, with a diameter of 2–2.5 cm. By T1WI, the central caseous necrosis of the lesion is demonstrated as low signal or equal low mixed signal, with surrounding low signal due to a large area of edema that shows space-occupying effect. By contrast imaging, the lesions are demonstrated with irregular ring-shaped enhancement and adjacent meningeal enhancement that indicates meningeal involvement Fig. 23.9. Intramedullary gumma neurosyphilis is manifested as swollen and thickened spinal cord, round-like or nodular lump that resembles to intracranial gumma, as well as enhancement and thickening of adjacent meninges.

Case Study 7

A male patient aged 53 years complained of dizziness with illusion for 1 month. He also experienced loss of memory, depression, and behavioral abnormalities. By laboratory tests, RPR was 1:8 and TPPA positive.

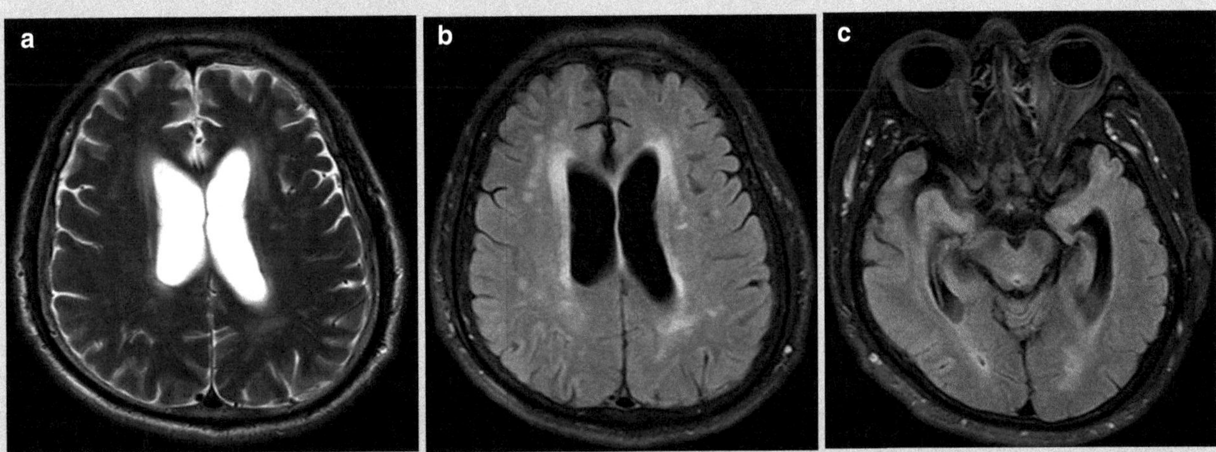

Fig. 23.5 Meningeal syphilis. (**a**, **b**) Transverse T2WI demonstrates multiple patches of long T1 long T2 signals at the bilateral semioval centrum and beside the bilateral lateral ventricles. By water and fat suppression T2WI, high signal can be observed. (**c**) The cortex at the inferior pole of bilateral temporal lobes and hippocampus is demonstrated to be thinner. (**d**, **e**) Contrast imaging demonstrates thickening and enhancement of the right temporal lobe and the meninges of brainstem; slight dilation of bilateral lateral ventricles

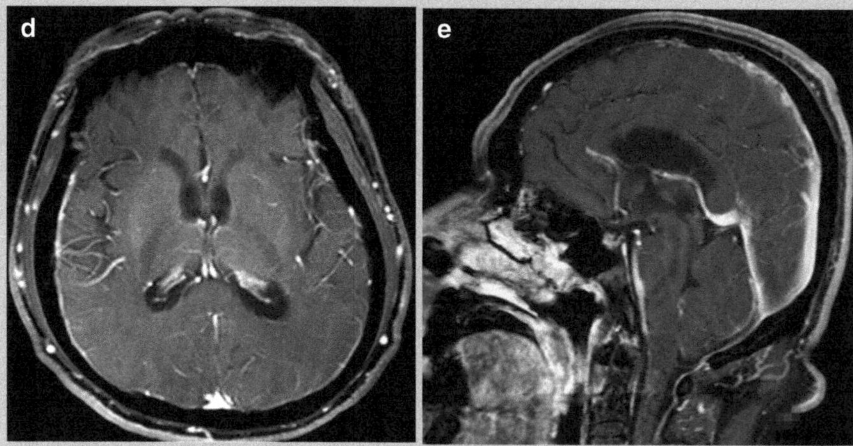

Fig. 23.5 (continued)

Case Study 8

A male patient aged 46 years experienced progressive instability of gait and dysuria. By physical examinations, deep reflex of both lower extremities was sensitive, bilateral Babinski sign was positive, and sensory disturbance was below L1. By laboratory tests, cell counts and protein level in the cerebrospinal fluid increased, while immunological assay of both cerebrospinal fluid and serum for syphilis was positive. The clinical diagnosis was syphilitic myelitis.

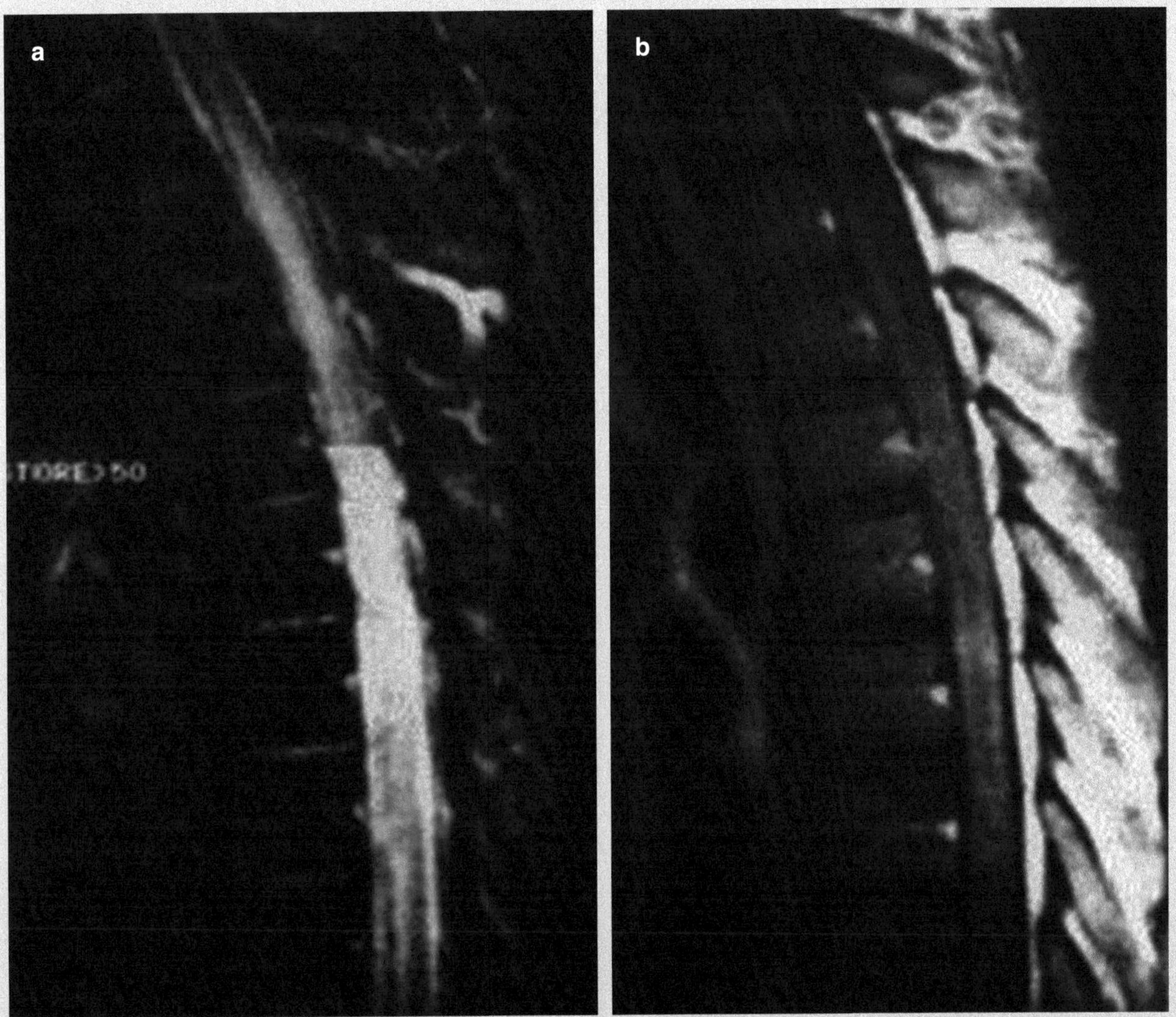

Fig. 23.6 Syphilitic myelitis. (**a**) Sagittal T2WI of MRI demonstrates high signal at the thoracic spinal cord. (**b**) Gd-DTPA contrast sagittal T1WI demonstrates uneven enhancement of the thoracic spinal cord, diffusive swelling of the spinal cord with internal low signal (Reprint with permission from H. Nabatame, et al. *Neuroradiology*, 1992, 34 (2): 105)

Case Study 9

A female patient aged 45 years complained of low back pain and upset with no known causes for 2 months that exacerbated for 2 weeks. The pain was especially obvious in the posture of supine at nights that affected her sleeping. In addition, she also experienced right lower-limb pain. By laboratory tests, RPR was positive, TPPA was positive, titer was 1:1,024, and HBV was positive. The pathological diagnosis was chronic inflammation with accompanying necrosis at T_{12}-L_1 spinal cord that is consistency with manifestations of syphilitic myelitis.

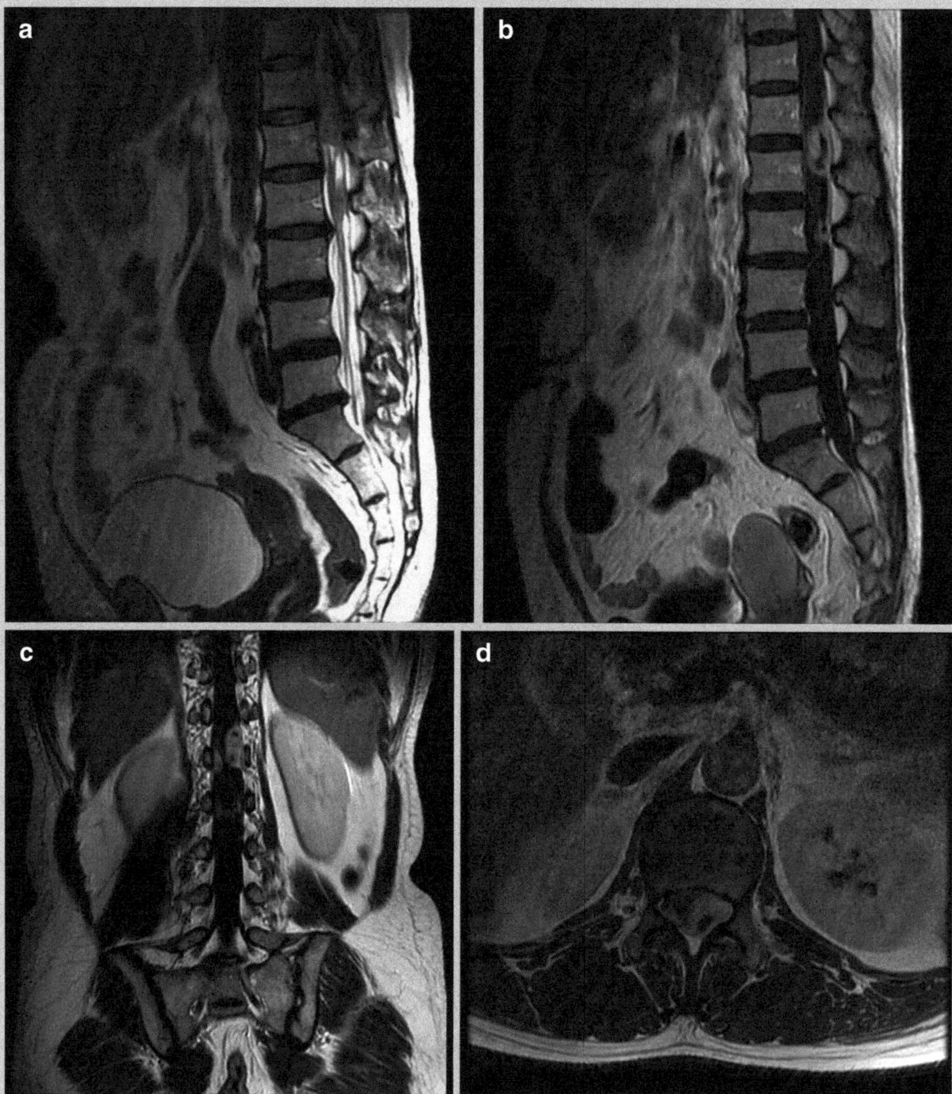

Fig. 23.7 Syphilitic myelitis. (**a**) T_2WI demonstrates heterogeneous signal shadows at the T_{12}-L_1 spinal cords. (**b–d**) Contrast imaging demonstrates the posterior wall of T_{12}-L_1 horizontal spinal canal with multiple lumps of ring-shaped enhancement, which adhere to dura mater at the posterior wall of spinal canal. The adjacent dura mater is also demonstrated with enhancement

(The case and figures were provided by Tang YH at Ruijin Hospital, Shanghai, China)

Case Study 10

A male patient aged 49 years experienced unclear language expressions, loss of memory, emotional instability, tremor of upper limbs, poor orientation, uncoordinated gait, hypermyotonia of the four limbs, and tendon hyperreflexia. By laboratory tests, serological test for TP antigen was positive; VDRL of the cerebrospinal fluid was qualitatively positive and quantitatively 1:8. The clinical diagnosis was paralytic dementia.

For case detail and figures, please refer to Peng FH et al. *Chinese Journal of Radiology*, 2005, 39 (9): 957 (In Chinese).

Case Study 11

A male patient aged 44 years was detected syphilis positive more than 1 month ago. He had histories of unhealthy sexual life and drug abuse. And he experienced psychiatric disorder, loss of memory, and intelligence decline. By laboratory tests, TPPA was positive and RPR was 1:32.

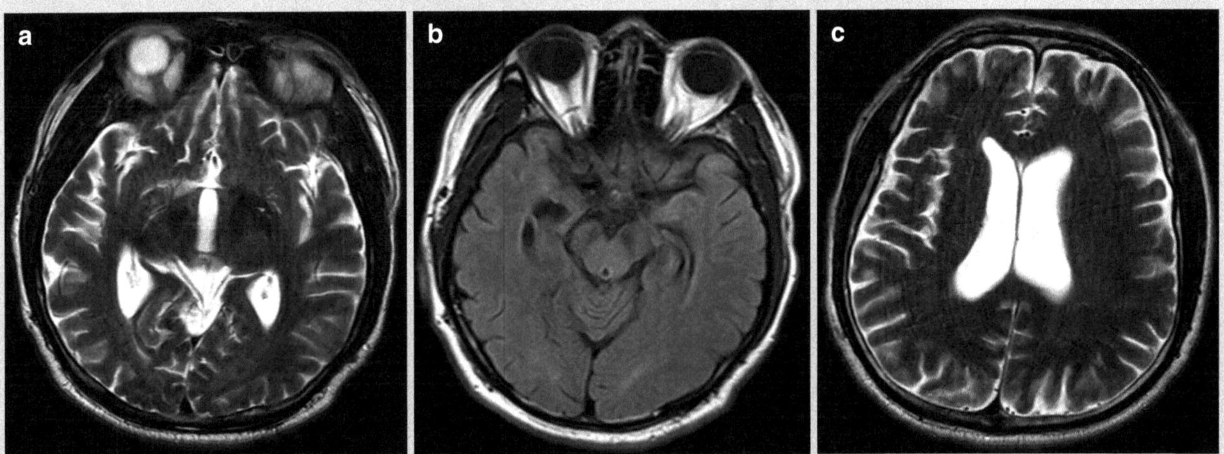

Fig. 23.8 Brain parenchymal syphilis. Transverse T2WI demonstrates multiple spots and strips of long T1 long T2 signals at the bilateral basal ganglia. (**b**) Atrophy of bilateral hippocampus and parahippocampal gyri is demonstrated. (**a**, **c**) Dilation of the bilateral lateral ventricle and the third ventricle is demonstrated

Case Study 12

A female patient aged 40 years complained of blurry vision for 1 month, with defects of bilateral lower right vision.

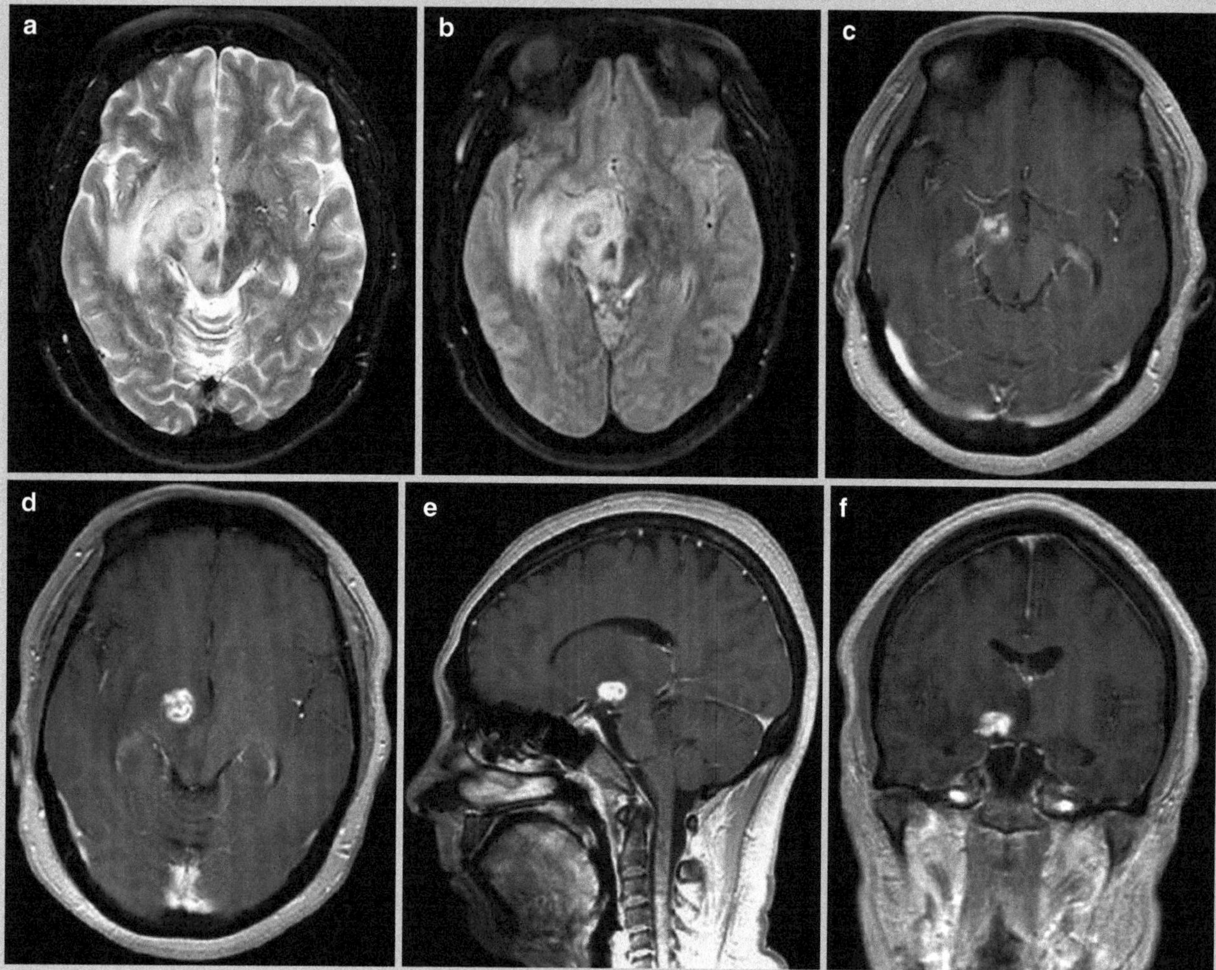

Fig. 23.9 Gumma neurosyphilis. (**a**, **b**) Transverse MR imaging demonstrates round-like long T2 signal at the right mesencephalon and cerebral peduncle, with internal uneven and mixed signals. The center of the lesion is demonstrated with slightly low signal. And the lesion is demonstrated with surrounding large flakes of high-signal edema. And the midline structure is demonstrated to shift slightly leftward. (**c**–**f**) Contrast imaging demonstrates obvious enhancement of the lesion, with well-defined boundary, and slight enhancement of the adjacent meninges

(Note: the case and figures were provided by Xia S at the Department of Radiology, the First Central Hospital, Tianjin, China.)

Case Study 13

A male patient aged 56 years experienced IV degree myodynamia of the left lower limb and hyperalgesia of the left lower limb. He had a history of unhealthy sexual life. By laboratory tests, RPR was negative and TPPA was 1:640 to be positive.

For case detail and figures, please refer to Liu H et al. *Journal of Clinical Radiology*, 2008, 27 (9): 1275 (In Chinese).

23.7.3 Cardiovascular Syphilis

23.7.3.1 Syphilitic Aortitis

Syphilitic aortitis is commonly complicated by incomplete closure of aortic valve, stenosis of coronary orifice, and other conditions. Ultrasonocardiography demonstrates dilated aorta, aortic regurgitation, and enlarged left ventricle.

23.7.3.2 Syphilitic Incomplete Closure of Aortic Valve

Ultrasonocardiography indicates abnormal enlargement of the aortic circle, dilated ascending aorta, different degrees of aortic regurgitation with following enlarged left ventricle, and widened outlet of the left ventricle. Color Doppler demonstrates colored regurgitation bundle during diastole from aortic circle to the outlet of left ventricle.

23.7.3.3 Syphilitic Aortic Aneurysm

X-ray demonstrates mediastinal mass shadow. Both CT scanning and MR imaging demonstrate the location, size, and morphology of aortic aneurysm, which is usually cystiform or spindle-shaped aortic aneurysm shadow (Figs. 23.10 and 23.11).

23.7.3.4 Syphilitic Stenosis of Coronary Orifice

The condition mainly involves the proximal coronary orifice. By coronary angiography, morphology of the coronary artery and the location, severity, and range of its obstructive lesion can be defined. And such an examination is currently the only way to observe the morphology of coronary artery. Coronary angiography can define the location and severity of stenosis of coronary orifice.

Case Study 14

A male patient aged 74 years experienced stable angina pectoris and accompanying aortic regurgitation. Ultrasonocardiography demonstrated dilated aortic root and obvious aortic regurgitation.

For case detail and figures, please refer to Pugh PJ et al. *N Engl J Med*, 2002, 346 (9): 676.

Case Study 15

A male patient aged 76 years experienced progressive dyspnea and accompanying swelling of the lower limbs. He had a history of chronic syphilis, but no history of receiving therapies.

For case detail and figures, please refer to Rajab TK et al. *N Engl J Med*, 2011, 364 (13): 1258.

Case Study 16

A male patient aged 57 years experienced chronic hypertension, lipid metabolism disorder, and a history of smoking and drinking. Ultrasonocardiography demonstrated dilated ascending aorta, normal diameter of aortic root, moderate hypertrophy of the left ventricle, and favorable ventricular systole. No lump in the cavity of aortic regurgitation and no communication between the atria and ventricles were found.

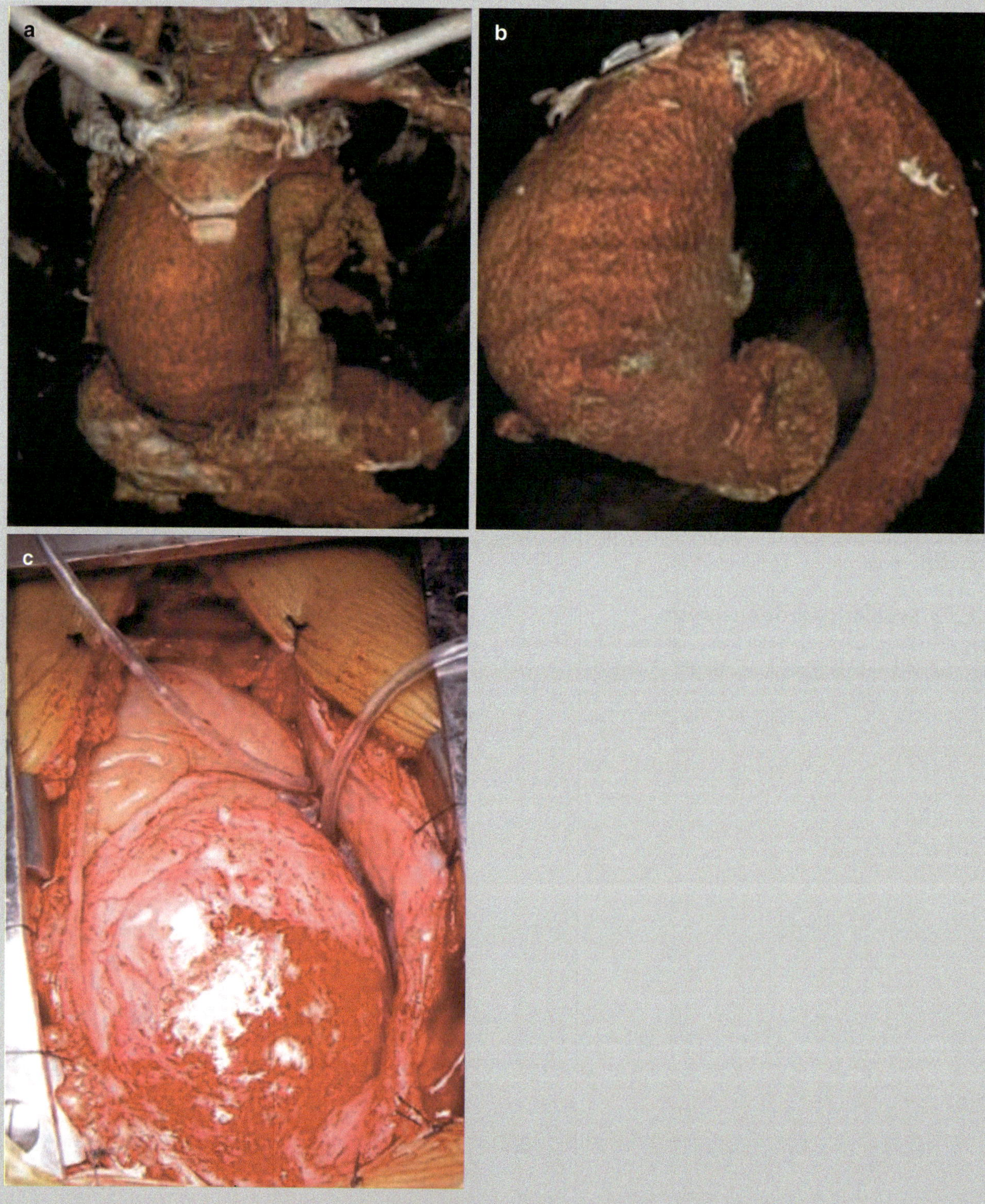

Fig. 23.10 Syphilitic aortic aneurysm. (**a**, **b**) VR of CT scanning demonstrates aneurysm at the ascending aorta. (**c**) Observations during surgery to remove the aneurysm (Reprint with permission from Paulo N, et al. *Interact Cardiovasc Thoracsurg*, 2012, 14 (2): 193)

Case Study 17

A male patient aged 38 years experienced sudden dyspnea, sharp stabbing pain at the chest, and cardiac shock.

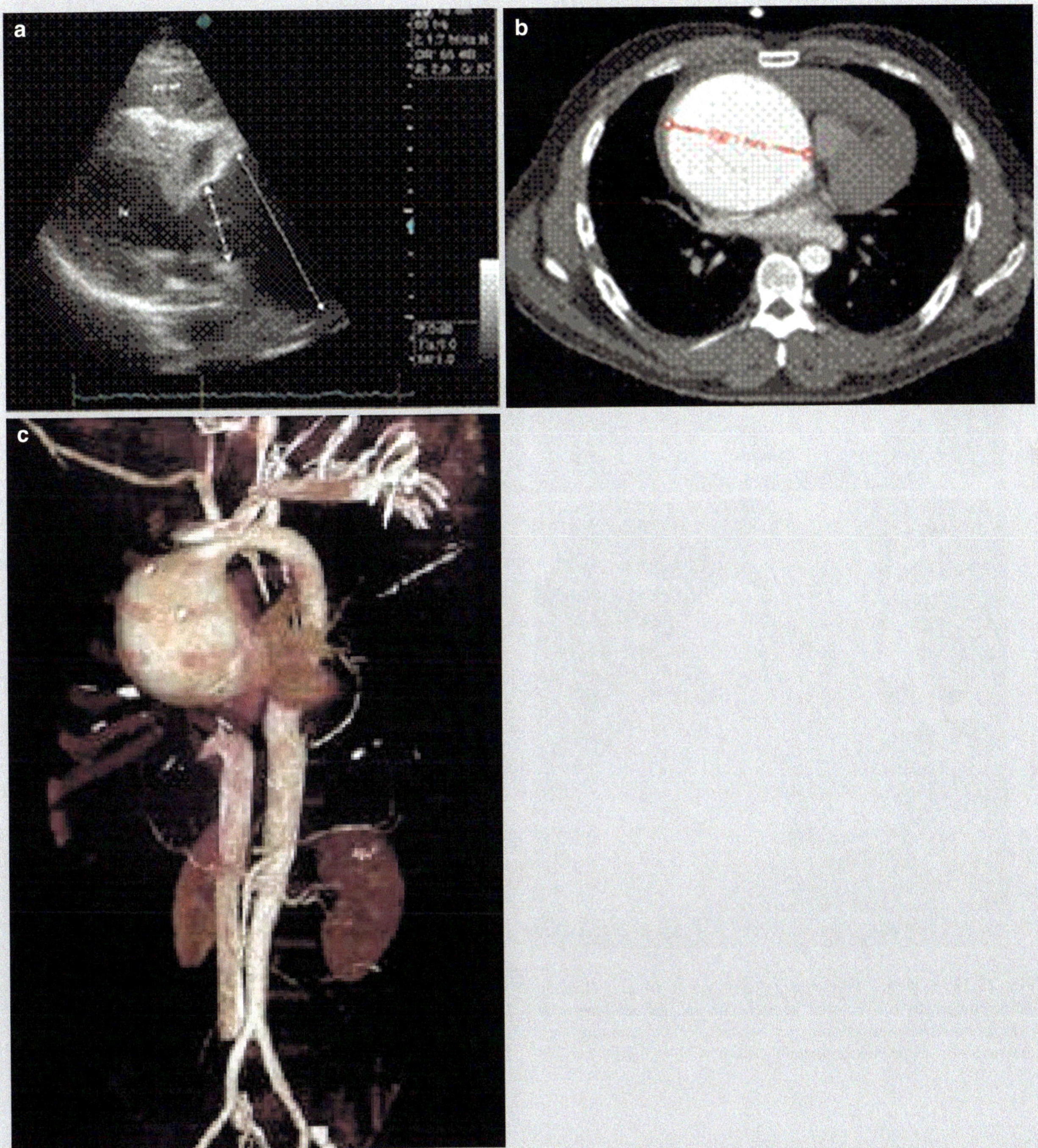

Fig. 23.11 Syphilitic aortic aneurysm. (**a**) Ultrasonocardiography demonstrates serious dilation of the ascending aorta and accompanying moderate incomplete closure of aortic valve. (**b**, **c**) CT scanning demonstrates dilated ascending aorta with a diameter of about 10 cm and compressed right atrium (Reprint with permission from Acar Z, et al. *J Am Coll Cardiol*, 2012, 59 (1): e1)

Case Study 18

A male patient aged 34 years experienced dyspnea and palpitation. By serological test for syphilis, TPHA was strongly positive and VDRL was strongly positive (Fig. 23.12).

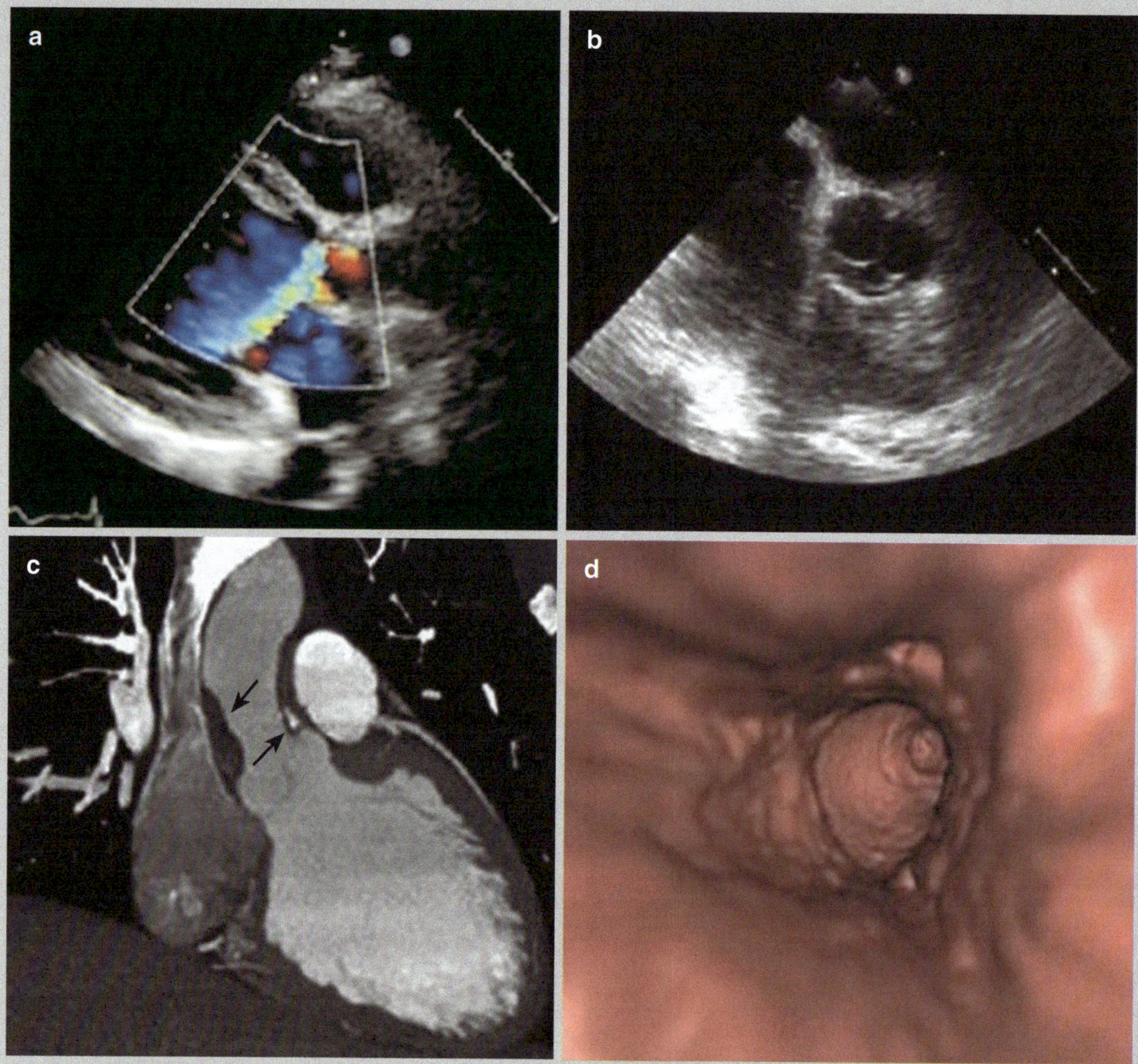

Fig. 23.12 Syphilitic inflammatory gumma. (**a**, **b**) Transthoracic echocardiography (TTE) and transesophageal echocardiography (TEE) demonstrate serious aortic regurgitation. (**c**) CT scanning demonstrates ring-shaped thickening of the aortic wall, with a thickness of about 8 mm (indicated by an *arrow*). (**d**) It is demonstrated that calcification of partial vascular wall causes stenosis of major artery lumen, with a diameter of 16 mm (Reprinted with permission from Bouvier E, et al. *J Am Coll Cardiol*, 2011, 57 (24): e375)

23.7.4 Ocular Syphilis

Case Study 19
A female patient aged 42 years complained of blurry vision of both eyes for 4 months. By examinations, the light sense of right naked eye was within 1 m, the vision of left naked eye was 0.08, both ciliary bodies were congested, the cornea was transparent, a small quantity of flocculent exudates from the right eye, PHA was (+), and RPR titer was 1:64.

For case detail and figures, please refer to Zhao Q et al. *Ophthalmologic Research*, 2009, 27 (4): 268 (In Chinese).

Case Study 20
A male patient aged 59 years had a history of unhealthy sexual life. He complained of painless blurry vision for 10 days. By examinations, the binocular vision was 0.5, there was no congestion of the bulbar conjunctiva, cornea was transparent, KP and vitreous opacity were positive, and crystalline lens was transparent. Primary screening test for syphilis was positive (++); antibody test for syphilis was positive (++) (Fig. 23.13).

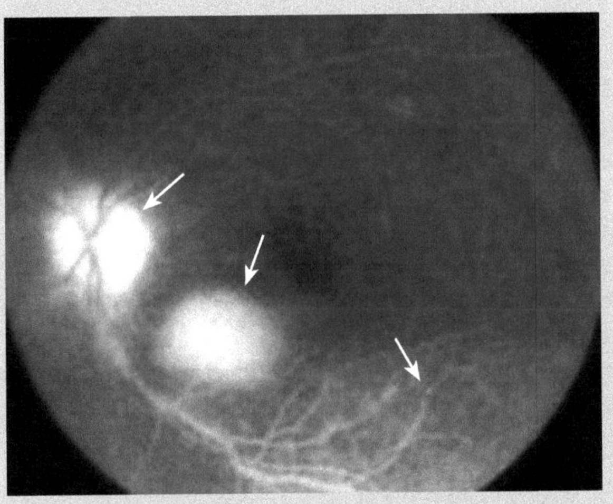

Fig. 23.13 Syphilitic neuroretinitis and uveitis. FFA of the left eye fundus demonstrates focal leakage of fluorescein at the retina, leakage at the venous wall, and leakage at the optic disk (indicated by *arrows*)

Case Study 21
A male patient aged 42 years had a past history of unhealthy sexual life. He complained of sudden decline of the right eye vision for 5 days. By examinations, the vision of right eye for counting fingers was 30 cm, and the vision of left naked eye was 1.0. By laboratory tests, the primary screening test for syphilis was positive (++), and the antibody test for syphilis was positive (++).

For case detail and figures, please refer to Cai QH et al. *Ophthalmologic Research*, 2005, 23 (6): 631. (In Chinese)

23.8 Diagnostic Basis

The definitive diagnosis of syphilis should be based on comprehensive analysis of the medical history, clinical manifestations, physical examination findings, and laboratory test findings.

23.8.1 Diagnosis of Syphilis

23.8.1.1 Primary Syphilis

Epidemiological History
The patients usually have multiple sexual partners and high-risk sexual behaviors. Otherwise, his/her sexual partner has a case history of syphilis infection.

Clinical Manifestations
The patients usually have singular painless caries callosa, which has an incubation period of 2–4 weeks, and has cartilage like hardness. The caries callosa is commonly found at the external genitals, with inguinal lymphadenectasis or lymphadenectasis around the lesion.

Laboratory Tests
By dark-field microscopy, patients with syphilis usually have lesions at the skin and mucosa. Otherwise, by puncture of lymph node, TP can be detected in the collected fluid.

After occurrence of caries callosa for 2–3 weeks, serological test for TP antigen turns to be positive.

23.8.1.2 Secondary Syphilis

Epidemiological History

The patients usually have multiple sexual partners and high-risk sexual behaviors. Otherwise, his/her sexual partner has a history of syphilis infection or the patient has a history of blood transfusion.

Clinical Manifestations

The patients may have a history of primary syphilis that lasted for less than 2 years. The patients with syphilis usually have various skin rashes, accompanying general upset and systemic superficial lymphadenectasis.

Laboratory Tests

The serological test for TP antigen is positive.

23.8.1.3 Tertiary Syphilis

Epidemiological History

The patients usually have multiple sexual partners and high-risk sexual behaviors. Otherwise, his/her partner has a history of syphilis infection.

Clinical Manifestations

The patients may have a history of primary or secondary syphilis that lasted for above 2 years. The typical manifestations include nodular syphilid, syphilitic gumma, perforation of palate and nasal septum caused by syphilitic gumma, saddle nose, bone syphilis, ocular syphilis, and other organ syphilis. Tertiary syphilis may involve respiratory tract, gastrointestinal tract, liver and spleen, urogenital system, endocrine glands, and skeletal muscles. Neurosyphilis and cardiovascular syphilis may also occur.

Laboratory Tests

(1) Serological test for non-TP antigen is positive, and serological test for TP antigen is also positive. (2) By examination of cerebrospinal fluid, the WBC count in the cases of neurosyphilis $\geq 10 \times 10^6$/L, the protein level >500 mg/L, and VDRL test was positive.

23.8.1.4 Latent Syphilis

Epidemiological History

The patients usually have multiple sexual partners and high-risk sexual behaviors. Otherwise, his/her sexual partner has a history of syphilis infection.

Clinical Manifestation

The patients usually have no symptoms and signs of syphilis.

Laboratory Test

Serological test for non-TP antigen is positive for at least twice. Otherwise, serological test for TP antigen is positive, with biologically false positive excluded.

Cerebrospinal Fluid Examination

By examination of the cerebrospinal fluid, the results are negative.

23.8.1.5 Congenital Syphilis

Epidemiological History

The biological mother is a patient with syphilis or TP infection.

Clinical Manifestation

The patients usually have typical symptoms and signs of syphilis.

Laboratory Test

By dark-field microscopy, TP is found at the lesions of skin and mucosa or at the placenta in baby patients. Serological test for non-TP antigen is positive and serological test for TP antigen is positive.

23.8.2 Diagnosis of Syphilis-Related Complications

23.8.2.1 Bone Syphilis

The diagnosis of bone syphilis should be comprehensively based on medical history, clinical manifestation, laboratory test findings, and radiological findings. Congenital bone syphilis is common in children, and the mother usually has a history of syphilis infection. X-ray commonly demonstrates metaphysitis, periostitis, and diaphysitis. The characteristic manifestation is multiple symmetric lesions, commonly at long bones of all four limbs, such as femur and tibia. Metaphysitis is manifested as concurrent osteoproliferation and bone destruction, in typical signs of hamburger sign, cat-bite sign, and Wimberger sign. And the lesions usually do not involve metaphysis. Periostitis is common in the cases of bone syphilis, with X-ray demonstrations of thickening of diaphysis and periosteum in various morphologies. In some serious cases, X-ray demonstrates sarcophagus-like sign. In the cases with lesions of periostitis at the tibia, the periosteum is demonstrated with laminar or lacelike proliferation, and the diaphysis is demonstrated to be thickened, with an appearance of a curved knife, which is typically saber tibia sign. Osteomyelitis is common at long bones, which is manifested as worm-bitten-like bone destruction, and accompanying osteoproliferation and osteosclerosis. By X-ray, diaphysis is demonstrated with transparent areas in different sizes. Based on the above characteristic demonstrations of bone syphilis by X-ray as well as the case history and positive finding by serologic test, the diagnosis can be defined.

23.8.2.2 Neurosyphilis

Currently, the diagnosis of neurosyphilis still has no golden standard. Therefore, its diagnosis is commonly based on comprehensive analysis of the case history, clinical manifestations, laboratory test findings, and radiological demonstrations.

The diagnostic criteria for syphilis implemented by CDC of the United States are (1) having evidence supporting TP-induced infection of the central nervous system; (2) a serological test for syphilis is positive and VDRL test of CSF for TP is positive; (3) suspected cases with syphilis at any stage having VDRL test of CSF negative plus the following two conditions, the increase of CSF protein and cells counts with no other known causes and symptoms and signs in consistency with neurosyphilis with no other known causes; and (4) definite cases with syphilis at any stage having laboratory findings in consistency with neurosyphilis.

The diagnostic criteria for syphilis are feasible and practicable, but with no criteria to exclude neurosyphilis. FTA-ABS test of cerebrospinal fluid has high specificity to neurosyphilis, and the cases with negative result can be excluded as non-neurosyphilis.

The radiological demonstrations of neurosyphilis are nonspecific. Contrast CT scanning and MR imaging demonstrate meningeal syphilis with linear enhancement of the meninges, swollen adjacent brain tissue, as well as widened cistern and sulcus. Contrast MR imaging demonstrates meningovascular syphilis with patches of enhancement of the lesion and gyrus-like enhancement of the cortex. CT scanning and MR imaging commonly demonstrate brain parenchymal syphilis with atrophy of brain parenchyma and dilated lateral ventricle, which are more common at the frontal and temporal lobes with accompanying edema of different degrees. Gumma neurosyphilis is commonly demonstrated with round-like lesions in the brain, which are surrounded by accompanying edema. By contrast scanning or imaging, the lesions may be demonstrated with irregular ring-shaped enhancement and adjacent meningeal enhancement. The adjacent meningeal enhancement indicates meningeal involvement.

23.8.2.3 Cardiovascular Syphilis

Syphilitic aortitis is usually manifested as dilated aorta, aortic valve regurgitation, and enlarged left ventricle. Syphilitic incomplete closure of aortic valve is manifested as enlarged aortic ring, dilated ascending aorta, and aortic valve regurgitation of various degrees. X-ray demonstrates syphilitic aortic aneurysm with mediastinal mass shadow, while CT scanning and MR imaging usually demonstrate cystiform or spindle-shaped aortic aneurysm shadow. Syphilitic stenosis of coronary orifice can be examined by coronary angiography to define the morphology of coronary artery as well as the location, severity, and range of the obstructive lesions.

23.9 Differential Diagnosis

23.9.1 Primary Syphilis

Caries callosa should be differentiated from soft chancre, fixed drug eruption, genital herpes, tuberculous ulcer, and Behçet disease.

23.9.2 Secondary Syphilis

The skin rashes are morphologically various, which may resemble to skin rashes of various skin diseases. The differential diagnosis should be comprehensively based on case history, clinical manifestations, and laboratory findings. Macular syphilis rash should be differentiated from pityriasis rosea. Other skin rashes should be differentiated from drug rash, lichen planus, pustule sore, and psoriasis.

23.9.3 Tertiary Syphilis

Nodular syphilitic rash should be differentiated from lupus vulgaris, rheumatic nodule, lepra lepromatosa, scrofuloderma, sporotrichosis, and chronic leg ulcer. Syphilitic gumma should be differentiated from lupus vulgaris, lepra lepromatosa, erythema induratum, and ulcers.

23.9.4 Neurosyphilis

23.9.4.1 Differential Diagnosis of Meningeal Syphilis

Meningeal syphilis should be differentiated from diseases with meningeal enhancement. The meningeal lesion at the skull base in the cases of meningeal syphilis is more serious than that in the cases of other diseases. By contrast imaging, meninges is demonstrated to be thickened with obvious enhancement, which are more obvious at the hypothalamus, brainstem, suprasellar cistern, and around the sylvian cistern.

23.9.4.2 Differential Diagnosis of Meningovascular Syphilis

Meningovascular syphilis should be differentiated from cerebral infarction. Generally, meningovascular syphilis has multiple asymmetric infarction lesions at the cerebral hemispheres, mainly located at the subcortex and deep cerebral white matter. CT scanning demonstrates patches of low-density areas. In some serious cases, the middle cerebral artery can be occluded. In addition, meningovascular neurosyphilis should also be differentiated from herpes simplex virus encephalitis. Meningovascular neurosyphilis has chronic onset, which is commonly manifested as slight atrophy of the temporal lobe and slight dilation of the temporal horns of cerebral ventricles. However, herpes simplex virus encephalitis has an acute onset, commonly with space-occupying effect.

23.9.4.3 Differential Diagnosis of Brain Parenchymal Syphilis

Paralytic dementia in the cases of brain parenchymal syphilis is often manifested as diffuse cerebral atrophy of different degrees, which is commonly located as the frontal lobe and temporal lobe. In addition, most cases have asymmetric cerebral atrophy of bilateral hemispheres and accompanying symmetric dilation of bilateral ventricles. In the cases of Alzheimer's disease, cerebral atrophy is commonly symmetric, with accompanying hippocampal atrophy.

23.9.4.4 Differential Diagnosis of Gumma Neurosyphilis

Gumma neurosyphilis should be differentiated from brain neoplasm, parasitic granuloma, and tuberculoma. Gumma neurosyphilis may be manifested as ring-shaped enhancement of the lesions adjacent to the meninges, with thickened adjacent meninges that can be observed with enhancement.

23.9.5 Cardiovascular Syphilis

23.9.5.1 Differential Diagnosis of Syphilitic Aortitis

Syphilitic aortitis should be differentiated from atherosclerosis. Syphilitic aortitis commonly occurs at the ascending aorta, with common complications of syphilitic aortic aneurysm, incomplete disclosure of aortic valve, and stenosis of coronary orifice. By X-ray, it is demonstrated with dilated ascending aorta, linear calcification, and irregular edge of vascular lumen. However, atherosclerosis usually does not involve the ascending aorta, which commonly involves the descending aorta with masses of calcification.

23.9.5.2 Differential Diagnosis of Syphilitic Aortic Aneurysm

Syphilitic aortic aneurysm should be differentiated from the diseases with intramediastinal lump, such as central lung carcinoma, lymphoma, and retrosternal thyroid. These diseases are usually not accompanied by shift of aorta. Aortic angiography can facilitate to define the diagnosis. Syphilitic aortic aneurysm usually occurs at the thoracic aorta, which is singular and commonly found at the ascending aorta and aortic arch.

23.9.6 Congenital Bone Syphilis

Congenital bone syphilis should be differentiated from late-onset congenital bone syphilis, congenital rickets, and pyogenic osteomyelitis. Late-onset congenital bone syphilis occurs at an elderly age, and periostitis commonly occurs at the tibia, which is usually confined at the anterior tibia in saber tibia sign. Pyogenic osteomyelitis is manifested as systemic toxic symptoms, confined bone destruction, obvious sequestration and osteoproliferation, rare simultaneous involvements of multiple bones, and even rarer occurrence of symmetric lesions. Congenital rickets is manifested as common osteoporosis of diaphysis, cup-shaped metaphysic, and serration-shaped metaphysis due to bone destruction. In addition, laboratory tests demonstrate abnormalities of calcium and phosphate concentrations in the blood. By physical examinations, typical signs of rickets, such as rachitic beads, cephalus quadratus, and hand-foot bracelets, can be found. However, bone changes are not definitely demonstrated by X-ray in the cases of neonatal congenital syphilis, especially those experiencing premature delivery and baby patients. In such cases, the metaphysis can be demonstrated normal by X-ray.

References

Acar Z, Ağaç MT, Demirbas M, et al. Giant syphilitic aortic aneurysm presenting with pericardial tamponade as an initial sign. J Am Coll Cardiol. 2012;59(1), e1.

Bouvier E, Tabet JY, Malergue MC, et al. Syphilitic aortic regurgitation and ostial coronary occlusion. J Am Coll Cardiol. 2011;57(24), e375.

Cai QH, Shen W, Li LB, et al. Syphilitic neuroretinitis. Opthalmol Res. 2005;23(6):631.

Liu H, Ji SP, You NX. MRI demonstrations of neurosyphilis and its SPECT demonstrations after brain perfusion: report of 3 cases. J Clin Radiol. 2008;27(9):1275–8.

Marks KL. Congenital syphilis diagnosed by bone changes. Br Med J. 1954;1(4869):1018.

Nabatame H, Nakamura K, Matuda M, et al. MRI of syphilitic myelitis. Neuroradiology.1992;34(2):105–6.

Paulo N, Cascarejo J, Vouga L. Syphilitic aneurysm of the ascending aorta. Interact Cardiovasc Thorac Surg. 2012;14(2):223–5.

Peng FH, Hu XQ, Qiu W, et al. MRI demonstrations of paralytic dementia. Chin J Radiol. 2005;39(9):956–8.

Peng F, Ma LB, Chen J. Diagnostic value of X-ray for early-onset congenital bone syphilis. J Med Radiol. 2011;21(6):911–3.

Pugh PJ, Grech ED. Images in clinical medicine. Syphilitic aortitis. N Engl J Med. 2002;346(9):676.

Rajab TK, Gallegos RP. Images in clinical medicine. Giant syphilitic aortic aneurysm. N Engl J Med. 2011;364(13):1258.

Zhang GY, Liu K, He JW. Early clinical manifestations and X-ray demonstration of bones in the cases of congenital syphilis. J Med Res. 2012;41(2):165–8.

Zhao Q, Zhang F, Cui YH, et al. Syphilitic uveoretinitis: report of 1 case. Opthalmol Res. 2009;27(4):268–9.

Suggested Reading

Barrera MV, Bosch RJ, Mendiola M, et al. Revival of syphilis in Malaga. Actas Dermosifiliogr. 2006;97(5):323–6.

Cheng J, Duan HY, Li AX. Epidemiological study of syphilis and its diagnosis and treatment. Inf Infect Dis. 2012;25(1):58–9.

Fu ZY. Recent studies on sexually transmitted diseases. Beijing: People's Military Medical Press; 2009.

Kodana K, Okada S, Komatsu N, et al. Relationship between MRI findings and prognosis for patients with General Paresis. J Neuropsychiatry Clin Neurosci. 2000;12(2):246–50.

Li HJ. Practical radiology of HIV/AIDS. Beijing: People's Medical Publishing House; 2012.

Saraiva RS, César CA, Mello MA. Syphilitic aortitis: diagnosis and treatment. Case report. Rev Bras Cir Cardiovasc. 2010;25(3): 415–8.

Singh AE, Romanowski B. Syphilis: review with emphasis on clinical, epidemiologic, and some biologic features. Clin Microbiol Rev. 1999;12(2):187–209.

Smith MM, Anderson JC. Neurosyphilis as a cause of facial and vestibulocochlear nerve dysfunction: MR imaging features. AJNR Am J Neuroradiol. 2000;21(9):1673–5.

Zhang LX, Zhou XZ. Modern studies of infectious diseases. Beijing: People's Military Medical Press; 2010.

Zhong WB. Color Doppler ultrasonographic study of syphilitic cardiovascular diseases. Chin Med J Coal Ind. 2002;6:622–3.

24 Typhoid and Paratyphoid Fever

Dongli Shi, Hongjun Li, and Ailin Cheng

Typhoid and paratyphoid fever are acute gastrointestinal infectious diseases caused by *Salmonella* typhi and *Salmonella* paratyphi. Main pathological changes of the diseases are continuous bacteremia and productive reaction of systemic monocyte-macrophages system, which is mainly characterized by proliferation and necrosis of lymphoid tissues in the lower ileum. Clinically, typhoid fever is characterized by persistent fever, relative bradycardia, systemic toxic and gastrointestinal tract symptoms, roseola, hepatosplenomegaly, and leucopenia, which are complicated by enterorrhagia and enterobrosis. Clinical manifestations of paratyphoid fever A and B are similar to those of typhoid fever but are mild with shorter courses. However, the clinical manifestations of paratyphoid fever C are special with acute gastroenteritis and pyemia.

24.1 Etiology

Typhoid fever and paratyphoid fever A, B, and C are caused by serogroup D and A, B, and C of salmonella, which is a gram-negative brevibacterium with a length of 1–3 mm and a width of 0.4–0.9 mm. Without spores and capsule, salmonella has bacterial flagellum all over the thallus. The aerobic or facultative anaerobic bacterium can move. The optimal environment for its growth includes a temperature of 37 °C and a pH value of 6.8–7.8. It can live in water for 2–3 weeks, in the feces for 1–2 months, in the frozen earth for half a year, but can be killed at a temperature of 60 °C for 15 min or in 5 % hydroxybenzene for 5 min. *Salmonella* typhi can live in normal medium but can live well in the medium with bile, for it provides lipoid and tryptophan for *salmonella* typhi as nutrients. Splitting of thallus can release endotoxin, which plays an important role in the course of typhoid fever.

Thallus (O), flagellum (H), and surface (Vi) antigen of *Salmonella* typhi and *Salmonella* paratyphi stimulate the human body to produce specific antibody IgM and IgG, in which O and H have solid antigenicity, so serum agglutination test (Widal reaction) can be used to measure the titer of antibody-O and antibody-H in serum in order to assist clinical diagnosis. The titer of antibody-Vi is low so that it has limited clinical diagnostic value. However, most carriers of *Salmonella* typhi test positive for antibody-Vi, so it is helpful for the test of chronic *Salmonella* typhi carriers.

24.2 Epidemiology

24.2.1 Source of Infection

Patients and carriers of typhoid fever and paratyphoid fever are the sources of infection. In the latent period, patients will excrete bacteria. The amount of bacteria becomes largest with the strongest contagiosity in 2–4 weeks after the onset, while in the recovery phase or after being cured, the excretion of bacteria will decrease. Patients with excretory phase less than 3 months are temporal excreters, but more than 3 months are chronic excreters, who are the main pandemic source of typhoid fever and make great contributions to epidemiology.

24.2.2 Route of Transmission

The human body is infected by *Salmonella* typhi and *Salmonella* paratyphi through fecal-oral route. Polluted water is the most important transmission route, which may often result in outbreaks of this disease. Polluted food is the main transmission route, which may cause food-based outbreaks. Besides, close contact in daily life is another transmission route of typhi fever. Media such as flies and cockroaches can mechanically carry *Salmonella* typhi, which will give rise to the prevalence of the disease.

D. Shi • H. Li (✉) • A. Cheng
Department of Radiology, Beijing You'an Hospital, Capital Medical University, Beijing, China
e-mail: lihongjun00113@126.com

H. Li (ed.), *Radiology of Infectious Diseases: Volume 2*, DOI 10.1007/978-94-017-9876-1_24

24.2.3 Susceptible Population

People are generally susceptible but can acquire strong immunity after recovery as well as not easily be susceptible to a secondary infection.

24.2.4 Epidemic Features

Men and women of all ages can be attacked by the disease, of which children are with high morbidity of paratyphoid fever, while adults are often present with paratyphoid fever A. Typhoid and paratyphoid fever have no seasonal changes, but often occur in summer and autumn. Outbreaking in sporadic, endemic, or pandemic, the diseases can occur all over the world, especially in tropics and subtropics.

24.3 Pathogenesis and Pathological Changes

24.3.1 Pathogenesis

Because most *Salmonella* typhi and *Salmonella* paratyphi are destroyed in the stomach after entering the alimentary canal, the onset of the disease is determined by the amount of bacteria entering to the intestines. If the amount of bacteria is large, the bacteria will enter the small intestines and invade lymphatic tissues of the intestinal wall, especially the aggregated or solitary lymphoid nodules in the distal ileum through epithelial cells in the intestinal mucosa. Then the bacteria will reach the mesentery lymphoid nodules along the lymphatic vessels, where *Salmonella* typhi is swallowed by macrophages and grows at the same time as well as enters the blood through the thoracic duct inducing bacteremia. Bacteria in the blood are soon swallowed by the systemic mononuclear phagocyte system such as the macrophage system in the liver, spleen, bone marrow, and lymphatic nodules as well as proliferate in quantity. During this period, though there is a mononuclear phagocyte system proliferative response, it is asymptomatic clinically, which is known as incubation period lasting about 10 days. Bacteria proliferating in the systemic mononuclear phagocyte system and endotoxins released by the bacteria enter the blood again, causing secondary bacteremia with fever, rash, hepatosplenomegaly, acute pyogenic osteomyelitis, nephrapostasis, cephalomeningitis, acute cholecystitis, and pericarditis.

24.3.2 Pathology

Typhoid fever, inflammatory proliferative response of systemic mononuclear phagocyte system, is mainly characterized by macrophages, that is, "typhoid cells" that have swallowed lymphocytes, red blood cells, *Salmonella* typhi, and necrotic debris which are demonstrated by microscopy. "Typhoid cells" clump together to form "typhoid nodules," which mainly occur in aggregated lymphatic nodules or solitary lymphoid follicles of the lower ileum.

Typhoid fever can be divided into four stages according to pathological changes of the intestines. The first week is called medullary swelling stage, which is characterized by medulla hyperplasia, mild swelling of lymphoid tissues in the lower ileum, infiltration and proliferation of large amount of macrophages seen under a microscope, and aggregated lymphatic nodules that are most typical. The second week is necrotic stage, in which mucosal lesions become necrotic. The third week is known as the ulcerative stage: the necrotic tissues fall off and ulcer forms, when enterorrhagia and enterobrosis may happen. The fourth week is healing stage, in which the ulcerative tissues heal gradually without leaving cicatrices or stenosis.

For organs outside the intestines, lesions of the spleen and liver are most obvious. Lesions of the spleen are splenomegaly, dilation, and congestion of the splenic sinus, obvious medulla hyperplasia, filtration of macrophages, and typhoid nodules. Lesions of the liver are obvious swelling, cloudy swelling and degeneration of hepatocytes, focal necrosis, dilation of the blood sinus, and typhoid nodules. In addition, mild inflammatory changes can be seen in the cholecyst. Patients with severe toxemia are present with opacity of the myocardia and kidney. Roseola is caused by congestion and dilation of capillaries on the surface of the skin as well as infiltration of monocytes, where *Salmonella* typhi can be found. Pathological changes of the respiratory system are chiefly bronchopneumonia as well as secondary bronchopneumonia or lobar pneumonia. Occasionally, metastatic abscess can be seen in the kidney, meninges, pericardium, lungs, and middle ear.

Pathological changes of paratyphoid fever A and B are similar to those of typhoid fever. Bowel lesions are not obvious in paratyphoid fever C. Also, there is no ulcer in the wall of the intestines. However, localized purulence will be seen in other organs.

24.4 Symptoms and Signs

24.4.1 Typhoid Fever

The incubation period of the disease generally ranges from 7 to 23 months. In most cases, it lasts for 10 to 14 days. The course of a typical typhoid fever lasts for 4–5 weeks, which can be divided into four stages clinically, that is, preliminary, critical, remission, and recovery stage.

24.4.1.1 Preliminary Stage (Invasion Stage)

In the first week, with slow onset and fever, patients' body temperature increases gradually and may feel chills before fever. Often, patients are present with general malaise, weakness, anorexia, and abdominal discomfort. The disease will progressively get worse.

24.4.1.2 Critical Stage

In the second to third week, specific symptoms and signs of typhoid fever will appear.

1. Persistent high fever: main types of the fever are high fever and continued fever. A few patients will be with remittent or irregular fever. Fever persists for 10–14 days.
2. Symptoms of digestive system: obvious anorexia, thick-coated tongue, abdominal discomfort, abdominal distension, constipation or diarrhea, and slight tenderness of the hypogastrium.
3. Symptoms of the cardiovascular system: relative bradycardia and dicrotic pulse.
4. Symptoms of nervous system: absentmindedness, apatheia, lags in response, hearing loss and even delirium, and coma or meningeal irritation sign in critical patients.
5. Hepatosplenomegaly: most patients are with splenomegaly that is soft with tenderness; some patients are with hepatomegaly, and when it is complicated by toxic hepatitis, there will be liver dysfunction or jaundice. Besides, in the sixth day, reddish stains and papule which blanch on pressure on the chest and abdominal skin, i.e., roseolas, can be seen. With the diameter of 2–4 mm and the number of less than 10, those roseolas appear in batches and disappear in 2–4 days. Also, enterorrhagia and enterobrosis often occur in this stage.

24.4.1.3 Remission Stage

In the third to fourth week, the body temperature will decrease with relieved symptoms, better appetite, disappearing abdominal distension, and hepatolienal retraction. Complications such as enterorrhagia and enterobrosis may occur in this stage.

24.4.1.4 Convalescence Stage

In the fifth week, the body temperature will become normal with disappearing symptoms and regained appetite. Generally, complete rehabilitation can be achieved in around a month. However, for weak patients or patients with chronic diseases, the course of disease often prolongs.

24.4.2 Paratyphoid Fever

24.4.2.1 Paratyphoid Fever A and B

Manifestations of paratyphoid fever A and B are very similar to those of typhoid fever, but with relatively mild condition and shorter course. Clinically, it can be divided into preliminary, critical, remission, and recovery stage. The incubation period of the disease ranges from 2 to 15 days. Generally, it lasts for 8 to 10 days. Symptoms of acute gastroenteritis may occur at the beginning of the disease, such as abdominal pain, vomiting, and diarrhea. After 2 to 3 days, clinical manifestations of typhoid fever such as fever will occur but the symptoms of gastroenteritis will relieve. In addition, roseola occurs earlier with more in the number, bigger in size, and darker in color. Bowel diseases are few and superficial, so enterorrhagia and enterobrosis are rare and the mortality is lower. The recurrence rate of paratyphoid fever A is higher than that of typhoid fever.

24.4.2.2 Paratyphoid Fever C

Clinical manifestations of paratyphoid fever C are complicated, which can be categorized into following three types.

Typhoid Type

The clinical manifestations of typhoid type are similar to paratyphoid fever A and B.

Acute Gastroenteritis Type

It is mainly characterized by the symptoms of gastroenteritis with short course.

Septicopyemia Type

This type often occurs in weak children with characteristics of acute onset, chill, high fever, and metastatic purulent complications in more than half of the patients.

24.5 Complications of Typhoid and Paratyphoid Fever

24.5.1 Enterorrhagia and Enterobrosis

Enterorrhagia and enterobrosis occur in the second to third week with symptoms of fecal occult blood and even hematochezia in large amounts. Enterobrosis is one of the most severe complications, which often occurs in the distal ileum. Because of the abundant lymphoid follicles and nodules on the intestinal wall, after the onset of the disease, bacteria will enter the lymphatic tissues through the small intestinal mucosa. Then the bacteria are swallowed by macrophages in the lymphatic tissues, which results in ulcers in the small intestinal mucosa to various degrees. Intestinal canal and ileocecal valve dysfunction with large amount of bacteria for a long term as well as hypertension of the intestinal canal will result in enterobrosis, which occurs in the second to third week of the course.

24.5.2 Pulmonary Infection

Symptoms of the lungs are bronchitis, pneumonia, pulmonary abscess, and adult respiratory distress syndrome, of which bronchitis is often seen in children. In the preliminary stage of the disease, it is characterized by slight cough with white phlegm. For the decreased body resistance, pulmonary infection often develops secondary to streptococcus pneumonia or other diseases caused by respiratory tract bacterial infections.

24.5.3 Others

Toxic myocarditis, hemolytic-uremic syndrome, osteomyelitis, sacroiliitis, nephropyelitis, and brain stem encephalitis are often seen and perforation of the gallbladder occurs occasionally.

24.6 Diagnostic Examination

24.6.1 Laboratory Tests

24.6.1.1 Blood Routine Examination

Low or normal white blood cell counts, decreased neutrophilic granulocytes, and decreased or disappearing eosinophilic granulocytes are valuable for diagnosis and observation of the conditions. Growth and decline of those indicators are consistent with the disease. Besides, blood platelets may decrease as well.

24.6.1.2 Bacterial Culture

As the golden standard of typhoid fever, the blood culture's positive rate reaches the highest value (80–90 %) in the first week and then decreases gradually. After antibiotic therapy, the positive rate decreases significantly. Sensitivity of bone marrow culture is 80–95 %, which still remains high in the late stage of the disease and after antibiotic therapy. Positive rate of stool culture in the acute stage is 30 %, which increases gradually in the second week of the course and reaches the highest rate, i.e., 75 % in the third to fourth week. It is often negative for urine culture in the early stage, while in the third to fourth week, it can be positive. Bile culture is significant to diagnose and find bacteria carriers in the late stage of the disease.

24.6.1.3 Widal Reaction

Antigens used in Widal reaction are antigen O, H, and flagellar antigen of paratyphoid fever. Antibodies in patients' serum are tested by agglutination reaction. Antibodies occur in the first week of the disease and their positive rate reaches higher than 70 % in the third to fourth week, which maintains several weeks in high titer. A few patients with typhoid fever always remain negative in Widal reaction.

24.6.1.4 Other Immunological Tests

Serologic tests studied at home and abroad in recent years such as dot-blot enzyme immunoassays and semiquantitative detection are controversial for the diagnostic value of sensitivity and specificity of typhoid fever.

24.6.2 Diagnostic Imaging

24.6.2.1 Ultrasonography

Ultrasound is often used to test for organs in the abdomen, such as the liver, cholecyst, spleen, etc.

24.6.2.2 X-Ray

X-ray is to detect combined pneumonia and other pulmonary lesions. The erect abdominal plain radiograph is to exclude intestinal obstruction and perforation, etc.

24.6.2.3 CT Scanning and MRI

CT scanning and MRI are used to further locate and determine the nature of intestinal perforation, bleeding, abscess formation, brain stem encephalitis, osteomyelitis, and nephropyelitis.

24.7 Imaging Demonstrations

24.7.1 Typhoid Fever

24.7.1.1 Abdominal Organs

Ultrasonography

Ultrasound demonstrates that the intestinal wall becomes thicker, some of which reach 9 mm, mainly at the terminal ileum and cecum or the whole colon but with the five layers intact: mesenteric lymphatic nodes become larger with the diameter of 8–34 mm in round or oval shape, and the hypoechoic parenchyma is with clear edge; echoes of the enlarged spleen's parenchyma are normal, and abscess or obstruction can be seen in a few cases; cholecyst dilates with thicker wall, cholestasis in some cases (i.e., there is echogenic mass or echogenic foci in the cholecyst), and ulcers in the cholecystic wall; and in some cases, the liver enlarges with normal echoes in the parenchyma (Fig. 24.1).

Case Study 1

A group of typhoid patients with fever and positive results in Widal reaction.

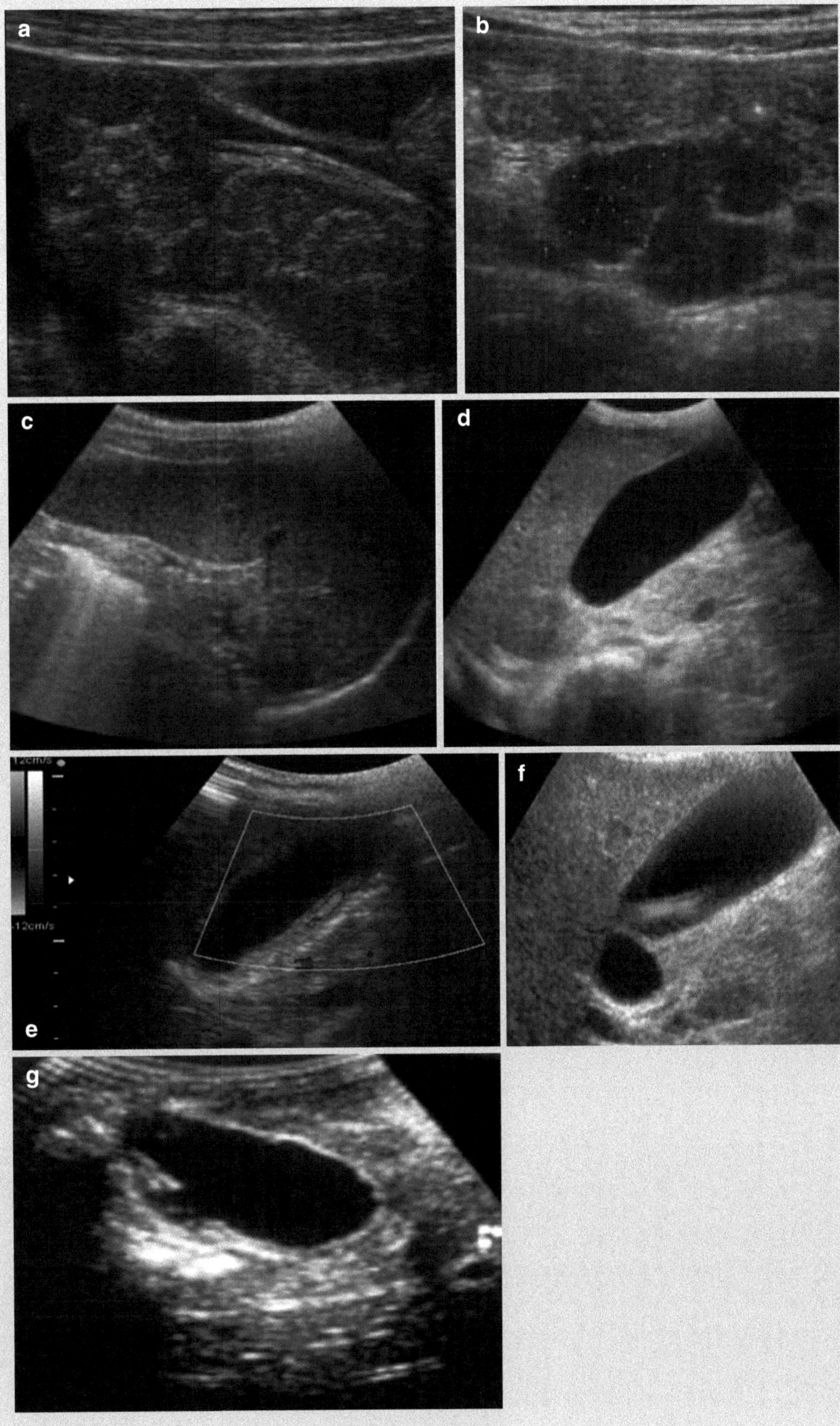

Fig. 24.1 Abdominal organs (ileum, spleen, and cholecyst) and lymphatic node lesions of typhoid fever. (**a–g**) Ultrasound demonstrates thicker wall of the ileum, enlarged mesenteric lymphatic nodes, enlarged spleen with normal echoic structure, enlarged cholecyst, thicker wall of the cholecyst with more blood vessels in it, cholestasis, and ulcers in cholecystic mucosa with interruption of its continuity (Reprint with permission from Mateen MA, et al. *Indian J Pediatr*, 2006, 73 (8): 681)

CT Scanning

CT scanning demonstrates enlarged lymphatic nodes and annular thickening of the intestinal wall, especially at the terminal ileum; diffuse enlargement of the spleen with uneven density of some nidi and sheet nidi with low density that reveal splenic abscess or destruction, which can be identified by enhancement scanning; moderate enlargement of the liver compared with enlarged spleen; and even thickening of the cholecystic wall with even low density by enhancement scanning. Some results show ascites and a few reveal intestinal perforation, bleeding, and abscess (Figs. 24.2, 24.3, and 24.4).

Case Study 2

A 29-year-old male with fever and right lower quadrant pain.

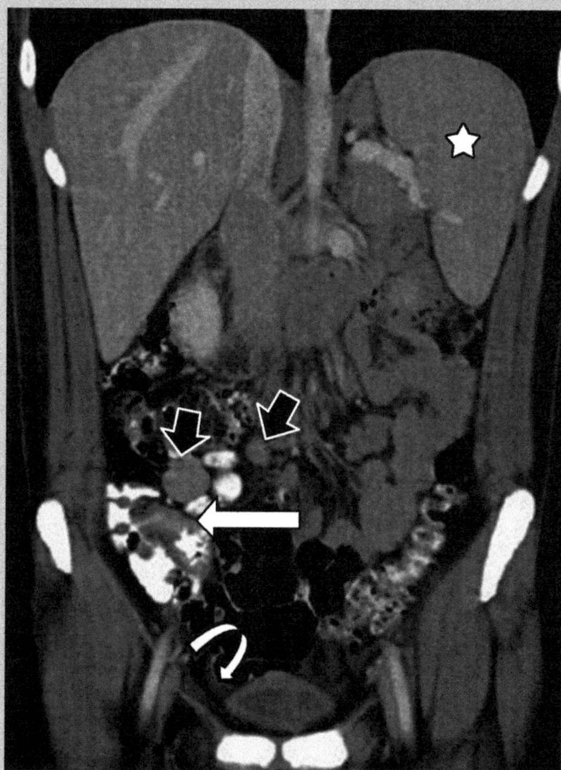

Fig. 24.2 Abdominal organs (ileum, spleen, and cholecyst) and lymphatic node lesions of typhoid fever. CT scanning of the abdomen demonstrates thickening of the distal ileum wall (*white arrows*), enlarged mesenteric lymphatic nodes (*black arrows*), enlarged spleen (*stars*), and effusions (*white curving arrows*)

Case Study 3

A 22-year-old male with clinical diagnosis of typhoid fever.

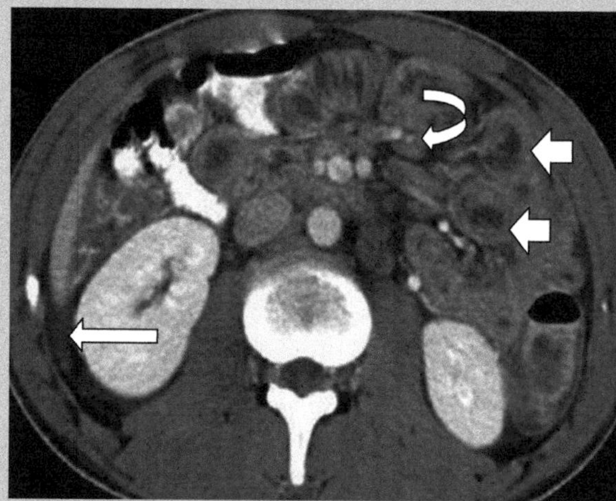

Fig. 24.3 Typhoid fever involving jejunum and lymph nodes. CT scanning demonstrates thickening of the jejunum wall (*short arrows*), enlarged lymphatic nodes (*curving arrow*), and ascites (*long arrow*)

Case Study 4

A 43-year-old male with abdominal distension.

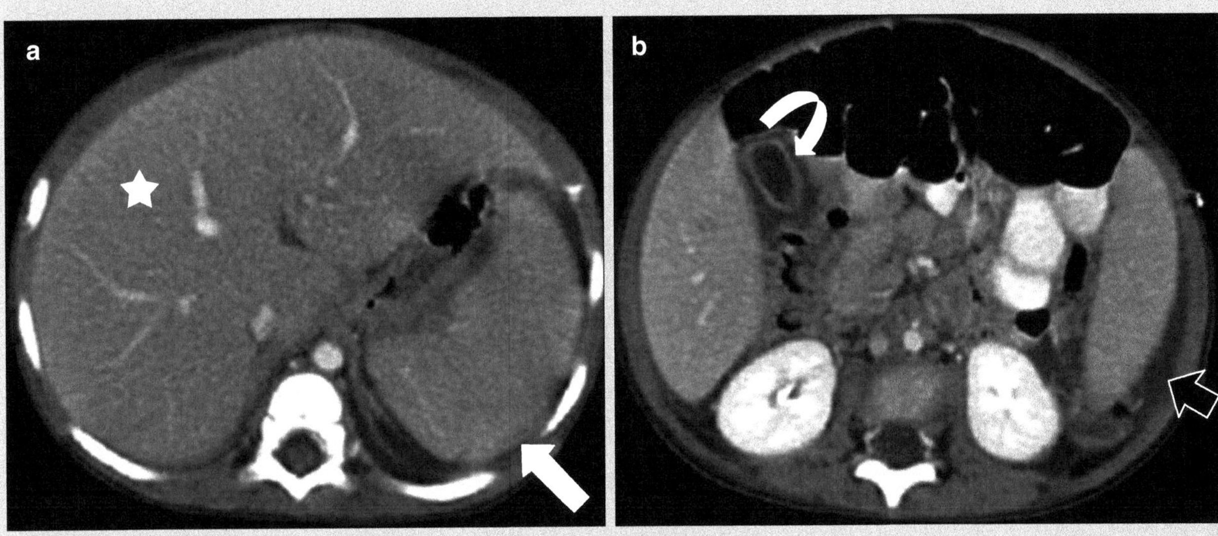

Fig. 24.4 Abdominal organs (ileum, spleen, and cholecyst) and lesions of typhoid fever. (**a**, **b**) CT scanning demonstrates enlarged liver (*star*) and spleen (*white arrow*), thickening of the cholecyst wall (*curving arrow*), and ascites (*black arrow*)

24.7.1.2 Typhoid Encephalopathy

Examinations reveal mild hydrocephalus, slightly expanded encephalocele but without sulcus and cistern expansion, localized and diffuse decrease of white matter density, and parts of enhanced nidi. In addition, enhanced meninx line and diffusely enhanced gyri are often seen, while basilar cistern and ependyma are rarely enhanced. CT scanning reveals common features of encephalitis, meningitis, and meningoencephalitis, which may exist together or solely.

24.7.1.3 Pulmonary Infection

Pulmonary infections often involve pulmonary mesenchyme, which is characterized by bronchial vascular bundles and interlobular and intralobular septum thickening. Reticular opacity and reticular nodes with clear edges and slightly high density can be seen in the lungs.

Case Study 5

A patient with typhoid fever with pulmonary infections.

For case detail and figures, please refer to Zou Jun. *Infection and Chemotherapy Journal of China*. 2008, 8 (3): 228.

24.7.2 Paratyphoid Fever

Imaging demonstrations of paratyphoid fever A, B, and some paratyphoid fever C are similar, which are generally characterized by annular thickening of the intestinal wall, especially the terminal ileum. Mesenteric lymphatic nodes, spleen, and liver enlarge. Some of the cases are present with ascites and a few with intestinal perforation, bleeding, and abscess. Septicopyemia caused by paratyphoid fever C can mainly induce suppurative inflammation, which is characterized by systemic suppurative metastatic nidi, of which localized suppurative inflammation in the lungs, bones, and joints, meningitis as well as endocarditis are the most common (Fig. 24.5).

Case Study 6

A 23-year-old male with paratyphoid fever A complicated by small intestinal perforation.

For case detail and figures, please refer to from Hennedige T, et al. *Ann Acad Med Singapore*, 2012, 41(7):281.

Case Study 7
A 28-year-old female who once worked in Indonesia for 3 months, present with fever and vomiting for one day, is diagnosed of paratyphoid fever A complicated by Bickerstaff's brainstem encephalitis.

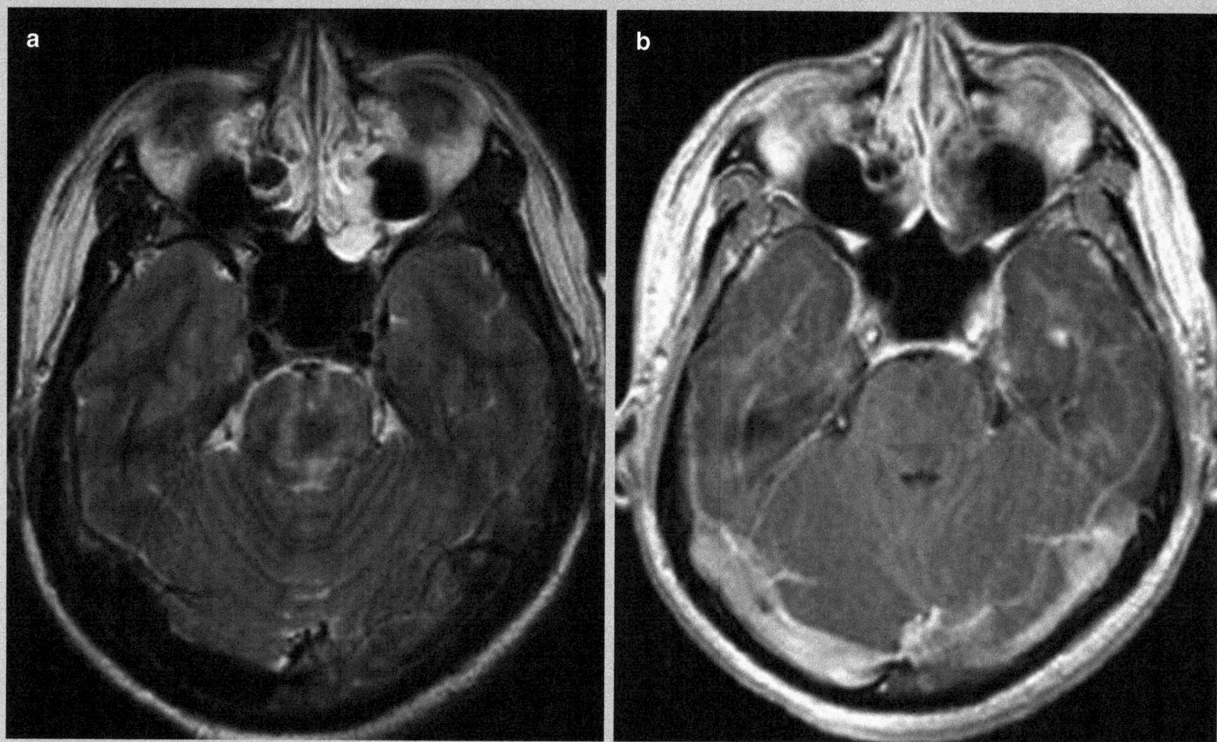

Fig. 24.5 Paratyphoid fever A involving the brainstem. (**a**, **b**) MRI demonstrates sheet high signal in the brainstem. (**a**) Enhancement canning reveals no obvious abnormal aggrandizement (Reprint with permission from Sheng B, et al. *Neurol Sci*, 2011, 302 (1-2):108)

Case Study 8
A 64-year-old male, hospitalized for pain in the back and loin, limitation of motion, chills, and fever for 19 days, was diagnosed of spinal osteomyelitis caused by paratyphoid fever C.

For case detail and figures, please refer to Wang XW, et al. *Chinese Journal of Reparative and Reconstructive Surgery*. 2012, 26(3): 382.

24.8 Diagnostic Basis

24.8.1 Epidemiology

Attention should be paid to if there is unclean food or the food from affected areas.

24.8.2 Clinical Manifestations

Patients with fever for more than one week and symptoms of systemic poisoning, dull expressions, anorexia, abdominal distension, constipation, diarrhea, roseola, and splenomegaly complicated by enterorrhagia and enterobrosis are more easily to be diagnosed.

24.8.3 Laboratory Test

Patients are present with decreased WBC counts, relatively increased lymphocytes, decreased or disappearing eosinophilic granulocytes, and positive Widal test. The golden diagnostic criterion is *Salmonella* typhi, which is tested by blood culture in the early stage. It is helpful to improve the positive rate by bone marrow culture for patients with negative blood culture results.

24.8.4 Imaging Demonstrations

Imaging demonstrations include enlarged mesenteric lymphatic nodes, ascites, enteritis, hepatosplenomegaly, brainstem encephalitis, and rachitis.

24.9 Differential Diagnosis

24.9.1 Cirrhosis

Cirrhosis is presented with hepatosplenomegaly, ascites, and thickening cholecystic wall. Enlarged liver occurs in the early stage of cirrhosis, but in the middle and late stage, hepatic lobes will be disproportionate with the enlarged left lateral and caudal lobes and atrophic right and quadrate lobes as well as diffusely or unevenly decreased hepatic density. Also, collateral circulation around the esophagus, fundus of the stomach, and hilus lienis demonstrated by CT scanning of portal veins is helpful for diagnosis.

24.9.2 Crohn's Disease of the Small Intestines

Lesions usually occur at the distal ileum. CT scanning demonstrates thickening intestinal wall caused by lymphedema. Intestinal wall becomes thickening periodically and double annular changes of the diseased intestinal canal can be demonstrated by enhancement scanning. In addition, abscess and fistula are formed in the abdominal cavity and wall. Crohn's disease of the small intestines is diagnosed by X-ray barium meal examination, periodic asymmetrical lesions, cobblestone, and longitudinal ulcer, characteristics of intestinal canal stenosis and internal and external fistula as well as clinical manifestations.

24.9.3 Small Intestinal Lymphoma

The intestinal canal with lesions is present with annular thickening, which is difficult being differentiated from the normal intestinal canal. Peripheral lymph nodes are enlarged and the involved intestines are long with multiple periodic nidi. Besides, aneurismal dilation is the characteristic of the disease.

24.9.4 Small Intestinal Tuberculosis

Small intestinal tuberculosis usually occurs at the ileocecal junction, which is characterized by thickening of the mucosal membrane around the intestinal wall. This disease is mainly diagnosed by radiography, which demonstrates irritation when barium is passing, thickening and disorder of mucosa membrane and small niche in the early stage of ulcerative type as well as thickening intestinal wall and lumen stenosis in the late stage. The disease is the transitional disorder, which has no clear boundaries with normal intestines.

24.9.5 Purulent Meningitis

CT scanning in the early stage has no specific demonstrations, but later may reveal communicating and obstructive hydrocephalus. Generally, dilation of the cerebral ventricle is obvious. Besides, the meninges and ventricle can be enhanced but with few nidi of low density in white matter unless abscess is formed, which shows annular enhancement.

References

Gali BM, Ali N, Agbese GO, et al. Gallbladder perforation complicating typhoid fever: report of two cases. Niger J Med. 2011;20(1):181–3.

Hennedige T, Bindl DS, Bhasin A, et al. Computed tomography features in enteric fever. Ann Acad Med Singapore. 2012;41(7):281–6.

Husain EH. Fulminant hepatitis in typhoid fever. J Infect Public Health. 2011;4(3):154–6.

Khan MI, Ochiai RL, Soofi SB, et al. Risk factors associated with typhoid fever in children aged 2–16 years in Karachi, Pakistan. Epidemiol Infect. 2012;140(4):665–72.

Li YL. Pathology. Beijing: People's Publishing House; 2006.

Mateen MA, Saleem S, Rao PC, et al. Ultrasound in the diagnosis of typhoid fever. Indian J Pediatr. 2006;73(8):681–5.

Mayer CA, Neilson AA. Typhoid and paratyphoid fever -prevention in travellers. Aust Fam Physician. 2010;39(11):847–51.

Neil KP, Sodha SV, Lukwago L, et al. A large outbreak of typhoid fever associated with a high rate of intestinal perforation in Kasese District, Uganda, 2008–2009. Clin Infect Dis. 2012;54(8):1091–9.

Ratnayake EC, Shivanthan C, Wijesiriwardena BC. Cholestatic hepatitis in a patient with typhoid fever – a case report. Ann Clin Microbiol Antimicrob. 2011;10:35. doi:10.1186/1476-0711-10-35.

Sheng B, Ho WS, Lau KK, et al. Bickerstaff's brainstem encephalitis complicating Salmonella Paratyphi A infection. Neurol Sci. 2011;302(1–2):108–11.

Wang XW, Lu JM. A case study of bone marrow spondylitis caused by Salmonella Paratyphi C. Chin J Reparative Reconstr Surg. 2012;26(3):382–3.

Wang LQ, Kan B, Zhang FN. Global epidemic overview and prevention of typhoid and paratyphoid fever. Dis Surveil. 2007;22(7):492–4.

Yu RH, Xue HM. Progress of laboratory diagnosis of typhoid fever. Int J Lab Med. 2009;30(11):1093–4.

Zou J. A case study of typhoid fever with the first clinical manifestation of interstitial pneumonia. Chin J Infect Chemother. 2008;8(3):228–9.

Part II

Radiology of Parasitic Infections

25 Filariasis

Jiangfeng Pan

Filariasis is a parasitic disease caused by the parasite of filaria. In China, the prevalent filariasis is commonly caused by the parasite of *Wuchereria bancrofti* and *Brugia malayi*. The early clinical symptoms of filariasis mainly include lymphangitis and lymphadenitis, while the advanced clinical symptoms include lymphatic obstruction and its related symptoms. In this chapter, we focus on filariasis caused by the parasite of *Wuchereria bancrofti* and *Brugia malayi*.

25.1 Etiology

Currently, eight types of filaria are known to parasitize in human bodies, including *Wuchereria bancrofti*, *Brugia malayi*, and *Brugia timori* that parasitize in the lymphatic system; *Onchocerca volvulus*, *Loa loa*, and *Mansonella streptocerca* that parasitize in the subcutaneous tissues; and *Filaria perstans* and *Filaria ozzardi* that parasitize in the cavities of the human body. Filariasis has a widespread prevalence. In China, filariasis caused by *Wuchereria bancrofti* and *Brugia malayi* are common.

25.1.1 Adult Filaria

Wuchereria bancrofti and *Brugia malayi* share certain morphological similarities. They are both slender and milky white in appearance, with smooth surface. Both are dioecious but commonly intertwined. In a size of 28–42 × 0.1 mm, the male *Wuchereria bancrofti* is slightly longer than male *Brugia malayi*, but their structures are almost the same. Being twice as long and wide as the male filaria, the female *Wuchereria bancrofti* and *Brugia malayi* have almost the same morphology and structure.

J. Pan
Department of Radiology, City Central Hospital,
Jinhua, Zhejiang, China
e-mail: panjiangfeng967@163.com

25.1.2 Microfilaria

Filaria is viviparous and the larva reproduced by a female filaria is known as microfilaria. Microfilaria is mainly found in peripheral blood with a filamentous activity. After its access into the blood flow from the lymphatic system, the microfilaria stays in microvascular vessels in the lungs during daytime and enters into peripheral blood circulation during nights, showing an obvious nocturnal periodicity. Microfilaria has an average life span of 2–3 months in a human host, but some can survive as long as several years.

25.1.3 Life Cycle

The life cycle of *Wuchereria bancrofti* and *Brugia malayi* can be divided into two stages: one stage in mosquitoes (the intermediate host) and the other in humans (the final host).

25.1.3.1 Life Stage in Mosquitoes

After the human blood containing microfilariae is sucked by a mosquito, the microfilariae gain their access into the mosquito and shed sheaths in the following 1–7 h to develop into parasitic microfilariae. After ecdysis for twice in the following 1–3 weeks, the parasitic microfilariae develop into infective microfilariae that can invade the human body via mosquito bites.

25.1.3.2 Human-Vector Cycle

After invasion of infective microfilariae into the human body, some of them may die during the processes of migration and development in the human tissue. And some others reach the lymphatic vessels or lymph nodes and develop there into adult filariae. *Wuchereria bancrofti* and *Brugia malayi* occupy different parts of the human body. *Wuchereria bancrofti* primarily parasitizes in the superficial lymphatic system and the deep lymphatic system in the lower extremities,

H. Li (ed.), *Radiology of Infectious Diseases: Volume 2*, DOI 10.1007/978-94-017-9876-1_25

scrotum, spermatic cord, inguinal canal, and abdominal cavity, while *Brugia malayi* occupies the superficial lymphatic system in upper and lower extremities. *Wuchereria bancrofti* spends 8–12 months progressing from infective microfilariae into their occurrence in peripheral blood in the human body, while *Brugia malayi* only spends 3–4 months for that. Both of them have an average life span of 4–10 years and some may survive as long as 40 years.

25.2 Epidemiology

Filariasis is a global health problem affecting many areas around the world. *Wuchereria bancrofti*-induced filariasis mainly prevails in Asia, Africa, Oceania, and parts of America, while *Brugia malayi*-induced filariasis only prevails in Asia. Filariasis prevails in 16 provinces, cities, and autonomous regions in mainland China. Shandong province and Taiwan only witness *Wuchereria bancrofti*-induced filariasis, while other 14 places witness both prevalences of *Wuchereria bancrofti*-induced filariasis and *Brugia malayi-induced* filariasis.

25.2.1 Source of Infection

Wuchereria bancrofti so far has been found to infect only humans, with persons with microfilaremia including patients and asymptomatic carriers as its only source of infection. *Brugia malayi* can parasitize not only in humans but also in other mammals such as cats, dogs, and monkeys. Therefore, the infected animals are also the source of *Brugia malayi* infection.

25.2.2 Route of Transmission

Filariasis can be transmitted via mosquito bites. The principal mosquito vectors of *Wuchereria bancrofti* infection include *Culex pipiens pallens* and *Culex quinquefasciatus*, followed by Anopheles sinensis. *Brugia malayi* infection is mainly transmitted via Anopheles sinensis bites.

25.2.3 Susceptible Population

Populations are generally susceptible and the occurrence has no significant gender difference. The population aged 20–25 years has the highest incidence as well as infection rate. Although certain immunity can be acquired after the infection is cured, it is not strong enough to prevent the following infection.

25.2.4 Epidemic Features

The mosquito-breeding seasons (from May to October) witness the highest incidence of filariasis because the climate is optimal for development of a microfilaria in mosquitoes. However, filariasis can be an epidemic disease all year round in the southern areas of China due to the warm weather all year round.

25.3 Pathogenesis and Pathological Changes

25.3.1 Pathogenesis

The occurrence and development of filariasis depend on the type of filaria, frequency of infection, the quantity of infective microfilaria entering human body, locations where adult filariae parasitize, immune responses of the human body, and the occurrence of secondary infection. The onset and lesions of filariasis are primarily caused by adult filariae, and infective microfilariae also play a role. During the development of infective microfilariae into adult filariae in the human body, the secretions and metabolites of both infective microfilariae and adult filariae may cause not only tissue reaction of the lymphatic system but also systemic allergic reactions. The symptoms, probably caused by type I or type III allergic reaction, include periodic filarial fever, lymphadenitis, and lymphangitis. Secondary infections and lesions caused by lymphatic obstruction occur in the late period, which is related to type IV allergic reaction.

25.3.2 Pathological Changes

Primarily caused by adult filariae, the basic pathological changes of filariasis are characterized by lesions in the lymphatic system. Symptoms of the acute stage include exudative inflammation, congestion of lymph nodes, swelling of lymph vessel wall, eosinophil infiltration, and fibrin deposition. As the disease develops, proliferative granulomas, with *degenerative* adult filariae and eosinophils at the center, can be gradually found in lymph vessels and nodes. The proliferative granulomas are surrounded by fibrous tissue and epithelioid cells. In addition, large quantities of lymphocytes and plasma cells cluster together to form tuberculoid nodules. In severe cases, eosinophilic abscesses can be found due to tissue necrosis, liquefaction, and a large quantity of eosinophils infiltration. During the chronic stage, occlusive endolymphangitis occurs due to proliferation of endothelial cells in the lymph vessels, thickened endothelium, and its fibrosis, as well as lumen stenosis. Lymphatic varices and rupture may occur due to increased internal pressure of the distal lymph vessels caused by obstruction of lymph nodes and vessels. Therefore, the lymph fluid flows into the neighboring tissues and organs to continually stimulate the local tissues. As a result, elephantiasis occurs since the fibrous tissues proliferate in a large quantity as well as the subcutaneous tissues thicken, wrinkle, and harden.

25.4 Clinical Symptoms and Signs

Clinical symptoms of filariasis vary in severity, with asymptomatic infection accounting for about 50 % of all the cases. *Wuchereria bancrofti* and *Brugia malayi* infections have an incubation period varying from 4 months to 1 year.

25.4.1 Acute Stage

25.4.1.1 Lymphadenitis and Lymphangitis

Lymphadenitis and lymphangitis commonly occur in extremities, especially in lower extremities. Lymphadenitis may occur alone, while lymphangitis always occurs along with lymphadenitis. Clinical symptoms are characterized by nonperiodic painful enlargement of lymph nodes in the groin and abdomen. As the disease develops, lymph vessels are painful and swollen, which extends along the medial thighs to form eccentrically distributed red lines and thus result in retrograde lymphangitis. Retrograde lymphangitis occurs once a month or once every several months, commonly lasting for 1–3 days with symptoms of aversion to cold, fever, and general fatigue.

25.4.1.2 Filarial Fever

Filarial fever is characterized by periodic onset of fever with accompanying aversion to cold, chills, and a body temperature up to 40 °C. Some patients may experience only fever but no chills. The fever commonly lasts for 2–3 days and filarial fever is very common in epidemic areas of *Wuchereria bancrofti*-induced filariasis.

25.4.1.3 Spermatocystitis, Epididymitis, and Orchitis

Spermatocystitis, epididymitis, and orchitis mainly occur in cases of *Wuchereria bancrofti*-induced filariasis. The manifestations include unilateral inguinal pain, swollen testicles, epididymides with tenderness, and palpable one or multiple nodules in the spermatic cord with obvious tenderness. After the inflammation is cured, the swollen tissues shrink and are hardened, which can be gradually enlarged after repeated onset.

25.4.1.4 Tropical Pulmonary Eosinophilia (TPE)

Tropical pulmonary eosinophilia (TPE) is also known as filarial eosinophilia. When filariasis affects the lungs, the manifestations include aversion to cold, fever, cough, asthmatic episodes, and enlarged lymph nodes. In the lungs, there are migratory infiltrative lesions. By chest X-ray, the lung markings are demonstrated to be thickened, with extensive military spots of opacities. In addition, eosinophils and Charcot-Leyden crystals can be detected in sputum. The eosinophil count in peripheral blood increases, accounting for 20–80 % of the total WBC count.

25.4.2 Chronic Stage (Lymphatic Obstruction Stage)

The chronic stage is primarily characterized by manifestations caused by proliferation and obstruction of the lymphatic system.

25.4.2.1 Lymphadenectasis and Lymphatic Varix

Lymphatic sinus dilates in the swollen lymph nodes, with neighboring lymphatic varix centripetally to form masses that can be observed in unilateral or bilateral groins and femoral regions. By palpations, the masses feel like spongy cysts with a solid center. By puncture, lymph fluid can be aspirated, sometimes with microfilariae. Lymphatic varix is commonly observed in the spermatic cord, scrotum, and medial thighs.

25.4.2.2 Hydrocele

Hydrocele commonly occurs in *Wuchereria bancrofti-induced* filariasis. It is caused by stagnation of lymph fluid in the urethral crest due to the lymphatic obstruction in the spermatic cord and testes. Microfilariae can be observed by centrifugal sedimentation of the fluid obtained by puncture.

25.4.2.3 Chyluria

Chyluria is one of the major advanced symptoms of *Wuchereria bancrofti*-induced filariasis. Lymphatic ruptures commonly occur in the renal pelvis and ureters, but rarely in the bladder. Clinically, it has a sudden onset with no prior symptoms or signs. However, in some cases, the prior symptoms may occur including aversion to cold, fever, and soreness in the lower back, pelvic cavity, and groin. Consequently, chyluria occurs.

25.4.2.4 Lymphatic Edema and Elephantiasis

Lymphatic edema is difficult to be clinically differentiated from elephantiasis and both conditions commonly concur. Lymph edema can be healed spontaneously after lymph reflux is improved. However, in the cases of continuous unsmooth lymph reflux, the condition may develop into elephantiasis, which is characterized by depressive but solid edema. The skin is thickened and coarse, with deepened skinfolds, wart-like and moss-like nodules. Secondary infection commonly occurs to form chronic ulceration. Elephantiasis commonly occurs in lower extremities, but rarely in the scrotum, penis, labium, upper extremities, and breasts.

25.4.2.5 Filarial Nodules in the Breast

Filarial nodules in the breast rarely occur, which are caused by the parasite of adult filariae in the breast tissues or in the dilated lymph vessels around the breast tissues. In most cases, the nodule is singular and located in superficial latero-superior breast, with a diameter of 1–2 cm. The intermediate hard immobile nodule develops slowly with unclearly defined boundary. The skin thickens like the manifestation of elephantiasis.

25.4.2.6 Filarial Pericarditis

Similar to acute pericarditis of other causes, the manifestations of filarial pericarditis include dyspnea, precordial pain, fever, and fatigue. The physical signs of the disease include distant heart sounds, enlarged heart boundaries, and occasional pericardial frictions. By pericardiocentesis, milky or bloody effusion can be found, with findings of microfilariae.

25.4.2.7 Filarial Arthritis

Filarial arthritis commonly invades unilateral knee joint, less commonly the ankle. Facet joints are hardly involved. With a benign progress, the disease usually lasts for a short period of time. Most patients experience painless swelling. But some patients may experience pain, swelling and fever, tenderness as well as limited movements. Its pathogenesis remains elusive. Microfilariae of *Wuchereria bancrofti* can be detected in the articular fluid.

25.5 Filariasis-Related Complications

The main complication of filariasis is secondary bacterial infection. Patients with filariasis with a long-term use of immunosuppressant are vulnerable to secondary bacterial infections, with symptoms of chills, high fever, and toxemia.

25.6 Diagnostic Examinations

25.6.1 Laboratory Tests

25.6.1.1 Routine Blood Test

In the cases with early allergic reactions, the WBC count commonly is $(10–20)\times10^9/L$, with a major increase of the eosinophil count that accounts for more than 20 % of the WBC count. In the cases with secondary infection, the neutrophil count may also increase significantly.

25.6.1.2 Etiological Tests

Peripheral Blood Test for Microfilariae

The finding of microfilariae in the blood specimen is important evidence for early diagnosis of filariae. The positive rate is relatively higher during 22:00 p.m. to 02:00 a.m. The etiological examinations include smearing, fresh blood examination, concentration method, daytime trapping method, and micropore filtration. Among all these methods, the micropore filtration witnesses a higher positive rate.

Body Fluid Test for Microfilariae

Microfilariae can be observed in the hydrocele fluid, chylous urine, lymph fluid, chylous ascites, and pericardial effusion.

25.6.1.3 Biopsy

Biopsy of suspected lesion tissues, such as subcutaneous nodules and epididymal nodules, should be performed to detect the adult filariae and to observe the related pathological changes.

25.6.1.4 Immunological Assays

Immunological assays include the intracutaneous test, indirect immunofluorescent assay (IFA), complement fixation test, and enzyme-linked immunosorbent assay. However, the specificity is low due to the cross-reaction with other nematodes.

25.6.1.5 Molecular Biological Examinations

Molecular biological techniques, such as DNA hybrid test and PCR, can be applied for the detection of microfilaremia. Such examinations are especially appropriate for the cases with a small quantity of microfilariae in the blood or for the cases which need identification of parasitic worms.

25.6.2 Diagnostic Imaging

25.6.2.1 Ultrasonography

Ultrasonography is commonly applied for the assessment of enlarged lymph nodes, lymphatic dilation, and hydrocele. The findings facilitate etiological diagnosis of filarial lymph edema and therapeutic following up. Ultrasound-guided puncture for biopsy is performed if necessary.

25.6.2.2 Lymphangiography

Lymphangiography is commonly applied to define the severity of lymphatic dilation. It can demonstrate the dilated afferent lymph vessels and the narrow efferent lymph vessels. Defects in the parenchymal lymph nodes can be demonstrated.

25.6.2.3 X-Ray Radiology and CT Scanning

X-ray radiology and CT scanning are commonly applied for the diagnosis of pulmonary and joint lesions for the cases of filariasis.

25.6.2.4 MR Imaging

MR imaging is commonly applied for the diagnosis of central nervous system lesions and filarial lymph edema for the cases of filariasis.

25.7 Imaging Demonstrations

25.7.1 Central Nervous System

Filariae rarely invade the central nervous system. Jing, XQ. reported a case of intraspinal filariasis. MR imaging demonstrated that semioval lesions with slightly low signal at the epidural T7–9 level, which have clearly defined boundaries and have wide fundus close to the posterior edge of the vertebral body, as well as narrowed subarachnoid space due to local compression.

Acute disseminated encephalomeningitis (ADEM) commonly occurs secondary to vaccination and virus infection. However, Paliwal et al. reported a case of ADEM caused by *Wuchereria bancrofti* infection. In their report, MR imaging demonstrated multiple round-like long-T1 and long-T2 signal lesions in bilateral semioval centrum. Contrast MR imaging demonstrated slight enhancement of the lesions. DWI demonstrated restricted diffusion of most lesions, ring-shaped high and even signals at the edges of the lesions, and no edema and space-occupying effect around the lesions (Fig. 25.1).

Case Study 1

A male patient aged 38 years, with acute filariasis in the left upper extremity for 2 months.

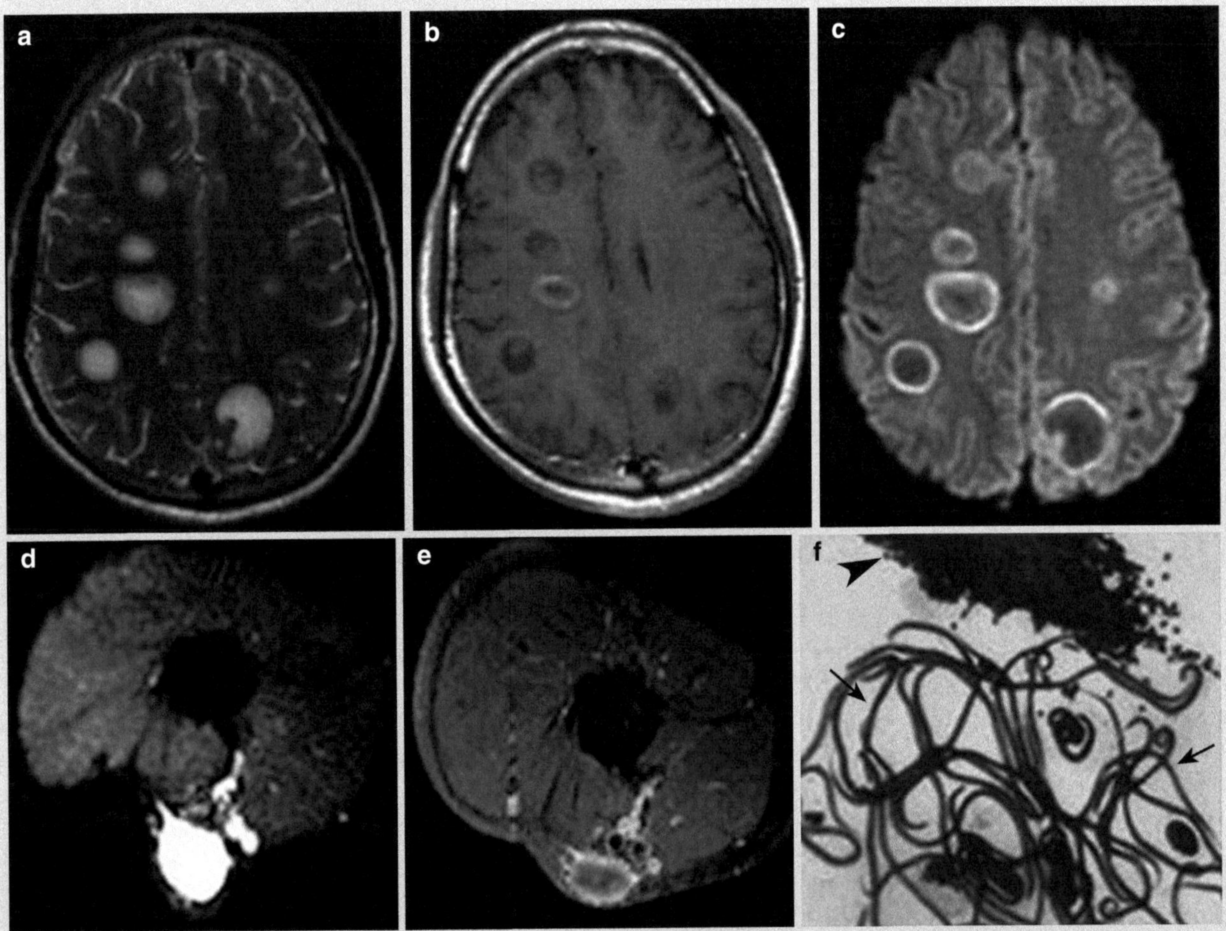

Fig. 25.1 Acute disseminated encephalomeningitis. (**a**) MRI T2WI demonstrates multiple round-like high-signal lesions in bilateral semioval centrum with different sizes and clearly defined boundaries. (**b**) Contrast imaging demonstrates slight enhancement of the lesions and some lesions in a ring-shaped enhancement. (**c**) DWI demonstrates restricted diffusion of the lesions. (**d**, **e**) T2WI demonstrates high signal in the subcutaneous swelling of the left upper extremity, which is demonstrated in a ring-shaped enhancement by contrast imaging. (**f**) Fine needle aspirate of arm swelling shows numerous microfilariae (*arrows*) of Wuchereria bancroftialong with adult female worm (*arrow head*) (Reproduced with permission from Paliwal VK, et al. *J Neurol Neurosurg Psychiatry*, 2012, 83 (3): 347)

25.7.2 Lymphatic System

Ultrasonography demonstrates obvious enlargement of lymph nodes with cystic changes. In the cases of filarial lymphangitis, peristalsis of filariae can be observed in the dilated lymph vessels. By following up some patients receiving medication therapy, the peristalsis of filariae in the dilated lymph vessels was found to be decreased or even disappeared. In the cases of filarial lymph edema, the skin layers and structures are unclearly defined, with thickened subcutaneous tissues and deep fascia as well as blurry subfascial muscular tissues and fibers. The echoes from subcutaneous tissue are subject to changes, with cracks and effusion of different severity. No blood flow signal is demonstrated in the thickened subcutaneous tissues. MRI T2WI favorably demonstrates extensive subcutaneous lymphatic dilation in the lower limbs of elephantiasis cases, with crude reticular high signal. Lymphangiography can demonstrate inflammations of the dilated afferent lymph vessel and the narrow efferent lymph vessel, as well as defective parenchyma of lymph nodes.

Case Study 2

A girl aged 12 years, with painless enlarged lymph nodes in the right groin for 4 months. She had no history of extremity abnormality or bacterial infection. By physical examination, three painless and movable lymph nodes can be palpated, which feel like elephant skin. The size of the largest lymph node is approximately 3.5 × 3.0 cm. There were no skin abnormalities and no extremity and vulva edema.

For case detail and figures, please refer to Dreyer G, et al. *Am J Trop Med Hyg*, 2001, 65 (3): 204.

25.7.3 Respiratory System

The lesions of the respiratory system are usually divided into two types. One type of the lesions is resulted from direct invasion of the pathogens into the lungs. These lesions are pulmonary infarction caused by stagnation of filariae in the pulmonary vein, with the most common manifestation of singular pulmonary nodule in a size of below 3 cm. The other types of lesions are pulmonary lesions caused by allergic reactions, with common clinical manifestations of tropical pulmonary eosinophilia (TPE) syndrome. Chest X-ray demonstrates thickened lung markings and extensive miliary spots of shadows. The typical manifestation of TPE is characterized by infiltration of the upper and middle fields of both lungs that is more obvious in the peripheral areas. The atypical manifestations include pulmonary cavity, small patches of inflammatory exudation, and pleural effusion, with occasional occurrence of large flakes of pneumonia lesions. Sandhu et al. reported a group of ten patients with filarial pulmonary lesions. In their report, X-rays and CT scanning demonstrated diffusive lesions in both lungs, with inferior lobes not involved in some cases. CT scanning more favorably demonstrated reticular nodular shadow, bronchiectasia, air-trapping sign, calcification, and mediastinal lymphadenectasis.

25.7.4 Scrotum

Ultrasonography is commonly applied for the examination of the scrotum, with clear demonstrations of the occurrence and severity of hydrocele as well as the cystoid structure in the testes and epididymis. The solid lesions are demonstrated as curve-shaped high echo. Real-time ultrasonography demonstrates irregular twist or snaking motion, which is known as the filaria dance sign. The sign indicates the activity of the pathogen. A dynamic monitoring of its activities can provide evidence for assessing the therapeutic effectiveness.

Case Study 3

A male patient aged 17 years, with swelling and dull pain of the scrotum for 3 months.

For case detail and figures, please refer to Shetty GS, et al. *Padiatr Radiol*, 2012, 42 (4): 486.

Breast filariasis has a characteristic manifestation of calcification of the mammary glands. The calcifications are in hollow-tube pattern and have a cluster-like distribution. The calcifications are mainly located around the mammary areola or at the posterior region of mammary glands, with a different running course from the mammary ducts. The real-time ultrasonography can also demonstrate filaria dance signs in the breast lumps. The lesions may also be in changes of mammary lobular hyperplasia, with ultrasound demonstrations of weak-echogenic masses with no capsule and clearly defined boundaries.

25.7.5 Filarial Pericarditis

X-ray demonstrates bilaterally enlarged heart and the heart in a shape like a triangle flask.

25.7.6 Filarial Arthritis

By X-ray, the swelling of soft tissues around the knee joint and the widened joint space can be observed.

25.8 Basis for the Diagnosis

25.8.1 Epidemiology and Clinical Diagnosis

The patients with filariasis commonly have a history of mosquito bites. The typical clinical manifestations include periodic fever, centrifugal lymphangitis, swollen and painful lymph nodes, chyluria, chorditis, and elephantiasis. In combination of the epidemiological history and typical clinical manifestations, filariasis can be diagnosed.

25.8.2 Laboratory Diagnosis

The diagnosis of filariasis can be defined after the detection of microfilariae in the peripheral blood.

25.8.3 Therapeutic Diagnosis

For the cases with suspected diagnosis of filariasis and no finding of microfilariae in the blood, diethylcarbamazine can be prescribed for the patients. After the medication, some patients experience lymphatic responses and lymphatic nodules within 2–14 days, which facilitates the diagnosis of filariasis.

25.8.4 Imaging Diagnosis

25.8.4.1 Lymphangiography

Lymphangiography commonly demonstrates the cases of filariasis with inflammations of the dilated afferent lymph vessel and the narrow efferent lymph vessel, with defective parenchyma of lymph nodes.

25.8.4.2 Ultrasonography

By ultrasonography, the location and morphology of adult filariae in the lymph vessel, scrotum, and mammary gland can be revealed.

25.8.4.3 X-Ray Radiology

Demonstrated by X-ray, thickened lung markings and extensive miliary spots of shadows facilitate the diagnosis of TPE syndrome.

25.8.4.4 MR Imaging

By MR imaging, ADEM can be demonstrated as multiple round-like long-T1 and long-T2 signals in the semioval centrum. By contrast imaging, the lesions are slightly enhanced. Filarial lesions in the spinal canal are demonstrated in low signals.

25.9 Differential Diagnosis

25.9.1 Bacterial Lymphangitis

Lymphadenitis and lymphangitis during the acute stage of filariasis should be differentiated from bacterial lymphangitis. Bacterial lymphangitis spreads to regional lymph nodes upwards from the bottom and the local lesions are commonly found. In the cases of bacterial lymphangitis, toxic symptoms are serious, local pain and tenderness are more obvious, and neutrophil count significantly increases.

25.9.2 Elephantiasis

Elephantiasis occurs following the repeated onsets of bacterial lymphangitis or following surgical removal of lymphatic tissues that obstruct lymphatic back flow due to local lesions or tumor compression. For the cases of elephantiasis, differential diagnosis should be made in combination to medical history. In addition, ultrasound demonstration of filariae peristalsis in the dilated lymph vessels facilitates the differential diagnosis.

25.9.3 Tuberculosis of Epididymis

Chorditis and epididymitis should be differentiated from epididymal tuberculosis. The medical history of tuberculosis facilitates the differentiation. Epididymal tuberculosis is characterized by swelling of hard nodules with slight tenderness. As the characteristic ultrasound demonstration of filarial epididymis, filaria dance sign facilitates the differential diagnosis. As for other signs, the tube-like twisted solid or calcified lesions support the diagnosis of filariasis, while spots and patches of calcification are lesions supporting the diagnosis of tuberculosis.

25.9.4 Pulmonary Nodules and Pneumonia

The diagnosis of filariasis with singular pulmonary nodule is difficult to be defined. Such cases should be differentiated from pulmonary nodules of other causes. TPE also should be differentiated from pulmonary eosinophilia of other causes. The clinical development of the conditions facilitates to define the etiological factors.

25.9.5 Breast Disease

Breast filariasis should be differentiated primarily from breast calcification and lumps of other causes. Special calcifications and ultrasound demonstration of filaria dance signs in the lumps facilitate to define the diagnosis of filariasis.

References

Dreyer G, Figueredo-Silva J, Carvalho K, et al. Lymphatic filariasis in children: adenopathy and its evolution in two young girls. Am J Trop Med Hyg. 2001;65(3):204–7.

Paliwal VK, Goel G, Vema R, et al. Acute disseminated encephalomyelitis following filarial infection. J Neurol Neurosurg Psychiatry. 2012;83(3):347–9.

Shetty GS, Solanki RS, Prabhu SM, et al. Filarial dance – sonographic sign of filarial infection. Pediatr Radiol. 2012;42(4):486–7.

Suggested Reading

Friedman PD, Kalisher L. Case 43: filariasis. Radiology. 2002;222(2):515–7.

Ma YL, Li LJ. Studies of infectious diseases. Shanghai: Shanghai Science and Technology Press; 2011.

Martínez S, Restrepo CS, Carrillo JA, et al. Thoracic manifestations of tropical parasitic infections: a pictorial review. Radiographics. 2005;25(1):135–55.

Ramzy RMR, EL Setouhy M, Helmy H, et al. Effect of yearly mass drug administration with diethylcarbamazine and albendazole on bancroftian filariasis in Egypt: a comprehensive assessment. Lancet. 2006;367(9515):992–9.

Sandhu M, Mukhopadhyay S, Sharma SK. Tropical pulmonary eosinophilia: a comparative evaluation of plain chest radiography and computed tomography. Australas Radiol. 1996;40(1):32–7.

Schick C, Thalhammer A, Balzer JO, et al. Cystic lymph node enlargement of the neck: filariasis as a rare differential diagnosis in MRI. Eur Radiol. 2002;12(9):2349–51.

Yang SJ, Ren H. Studies of infectious diseases. Beijing: People's Medical Publishing House; 2011.

Hydatidosis

26

Wenxiao Jia and Hong Wang

Hydatidosis or hydatid disease, also known as echinococcosis, is a parasitic zoonosis caused by parasitism of echinococcus larva in humans or animals. The main manifestations include space-occupying lesions and compressive symptoms of the involved organs. In China, two types of hydatidosis occur, cyst echinococcosis (CE) caused by *Echinococcus granulosus* and alveolar echinococcosis (AE) caused by *Echinococcus multilocularis*. Hydatidosis is an important parasitic disease threatening health of humans and farm animals in northern and southwestern China, which has been legally listed as one of the class C infectious diseases.

26.1 Etiology

Echinococcus has various species and four species have been generally recognized: *Echinococcus granulosus* (E.g.) (Batsch 1786), *E. multilocularis* (E.m.), *E. oligarthrus* (E.o.) (Diesing 1863), and *E. vogeli* (E.v.) (Rausch and Bernstein 1972). The former two species are pathogenic in China. The larvae of the latter two species are categorized into polycystic echinococcosis.

26.1.1 *Echinococcus granulosus* (E.g.)

26.1.1.1 Adult Worm

The adult worm of E.g. is parasitic in the small intestines of the terminal hosts, such as dogs, wolves, and other predators. The worms are fine with a length of about 2–7 mm, composed of one scolex, one collum segment, one mature proglottid, and one gravid proglottid and are the smallest species in tapeworms. The scolex is almost in the shape of a pear, including rostellum and four sucker apparatuses (Fig. 26.1). The uterine of the gravid proglottid is filled with eggs.

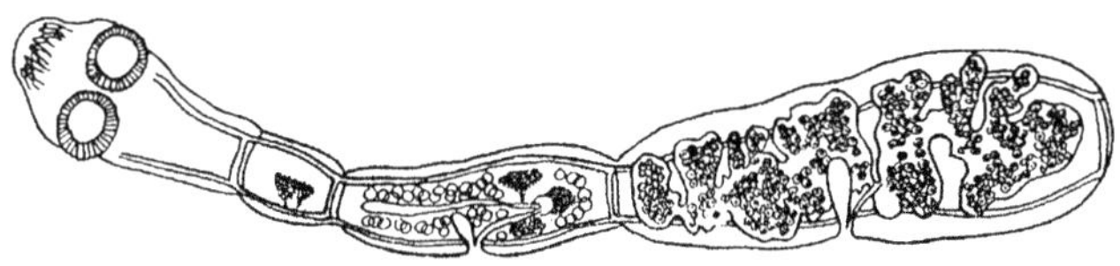

Fig. 26.1 Adult *Echinococcus granulosus*

26.1.1.2 Egg

The egg of E.g. resembles to the egg of *Taenia saginata* parasitic to cows and pigs. They are wide oval in a color of yellowish brown, with two layers of embryonic membrane and inner radiating ridge (Fig. 26.2). After maturation, just before or after discharge of the gravid proglottid via the intestinal canal of the host, its uterine ruptures to discharge eggs. The eggs have strong resistance to external environment, which can survive for above 2.5 years in water at 2 °C. However, the eggs are heat intolerant and can be killed at a temperature of 80 °C. The eggs can survive for 6–24 h in common disinfectants and chemical agents, such as 20 % Lysol, and can survive for 24 h in 20 % formaldehyde.

26.1.1.3 Larva

The larva of E.g. is echinococcus, which is a round or round-like cystid. The cystid wall is composed of an external transparent cuticle and an internal germinal layer, which is enveloped by a fibrous capsule formed by host tissue response (Fig. 26.3). The germinal layer is embryonic membrane tissue capable of reproduction, with its lining capable of budding many small projections. These projections gradually develop into germinal cysts and then daughter cysts after shedding. In the daughter cysts, several scolices can be produced, which are known as protoscolices. In the daughter

W. Jia (✉) • H. Wang
Department of Radiology, The Second Affiliated Hospital, Xinjiang Medical University, Urumqi, Xinjiang Uygur Autonomous Region, China
e-mail: jwxxj@sina.com

H. Li (ed.), *Radiology of Infectious Diseases: Volume 2*, DOI 10.1007/978-94-017-9876-1_26

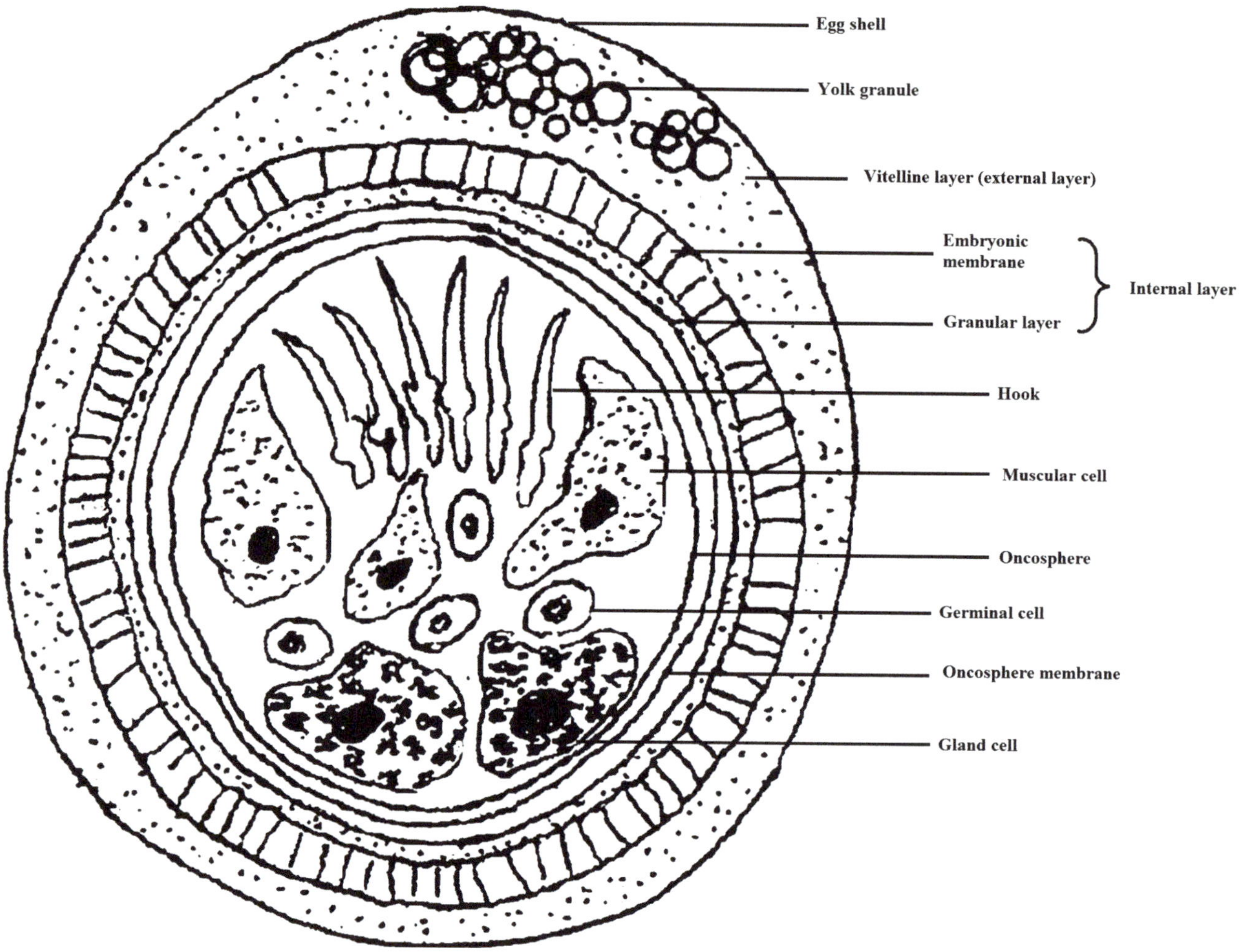

Fig. 26.2 An egg of *Echinococcus granulosus*

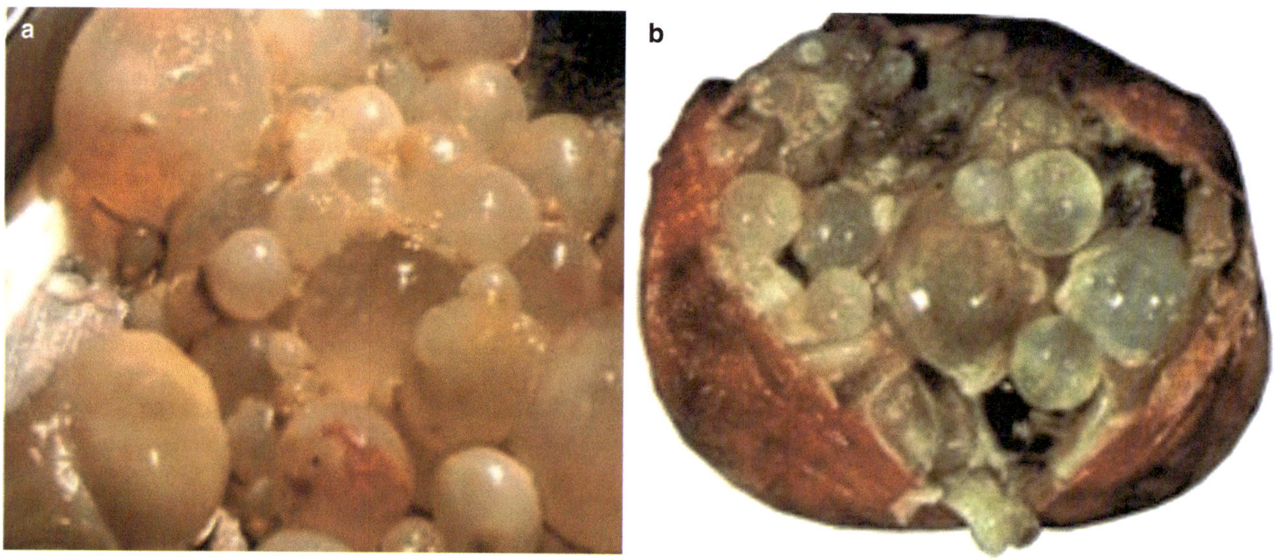

Fig. 26.3 Specimens of Echinococcus granulosus

cysts, the granddaughter cysts can be produced. The cyst is filled with hydatid fluid. The size of echinococcus is related to the parasitic time, parasitic position, and host, which ranges from less than 1 cm to more than 10 cm. The large echinococcus contains more than 1,000 ml hydatid fluid. And echinococcus can survive in the body of its host for several years or even 20 years.

26.1.2 *Echinococcus multilocularis* (E.m.)

26.1.2.1 Adult Worm

The adult worm resembles to that of E.g. but with an even smaller size (1.2–4.5 mm). The size of its egg is (30–38) μm × (29–34) μm.

26.1.2.2 Egg

The shape and size of E.m. eggs are similar to those of E.g., presenting difficulties for their differentiation.

26.1.2.3 Larva

E.m. is commonly parasitic in the liver and sometimes in the lungs and brain. Generally, it is a single giant vesicular mass like in the color of light yellowish or whitish. Sometimes, it is nodular. Otherwise, vesicular and nodular masses concur. E.m. reproduces in ways of budding or infiltration, with continuous production of new vesicles to grow into the tissues like neoplasms. It mostly grows outward, with rare occurrence of inward growth to form septum. Therefore, the cystid is separated into multiple small cysts. The new vesicles may invade the vascular or lymphatic vessels to metastasize into the lungs, brain, spleen, kidney, adrenal gland, heart, and even occasionally portal lymph nodes. Therefore, by naked eyes, the conditions may be misdiagnosed as hepatic carcinoma. Generally within 1–2 years, the parasitized organs are occupied by vesicles in different sizes. The grape cluster-like vesicles may spread from the organ surface into body cavities, which appear like carcinoma. Therefore, it is referred to as worm cancer.

26.2 Epidemiology

26.2.1 The Source of Infection

House dogs are the terminal host of E.g., which is also the most important source of infection. The adult worms parasitic in the intestines of dogs experience maturation of eggs and shedding of gravid proglottid in a cycle of 7–14 days. Continual egg excretion can be found in the feces of infected dogs.

26.2.2 Route of Transmission

Due to close contacts to dogs, the eggs of E.g. infect humans via contaminated hands and oral intake. The worm eggs in dog feces may contaminate vegetables and water sources, especially sharing water source in humans and animals, which also causes infection.

26.2.3 Susceptible Populations

The susceptible populations are mainly farmers, peasants, and the fur workers. However, because increasingly more people raise dogs in urban areas, the urban residents are also at high risk of infection. Most patients are infected during childhood and show the obvious symptoms after they develop into young or middle-aged adults.

26.2.4 Epidemiological Features

Cyst echinococcosis is distributed worldwide, but is more common in countries and regions with dominant industry of stockbreeding such as Australia, New Zealand, Argentina, Uruguay, South Africa, and Asia. In China, cyst echinococcosis mainly prevails in northwestern farming areas such as Xinjiang Wei Autonomous Region, Ningxia Hui Autonomous Region, Tibet, and Gansu, with sporadic cases in other regions.

Alveolar echinococcosis is sporadic, which is mainly distributed in Middle and South Europe, North America, and Britain. In China, the cases are reported in Qinghai, Ningxia Hui Autonomous Region, and Xinjiang Wei Autonomous Region.

26.3 Pathogenesis and Pathological Changes

26.3.1 Pathogenesis

After the eggs of E.g. enter the human body along with food intake, they are incubated into oncospheres under the effects of digestive juice. Some oncospheres invading into the tissues are surrounded by local cells and eliminated, with some other oncospheres surviving and developing. The oncospheres firstly invade the liver along with blood flow in the portal vein, with most forming hydatid cysts in the liver and rarely others invading the lungs via the hepatic sinusoid, hepatic vein, and right heart. The cases with following invasion of hydatid cysts into the systemic circulation via pulmonary microvascular vessels and the left heart show systemic involvements of organs. Therefore, it has been known that hydatid can be parasitic at any part of human body. The infective rate of each organ is directly related to the blood flow volume of each organ and the sequence of oncosphere invasion along with blood flow. Therefore, the organ with the highest to the lowest incidence rate is sequentially the liver, lungs, abdominal cavity, pelvic cavity, spleen, kidneys, and brain. The pathogenesis of CE is predominantly mechanic compression, and the other etiological factor is rupture of E.g. cyst-induced homologous protein allergy. E.g. grows very slowly and it usually lasts for about 10 years from infection to onset of symptoms.

After intake of food contaminated by worm eggs, oncospheres are inoculated in the intestines of humans, which then penetrate intestinal mucosa into the portal vein. After their arrival at the liver, they develop into hydatid.

26.3.2 Pathological Changes

The pathological changes of hydatidosis include space-occupying growth of the cysts and the consequent compression to the adjacent organs. E.g. gradually grows and matures in the liver, with intrahepatic cholangioles compressed and imbedded into the external cyst wall. Sometimes, the cholangioles penetrates into the cystic cavity due to compressive necrosis to stain the daughter cysts and the cyst fluid into yellow and to cause secondary bacterial infection. The hydatid cysts of lungs can penetrate into the bronchi. Occasionally, the germinal layer, scolex, and cyst fluid can be coughed up altogether, with complication of bacterial infection. If the hydatid cyst penetrates into the bronchioles, air fills in the space between internal and external cyst to show crescent air-containing area. If hydatid cysts of the liver rupture with the fluid flowing into the abdominal cavity, allergic shock may occur. The access of scolex into the abdominal cavity can cause multiple hydatidosis.

E.m. is in multilocular growth, with virtually all of its primary focus originating from the liver, and the foci in other organs are metastatic from the liver. The liver lesions are scattered light grayish-white nodules in different sizes on the liver surface, which are hardened with no envelope and poorly defined boundaries with surrounding liver tissues. On the cross sections of the lesions, there are necrotic tissues and cavities. Microscopy demonstrates vesicles in irregular shapes and different sizes, which are surrounded by infiltration of eosinophils granulocytes, lymphocytes, plasmocytes, and other inflammatory cells. E.m. surviving for several years is commonly surrounded by a thick layer of fibers, with no or small quantity of fluid in the cyst. At the cystic wall, there are calcium depositions, which are granular in amorphous calcification.

26.3.3 Types of Hydatidosis

26.3.3.1 Singular and Multiple Hydatidosis

Singular hydatidosis refers to infection of only one hydatid. Multiple hydatidosis refers to concurrent infection of at least two hydatids in one or more organs.

26.3.3.2 Primary and Secondary Hydatidosis

Primary hydatidosis is the infection of E.g. eggs, which grow and develop parasitically in host. Primary hydatidosis accounts for most of the hydatidosis cases. Secondary hydatidosis is infection of newly developed hydatid from transplanting germinal cyst, daughter cyst, or protoscolex as well as from asexual reproduction of primary hydatid cyst.

26.3.3.3 In Situ Relapse of Hydatidosis

After surgical removal of the hydatid, the residual daughter cyst or protoscolex in the external cystic cavity continues its growth into new hydatid that causes in situ relapse of hydatidosis.

26.3.3.4 Recurrent Hydatidosis

After hydatidosis is healed, a repeated infection of hydatid eggs causes hydatidosis again, which is known as recurrent hydatidosis.

26.4 Clinical Symptoms and Signs

In the early stage of the disease, the patients may have no subjective symptoms. The clinical manifestations are related to the parasitic site, size, and quantity of echinococcus as well as host responses and complications. Hydatidosis has a long incubation period, commonly 10–20 years or even longer from the infection to the onset of symptoms.

26.4.1 Hepatic Hydatidosis

26.4.1.1 Hepatic Cystic Hydatidosis

This type is the most common, with lesions commonly located in the right liver lobe. The patients may experience hepatic upset, dull pain or distended pain, enlarged liver, and protruding liver surface. Painless mass can be palpated that has smooth surface and is mobile along with breathing. By percussion, the mass feels trembling, which is known as hydatid thrill sign. The hydatid adjacent to hepatic hilum can compress the bile ducts to show jaundice. It can also compress the portal vein to cause portal hypertension. In the cases with complicated infections, lesions resembling to hepatic abscesses can be found. And its penetrating into abdominal cavity can cause diffuse peritonitis and allergic responses. In some serious cases, allergic shock occurs. Secondary abdominal or thoracic hydatidosis may occur due to dissemination of hydatid into abdominal or thoracic cavity along with cystic fluid.

26.4.1.2 Hepatic Alveolar Hydatidosis

In its early stage, the patients experience no upset. Along with progress of the conditions, the patients experience hepatic pain, poor appetite, abdominal distension, and other symptoms. In its late stage, the patients experience jaundice, cachexia, itchy skin, ascites, and other signs of portal hypertension. By physical examination, hardened painless mass can be palpated, which has smooth or nodular surface and tends to be misdiagnosed as hepatic carcinoma.

26.4.2 Pulmonary Hydatidosis

Pulmonary hydatidosis commonly occurs in the right lung, especially middle and lower lobes of the right lung. In the early stage, the patients commonly have no subjective symptoms and its early detection depends on physical examinations. The patients may complain of chest dull pain or stabbing pain, irritating cough, and hemoptysis. In the cases with hydatid cyst penetrating into the bronchus, the patients experience sudden dyspnea and paroxysmal cough with large quantity of watery cystic fluid along with sheet jellylike cystic wall and cystic sands. Occasionally, suffocation occurs due to overflow of cystic fluid and occlusion. In the cases with secondary infection, the patients experience high fever, chest pain, and cough with thick sputum.

26.4.3 Brain Hydatidosis

Its incidence rate is low, with more common occurrence in children. The lesion is commonly located at the parietal lobe, with accompanying hepatic and/or pulmonary hydatidosis. The clinical symptoms include headache, papilledema, and other symptoms of intracranial hypertension, with accompanying epilepsy attacks.

26.4.4 Spleen Hydatidosis

The patients experience falling pain, distension, and upset of the left epigastrium. The lesion commonly compresses the gastric fundus and the greater curvature of the stomach to cause abdominal distension, nausea, hiccups, poor appetite, and other digestive symptoms after food intake. However, complications rarely occur. The typical cases have palpable painless half sphere-shaped tough mass at the left epigastrium, which has smooth surface and feels elastic by pressure touch. By percussion, hydatid thrill sign can be found.

26.4.5 Kidney Hydatidosis

The patients experience dull pain of the lower back with falling pain, distension, and upset. The patients with long illness course commonly pay their clinic visit due to touchable painless mass at the epigastrium or lower back.

26.4.6 Abdominal and Pelvic Cavity Hydatidosis

Abdominal and pelvic hydatidosis can be divided into primary and secondary, with secondary cases being more common, which is secondary to rupture of hepatic hydatid or surgeries removing hepatic hydatid. Clinically, the common symptoms include abdominal distension, abdominal falling pain, poor appetite, and emaciation. The lesion compresses the intestinal canal to produce mechanical incomplete intestinal obstruction. The lesion compresses the diaphragm to elevate it and confine its movements, with consequent occurrence of shortness of breath and inability of supine position. The lesion may also compress the inferior vena cava to cause edema of lower limbs. Pelvic hydatid may compress the rectum and bladder to cause symptoms during defecation or urination. Hydatid in female reproductive organs may invade and compress the uterine and/or fallopian tubes to cause falling pain and distension of the lower abdomen as well as dysmenorrheal. After pregnancy, the hydatid can also be compressed with complicated hydatidosis by rupture of hydatid or infection.

26.4.7 Bone Hydatidosis

The patients may have painless mass or only local soreness and pain. The conditions tend to be misdiagnosed as chronic pain of soft tissues.

26.4.8 Cardiac Hydatidosis

Cardiac hydatidosis rarely occurs, with hydatid commonly parasitic in the left ventricle (accounting for about 50–60 % of cardiac hydatidosis cases). Other parasitic positions include the interventricular septum, right ventricle, pericardium, and left and right atrium according to the respective incidence rate. The parasitic position of cardiac hydatid is related to the route of infection and the blood supply of each part. In the early stage, X-ray commonly detects confined protrusion at the cardiac margin. With progress of the conditions, the patients experience symptoms of chest distress, palpitation, and arrhythmia.

26.4.9 Hydatidosis of Other Body Parts

Hydatidosis can also be found at the eye socket, mammary gland, subcutaneous tissues, muscles, pancreas, and thyroid gland.

26.5 Hydatidosis-Related Complications

26.5.1 Complications of Hepatic Hydatidosis

26.5.1.1 Hepatic Cyst Rupture

Hepatic hydatid can penetrate into the abdominal cavity to cause sudden severe abdominal pain and sudden shrinkage or disappearance of abdominal mass, with accompanying itchy skin, urticaria, dyspnea, cyanosis, vomiting, diarrhea, and other allergic responses. In some serious cases, shock and even death occur.

26.5.1.2 Secondary Infection

Secondary infection is commonly caused by penetration of the cyst into the bile duct. Clinically, its manifestations resemble to bacterial hepatic cyst and cholelithiasis. Due to ruptured cystic membrane or occlusion of daughter cyst, secondary infection occurs to cause purulent angiocholitis.

26.5.2 Complications of Pulmonary Hydatidosis

The incidence rate of secondary infection is 10–15 %, with concurrent infection and rupture, which are mutually cause and effect. Secondary infection occurs due to rupture. Occasionally, patients have no case history of rupture symptoms before the infection. Therefore, the infection is primary. After infection, hydatid cyst-bronchus fistula forms. Regardless of the formation of bronchial fistula, symptoms of pulmonary abscess occur, including chest pain, fever, emaciation, cough, and purulent sputum, which persist for a long period of time. In the cases with accompanying bronchial fistula, the patients experience coughing up purulent sputum with daughter cyst or internal cyst fragments and no hemoptysis when infection is not serious. When the bronchial fistula is smoothly drained, more purulent sputum is coughed up, followed by a decrease of body temperature and alleviated symptoms.

26.5.3 Complications of Abdominal Hydatidosis

26.5.3.1 Intestinal Obstruction

During the development of parasitic hydatid in the host abdominal cavity, the parasitized organ show fibrous tissue hyperplasia to surround the hydatid. Therefore, the external cyst is formed and its surrounding serous tissues response to exudate fibrin to form membranous or cord-like adhesion. Mechanical incomplete intestinal obstruction is resulted in, which may repeatedly occur with aggravated conditions.

26.5.3.2 Abdominal Infection

Its incidence rate is lower than that of hepatic hydatidosis, accounting for about 10 % of the cases with abdominal hydatidosis. It mainly occurs in the cases with multiple hydatidosis and a long history of illness. The external cyst of abdominal hydatid is thick and plays a role of barrier to confine the inflammation within the cyst. Therefore, the systemic inflammation is mild and the patients experience only dull pain, long-term low-grade fever, poor appetite, anemia, and emaciation.

26.6 Diagnostic Examinations

26.6.1 Laboratory Tests

26.6.1.1 Casoni Test

The operational procedures are simple and the test results can be obtained within 15 min. Casoni test has a positive rate of 68–100 %, which can be applied for primary screening.

26.6.1.2 Indirect Hemagglutination Test (IHA)

The operational procedures are quite simple and the test has a high specificity. It has a positive rate of about 82 % for hepatic hydatidosis.

26.6.1.3 Enzyme-Linked Immunosorbent Assay (ELISA)

Its sensitivity and specificity exceed IHA, with rare false-positive results.

26.6.1.4 Dot-ELISA

Its operational procedures are simple and the test results are directly observable. And the test is applicable in community-based hospitals.

26.6.1.5 ABC-ELISA

The sensitivity is the highest in these laboratory tests, being about four to six times as high as routine ELISA.

26.6.1.6 Detection of Specific Antibody of Hydatidosis

In April 2011, the specific antibody test kit for the diagnosis of hydatidosis was successfully developed in Xinjiang

Medical University, China. The kit is for the diagnosis of hydatidosis with advantages of being fast, simple, specific, and accurate. It can be applied both in clinical diagnostic trials and field epidemiological investigations, functioning in both diagnosis and differential diagnosis (between CE and AE). The kit is the first serologic test for the diagnosis of hydatidosis, which standardizes the diagnostic criteria of hydatidosis. It is a favorable diagnostic tool for early diagnosis, differential diagnosis, and epidemiological studies of hydatidosis.

26.6.2 Radiological Examinations

26.6.2.1 Ultrasound

Ultrasound examination is a noninvasive and safe radiological technology, which renders direct observation for diagnosis and assessment of the diseases. It can clearly demonstrate the space-occupying lesion of hydatidosis, which provides repeated and dynamic observation of the lesions and can be operated conveniently.

26.6.2.2 X-Ray Radiology

X-ray radiology is the examination of choice for the diagnosis of pulmonary hydatidosis and bone hydatidosis. Due to the distinct contrast of density between lungs and bone tissues to hydatid cysts, their respective locations, quantity, size, properties, and complications can be well defined by X-ray.

26.6.2.3 CT Scanning

CT is an important examination for the diagnosis of hydatidosis, which is applicable to all organs of human body.

26.6.2.4 MR Imaging

For the diagnosis of complex hydatidosis, MR imaging is superior, especially magnetic resonance hydrography and magnetic resonance angiography which play important roles in the diagnosis of hydatidosis.

26.7 Imaging Demonstrations

26.7.1 Hepatic Hydatidosis

26.7.1.1 Hepatic Cystic Hydatidosis

Ultrasound

Based on the natural development of hepatic hydatid, different stages of pathological changes, and pathological changes of various complications as well as their sonogram, hepatic cystic hydatidosis can be divided into seven types.

Singular Type

Because the hydatid cyst is filled with watery cystic fluid, both real-time linear array and fan-shaped scanning demon-

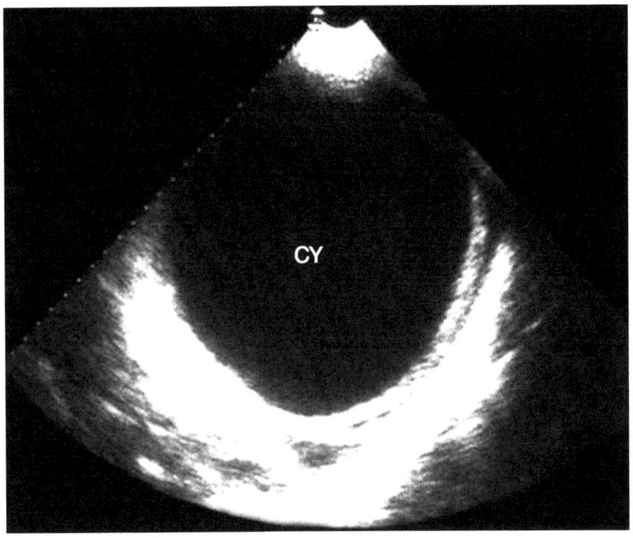

Fig. 26.4 Singular type of hepatic cystic hydatidosis. Ultrasound demonstrates liquid dark area in the left liver lobe (*CY*), with space between lateral wall of the internal cyst and external cyst and posterior enhancement effect

strate round or oval singular liquid dark area with no echo. However, small hydatid cysts have less tension and some of them may fail to show a round lesion area (Fig. 26.4). In the cases with the hydatid cyst located inferior to the hepatic capsule to form hump-like change, the cyst may compress the intrahepatic duct system and the adjacent right kidney and gallbladder. The smooth and thick hydatid cystic wall has obvious acoustic impedance different from hepatic parenchyma to form bright boundary. The large hydatid cysts has double-layered cystic wall (internal cystic wall and external cystic wall) that produces strong echo, which shows well-defined bright boundary from the organ tissues. The hydatid cystic wall is far thicker than other cysts. The ultrasound is reflected by the lateral margin of thick cystic wall to produce acoustic shadow at the lateral wall. Ultrasound demonstrates no echo area or no reflection area for liquid-contained hydatid cyst. Its demonstration depends on the potential space between the internal cyst wall and the external cyst wall as well as small quantity of liquid. Therefore, a fine dark interface is commonly demonstrated to show double-wall sign, which is characteristic at sonogram of hydatidosis. The ultrasound bundle produces acoustic energy via hydatid cystic fluid to increase the adduction, which shows the enhancement effect of the posterior wall of hydatid cyst. When the probe pressed, the hydatid cyst may be deformed. It should be cautious to avoid rupture of the hydatid cyst. When the hydatid cyst is vibrated with the ultrasound probe, there are floating fine light spots posterior to the cyst, which are stirred protoscolex to show reflected light spots that deposited at inferior to the cyst, which are known as cystic sands.

Multiple Type

In the liver, at least two round or oval cysts are probed, which are in different sizes but with characteristic sonogram of hydatid and septum of liver tissues or cystic wall of the hydatid.

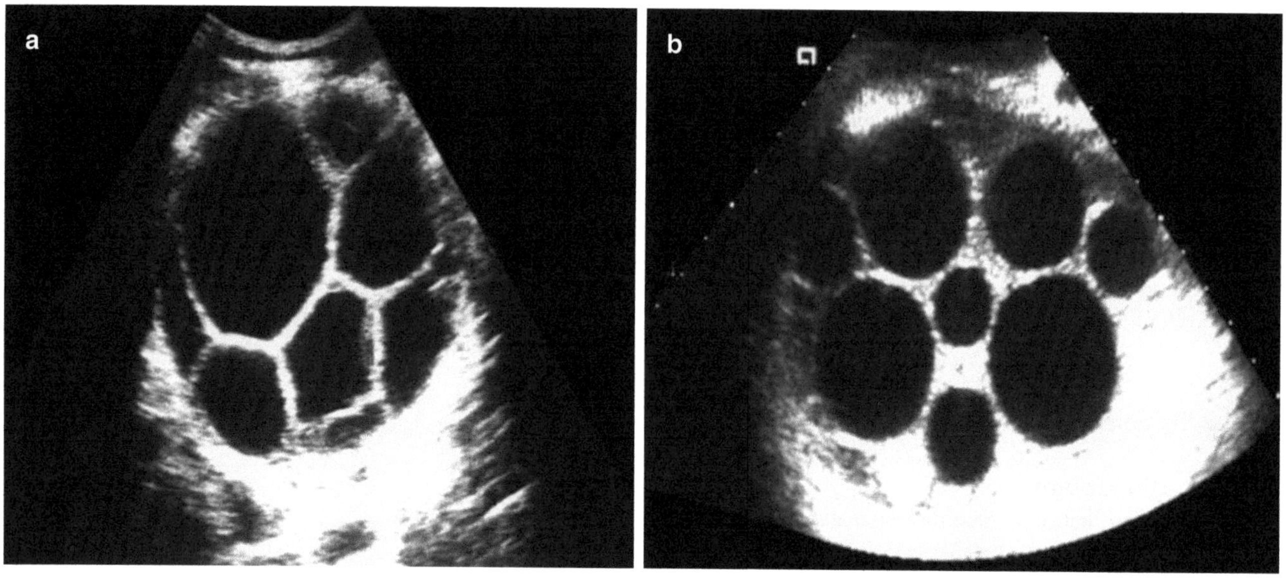

Fig. 26.5 Hepatic cystic hydatidosis (daughter cyst type). (**a**, **b**) Ultrasound demonstrates dark areas of small sphere-shaped daughter cysts with different sizes in the mother cyst, with their echo being lower than that of the mother cyst fluid

Daughter Cyst Type

In the dark liquid area of the mother cyst, there are sphere-shaped dark light rings in different sizes and different quantities, namely, characteristic cyst-in-cyst sign of hydatidosis. In the cases with rare daughter cysts, the daughter cysts are arranged close to the mother cyst wall. In the cases with more daughter cysts, the mother cyst can be filled up, with the daughter cysts clinging and overlapping to form large quantity of small round light rings or dense short light strips, namely, honeycomb sign or grape cluster sign. In the cases with daughter cysts growing up to filling in the mother cyst, the daughter cysts compress to each other to transform the daughter cysts from sphere shape into polyhedron shape, namely, the wheel sign or honeycomb sign (Fig. 26.5).

Calcification Type

Hydatidosis with a long illness course is demonstrated with thickened and rough external cyst wall and calcium deposition. By ultrasound, it is demonstrated as spotlike strong echoes at the hydatid cyst wall. In the cases with partial calcification, the sonogram shows arch-shaped light bands with strong echoes. In the cases with complete calcification of the hydatid cyst wall, the sonogram shows eggshell-like change, with obvious acoustic shadow at the lateral wall. Along with the severity of calcification, the acoustic shadow at posterior cyst is increasingly obvious, indicating decline or even death of the hydatid.

Consolidation Type

During the long illness course of hydatidosis, the cyst is gradually subject to degeneration, necrosis, lysis, and shrinkage into cheese appearance due to decreased and absorbed cystic fluid. In the cyst, consolidation mass is demonstrated with uneven intensity of echoes, which is typically gyrus like. The consolidated space-occupying lesion occurs due to collapse and folding of the mother cyst after absorption of cystic fluid as well as degeneration and necrosis of the daughter cysts. Its sonogram resembles to benign tumor with homogeneous echo.

Infective Type

Secondary infection occurs in the hydatid cyst to form pus, with collapse, necrosis, and decreased tension of the mother cyst. The mother cyst, therefore, deforms with unevenly thickened and coarse cystic wall. The internal cyst sheds off in the external cyst, which is twisted and irregular. The daughter cyst also deforms or is dried up, with uneven echoes of cotton-like light spots, light strips, and small light masses in different intensities filling up the cyst.

Rupture Type

The hydatid cyst sheds off from the external cyst wall, with collapsed, shrunk, and invaginated cyst wall that is twisted and folded, floating in the cystic fluid. In the liquid dark area, it is demonstrated with arch and folded cord-like strong echo band. When the posture is changed, the echo band may be floating and deformed.

X-Ray Radiology

Liver

The contour is enlarged. In the cases with giant hydatid in the right liver lobe compressing the right diaphragm, the diaphragm is observed to be elevated to cause limited breathing

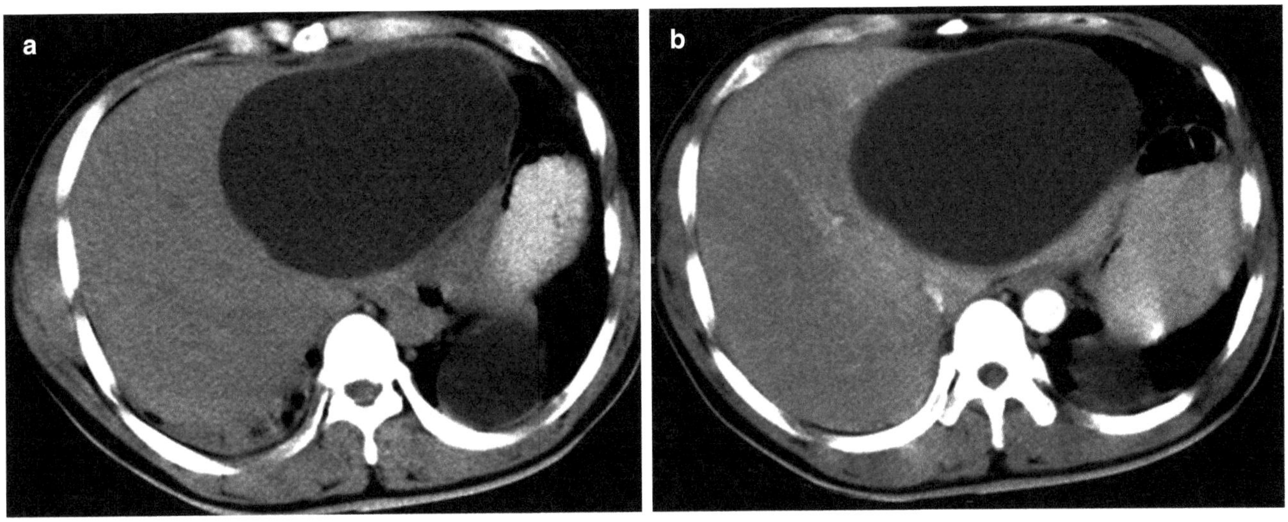

Fig. 26.6 Hepatic cystic hydatidosis (simplex cystic type). (**a**) Plain CT scanning demonstrates oval-shaped low-density shadow in the left liver lobe, with smooth and sharp margin and even density. The cystic wall is observed to be thin; (**b**) contrast CT scanning demonstrates no intracystic enhancement

movement and even left shift of the heart. In children patients, the right lower thorax protrudes with widened intercostal space.

Calcification

Calcification can be found in the hepatic area. The ring-shaped, semiring-shaped, or eggshell-like calcification indicates cystic wall calcification. Intracystic calcification is demonstrated with round or round-like nodular calcification or stratified calcification.

Complications

Signs of hepatic abscess can be observed. The patients are demonstrated to have elevated right diaphragm, blurry diaphragmatic surface, and limited breathing movement. Otherwise, the complications may be demonstrated with right pleural inflammatory responses and effusion, blurry costophrenic angle and cardiodiaphragmatic angle, and poorly defined boundary between right lower chest and hepatic area. By pneumoperitoneography, left subphrenic inflation occurs due to right phrenic adhesion with no inflation.

Penetration Into Lungs

After infections occur to complicate hydatidosis at the top of right liver lobe, the hydatid may penetrate the diaphragm into the lung, which commonly causes pulmonary abscess at the anterior or posterior fundus segment in the right lower lung lobe. It is demonstrated as elevated right diaphragm or local protrusion of the right diaphragm, decreased breathing movement, inflammatory mass or lump in the right lower lung field, thickened pulmonary markings, and cord-like shadows extending toward the pulmonary hilum.

Penetration Into Thoracic Cavity

The hydatid cyst at the top of right liver lobe can penetrate into the right thoracic cavity to cause acute pleural effusion, with the lung compressed. In the cases with complicating bronchial fistula, hydropneumothorax can be demonstrated.

CT Scanning

By CT scanning, hydatidosis can be divided into cystic type, cystic calcification type, consolidation type, and mixed type. The former three types are basically corresponding to the germination, development, degeneration, and death of hepatic hydatid.

Cystic Type

In the liver, there are singular or multiple cysts that are round or round-like in shape with well-defined boundaries and smooth margins. Their densities are even and homogeneous, being close to the density of water. The cystic wall is thin and even, with no nodules. The intrahepatic bile ducts, vascular vessels, and adjacent organs are compressed with shifts. By contrast scanning, the cystic fluid and the cystic wall are demonstrated with no enhancement.

Simplex Cystic Type

In the liver, the cyst has smooth and sharp margin, which is singular or multiple round- or oval-shaped shadows with different sizes and even densities. The cystic wall is demonstrated as linear dense shadow in a thickness of 1–5 mm. By contrast scanning, no obvious enhancement is observed in the cyst (Fig. 26.6).

Multiple Daughter Cyst Type

Emergence of multiple daughter cysts in the mother cyst is one of the characteristic manifestations of hepatic hydatidosis.

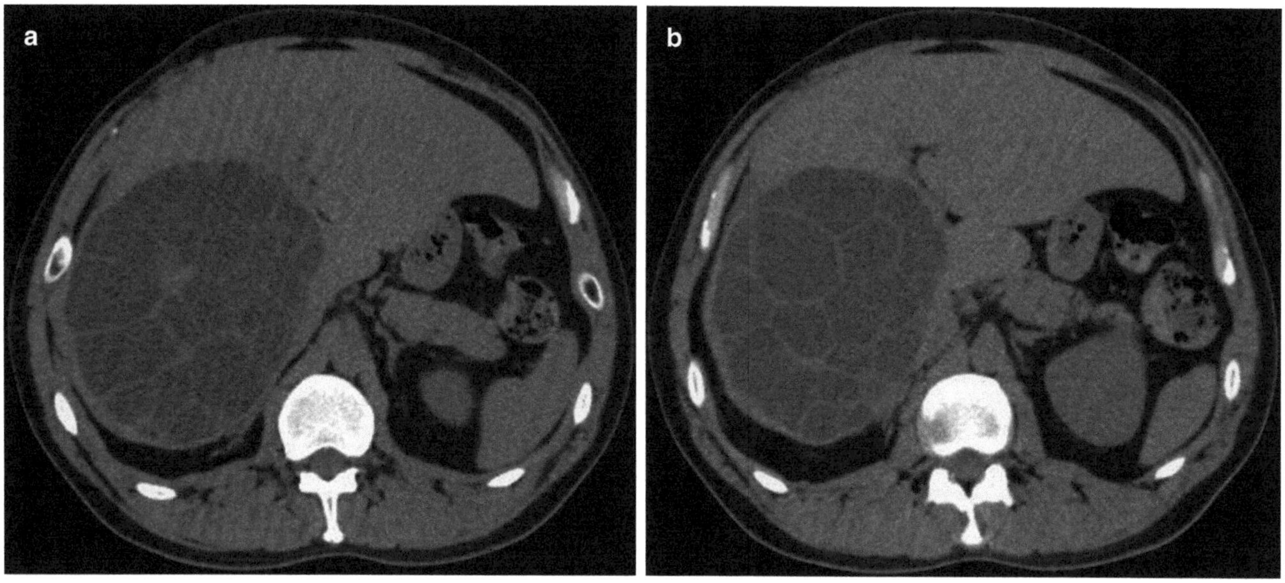

Fig. 26.7 Hepatic cystic hydatidosis (multiple daughter cyst type). (**a**, **b**) Plain CT scanning demonstrates hydatidosis at the right liver lobe, with multiple daughter cysts filling up the mother cyst that compress each other in honeycomb sign

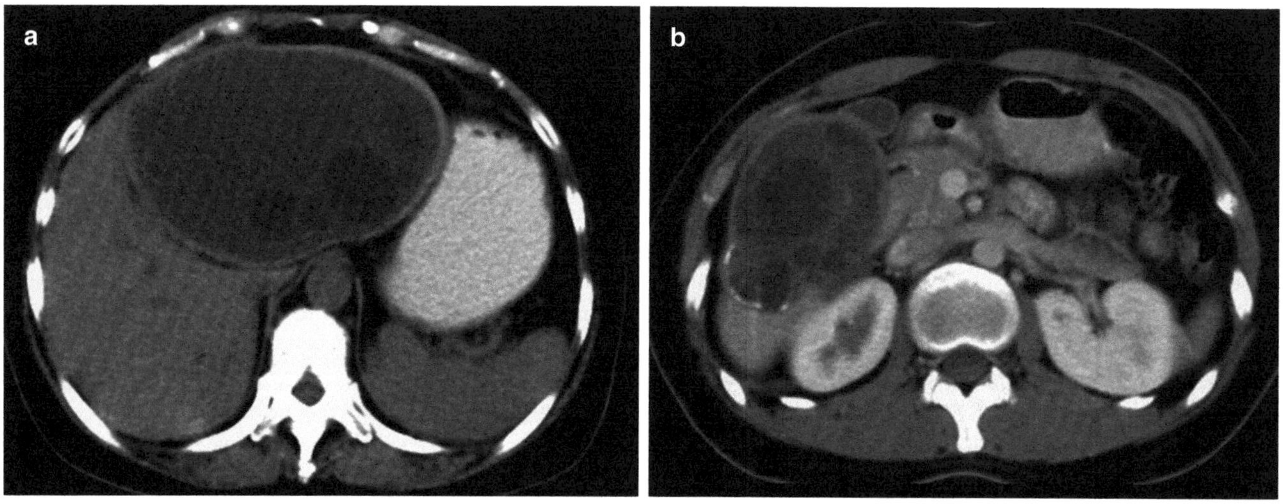

Fig. 26.8 Hepatic cystic hydatidosis (multiple daughter cyst type). (**a**, **b**) Plain CT scanning demonstrates multiple round low-density shadows in the liver, with internal multiple lower-density round-like shadows of daughter cysts. The shadows are well defined, with smooth and sharp margins. Calcification can be observed at the posteroexterior margin of the lesion in the right liver lobe. By contrast scanning, no obvious enhancement is observed

There may be daughter cyst shadows in the mother cyst in different quantities and sizes and in round or irregular shape. The fibrous septum has different thicknesses. The daughter cysts are arranged around the mother cyst-like honeycomb or wheel, with their density being lower than their mother cyst. Along with increases of daughter cysts in quantity and size, the daughter cysts compress each other to be deformed into round shape, diamond shape, or polygon shape, which are distributed in the mother cyst-like grape cluster. The mother cyst fluid scatters between the daughter cysts, with higher density than daughter cyst fluid (Fig. 26.7). In the other cases, the daughter cysts are small in size and quantity. In the early stage, the small and round daughter cysts are arranged close to the mother cyst wall, with their density being close to the mother cyst (Fig. 26.8).

Secondary Infection Type

The cystic wall is subject to irregular thickening, with poorly defined boundaries. In some cases, the cystic wall is imperfect, with increased but uneven intracystic density. The boundary of the cysts is poorly defined, sometimes with fluid level observed. By contrast scanning, the thickened cystic wall can be demonstrated with enhancement.

Rupture Type

David further divided the rupture type into two subtypes, internal cyst rupture and direct rupture. The subtype of internal cyst rupture is demonstrated with ruptured internal cyst but with its content within the external cyst. The cystic fluid gains its access into the external cyst and the internal cystic wall stripped partially or completely off the external cyst. By CT scanning, it is demonstrated as cyst bilateral sign or ribbon sign with wavy internal cyst membrane in the cystic lumen (Fig. 26.9). The completely separated internal cyst is subject to collapse and curling like a small lily. The subtype of direct rupture refers to rupture of both internal and external cysts, with the cystic fluid and their contents being directly drained into the abdominal cavity, ?? cavity or position inferior to the hepatic capsule. At this time, the hydatid cyst collapses and is deformed, with effusion at the abdominal cavity and the hepatic periphery as well as the daughter cyst shadows (Figs. 26.10 and 26.11). The rupture of hydatid cyst at the top of liver may cause intrathoracic complications or wrapping pleural effusion.

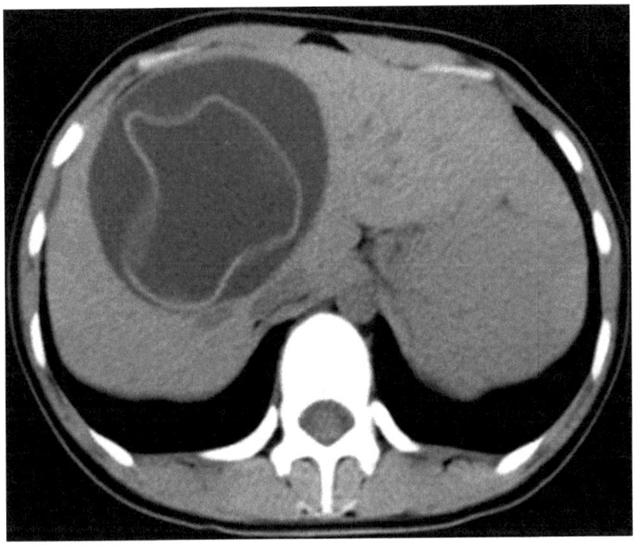

Fig. 26.9 Hepatic hydatid rupture. Plain CT scanning demonstrates collapse and shrinkage of the ruptured hydatid cystic wall, which is floating in the cystic fluid to form typical ribbon sign

Cystic Calcification Type

Based on the position of cyst calcification, cystic calcification can be further divided into two subtypes, cystic wall calcification and intracystic calcification. Cystic wall calcification is arch-shaped continuous or continual calcification along the cystic wall. Otherwise, the calcification may be shell-like or spotlike calcifications. The cystic wall is demonstrated to be thickened, with even intracystic density that is close to water density. Sometimes, gas-fluid level can be observed in the cyst, which shows no enhancement by contrast scanning. Intracystic calcification is demonstrated with patches or spots of calcification shadows or intracystic linear high but even density shadow. The cystic fluid has high density, but with no enhancement by contrast scanning.

Consolidation Type

Due to the long illness course, the hydatid shows decreased activity to result in degeneration and necrosis. The absorption and condensation of cystic fluid cause caseous change, which is mixed with softened internal cyst or daughter cyst to increase the CT value. The CT value is also uneven, being close to that of consolidation tumor density shadow.

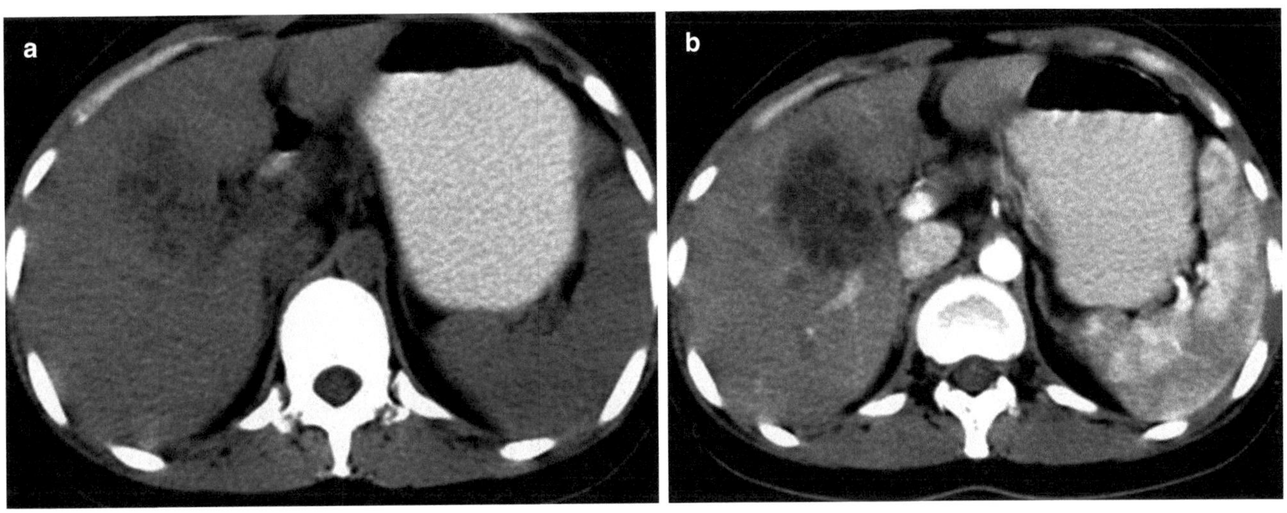

Fig. 26.10 Hepatic hydatid rupture. (**a**, **b**) Plain CT scanning demonstrates increased uneven density of intrahepatic cyst with poorly defined boundary. The intrahepatic bile ducts around the lesion are demonstrated to be slightly dilated. The lesion is not enhanced by contrast scanning

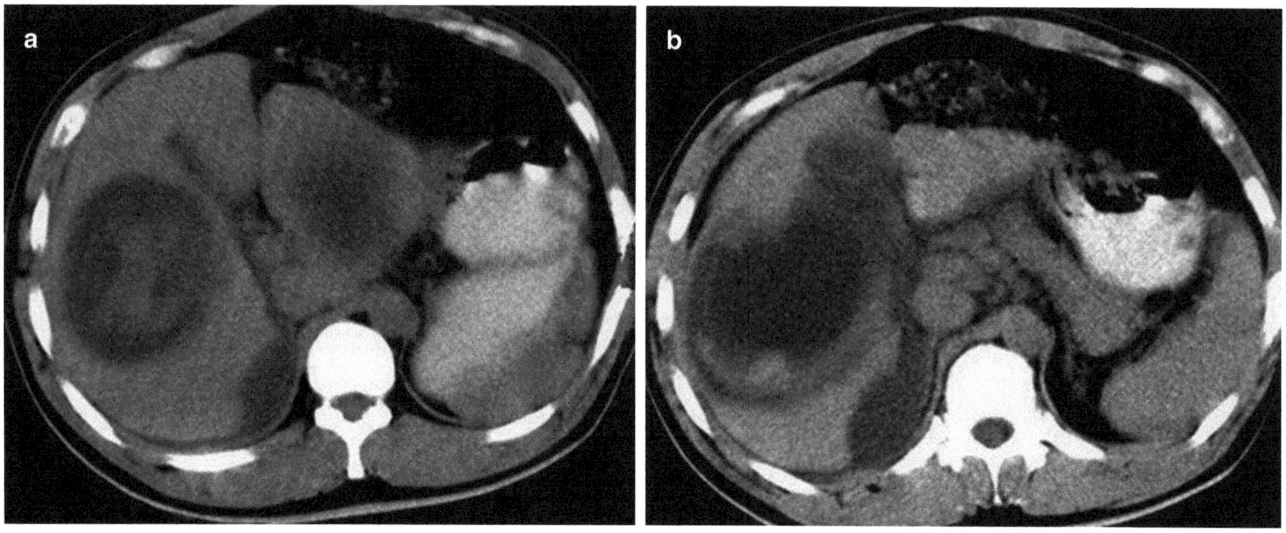

Fig. 26.11 Hepatic hydatid rupture. (**a**, **b**) Plain CT scanning demonstrates cyst rupture in the right liver lobe. The lesion has poorly defined boundary. In the cystic lumen, the density is increased. In the gallbladder fossa and around the liver, effusion is observable

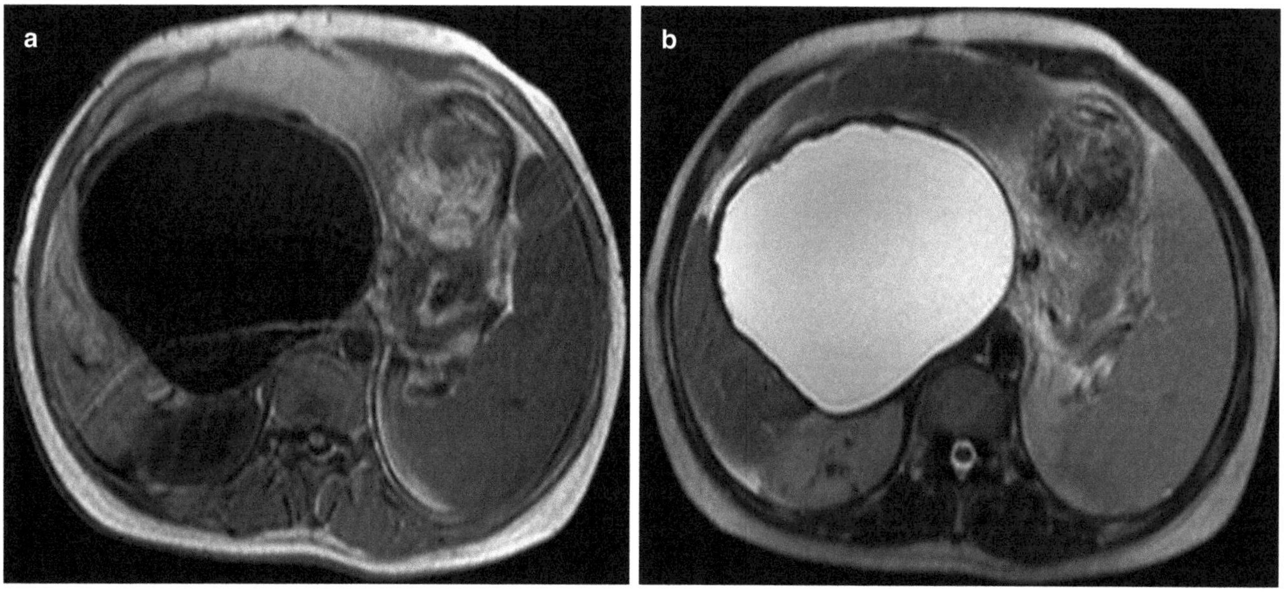

Fig. 26.12 Hepatic cystic hydatidosis (singular type). (**a**, **b**) MR imaging demonstrates round-like lesion in the right liver lobe, with well-defined boundary as well as smooth and sharp margin. By T1WI, it is at low signal; by T2WI, high signal

Mixed Type

In just one case, at least the above two types of lesions coexist, with CT scanning demonstrating characteristic lesions of different types.

MR Imaging

Singular Type

The typical demonstration by MR imaging is round-like lesion with well-defined boundary as well as smooth and sharp margin. By T1WI, low signal is demonstrated, while by T2WI, high signal is demonstrated. The cystic wall is in even and homogeneous thickness. Especially, low signal by T1WI is its characteristic demonstration. Contrast imaging demonstrates no enhancement of the cyst (Fig. 26.12).

Multiple Type

There are multiple lesions in the liver. MR imaging demonstrations are similar to those of singular type, only with difference in quantity.

Daughter Cyst Type

In the cases of daughter cysts contained in the mother cyst, it is demonstrated as rose petal sign, which is characteristically

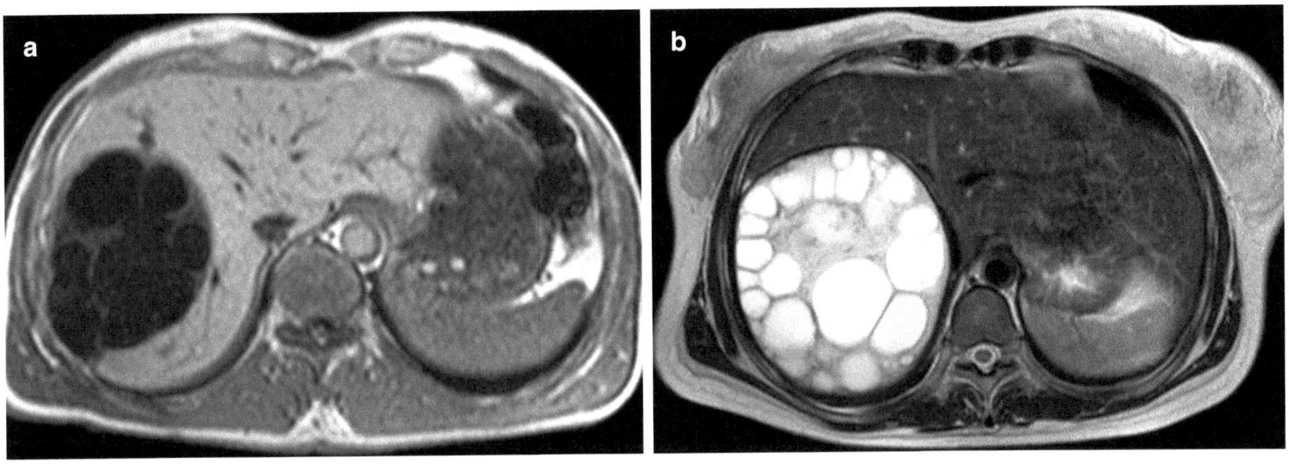

Fig. 26.13 Hepatic cystic hydatidosis (multiple daughter cyst type). (**a**) By T1WI of MR imaging, hepatic cyst is demonstrated in the right liver lobe, with daughter cysts arranged along the mother cyst wall in rose petal sign. (**b**) MR hydrography provides more direct view of the lesion

hepatic cystic hydatidosis. By MR hydrography, it is more clearly demonstrated. Moreover, MR hydrography demonstrates its relationship with the bile ducts (Fig. 26.13).

External Cyst Calcification Type

The calcification is demonstrated as low signal by both T1WI and T2WI.

Consolidation Type

MR imaging demonstrates parenchyma lesion with smooth and sharp margin, which resembles to benign tumor.

Infection Type

The cystic wall is in uneven thickness and the cystic contents are thick. By T1WI, the signal increases, with uneven internal signal. After injection of paramagnetic reagent, the surrounding area of the cystic wall is abnormally enhanced.

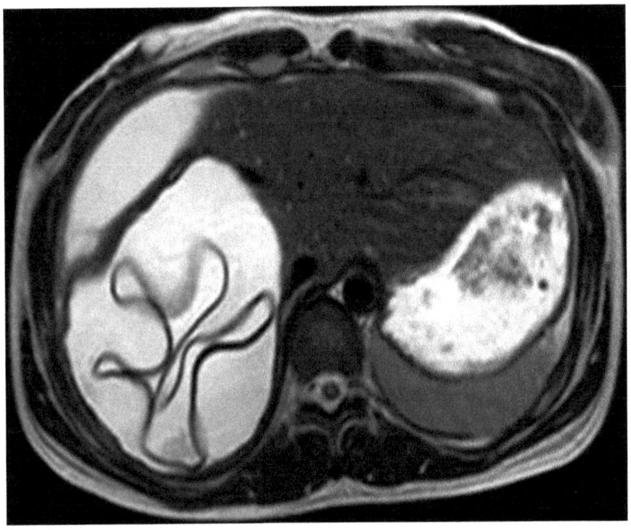

Fig. 26.14 Rupture of hepatic hydatid. T2WI of MR imaging demonstrates collapse and shrinkage of ruptured hydatid cystic wall, which floats in the cystic fluid in ribbon sign

Rupture Type

The intracystic signal is uneven, with separation of the internal cyst from the external cyst. The ruptured internal cyst can be observed floating in the cystic lumen in ribbon sign (Fig. 26.14). MR hydrography more clearly demonstrates the rupture of hydatid cyst and its penetration into the bile duct. With the invasion of hydatid into the bile duct, the cystic fluid leaks into the bile duct. The mother cyst has decreased tension with shrinkage of the cyst or deformation of the cyst into irregular oval shape. In the cases with fragments of small daughter cysts or hydatid into the bile duct, bile duct occlusion occurs. MR hydrography can clearly demonstrate the location of occluded bile duct, dilated bile duct, and the fragmented structures (Fig. 26.15).

The external cyst of hydatid is an envelope membrane of fibrous connective tissues, with obviously confined water molecules movement. However, no water molecule can be found in calcification. Therefore, both external cyst and calcification are demonstrated with low signal regardless of their b value. The cystic fluid in the hydatid cyst has relatively free water molecule movement. Along with the increase of b value, the lesion containing cystic fluid shows the most obvious decrease of the lesion signal. The simplex type or multiple daughter cyst type with no calcification demonstrates more obvious hydatid cyst. In the cases with the lesion of hydatid cyst filled with degeneration, necrosis, and calcified daughter cysts, there is basically no movement of water molecules. Therefore, the lesion signal shows no obvious change and is low signal by DWI. In the cases with collapsed internal cyst floating in the cystic fluid, along with the illness course, the collapsed internal cyst is subject to calcification. Due to the residual cystic fluid,

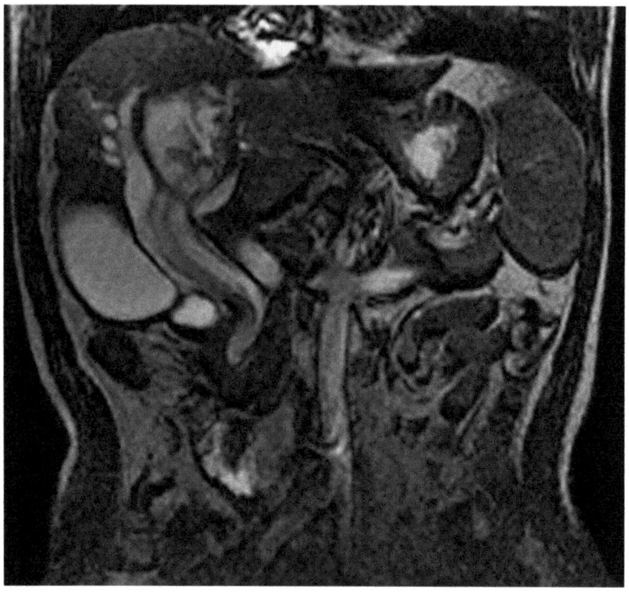

Fig. 26.15 Rupture of hepatic hydatid. MR imaging demonstrates rupture of hepatic hydatid

along with the increase of b value, the lesion signal gradually decreases. And the degree of decrease is lower than that in singular type and multiple daughter cyst type. In the cases of infective type, due to concurrent rupture of external and internal cysts and the large quantities of proteins and scolex in the cystic fluid, the lesion signal shows insignificant decrease along with the increase of b value, but high signal by DWI and obviously lower ADC value than that of other types.

By DWI, large b value indicates more serious phase discrete of water molecules, with more obvious decrease of the signal. When B value is 100 s/mm^2, the signal decrease of the hydatid cyst is not obvious, with poorly defined intracystic septum and fluctuating ADC values in different areas of interesting. When b value is 1,000 s/mm^2, the signals of hydatid cyst and hepatic tissue show obvious decreases, with more obvious artifacts. When b value is 500 s/mm^2, the external cyst and the intracystic septum are best defined, with the most stable ADC value.

26.7.1.2 Hepatic Alveolar Hydatidosis

Ultrasound

Based on the ultrasound findings about pathomorphology, histology, and pathological development of alveolar hydatidosis, hepatic alveolar hydatidosis can be relatively divided into three types. In one lesion, pathological changes of two or three types can be simultaneously observed. In different lesions, pathological changes of two or three types can also be simultaneously observed.

Infiltrative Proliferation Type

Light mass with strong echo can be demonstrated in the liver, which has irregular shape and poorly defined boundary. Its surrounding area shows low-echo halo zone, with uneven internal echoes. In the area close to the center of lesion, dense small light spots with strong echoes are observable, with obviously decreased echo bundle at the posterior lesion. In the cases with giant lesion to enlarge the liver volume, flakes and nodular nodules with moderate or strong echo scatter in the liver, which are in different sizes with uneven echo. In the cases with the lesion invading or compressing the hepatic ducts, the hepatic ducts are shown to be dilated.

Fibrous Calcification Type

Along with the invasion of alveolar hydatid into the liver tissue, the lesion is subject to fibrosis and calcium deposition. Ultrasound demonstrates spots of strong echo calcification, which extend to fuse into irregular flakes of calcification lesions with strong echoes, with accompanying posterior acoustic shadows. An acoustic halo zone surrounding the lesions is observable with low echo.

Liquefaction and Cavity Type

The light heterogeneous mass with strong echo is demonstrated with irregular liquid dark area, with enhanced echo at its posterior part, in hollow hole sign. Surrounding the hollow hole is demonstrated with unsmooth calcification wall with strong echo, which protrudes into the hollow hole to form cave sign or peninsular sign. The lesion has a halo zone with low-intensity echo.

Ultrasonography demonstrates hepatic alveolar type, with no inflow of the contrast agent into the hydatidosis mass during the arterial phase, portal phase, and delayed phase. During the arterial phase, negative development is rapidly demonstrated, which extends into the portal vein phase and the delayed phase.

DSA

1. During the arterial phase, the hepatic artery is demonstrated to be thickened, with a twisted course to surround the lesion in embracing ball sign. The consolidated mass in the liver may cause shift of and surrounded intrahepatic vascular vessels.
2. During the capillary phase, the lesion is stained in a ring shape, with no central staining. Due to infiltrative extension of the lesion margin, the capillaries are subject to proliferation to produce surrounding staining. Due to large quantities of fibrous tissue, necrotic and liquefied tissue, and calcium deposition at the central area, there is no central staining of the lesion.
3. Indirect portography demonstrates shift of the branches of portal vein due to compression.

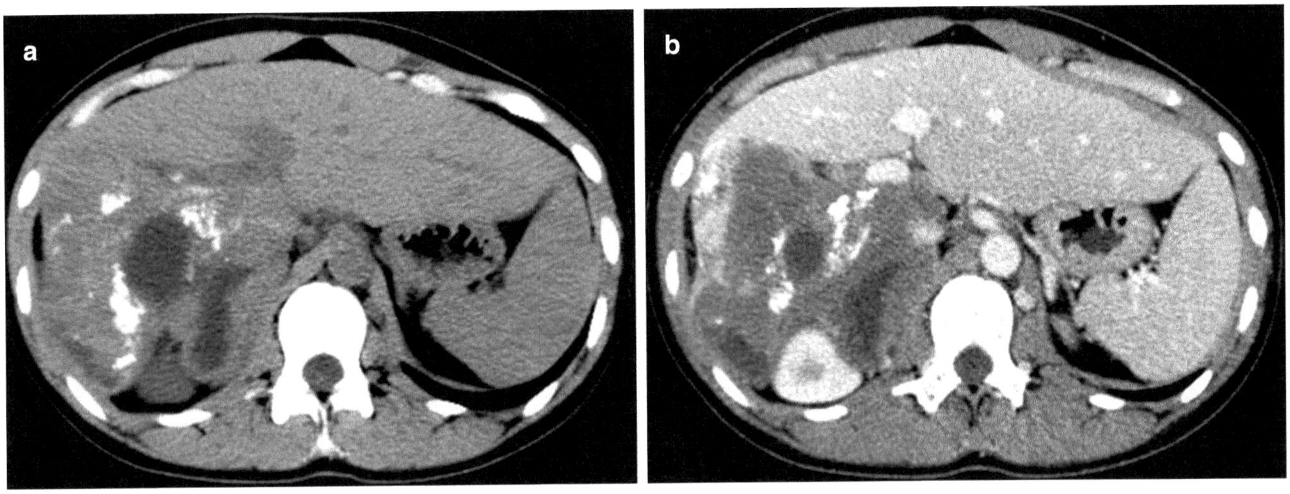

Fig. 26.16 Hepatic alveolar hydatidosis. (**a**) Plain CT scanning demonstrates low-density lesion with irregular shape and poorly defined boundary in the right liver lobe. In the lesion, multiple calcification lesions and cystic areas can be observed. (**b**) Contrast CT scanning demonstrates no obvious enhancement of the lesion, which has well-defined boundary

CT Scanning

Plain CT scanning demonstrates round-like or irregular shadows with mixed densities and poorly defined boundaries. In the lesion, dense small spots of calcification shadows scatter in different quantities. Otherwise, there are cyst-like low-density shadows in different sizes, possibly with irregular calcification at the cystic wall. Small spots of calcification with multilayered concentric round shape are the characteristic CT demonstration of hepatic alveolar hydatidosis. In some cases, flakes of calcification can be observed, which are surrounded by moderate- or low-density shadow in different widths to separate the lesion from normal liver tissue. At the center of the lesion, shadow in water density is demonstrated. By contrast CT scanning, irregular enhancement is demonstrated at the margin of the lesion. However, due to the enhancement of its surrounding hepatic parenchyma, the lesion is well defined in maplike sign, with the lesion range being slightly larger than the lesion range demonstrated by plain scanning. The lesion may penetrate the hepatic capsule for its growth to invade the adjacent organs and tissues. Meanwhile, the lesion may involve intrahepatic bile ducts to cause stenosis and obstruction of the local bile duct, with consequent dilation of intrahepatic bile ducts in different degrees.

CT perfusion demonstrates extremely low blood perfusion value in the lesion, which may even be 0. The margin of the lesion has uneven width, with unstable blood perfusion. The perfusion values of BF, PEI, TTP, and HAP are higher than that of the necrotic area in the lesion, but are lower than that of the normal liver tissue. Surrounding the lesion, accumulated blood vessels such as the hepatic artery and the portal vein can be observed due to compression to form false appearance of marginal enhancement of the lesion.

Most scholars consistently divide the hepatic alveolar type into three subtypes, including maplike type, pseudocyst type, and consolidation type.

Maplike Type

CT scanning demonstrates low-density lesions with different sizes, uneven density, irregular shape, and poorly defined boundaries in maplike sign. In the lesion, multiple patches of calcification can be observed in different sizes (Fig. 26.16).

Pseudocyst Type

The lesion is incompletely surrounded by high-density shadow, with a CT value of 71–100 Hu. At the center of the lesion, water density area is demonstrated with a CT value of −10 to 18 Hu. It is demonstrated to be an irregular pseudocystic cavity.

Consolidation Type

The flake of calcification plaques of the lesion is separated from the normal liver tissue by a low-density area, which infiltrates the liver parenchyma with no defined interface.

MR Imaging

Infiltrative Lesion

MR imaging demonstrates irregular mass-like lesion in the liver parenchyma, which has poorly defined boundary and uneven internal signal. It has no envelope, just like a raw marble inlaying in the liver tissue with an inlaying sign. The lesion is demonstrated with slightly high signal by T1WI and mixed low signal by T2WI. The internal liquefied necrotic lesion is morphologically irregular, like fulgurite or map, and is demonstrated with low signal by T1WI and high signal by

T2WI (Figs. 26.17, 26.18, and 26.19). Surrounding the mass, small alveolar hydatids still reproduce and extend the lesion to invade the liver tissue to cause low-signal halo sign, which is corresponding to the infiltrative area demonstrated by pathological examination. MR hydrography clearly demonstrates countless small alveoli and alveolar nest structure of the alveolar hydatid. By contrast imaging, the mass is demonstrated with no enhancement.

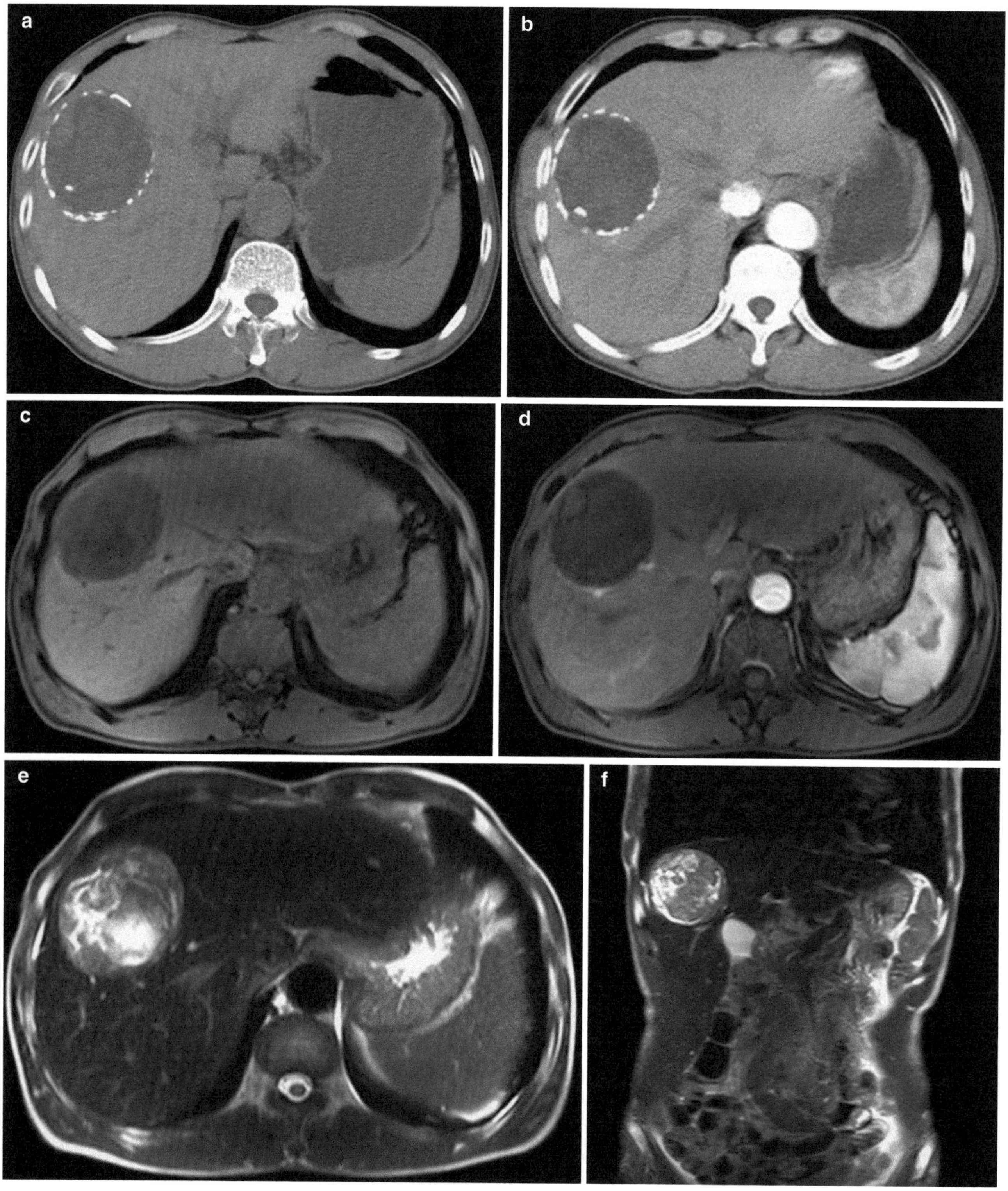

Fig. 26.17 Hepatic alveolar hydatidosis. (**a**, **b**) CT demonstrates round-like low-density lesion in the right liver lobe. In the lesion, there are uneven density, spots of calcification, and lower-density area. The alveolar wall is demonstrated with incomplete ring-shaped enhancement. By contrast scanning, the lesion is demonstrated with no enhancement. (**c**, **d**) T1WI of MR imaging demonstrates the lesion with uneven low signal. By contrast imaging, the lesion is demonstrated with no enhancement. (**e**, **f**) T2WI of MR imaging demonstrates the lesion with mixed high and low signals, with observable ribbon sign

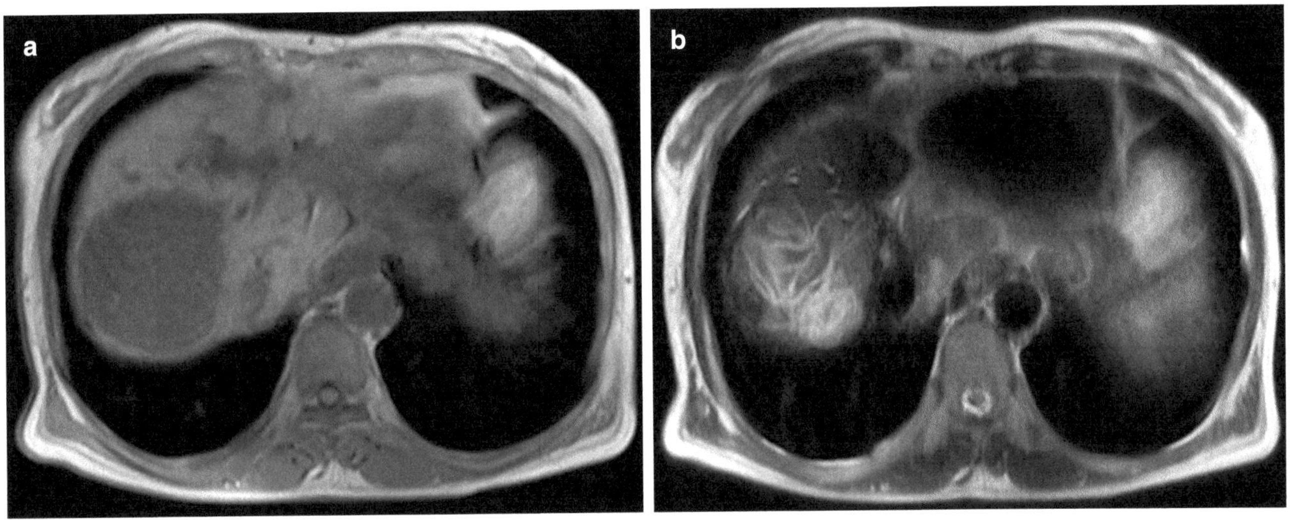

Fig. 26.18 Hepatic alveolar hydatidosis. (**a**, **b**) MR imaging demonstrates round-like lesion in the liver, with low signal by T1WI, uneven signal by T2WI, and observable ribbon sign

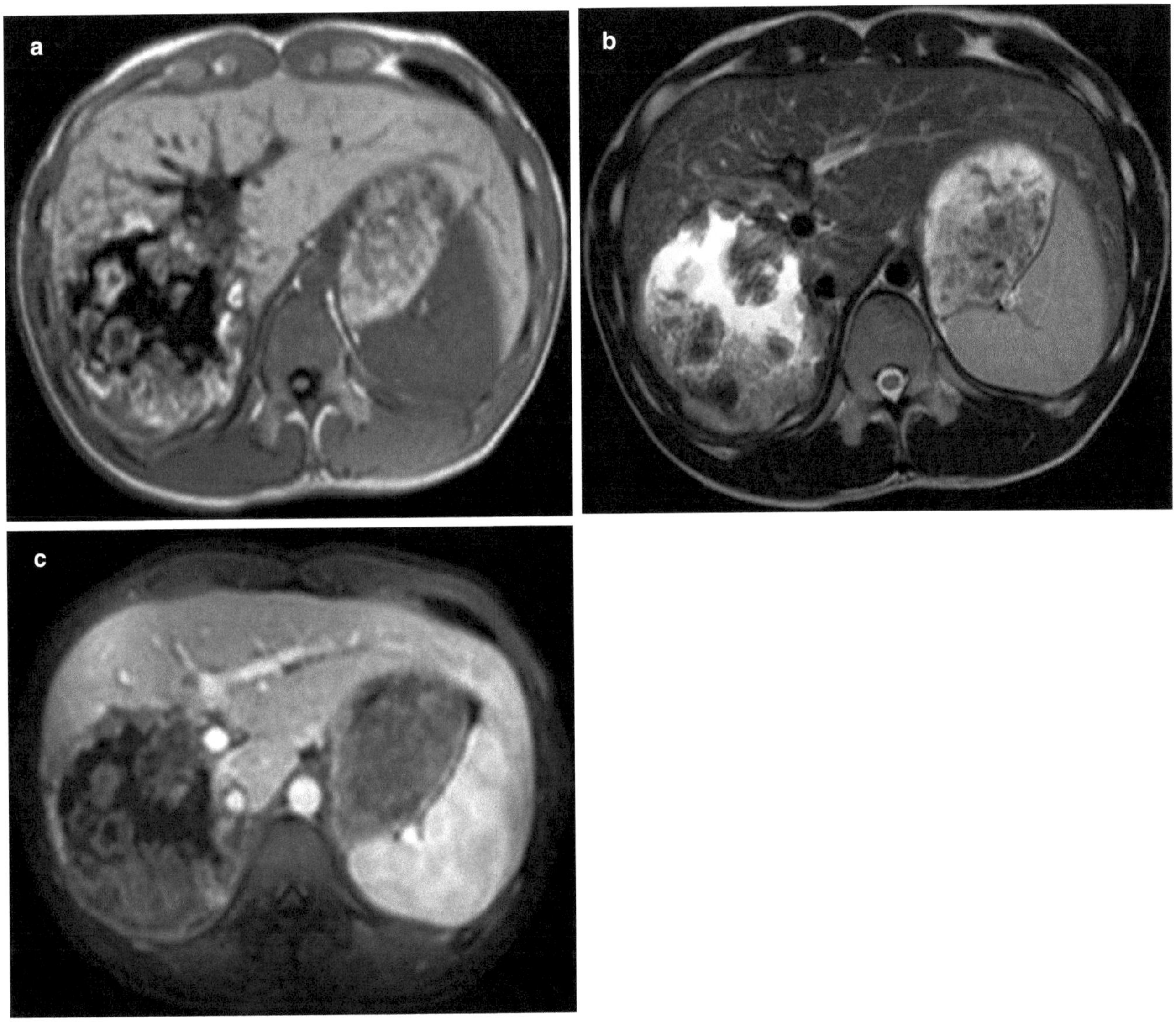

Fig. 26.19 Hepatic alveolar hydatidosis. (**a**, **b**) MR imaging demonstrates alveolar hydatidosis lesion in the right liver lobe, with uneven signal, irregular shape, and blurry boundary. In the lesion, there are patches of calcification. (**c**) Contrast imaging demonstrates well-defined boundary of the lesion and no enhancement of the lesion

Calcification Lesion

During the invasion of alveolar hydatid into the liver tissue, calcium deposition occurs, with formation of particle calcification in the early stage. Along with the illness course, the particles fuse into cotton-like or irregular large flake of calcification. MR imaging demonstrates reproduction of alveolar hydatid to extend the lesion, with consequent demonstration of low-signal infiltrative area or halo sign. The reproduced layer gradually declines and degenerates, with calcium deposition to form calcified area. The two pathological changes alternatively occur and repeatedly extend the lesion to produce multilayer ring sign. Fast spin echo or fat suppression sequence optimally demonstrates the lesion in multilayer ring sign with alternative high and low signal. MR imaging demonstrates the calcification with uneven signal, with typical calcification in low signal by both T1WI and T2WI.

Liquefaction Lesion

Alveolar hydatid reproduces into giant mass of the lesion, with internal consolidation, occlusive vascular vessels, ischemia and necrosis, and liquefaction into jellylike texture to form fulgurite-like lesion with indefinite location and irregular shape. The lesion is at even longer T1 and longer T2 signal, namely, lower signal by T1WI and higher signal by T2WI (Fig. 26.20). The hydatid is subject to degeneration and following necrosis, infection, and liquefaction to form larger liquefied necrotic cavity.

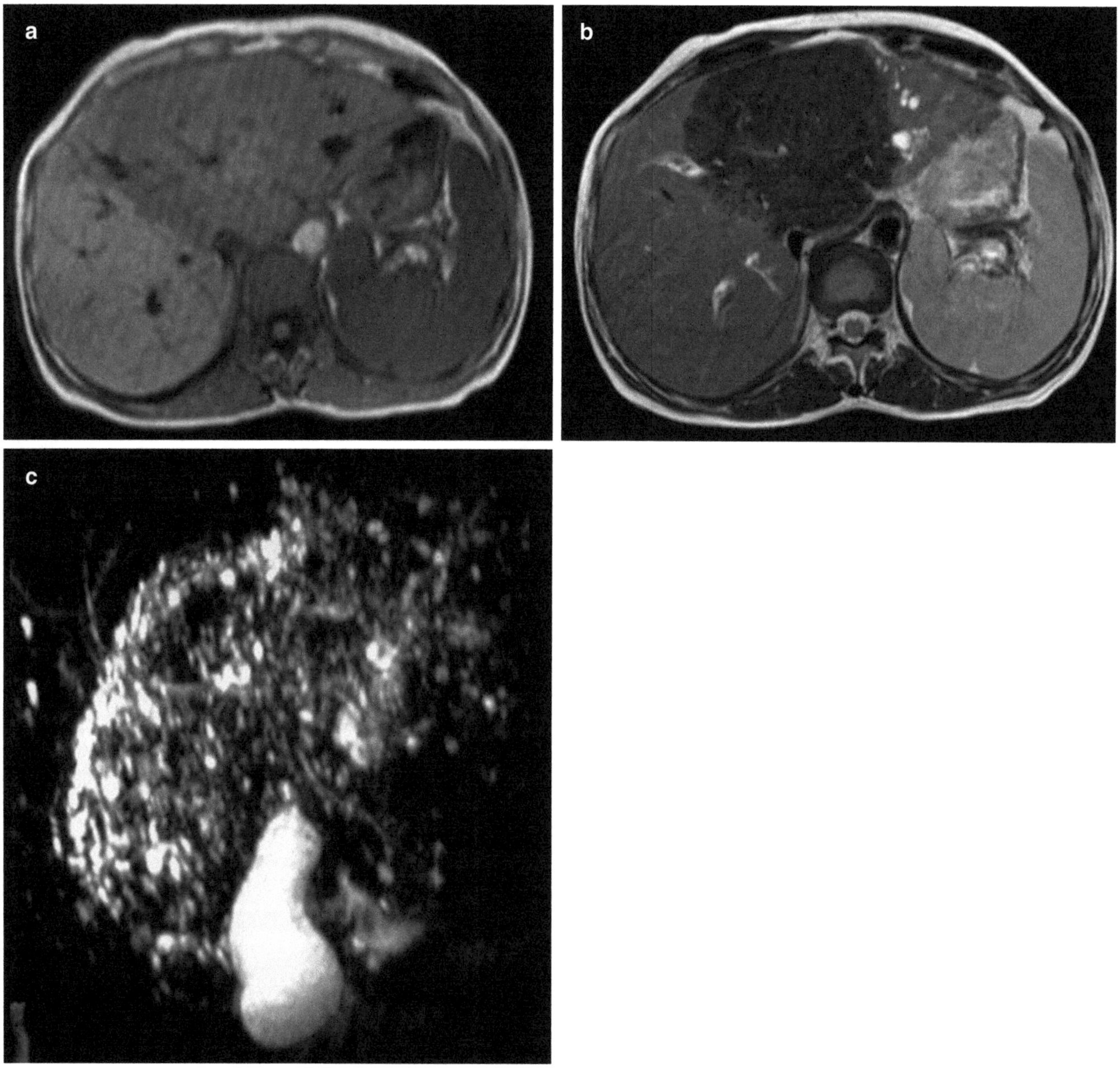

Fig. 26.20 Hepatic alveolar hydatidosis. (**a–c**) MR imaging demonstrates large flakes of lesion in the liver, with internal liquefied fulgurite-like area. The lesion is demonstrated with low signal by T1WI and even lower signal by T2WI

Complex Type of Complications

Necrosis in the lesion and shrinkage of the fibrous tissue can cause collapse of the lesion margin. The adjacent liver tissue and ductile structure may be subject to shift or deformation due to compression, with compensatory growth of the tissue in the normal liver lobe. MR hydrography more clearly demonstrates the small alveoli of alveolar hydatid. In addition, it can demonstrate the invasion of the lesion into the bile duct to cause its occlusion and shift of adjacent bile ducts due to compression. MRA can clearly demonstrate the involvement of the lesion into the portal vein, the inferior vena cava, and the hepatic artery. After injection of paramagnetic contrast agent, the contrast imaging demonstrates the lesion with no enhancement.

Kadama et al. divided hepatic alveolar hydatidosis into five subtypes based on the MR imaging demonstrations. Subtype I is demonstrated with multiple small cysts but no consolidation. Subtype II is demonstrated with concurrent small cysts and consolidation. Subtype III is demonstrated with large and small cysts in the large consolidated lesion. Subtype IV is demonstrated with consolidated lesion but no cysts. Subtype V is demonstrated with large and small cysts only but no consolidated lesion. Clinically, the subtypes of II and III are more common.

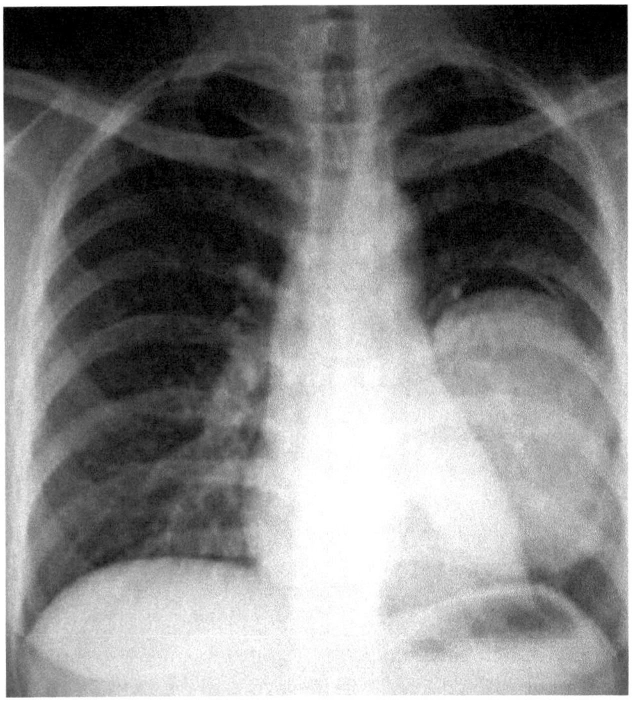

Fig. 26.21 Pulmonary hydatid X-ray demonstrates round shaped lesion in the left lower lung with regular margin, well defined boundary, and even density

26.7.2 Pulmonary Echinococcosis

26.7.2.1 Ultrasound

Successful detection by ultrasound for pulmonary echinococcosis depends on growth of hydatid protruding the lung surface and its adhesion to pleura or diaphragm. With pleura or diaphragm as the acoustic transparency window and with the ultrasonographic approach for lung gas avoided, the hydatid cyst can be echographically detected, as well as gas echoes from surrounding lung tissues. Otherwise, ultrasound detection of hydatid cyst can be interfered by multiple echo reflections via gas-containing alveolae.

26.7.2.2 X-Ray Radiology

Simplex Pulmonary Echinococcosis

Typical Signs of Pulmonary Hydatid Cyst

It is demonstrated as round- or oval-shaped lesion with regular margin, well-defined boundary, and even density. Otherwise, incisura at the margin can be demonstrated. The lesion is demonstrated to be singular or multiple isolated consolidation shadow that is lobulated, with higher central density than peripheral tissue. However, encapsulated by fibrous tissue at the external cyst wall, the margin is demonstrated to be dense, clear, and sharp (Fig. 26.21). The upper lung lobe is demonstrated with compressed mediastinum by huge hydatid cyst, and tracheal shift toward the contralateral normal counterpart can be observed.

Ball Embracing Sign

Due to explosive growth of the hydatid, the bronchus and lung tissues are pushed to the peripheral area of hydatid cyst, which is demonstrated as dense arch-shaped trips of lung markings around the hydatid.

Atelectasis

Gradual growth of pulmonary hydatid with large hydatid to compress the small bronchi further causes focalized atelectasis of pulmonary segment.

Multiple Pulmonary Echinococcosis

It refers to the above two typical hydatid cysts in the lung. The quantity of pulmonary hydatid can be up to more than ten or dozens.

Calcification of External Cyst

The external cyst of pulmonary hydatid is thin and soft. Its calcification is far rarer than calcification of external cyst of hepatic hydatid. Calcification of external cyst is demonstrated with shell-like calcification ring at the margin of oval-shaped space-occupying lesion.

Pulmonary Echinococcosis Complicated by Infection

Pulmonary echinococcosis complicated by infection accounts for 10–15 % of the total cases of pulmonary echinococcosis. Purulent fluid is found in the hydatid cyst, indicating loss of typical sign of simplex echinococcosis. The demonstrations

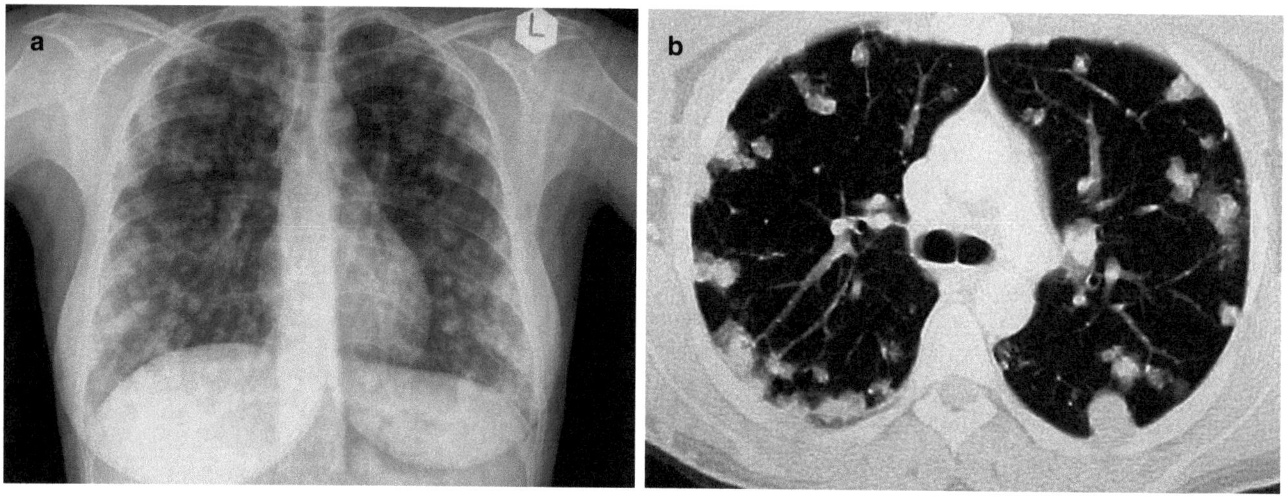

Fig. 26.22 Alveolar echinococcosis. (**a**) X-ray demonstrates diffuse patches of shadows in both lungs, with irregular and poorly defined boundaries. (**b**) CT scanning demonstrates plum blossom-like nodules with increased density and different sizes in both lungs

include rough margin, poorly defined boundary, increased density, thickened lung markings, cord-like shadows extending toward the hilum, and other lesions of pulmonary abscess. Pulmonary echinococcosis complicated by infection or its rupture with secondary infection develops into bronchial fistula, and the patients cough up some purulent cyst fluid. In the cases with air breaking into the cyst, the external cyst wall is demonstrated to be thickened and rough, with occurrence of transparent area and gas-fluid level in the cyst.

Pulmonary Echinococcosis Complicated by Its Penetration into the Bronchus

Pulmonary echinococcosis complicated by its penetration into the bronchus accounts for about 10–15 % of the cases with pulmonary echinococcosis. The external cyst of pulmonary hydatid is thin and soft and, therefore, is vulnerable to rupture. In the cases with fine rupture at the external cyst and intact internal cyst, a small quantity of gas may break into the space between external and internal cyst walls to cause a narrow and long crescent-shaped gas strip at the posterior hydatid cyst, namely, the sickle sign, which is typical but rare sign of the complication. In the cases with the hydatid penetrating into the third or fourth tier bronchus or in the cases with large rupture at the external cyst, the internal cyst fails to keep intact and is vulnerable to rupture with cyst fluid breaking into the bronchus to cause severe cough. Some cyst fluid may be coughed up. The air may break into the external cyst, with collapsed internal cyst floating at the cyst fluid level, which is floating lotus sign.

26.7.2.3 CT Scanning

Pulmonary Cystic Echinococcosis

It is demonstrated with singular or multiple low-density liquid lesions, with its CT value being close to water density. The lesion is demonstrated in round or round-like shape, occasionally lobulated. The cystic wall is demonstrated to be extremely thin, partially with calcification. By contrast scanning, the lesion is demonstrated with no enhancement (Fig. 26.22). It rarely contains daughter cysts, which is characterized by lower density of the daughter cysts than fluid in the mother cyst. In the cases with small daughter cysts distributed along the margin of mother cyst, the whole lesion is demonstrated with rose petal sign. In the cases with multiple large daughter cysts filling in the mother cyst, the whole lesion is demonstrated with mulberry sign or honeycomb sign. After the cyst ruptures, the following signs can be demonstrated.

The Crescent Sign (The Sickle Sign)

In the cases with ruptured external cyst but intact internal cyst wall, a small quantity of air enters into the space between the external and internal cysts to form smooth transparent strip in a shape of crescent. Such a transparent strip can change along with posture changes. In the cases with continuing expansion of the air space, the internal cyst can be completely isolated from the external cyst, with halo sign around the internal cyst.

The Double-Moon Sign

In the cases with ruptured internal and external cysts, some of the cystic fluid can be coughed up, with air entering into the space between the external and internal cysts. Therefore, two layers of transparent arch-shaped air strip shadow can be observed above the fluid level, which is known as the double-moon sign.

The Floating Lotus Sign

In the cases with ruptured external and internal cysts, some of the cystic fluid can be coughed up. The collapsed or fragmented internal cystic wall can be observed floating on the fluid level, which is a characteristic sign of the disease. In the cases with atypical manifestation, the fluid level is demonstrated with wavelike change.

The Rocks Emerging After Water Subsiding Sign
After the external and internal cyst rupture, most cystic membrane and fluid are coughed up, with air flowing into the cyst. After that, some cystic membrane and daughter cysts emerge at the inferior cystic cavity, just like the rocks emerging after water subsides.

The Ribbon Sign
The internal cystic membrane sheds off from the external cyst, which floats in the cystic fluid, just like ribbons floating in the air.

The Ring Shaped Cavity
After simultaneous rupture of both external and internal cysts, the cystic fluid and the contents in the cystic cavity are all coughed up, which results in ring-shaped thin-walled cavity. The cavity can be completely closed and the lesion self-healed.

The Annular Eclipse Sign
After the rupture of external and internal cysts, the cystic fluid is coughed up. The internal cyst adheres to the external cystic wall, with no occurrence of collapse.

The Floral Hoop Sign
The sign is demonstrated after rupture of both external and internal cysts with complicating slight infection. The external cyst and internal cyst adhere to each other and most of cystic fluid is coughed up. However, the cystic wall of both external cyst and internal cyst keeps intact, with no occurrence of collapse. The air flows into the internal cyst, with adhered daughter cysts in the cystic cavity there, just like a floral loop.

The Air Containing Lump
After rupture of both external and internal cysts, a small quantity of cystic fluid is coughed up, with air flowing into the cystic cavity. Due to the small quantity of air, fluid level is absent. Only patches of gas shadow are demonstrated in the lump.

Lung Abscess Like Change
Infection caused by rupture of hydatid further leads to thickened cystic wall, with fluid level in the cyst, and inflammatory infiltration shadow or edema strip out of the cyst.

Alveolar Echinococcosis
Multiple lesions can be demonstrated in the lung, which are mostly located at the lateral part of the lung field in small nodular or small patches of soft tissue density shadows. The shadows are slightly poorly defined, with calcification, liquefaction, and cavity in the lesions. The lesions develop upward from the lung apex to penetrate the diaphragm, with demonstrations of pneumonia-like blurry shadow and accompanying pleural effusion.

26.7.2.4 MR Imaging

Pulmonary Cystic Echinococcosis
Singular pulmonary hydatid cyst is demonstrated as low T1WI signal and high T2WI signal, with homogeneous internal signals. The cyst is characteristically demonstrated as low T1WI signal. Contrast imaging demonstrates no abnormal enhancement. The hydatid mother cyst containing daughter cysts is demonstrated with multiple daughter cysts in different sizes, which morphologically resembles to rose petals. More daughter cysts can be demonstrated like mulberry. The daughter cysts have lower signals than the mother cyst, with cyst-in-cyst sign. In the cases with ruptured cyst, infection is demonstrated as uneven signal and unevenly thickened cystic wall. The lesions compressing and penetrating into the bronchus are favorably demonstrated by coronal and sagittal MR imaging. In the cases with rupture of hydatid cyst complicated by infection, the lesions are demonstrated as follows by MR imaging.

The Ring Shaped Cavity Sign
After simultaneous rupture of external and internal cysts, most or all of the cystic fluid is coughed up to cause ring-shaped thin-walled cavity or ring-shaped cavity with no wall. The lesion is demonstrated as ring-shaped cavity with low signal by T1WI and T2WI.

The Crescent Sign
Local rupture is demonstrated at the external cyst, with intact internal cyst. The air flows into the space between the external and internal cysts. The air filling space is demonstrated as crescent sign with low signal by T1WI and T2WI.

The Ribbon Sign
The internal cyst ruptures and sheds off from the external cyst. The cystic membrane is demonstrated as equal signal by T1WI and low signal by T2WI, which floats in the cystic fluid like a ribbon. With the cystic fluid in high T2WI signal as the background, the ribbon sign can be more favorably demonstrated.

The Floating Lotus Sign
After rupture of both external and internal cysts and collapse of the internal cyst wall, the fragmented cystic membrane floats in the cystic fluid to show characteristic sign, which is more favorably demonstrated by coronal and sagittal MR imaging.

The Rocks Emerging After Water Subsiding Sign

The old lesions are demonstrated with absorbed cystic fluid. The cystic membrane folds and solidifies into caseous appearance with calcification, just like the rocks emerging after water subsides.

Alveolar Echinococcosis

Primary alveolar echinococcosis rarely occurs, which is commonly secondary to hepatic alveolar echinococcosis. By T1WI and T2WI, the lesions are demonstrated with equal signal, with heterogeneous internal signal as well as internal liquefaction and necrosis.

26.7.3 Abdominal, Pelvic, and Retroperitoneal Echinococcosis

26.7.3.1 Ultrasound

Abdominal and pelvic echinococcosis can be categorized into two types: primary and secondary echinococcosis. Secondary echinococcosis often develops from ruptured hepatic or abdominal hydatid cyst and surgical implantation. Therefore, multiple abdominal hydatid cysts are more commonly found than singular abdominal hydatid cyst, and more cases have daughter cysts. By radiological examinations, cyst-connecting-to-cyst sign or cyst-in-cyst sign is commonly demonstrated. Therefore, for patients receiving follow-up examinations, routine abdominal ultrasound should be performed to avoid misdiagnosis. Due to adhesion of abdominal or pelvic hydatid cyst to the surrounding organs and tissues as well as its peripheral gastrointestinal gas, ultrasound commonly demonstrates less favorably defined thick wall of hydatid cyst than the liver.

26.7.3.2 X-Ray Radiology

Abdominal echinococcosis is commonly demonstrated with no direct abnormalities by X-ray, but commonly with indirect signs. The indirect signs include compressed, migrated, and deformed adjacent gastrointestinal tract. Cases with multiple abdominal hydatids or giant abdominal hydatid demonstrate compressed bilateral diaphragm, elevated diaphragm, and restricted motion. In the cases with long-term case history of echinococcosis, calcification of external cyst can be demonstrated.

26.7.3.3 CT Scanning

The lesions of abdominal and pelvic cystic echinococcosis are distributed in the space between abdominal and pelvic organs or in the space adjacent to the pelvic wall. All the lesions compress the adjacent organs to complicate the conditions by occurrence of cystic hydatid lesions at the abdominal organs (Fig. 26.23). According to morphological demonstrations of abdominal and pelvic lesions, it can be categorized into five types.

Simplex Cystic Echinococcosis

The abdominal or pelvic cavity can be demonstrated with singular or multiple round or round-like cystic low-density lesions. The CT value of cystic fluid is 18–29 HU, with no enhancement by contrast scanning. The lining of cystic wall is demonstrated to be smooth, with uneven thickness between 1 and 4 mm.

Multiple Daughter Cyst Echinococcosis

In the cystic lump, the daughter cysts are demonstrated with different sizes and even lower density, which are in the mother cyst or concentrated unilaterally or scattering in the mother cystic fluid. Otherwise, the daughter cysts are demonstrated to occupy all the space in the mother cyst cavity to confine the small quantity of mother cystic fluid at the cystic center or between the daughter cysts. The whole lesion is demonstrated as likely to be separated by thick septum, with an appearance like rose petals or mulberry.

Cystic Wall Calcification

Calcification of cystic hydatid is demonstrated as curve-shaped calcification of the cystic wall.

Echinococcosis Complicated by Cyst Rupture or Infection

After rupture of a hydatid cyst, some shedded internal cyst is separated from the external cyst by a space to form a double-wall sign. The completely shedded internal cystic membrane is subject to folding and curving, which floats in the cystic fluid like a water snake or ribbon. In the cases with secondary infection, the cystic fluid is demonstrated with increased density.

Retroperitoneal Space Echinococcosis

Cystic echinococcosis may involve retroperitoneal space. CT scanning demonstrates calcified lump at the retroperitoneal area.

26.7.3.4 MR Imaging

Singular Cyst

Singular cyst is demonstrated as low T1WI signal and high T2WI signal. The internal signal is demonstrated to be homogeneous and the capsule is demonstrated with low T1WI signal, which is the characteristic demonstration of singular cyst. By contrast imaging, the cyst is demonstrated with no enhancement.

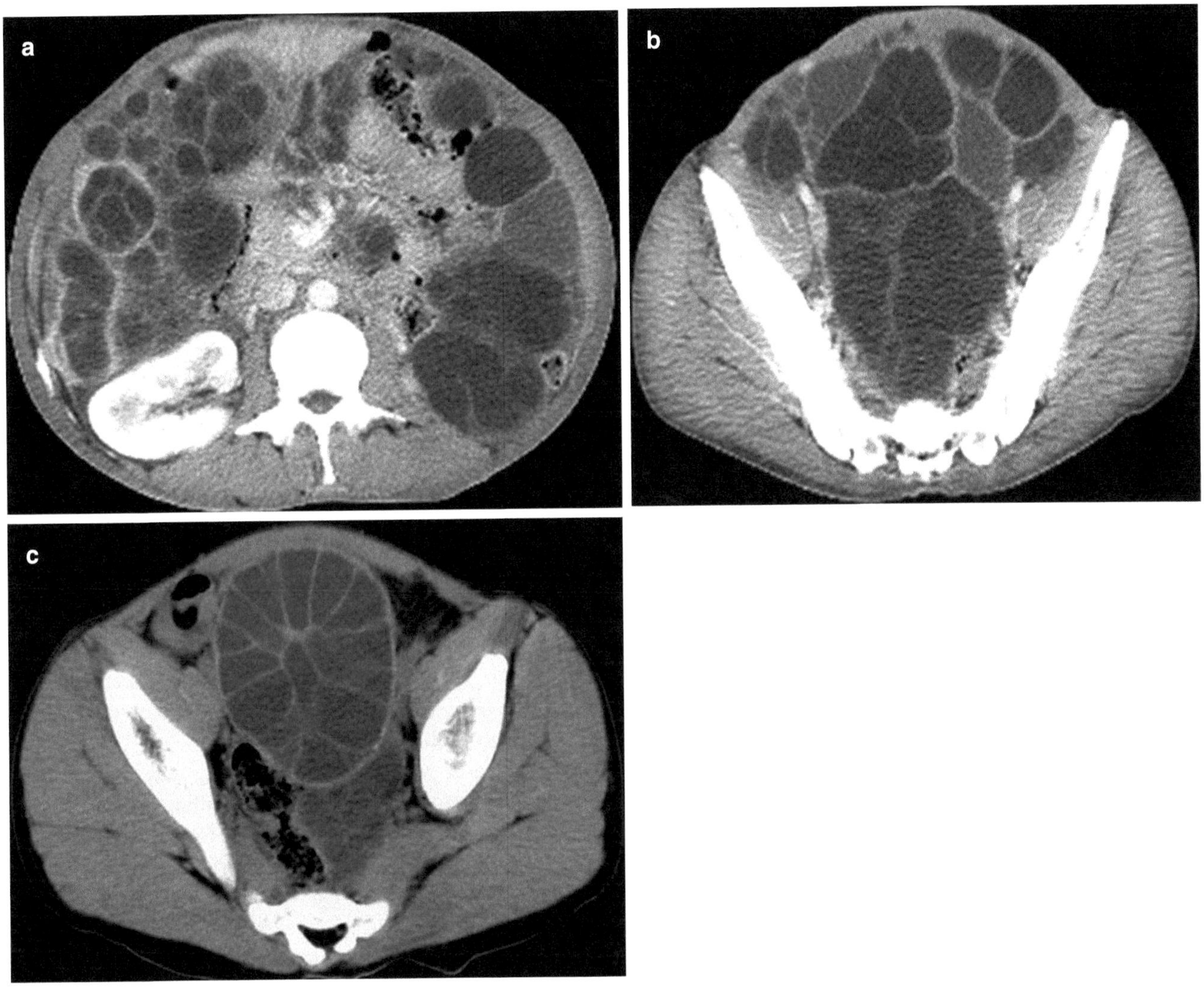

Fig. 26.23 Abdominal and pelvic cystic echinococcosis. (**a**, **b**) CT scanning demonstrates multiple round or round-like low-density lesions between abdominal intestinal loops, at the colonic ditch and at the retroperitoneum. By contrast scanning, the lesions are demonstrated with no enhancement. The cystic wall is demonstrated to be smooth with even thickness. (**c**) The daughter cysts are demonstrated to occupy all the space in the mother cyst, with a small quantity of mother cystic fluid between the daughter cysts. The whole lesion is demonstrated like to be separated by thick septum with rose petal sign

Cyst Containing Daughter Cysts

In the mother cyst, there are multiple daughter cysts with different sizes, with an appearance of rose petals. The signal of daughter cysts is lower than that of the mother cyst by T1WI, sometimes with pseudo-septum.

Cyst Complicated by Rupture and Infection

The cystic wall is demonstrated to be unevenly thickened with heterogeneous signal. By T1WI, the signal is demonstrated to be increased, with observable ribbon sign. For the cases with complex conditions, MR imaging can more clearly and accurately demonstrate the lesion. MR hydrography demonstrates small daughter cysts in the lesion and their relationship with surrounding organs containing water. MRA demonstrates its relationship with adjacent vascular vessels.

26.7.4 Splenic Echinococcosis

26.7.4.1 Ultrasound

The ultrasound diagnosis of splenic echinococcosis is almost the same as that of hepatic echinococcosis, but with slightly weaker echoes than the liver.

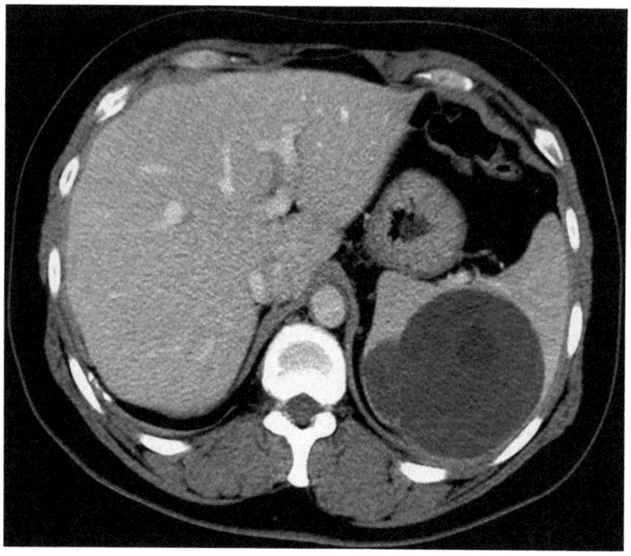

Fig. 26.24 Splenic echinococcosis. CT scanning demonstrates round-like cystic lesion in the spleen with well-defined boundary. Contrast scanning demonstrates no enhancement and internal daughter cysts with even lower density

26.7.4.2 CT Scanning

The demonstrations resemble to those of hepatic echinococcosis, and both are space-occupying lesions in the parenchymal organs (Fig. 26.24).

26.7.4.3 MR Imaging

The cysts in the cases of splenic echinococcosis and hepatic echinococcosis are the same, being space-occupying lesion in the parenchymal organs. MR imaging demonstrations of splenic echinococcosis resemble to those of hepatic echinococcosis.

26.7.5 Renal Cystic Echinococcosis

26.7.5.1 Ultrasound

Renal cystic echinococcosis commonly occurs at the renal parenchyma and collecting system. Ultrasound demonstrates singular or multiple round-like dark areas in the kidney, with certain tension and thicker cystic wall than other common cysts. Different compression signs can be demonstrated at different locations of hydatids. In the cases with hydatid at the renal pelvis, the collecting system is compressed to cause calyceal or renal pelvis effusion.

26.7.5.2 X-Ray Radiology

By X-ray, simplex renal cystic echinococcosis is demonstrated as enlarged kidney and arch-shaped shadow of protruding hydatid cyst. Giant hydatid at the right kidney can compress the right diaphragm to protrude to the thoracic cavity in arch shape, which tends to be misdiagnosed as echinococcosis at the right liver lobe. Perirenal pneumography more clearly demonstrates the enlarged kidney and protruding hydatid. Although the cystic wall of renal hydatid is comparatively thick, it is still thinner than the external cyst of hepatic hydatid. Therefore, calcification of the cystic wall is rarely demonstrated. Retrograde pyelography demonstrates compressed renal pelvis and calyces and their inward shift and longer and thinner calyces with arch-shaped separation in embracing ball sign, but no sign of destruction. Due to long-term compression, the renal parenchyma is demonstrated to be thinner with atrophy, with renal dysfunctions or no renal functions. Excretive pyelography usually fails to demonstrate the calyces.

In the cases with hydatid cyst penetrating into the renal pelvis, the cystic fluid partially leaks out, with shrinkage of hydatid shadow. Retrograde pyelography demonstrates filling of contrast reagent in the renal pelvis and its leakage into the hydatid cyst, with deformed renal pelvis and ball-shaped cyst. In the cyst, multiple daughter cysts are demonstrated in small round grape appearance with filling defect. In the cases with leakage of daughter cysts into the ureter, the dilated ureter is demonstrated with honeycomb-like filling defects. During surgical operation, the whole renal parenchyma is subject to atrophy. By incision of the hydatid cyst, it is demonstrated to be filled by daughter cysts.

In the cases with hydatid penetrating into renal calices, retrograde pyelography demonstrates filling of the contrast agent in the renal pelvis and its leakage from the renal calices into hydatid cyst. The contrast agent continually flows along daughter cysts, appearing like waterfall. The penetration site and its conducting state can be well demonstrated. Such rare typical radiological demonstration can only be temporarily demonstrated during rupture of hydatid, which fails to be observed after secondary infection of hydatid cyst and collapse of daughter cysts.

26.7.5.3 CT Scanning

The CT scanning demonstrations of renal cystic echinococcosis resemble to those of hepatic cystic echinococcosis.

Simplex Type

CT scanning demonstrates round or round-like cystic lesions in the kidney with smooth and intact margin as well as watery density. The cystic wall is demonstrated to be thick, with arch-shaped calcification. By contrast scanning, it is more clearly demonstrated.

Multiple Daughter Cyst Type

CT scanning demonstrates multiple small round or irregular daughter cyst shadows in the mother cyst and lower density of daughter cyst shadows than the mother cyst. In some cases, multiple large irregularly shaped daughter cysts are demonstrated, which is separated by a pseudo-septum. The

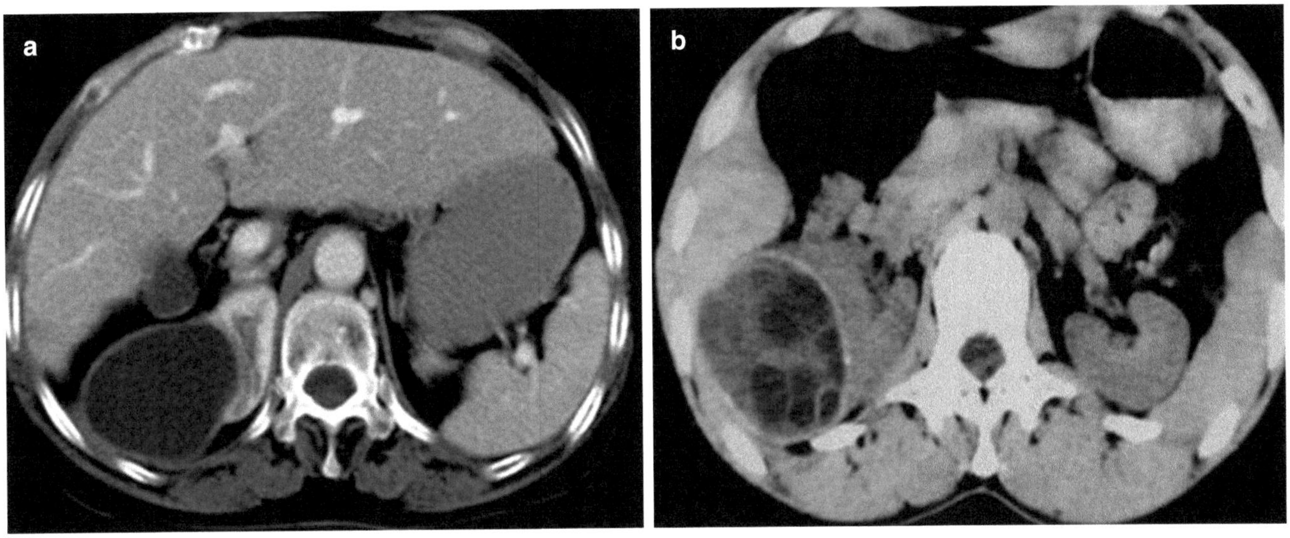

Fig. 26.25 Renal cystic echinococcosis. (**a**) CT scanning demonstrates round-like cystic lesion in the right kidney parenchyma with smooth and intact margin. The lesion is demonstrated with no enhancement. (**b**) Multiple hydatid cysts in the right kidney are demonstrated with multiple daughter cysts in the mother cyst and pushing of daughter cysts to each other to form mulberry sign

cystic cavity is filled with daughter cysts, appearing like with thick septum (Fig. 26.25).

Rupture and Infection Type

CT scanning demonstrates separated internal and external cysts, with folded and shrinkage of the internal cyst to form a double-ring sign. The external cystic wall is demonstrated with irregular calcification. CT scanning demonstrates shedding of internal cyst off the external cyst, with collapse of the internal cystic membrane into the cystic cavity to form wave-like curves of the membrane. Edema can be demonstrated around the cyst. By contrast scanning, marginal enhancement can be demonstrated at the hydatid cyst.

26.7.5.4 MR Imaging

Typical cystic hydatid is demonstrated with low T1WI signal and high T2WI signal. Cystic hydatidosis complicated by infection is demonstrated with corresponding change. The cystic wall of cystic echinococcosis has even thickness, with low T2WI signal, which is its characteristic demonstration. In the cases with complication of rupture, the external cystic wall is demonstrated to be thickened, with uneven density inside. The ruptured internal cyst is demonstrated to float in the cystic cavity to form ribbon sign. In the cases with a mother cyst containing daughter cysts, the characteristic rose petal sign is demonstrated. Contrast imaging for the cases of renal cystic echinococcosis demonstrates no enhancement of the cystic wall. In the cases complicated by infection, the cystic wall and its surrounding tissues are demonstrated with enhancement. MRU can clearly demonstrate the cystic hydatid, its rupture, and penetration into the ureter.

26.7.6 Cerebral Echinococcosis

26.7.6.1 CT Scanning

Cerebral Cystic Echinococcosis

Simplex Type

Singular hydatid cyst is more common, and multiple hydatid cysts are rare. By plain CT scanning, round- or oval-shaped cystic lump can be demonstrated, with even density that is close to the density of cerebrospinal fluid. The lesion has smooth and clearly defined boundary, with no surrounding edema. In some individual cases, edema around the lesion can be observed. The cyst can be demonstrated with accompanying space-occupying effect, with manifestations of compressed, deformed, or occluded local cerebral ventricle. Contrast scanning demonstrates mostly no marginal enhancement of the cyst or rarely slight ring-shaped enhancement at the margin of lesion (Fig. 26.26). These demonstrations are possibly related to soft brain tissues, their rich blood supply, and destructed blood-cerebral barrier at the margin of lesion.

Daughter Cyst Contained Type

Daughter cysts in different quantities can be observed in the hydatid cyst, with cystic, daughter cystic, or intracystic septum. The density of daughter cysts is lower than the mother cyst.

Degeneration of Hydatid Cyst

The cystic wall is demonstrated to be thickened due to degeneration, with occurrence of calcification.

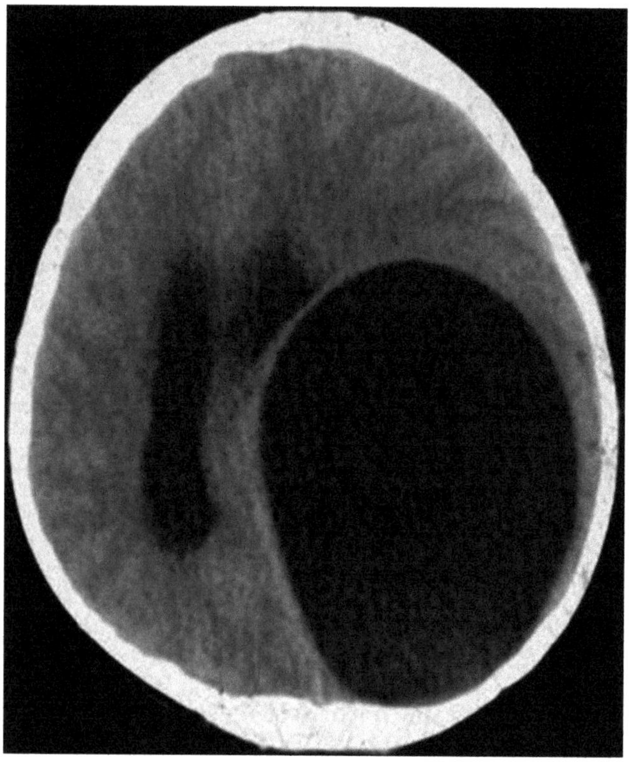

Fig. 26.26 Cerebral cystic echinococcosis. CT scanning demonstrates giant cystic space-occupying lesion in the brain, with smooth and regular cystic wall, homogeneous intracystic density, rightward shift of the midline structures, dilated bilateral ventricles, deformed left ventricle due to compression, and no obvious edema around the lesion

Rupture and Infection of Hydatid Cyst

The cystic wall is demonstrated with obvious ring-shaped enhancement, with increased density of cystic fluid. The ruptured cyst in the brain tissue can cause extensive edema of the surrounding brain tissue, with honeycomb-like low-density area and marginal ring-shaped enhancement.

Intracranial Extracerebral Echinococcosis

The hydatid cyst is located at the cranium or epidural space, with the broad base connecting to the cranium. In patients with long-term illness, the hydatid cyst may be demonstrated to compress the cranial inner plate to cause its depression or even bone destruction. Daughter cysts can be observed in the lesion.

Cerebral Alveolar Echinococcosis

Almost all cases of cerebral alveolar echinococcosis are secondary to hepatic alveolar echinococcosis due to its hematogenous spread. Due to soft brain tissue and its rich blood supply, cerebral alveolar echinococcosis develops rapidly, with clinical manifestations resembling to brain neoplasm. CT scanning demonstrates nodules in soft tissue density, with internal calcification. By contrast scanning, the nodules are demonstrated with enhancement, with marginal small cyst shadows. Otherwise, contrast scanning demonstrates marginal enhancement and no central enhancement (or calcification) to form a target sign resembling to tuberculoma. Uneven enhancement resembles to neoplasm, with obvious edema and space-occupying effect around the lesion.

26.7.6.2 MR Imaging

Cerebral Cystic Echinococcosis

The brain tissue is soft, with rich blood supply, which provides favorable environment for growth of hydatid. In the cases with large lesion, space-occupying effect and surrounding edema can be demonstrated. The internal cystic wall of cystic echinococcosis is actually the hydatid itself, while the external cystic wall is an extremely thin pseudocapsule formed by gliocyte proliferation, which is poorly demonstrated by MR imaging. Cerebral cystic echinococcosis is mostly demonstrated as singular lesion, with singular or multiple cystic lesions. The lesion is demonstrated with low T1WI signal and high T2WI signal, and the cystic wall is demonstrated as persistently homogeneous low-signal shadow. Contrast imaging demonstrates no enhancement (Fig. 26.27). In the cases with multiple daughter cysts, they are arranged along the periphery of the mother cyst, demonstrated as rose petals or wheel sign. Its T1WI signal is low and T2WI signal is high, with lower signal of the daughter cysts than the mother cyst by T1WI that resembles to water signal with no demonstration of the daughter cystic wall. However, due to the difference between signals from the mother cyst and daughter cyst, the arrangement of daughter cysts in the mother cyst can be demonstrated. Contrast imaging demonstrates slight marginal enhancement of the lesion. In the cases with ruptured cyst and infection, the cystic wall is demonstrated to be irregularly thickened; the cystic fluid is demonstrated with increased signal. Contrast imaging demonstrates obvious ring-shaped enhancement.

Cerebral Alveolar Echinococcosis

The lesion is demonstrated with infiltrative growth with poorly defined boundary. The lesion is commonly demonstrated with space-occupying effect and surrounding edema. The lesion is demonstrated with equal T1WI signal and low T2WI signal. By T2WI, the small cyst or cystic nest is demonstrated with slightly high signal with poorly defined boundary, but is well defined by hydrography (Fig. 26.28). In some cases, multiple sand like low signals demonstrate calcification. Being different from alveolar echinococcosis in other body parts, contrast imaging for the cases of cerebral alveolar echinococcosis demonstrates irregular enhancement, which is characteristic imaging demonstration of cerebral alveolar echinococcosis.

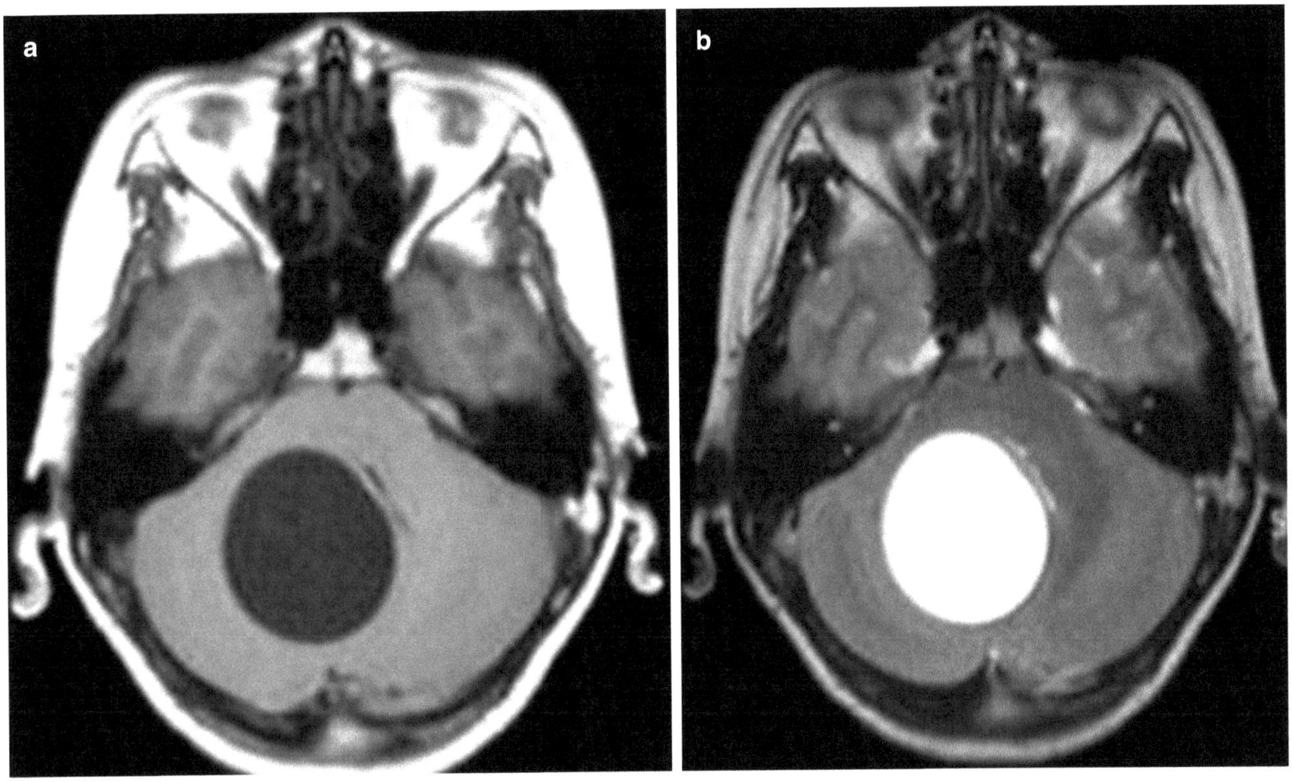

Fig. 26.27 Cerebral cystic echinococcosis. (**a**, **b**) MR imaging demonstrates cystic space-occupying lesion in the cerebellum with watery density, well-defined boundary, and intact capsule

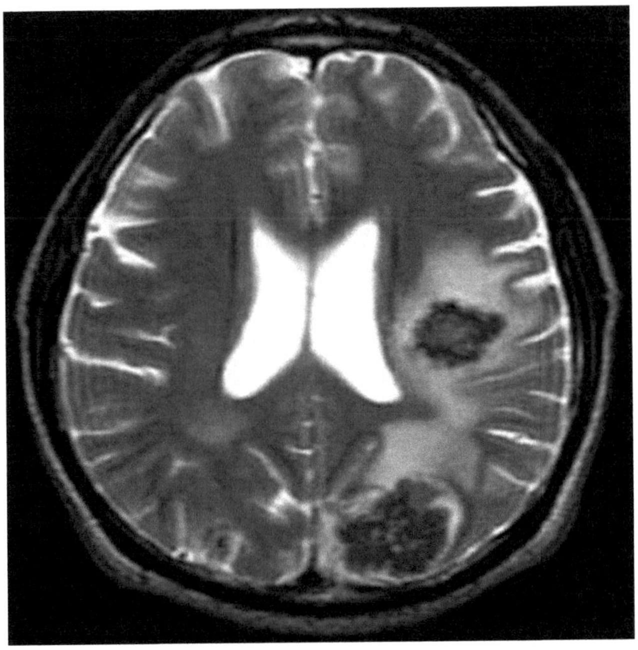

Fig. 26.28 Cerebral alveolar echinococcosis. MR imaging demonstrates multiple irregularly shaped lesions in the brain, mostly with low T2WI signal and surrounded by edema with high signal

26.7.7 Bone Echinococcosis

26.7.7.1 X-Ray Radiology

The Early Stage

X-ray demonstrates only sparse bone due to intramedullary confined absorption of bone pattern, bone destruction, decreased density, and confined round-like cavity. The lesion gradually develops into multiple interconnected round or irregular cystic transparent areas, with thick bone patterns between cystic cavities but no erosive destruction, no periosteal reaction, and no newly formed bone. In the early stage, the appearance of a bone is demonstrated with no obvious change.

The Middle Stage

The honeycomb-like cystic bone defect continuously extends with an extensive distribution but no normal bone pattern. The marginal bone pattern at the cystic transparent cavity is demonstrated to be thickened and deranged, with osteosclerosis of the cystic wall. The centrally hollow cystic bone shell is demonstrated with clearly defined margin and sharp boundary. The gradually enlarged cystic cavity compresses the bone cortex to cause its atrophy, which is thinner with unsmooth surface. The long tubular bone is demonstrated to be thickened with irregular protrusion. The flat bone is demonstrated to be thickened with protruding surface that appears like a broken fishing net and with thickened, hardened, and deranged bone shell and cystic cavities in different sizes.

The Advanced Stage

The cystic cavity is demonstrated to be enlarged and increased in quantity to involve the whole bone. On the surface of the bone cortex, a large bubble-like protrusion is especially obvious. Bone fragments with irregular boundary may be formed. Due to enlarged cystic cavity and increasingly less bone, the patients are susceptible to pathological fracture. In the cases with joint involved, the lesion may develop into the whole joint and contralateral bone. Destructed joint surface may cause pathological joint dislocation. Vertebral echinococcosis is demonstrated as transparent area with bone destruction, deformed vertebra due to compression, and even thinner and absence of major vertebra. In the cases with hydatid protruding from the vertebra and growing continually, the demonstration resembling to paravertebral abscess can be observed, which tends to be misdiagnosed as cold abscess of spinal tuberculosis. In the cases of cranial echinococcosis, the patients with long-term case history can be demonstrated with thinner cranial inner plate with arch-shaped regular impression resembling to a gyrus or mass. Even cranial inner plate is demonstrated with confined round defect, with no peritoneal reaction but possibly with intracranial hypertension. Children patients are demonstrated with enlarged skull and widened cranial suture. In the cases with giant cerebral hydatid, the affected cranial cavity is dilated. Due to its long-term compression to the skull, the cranial inner plate is demonstrated with confined depression and thinning. Cranial dipole echinococcosis is demonstrated as a honeycomb-like cavity defect at the bone plate, which may protrude inward or outward to involve the surrounding tissue. In some cases, X-ray demonstrates arch-like, ring-shaped, or eggshell-like calcification.

CT Scanning

Bone cystic echinococcosis is distinct from cystic echinococcosis at other parts of human body by CT scanning due to dense and hard bone tissue as well as small bone trabecular space. Cystic hydatid can only grow in a space that has the lowest resistance to finally form incomplete cystic destruction area with internal separations into honeycomb-like or grape-like appearance, resembling to alveolar echinococcosis. Due to no fibrous capsule around the bone, bone echinococcosis is demonstrated with no external cyst.

CT scanning demonstrates local bone destruction in the spongy bone with well-defined boundary and surrounding sclerosis. In the lesion, there are incompletely arch- or ring-shaped high-density linear crests to separate the lesion into honeycomb-like or multilocular appearance. In the cases with the hydatid penetrating the envelope into the surrounding soft tissue, the soft tissue can be demonstrated with cystic low-density area (Fig. 26.29).

26.7.7.2 MR Imaging

Spinal Echinococcosis

It mostly occurs at the lumbar spine, with explosive growth of the lesions to involve multiple vertebrae. The vertebral bone is demonstrated with eccentric destruction, which can compress and destroy the bone cortex to penetrate into the chest, abdominal cavity, or pelvic cavity for its persistent development into a soft tissue lump. The hydatid may also invade the psoas major muscle and other paravertebral tissues. The cases with singular cyst are demonstrated with round-like cystic lesion with smooth and sharp margin in long T1 and long T2 signals. The lesion at the paravertebral soft tissue is demonstrated with multiple daughter cysts with different or similar sizes in the mother cyst, which are arranged like rose petals or mulberry. By T1WI, the signal of the mother cyst is higher than that of the daughter cysts (Fig. 26.30). The cases with ruptured cyst and infection are demonstrated having morphologically irregular lesion with blurry boundary and increased signal due to generally increased content of protein in the cyst.

Flat Bone Echinococcosis

It commonly occurs at the ilium, skull, and rib. In the early stage, due to the limitation by bone tissue, the lesion has incomplete external wall and cannot expand into ball shape, but only grows along the bone marrow and spongy bone tissue for infiltration and destruction. In the spongy bones, the lesion causes cysts in different sizes, thinner bone cortex, or expanded bone cortex. MR imaging demonstrates multiple round-like lesions in the flat bones with well-defined boundary, low T1WI signal, and high T2WI signal. In the advanced stage, the hydatid cyst may penetrate the bone tissue into the surrounding soft tissue to form a lump. Otherwise, it expands out of the skin to cause its rupture and incurable fistula. In some cases, daughter cysts can be demonstrated to flow out. MR hydrography can favorably demonstrate the sinus tract, sometimes with visible daughter cysts and fragmented structures.

Tubular Bone Echinococcosis

It commonly occurs at the femur. Once the lesion invades into the tubular bone, the destruction begins at the epiphysis. In the spongy bones, round-like or irregular cavities are formed with honeycomb-like or multilobular appearance. It mainly destructs the margin and adjacent tissue, with no defined boundary. In the advanced stage, multilobular appearance disappears. In the cases with the lesion developing toward the diaphysis, the diaphysis is subject to slight dilation and cortex thinning. The lesion may even penetrate

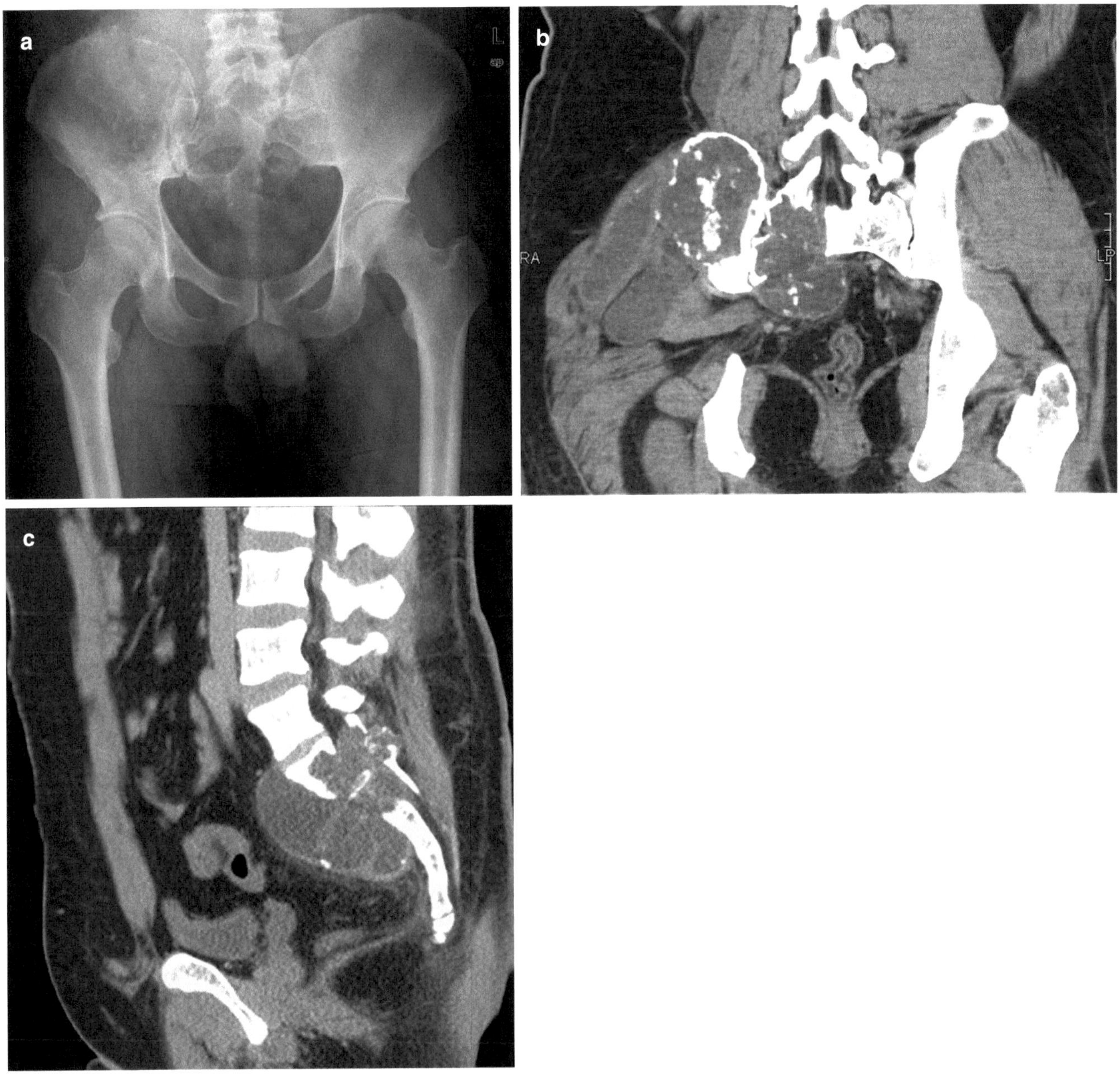

Fig. 26.29 Bone cystic echinococcosis. (**a**) X-ray demonstrates bone destructions at the right ilium and the sacrum, with well-defined lesions. (**b**, **c**) CT scanning demonstrates explosive bone destruction at the ilium and the sacrum with well-defined boundary and with inner patches of ossification shadows

the bone cortex to form cyst in soft tissue with septum and different-sized fluid levels. The lesion is demonstrated with low T1WI signal and high T2WI signal.

26.7.8 Cardiac Echinococcosis

26.7.8.1 X-Ray

Cardiac margin is subject to local protrusion. X-ray demonstrates the lump with no movements along with cardiac beat, but capable of being pushed during heartbeats. A multi-perspective observation demonstrates that the lump is inseparable from the heart, which facilitates the location of the lesion and the differentiation from pulmonary echinococcosis.

26.7.8.2 CT Scanning

CT scanning can facilitate to define the type and characteristic radiological demonstrations of hydatid lesion. Contrast scanning demonstrates obvious enhancement of the heart but no enhancement of the hydatid lesion. Therefore, the location of the lesion and its quantitative diagnosis can be defined. The cystic lesion is demonstrated with septum or daughter cysts, which is characteristically cystic echinococcosis. In individual cases, cardiac cystic echinococcosis

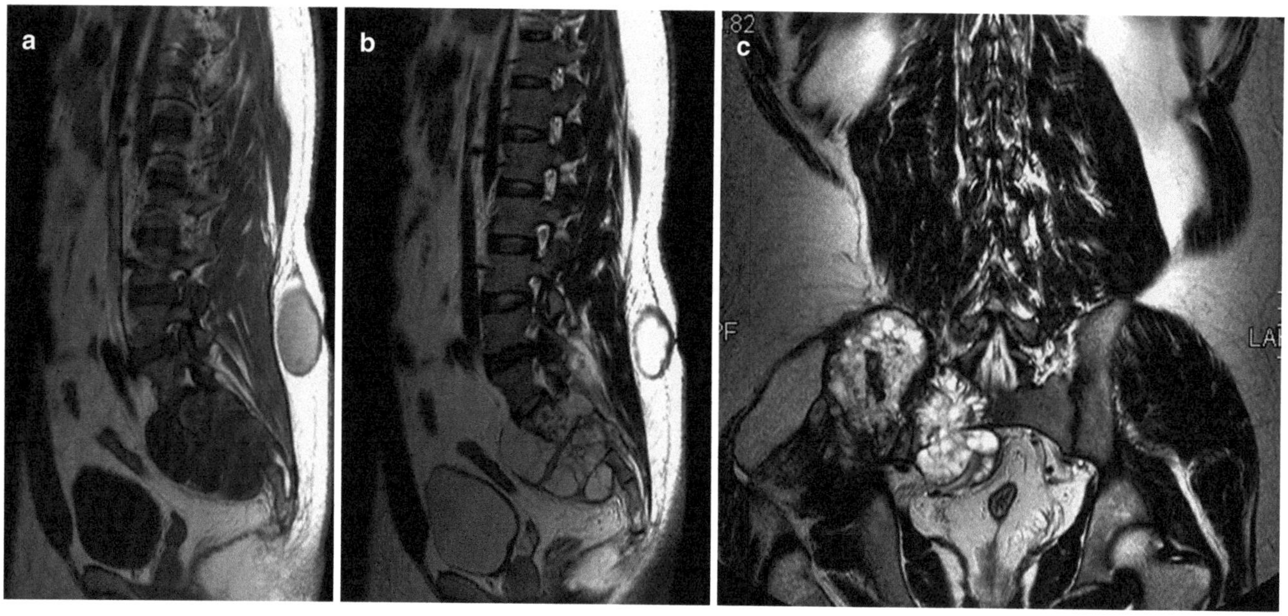

Fig. 26.30 Spinal echinococcosis. (**a–c**) MR imaging demonstrates bone destruction at the ilium, which is composed of multiple vesicles, with lower T1WI signal and high T2WI signal as well as internal septum. The dorsal soft tissue at about L4–L5 level is demonstrated with an oval-shaped lesion with long T1 and long T2 signal

should be differentiated from pericardial cyst or pericardial effusion. Cardiac alveolar echinococcosis is demonstrated as solid lump with internal calcification, whose diagnosis can be defined based on the finding of alveolar echinococcosis lesion at liver or other body parts.

26.7.8.3 MR Imaging

In addition to accurate location of the lesion, MR imaging can clearly demonstrate the hydatid cyst itself and its relationship with adjacent structures (Fig. 26.31). By electrocardiography or respiratory gating, MR imaging can also demonstrate accurately the cardiac valves, atrioventricular septum, and myocardium.

26.8 Diagnostic Basis

The clinical diagnosis can be made based on epidemiological history, major clinical symptoms and signs, radiological demonstrations, and serological test positive for specific antibody. The definitive diagnosis should be based on etiological examination or pathological examination.

26.8.1 Hepatic Echinococcosis

26.8.1.1 Epidemiological History

The patients usually have a life history in a farm or have a history of contact to farming animals, such as cattle, sheep, or dogs.

26.8.1.2 Clinical Manifestation

The patients experience clinical symptoms of hepatic upset with dull pain or distension pain and palpable painless cystic lump with smooth surface at the upper right abdomen.

26.8.1.3 Radiological Demonstration

Hepatic cystic echinococcosis is demonstrated as unilobular or multilobular cyst with no echoes, liquid density, or long T1 and long T2 signals. The margin of the lesion is demonstrated to be smooth and the cystic wall is demonstrated with even thickness. By T2WI, low signal is demonstrated, with calcification of the cystic wall. The type of multiple daughter cysts is demonstrated with rose petal sign. The cases with internal cyst shedding off the external cyst and with rupture are demonstrated with ribbon sign.

Hepatic alveolar echinococcosis is demonstrated as high density in the liver or space-occupying lesion with slightly long T1 and slightly long T2 signal, irregular necrotic liquefaction cavity, and scattering or irregular flakes of calcification lesions.

26.8.2 Pulmonary Echinococcosis

26.8.2.1 Epidemiological History

The patients usually have a life history in a farm or have a history of contact to farming animals, such as cattle, sheep, or dogs.

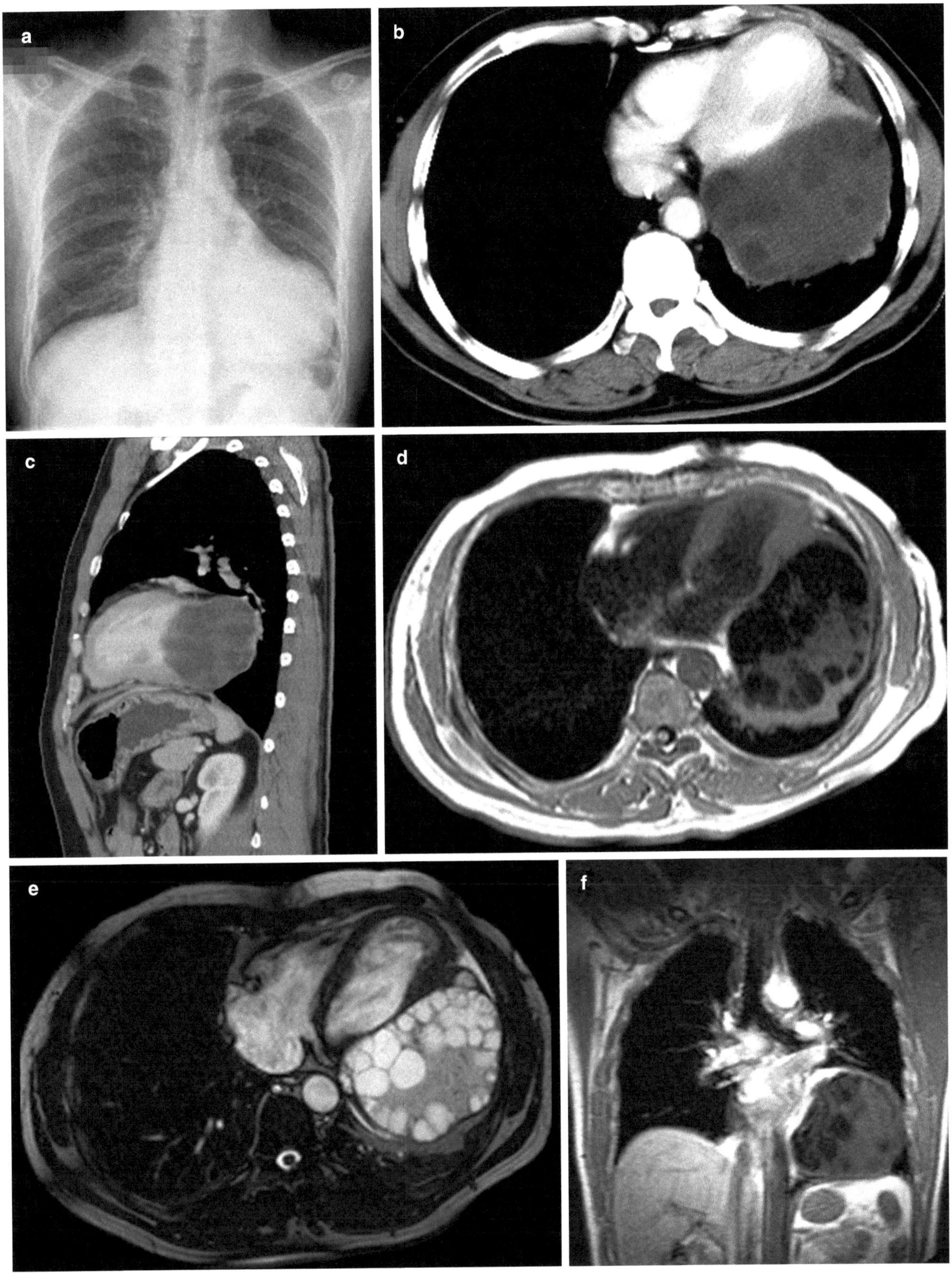

Fig. 26.31 Cardiac echinococcosis. (**a**) X-ray demonstrates enlarged heart shadow with increased density, which is mainly expansion of the left ventricle leftward. (**b**, **c**) CT scanning demonstrates cystic lump at the left ventricular wall with inner daughter cysts in different sizes scattering in the mother cystic fluid and higher density of mother cystic fluid than daughter cysts. (**d**–**f**) MR imaging demonstrates multiple cystic lesions at the left ventricular wall with well-defined boundaries, watery signal of the daughter cysts, and equal signal of the mother cyst

26.8.2.2 Clinical Manifestation

The clinical symptoms include chest pain and coughing up of salty fluid or sheet jellylike substance.

26.8.2.3 Laboratory Test

In the sputum, fragments of echinococcus are detected. Casoni test or serum immunological assay is positive. Routine blood test shows increased count of eosinophil granulocytes.

26.8.2.4 Radiological Demonstration

Ultrasound demonstrates acoustic transparent dark area of water-containing cyst in ball shape or oval shape, with smooth, regular, and well-defined boundary. The echo from posterior wall has enhancement effect. X-ray and CT scanning demonstrate singular or multiple round cystic lesion in the lung, with internal even density. For the type of daughter cysts, cyst-in-cyst sign can be demonstrated. In the cases with cyst rupture, the typical signs, such as air-crescent sign, floating lotus sign, rocks-emerging-after-water-subsiding sign, and floral hoop sign, are demonstrated.

26.8.3 Cerebral Echinococcosis

26.8.3.1 Epidemiological History and Clinical Manifestation

In children or young adults of farming area, symptoms of progressively severe intracranial hypertension or episodes of epilepsy with no known causes occur, which persist for 1–6 months.

26.8.3.2 Radiological Demonstration

The brain is demonstrated with round or round-like cyst. The cystic content has water-like density or is demonstrated with long T1 and long T2 signals. The density or signals of daughter cysts are demonstrated to be lower than the mother cyst, possibly with space-occupying effect.

26.8.4 Bone Echinococcosis

The diagnosis of bone echinococcosis mainly depends on the radiological demonstrations and serological test findings.

26.8.4.1 X-Ray and CT Scanning

X-ray and CT scanning demonstrate expansive lesion of singular cyst or multiple cysts that have spongy, grape-like, and soap-bubble-like appearance and fishing netlike bone scaffolds. The lesion is demonstrated with surrounding slight or no osteoproliferation and generally no periosteal reaction.

26.8.4.2 MR Imaging

MR imaging demonstrates the hydatid cyst as cystic multilobular low T1WI signal and high T2WI signal. In the lesion, daughter cysts are demonstrated with obviously low signal. In the cases with hydatid cyst complicated by infection, both T1WI and T2WI signals are obviously increased, especially T2WI signal.

26.9 Differential Diagnosis

26.9.1 Hepatic Echinococcosis

26.9.1.1 Hepatic Cystic Echinococcosis

Hepatic Abscess

CT scanning demonstrates simplex type of hepatic cystic echinococcosis with similar lesions to simplex hepatic abscess. However, the wall of simplex hepatic abscess is extremely thin, rarely with calcification. Contrast scanning demonstrates no enhancement of the cystic wall. However, hepatic cystic echinococcosis is demonstrated with clearly defined wall, which has higher density than its surrounding liver tissue. Calcification of cystic wall is common. Contrast scanning for the cases complicated by infection demonstrates enhancement of the cystic wall with different degrees. In combination with the clinical data and immunological assays, the differential diagnosis can be defined.

Bacterial Hepatic Abscess

Hepatic abscess is commonly demonstrated with uneven internal density, with fluid-gas level in the lesion. The solid part is demonstrated with calcification and small cysts. Contrast scanning demonstrates no internal enhancement of the lesion, but obvious enhancement of the hepatic abscess wall and its septum, and peripheral low-density edema around the abscess wall. However, hepatic cystic echinococcosis is demonstrated with no obvious enhancement of the cystic wall by contrast scanning and the lesions are commonly multiple. In the adjacent liver tissue and abdominal cavity, hepatic hydatid and its related signs are demonstrated, commonly with calcification of the cystic wall. In addition, systemic toxic symptoms in the cases of hepatic abscess are demonstrated to be severe, with obviously increased WBC count. And Casoni test shows negative in the cases with hepatic abscess.

Amebic Hepatic Abscess

At the wall of amebic hepatic abscess, calcification is demonstrated, which resembles to calcification at the cystic wall in the cases of hepatic cystic echinococcosis. The wall with calcification in the cases of amebic hepatic abscess is commonly thick, and the cystic fluid is demonstrated with high density. The wall with calcification in the cases of hepatic cystic echinococcosis is comparatively thin, and the cystic fluid is demonstrated with low density and with visible multiple cysts or multiple daughter cysts.

26.9.1.2 Hepatic Alveolar Echinococcosis

Liver Cancer

Alveolar hydatid and liver cancer show infiltrative growth in the liver to form a solid lump. The lesion is demonstrated to be an irregular solid space-occupying lesion, and the key points for their differentiation are as follows.

Ultrasound

Hepatic alveolar echinococcosis is demonstrated with moderate to strong echo, while liver cancer is demonstrated with moderate echo. Color Doppler ultrasonography demonstrates colored blood flow signal in the lump and typical flower-basket sign. The posterior echo attenuation at the lesion of hepatic alveolar echinococcosis is greater than that at the lesion of liver cancer. At the center of the lesion, hepatic alveolar echinococcosis is demonstrated with liquefaction and karst-cave sign, while the dark area of necrosis in the cases of liver cancer is demonstrated with no echo from liver parenchyma. At the peripheral lesion, hepatic alveolar echinococcosis is demonstrated with continuous and short line like vascular vessels that are interrupted at the peripheral lesion. No blood flow signal is demonstrated in the lesion. However, liver cancer is demonstrated with rich blood supply.

CT Scanning and MR Imaging

The lesion of hepatic alveolar echinococcosis is demonstrated with slightly high T1WI signal and mainly low T2WI signal. By CT scanning, the lesion is demonstrated with low density. The lesion of liver cancer is mostly demonstrated as long T1 and long T2 signal with low density. The lesion of hepatic alveolar echinococcosis has well-defined boundary with no surrounding edema. The lesion of liver cancer is demonstrated with poorly defined boundary, commonly with surrounding edema. The necrotic liquefaction area in the cases of hepatic alveolar echinococcosis is irregular with karst-cave-like or maplike appearance. The necrotic area in the cases of liver cancer is mostly located at the center of the lesion. Contrast scanning/imaging demonstrates no enhancement of the lesion in the cases of hepatic alveolar echinococcosis, but obvious enhancement of the lesion in the cases of liver cancer, with dynamic enhancement of rapid in and rapid out. Clinically, these radiological demonstrations should be combined with results by AFP examination for differentiation.

Angioma

Ultrasound demonstrates angioma as round or round-like lesion with sharp margin or strong light mass. Contrast CT scanning and MR imaging demonstrate persistent enhancement of the lesion. Casoni test shows negative result.

26.9.2 Pulmonary Echinococcosis

26.9.2.1 Pulmonary Abscess

The clinical symptoms are serious. CT scanning demonstrates uneven thickness of the abscess wall and no lacelike change in the abscess.

26.9.2.2 Cavity Type of Pulmonary Tuberculosis

Tuberculoma in most cases is located at the posterior segment of superior lobe and the dorsal segment of inferior lobe, with surrounding satellite lesions. The lesion is demonstrated with uneven density and internal spots of calcifications. Cystic echinococcosis may occur at any part of the lungs, more commonly at the lateral lung field of the inferior lung. The lesion is demonstrated with even density. Along with the development of the lesion, the diagnosis can be defined.

26.9.2.3 Bronchial Cyst

Simplex cystic echinococcosis should be differentiated from bronchial cyst. Bronchial cyst is commonly demonstrated as gas-containing cystic lesion. After occurrence of secondary infection, the intracystic density increases. Its connection with the bronchus causes the formation of fluid level. The lesion of simplex cystic echinococcosis is demonstrated to be cystic lump with water-like density and smooth margin. The formation of fluid level is commonly accompanied by floating lotus sign.

26.9.3 Cerebral Echinococcosis

26.9.3.1 Epidermoid Cyst

Epidermoid cyst is commonly demonstrated as low-density shadow, with its CT value being close to fat density. In the cases with intracystic hemorrhage or calcification deposition, the lesion can be demonstrated with high density. In some cases, the cystic wall is demonstrated with archlike calcification. The location of the lesion also facilitates the differential diagnosis. Epidermoid cyst commonly occurs at the cerebellopontine angle, the sella area, and the middle fossa. Its occurrence at the cerebral hemisphere accounts for less than 10 % of the cases with epidermoid cyst.

26.9.3.2 Brain Metastasis

Brain metastasis is mostly distributed in the areas supplied by the middle cerebral artery and in the subcortex. The lesion is demonstrated with high T2Wi signal. Contrast imaging demonstrates even enhancement, but no enhancement of the necrotic liquefaction area and no change of multiple small cysts. In combination with the clinical case history, the differential diagnosis can be made.

26.9.3.3 Arachnoid Cyst

About 2/3 of the cases with arachnoid cyst are demonstrated with the lesion at the lateral fissure and rarely at the convex of the brain. The lesion is demonstrated with semicircle or biconvex shape with its density being close to the cerebrospinal fluid. The cystic wall is thin. The lesion has smooth and regular margin. Contrast imaging demonstrates no enhancement. All the cases are accompanied by localized thinning or outward protrusion of the inner plate.

26.9.4 Bone Echinococcosis

26.9.4.1 Bone Giant Cell Tumor

Giant cell tumor of the bone commonly occurs at the epiphysis of the long bones, which is characterized by eccentric expansive osteolytic destruction. The lesion is demonstrated with soap-bubble-like fibrous bone septum. The hydatid cyst develops in the bone toward the part with the lowest growth resistance, commonly from the metaphysis to diaphysis. The cystic destruction area has sharp margin and irregular shape. Bone giant cell tumor is demonstrated with moderate T1WI signal and high or equal T2WI signal.

26.9.4.2 Vertebral Tuberculosis

The vertebra and the appendices with hydatidosis are demonstrated to be multi-cystic. In the cases with no severe lesions, the vertebra cannot collapse, with commonly unilateral paravertebral soft tissue lump. The intervertebral disc generally keeps intact with no stenosis. When vertebral tuberculosis invades the adjacent vertebra and corresponding intervertebral disk, bilateral paravertebral soft tissue lump shadows are demonstrated.

26.9.4.3 Bone Cyst

Bone cyst is demonstrated as an oval-shaped transparent area with well-defined boundary. By MR imaging, the lesion is demonstrated with moderate T1WI signal and high T2WI signal, with no low signaling external cyst and daughter cyst in the cases of cystic echinococcosis.

26.9.4.4 Aneurysmal Bone Cyst

The vertebra can be demonstrated with expansive polycystic bone destruction, with common involvement of the vertebral arch, which can be hardly differentiated from bone echinococcosis. However, the MR imaging demonstrations are totally different between the two diseases. Aneurysmal bone cyst is demonstrated with ladderlike fluid-fluid level, with multiple diverticular knobs in different sizes.

Suggested Reading

Ding GC, Wang J, Huang SQ. CT diagnosis and interventional therapy for hepatic hydatidosis. Chin J Int Radiol Ther. 2006;3(6):445–7.

Li T, Huang JQ. Ultrasound demonstrations alveolar hydatidosis. Chin J Ultrason. 1996;5(4):36–8.

Li T, Li Q, Yan XR. Ultrasound demonstrations of hydatidosis and their classification. Chin J Med Radiol. 2000;8(5):363–5.

Ren YF, Zhang LC, Jiang J, et al. Quantitative analysis of MR diffusion weighted imaging for hepatic echinococcosis. Pract Radiol. 2008;23(7):785–6.

Tevenet PS, Jensen O, Drut R, et al. Viability and infectiousness of eggs of Echinococcus granulous aged under natural conditions of inferior arid climate. Vet Parasitol. 2005;133(1):71–7.

Wen H, Xu MQ. Practical studies of echinococcosis. Beijing: Science Press; 2008.

Xiao N, Qiu JM, Nakao M, et al. Echinococcus shiquicus n.sp.a taeniid cestode from Tibetan fox and plateau pika in China. Int J Parasitol. 2005;35(6):693–701.

Xu MQ, Ha DE, Sun CQ, et al. Imaging diagnosis and typing of hepatic cystic echinococcosis. Chin J Med. 2002;82(3):176–9.

Zhang JX, Gao XZ. Clinical parasitology. Beijing: People's Medical Publishing House; 2009.

Zhang YL, Jean Mathieu B, Wen H, et al. Molecular evidence of sheep (G1) and camel (G6) strains of echinococcosis granulosus in domestic dogs. Chin J Parasit Dis Control. 2005;18(5):333–5.

Zheng H, Wen H, Xu ZX, et al. Experimental observation of anaphylaxis induced by echinococcus infection in meriones unguiculatus. Chin J Parasit Dis Control. 2004;18(2):109–12.

Zhou DH, Zhou HX, Lei JQ, et al. Diagnostic value of MRI for hepatic echinococcosis. Chin J Clin Radiol. 2006;17(7):381–4.

Kala-Azar

27

Yuxin Yang

Kala-azar is also known as visceral leishmaniasis, which is a chronic endemic infectious disease caused by *Leishmania donovani* and transmitted by sandfly. Clinically, it is characterized by persistent irregular fever, progressive hepatosplenomegaly, emaciation, anemia, pancytopenia, and increased plasma globulin. In the advanced stage of the disease, edema, jaundice, abdominal wall varicosis, and ascites may occur.

27.1 Etiology

Leishmania donovani is an intracellular parasitic flagellate, which is categorized into the family of trypanosomatidae. It has two variants, promastigote that is found in sandflies or culture medium and amastigote that can be found in its hosted mammals. The promastigote is cone shaped with a size of 15–25 × 1.5–3.5 μm. It has a wide head and a fine-pointed posterior end, with a flagellum projecting outward from the head, central nucleus, and anteriorly located kinetoplast body. The amastigote is also known as Leishman-Donovan body, which is oval in shape, with a size of 2.9–5.7 × 1.8–4.0 μm and with nucleus and kinetoplast body inside it. By Wright-Giemsa staining, Leishman-Donovan body is found to have a round or oval shape, with slightly blue-stained cytoplasm and a clearly defined cell body with a diameter of 1–3 μm. In addition, a large purplish red stained nucleus can be found, with a round-liked shape and a kinetoplast body in rod shape that is obviously smaller than the nucleus. The kinetoplast body is also stained purplish red, but much deeper that the stained color of the nucleus, with a compact structure. Leishman-Donovan body can be found with a scattering distribution or in a cluster. The scattering Leishman-Donovan body can be missed during observation. However, Leishman-Donovan body in phagocytes can be identified without any difficulty.

When a female sandfly stings and bites the infected animals and persons, blood containing Leishman-Donovan body is sucked into the stomach of sandfly, which then develops into mature promastigotes in 2–3 days and further multiply rapidly by dichotomy. About 1 week later, a large quantity of promastigotes accumulate at the buccal cavity and mouthpart of sandfly. When such sandflies sting and bite animals or persons, the promastigotes can invade these organisms, shedding off the flagellum to transform into amastigotes. The amastigotes multiply in a large quantity in the phagocytes to produce distension and rupture of phagocytes and release of *Leishmania donovani*, which are then swallowed by other phagocytes. Such a continual reproduction of *Leishmania donovani* in phagocytes leads to hyperplasia of the mononuclear phagocyte system. Consequently, the organs containing large quantity of phagocytes, such as the liver and spleen, are obviously enlarged.

27.2 Epidemiology

27.2.1 Source of Infection

The patients and infected dogs are the main source of infection. In China, the patients are the common source of infection in northern Anhui province and in the plain area north to eastern Henan province, while infected dogs are the common source of infection in the mountain areas of Northwest plateau. In desert areas like Xinjiang Uygur Autonomous Region and Inner Mongolia, wild animals are the major source of infection, also referred to as natural source or wild animal source.

27.2.2 Route of Transmission

Phlebotomus chinensis is the major transmitting vector responsible for spread of visceral leishmaniasis in China.

Y. Yang
Department of Radiology, The Sixth People's Hospital, Urumqi, Xinjiang Uygur Autonomous Region, China
e-mail: yangyuxin6068@163.com

H. Li (ed.), *Radiology of Infectious Diseases: Volume 2*, DOI 10.1007/978-94-017-9876-1_27

The disease is transmitted commonly via stings and bites by sandflies. Occasionally, the disease spreads through defective skin or mucosa, placenta or blood transfusion, accidental needlestick in laboratories, and sharing needles or syringes for intravenous drug abuse.

27.2.3 Susceptibility of Population

Populations are generally susceptible, with decreased susceptibility along with age. The infected persons can produce specific immune responses in their bodies, which generates antibodies without protective immunity. Specific therapy is required to eliminate Leishman-Donovan body for cure. After recovery, patients acquire persistent immunity against the disease. Healthy people can also have natural immunity of different degrees.

27.2.4 Epidemic Characteristics

Visceral leishmaniasis is widely distributed across the world, including Mediterranean region, North Africa, Central Africa, the Middle East, Central and Western Asia, Indian subcontinent, and America. In China, the disease is prevalent in 17 provinces, cities, and autonomous regions north to the Yangtze River. Due to its chronic onset, the occurrence of visceral leishmaniasis has no obvious seasonal changes. Visceral leishmaniasis is more common in populations of children under the age of 10 years, males, and residents living in rural areas.

27.3 Pathogenesis and Pathological Changes

27.3.1 Pathogenesis

When people are bitten by infected sandfly, promastigotes of *Leishmania donovani* invade the human body. Glycoprotein (gp63) and phosphate lipopolysaccharide on the surface of the promastigotes bind to complement C3 in the blood serum, with continuing binding to complement C3 in macrophages. After that, the promastigotes are attached to phagocytes, which are then swallowed into the phagocytes by receptor-mediated phagocytosis. There the promastigotes are transformed into Leishman-Donovan bodies to grow and replicate inside the sack formed by binding of their phagocytic vesicle to lysosome. Due to repeated multiplication, the host phagocytes are subject to ruptures to release the Leishman-Donovan bodies, which are then swallowed by other phagocytes for continuing growth and replication. As a result, proliferation occurs in the mononuclear phagocyte system, leading to pathological changes of the liver, spleen, bone marrow, and lymph nodes. The basic pathological changes of visceral leishmaniasis are proliferation of macrophages and plasma cells.

27.3.2 Pathological Changes

One of the common pathological changes of the disease is enlarged liver, with proliferation of Kupffer cells, a large quantity of Leishman-Donovan bodies filling in the cytoplasm, and accompanying infiltration of plasma cells. Another common pathological change is enlarged spleen, with massive proliferation of phagocytes and reticulocytes in the medullary cord, infiltration of plasma cells, proliferation of endothelial cells in the splenic sinus, and a large quantity of Leishman-Donovan bodies in the phagocytes. In addition, there is a significant decrease of splenic nodules that have unclearly defined structure and obvious atrophy. The small lymphocytes are hardly found in the thymus dependent area of lymphatic sheath surrounding the central artery. The decreases of various hemocytes are related to hypersplenism. The bone marrow tissues are found to be highly hyperplasic, with fillings of Leishman-Donovan bodies in the phagocytes and significantly increased plasma cells by microscopy. The lymph nodes are mildly or moderately enlarged, with proliferation of Leishman-Donovan body-filled phagocytes in the lymphatic cortex, medulla, and sinus tract. Small lymphocytes decrease or are absent. Phagocytes filled with Leishman-Donovan bodies proliferate in such organs as the small intestine, lungs, kidneys.

27.4 Clinical Symptoms and Physical Signs

27.4.1 Incubation Period

The incubation period of the disease generally ranges from 3 to 6 months. In some cases, it lasts only for about 10 days or even for about 9 years.

27.4.2 Typical Clinical Manifestations

The common symptom is long-term irregular fever, which is typically double-peaked fever. In some cases, it can be remittent fever or continued fever. Patients commonly sustain symptoms of sweating, fatigue, weakness, and general upset. In the advanced stage of the disease, patients can have anemia and malnutrition. Thrombocytopenia-induced hemorrhinia, gingival bleeding, and bleeding spots in the skin may also occur. In some serious cases, the skin of patient's face and extremities may turn into dark black. Therefore, the disease is also known as black fever.

In addition, mild systemic lymphadenectasis along with enlarged liver and spleen occurs in clinical settings. The spleen is progressively enlarged, with the spleen palpably soft within 2–3 weeks after onset of the disease. Along with progress of the illness course, the spleen is increasing hard, which can reach the umbilical level in 6 months and reach the pelvic cavity in 1 year. In the cases of intrasplenic embolism and bleeding, spleen pain and tenderness can be found.

Relief and exacerbation of symptoms can occur alternatively during the course of disease. Generally, the disease is in remission period in 1 month after onset of the disease, with decreased body temperature, relieved symptoms, reduced size of the affected spleen, and improved hemogram. After several weeks remission, the conditions can be exacerbated. In such a way, the course of the disease may persist for several months.

27.4.3 Special Clinical Types

27.4.3.1 Post-Kala-Azar Dermal Leishmaniasis

Post-kala-azar dermal leishmaniasis occurs mostly in patient with a history of visceral leishmaniasis. It can also present during the course of visceral leishmaniasis. In some rare cases, dermal leishmaniasis is primary in patients with no history of visceral leishmaniasis. The skin lesions occur years after the recovery of visceral leishmaniasis, which is therefore known as post-kala-azar dermal leishmaniasis. The skin lesions are mostly nodular type and rarely depigmented type. Compared to skin macula and papule, these nodules cover larger and deeper areas of the skin, commonly involving deep dermis layer and even involving subcutaneous tissues in some serious cases. The nodules are granulomas of varied sizes or dark-colored papules, commonly found on the face and neck. Amastigotes can be detected from tissues inside the nodules.

27.4.3.2 Lymphatic Visceral Leishmaniasis

The patients with lymphatic visceral leishmaniasis usually have no history of visceral leishmaniasis. The clinical manifestations include local superficial lymphadenectasis, especially in the inguinal region. The enlarged lymph nodes are in different sizes, with no tenderness and reddish swelling. Eosinophilic granulocyte count increases. By lymph node biopsy, amastigotes can be found in epithelioid cells.

27.4.3.3 Kala-Azar Complicated by AIDS

Patients infected with both *Leishmania donovani* and HIV can be another important source of infection for visceral leishmaniasis. Due to highly serious leishmaniaemia, sandfly is most likely to be infected after stings or bites of the patients, which reinforces the spread of *Leishmania donovani*. Its transmission is mainly via sharing syringes among intravenous drug users.

27.5 Kala-Azar-Related Complications

27.5.1 Secondary Bacterial Infection

Kala-azar can be complicated by secondary bacterial infections, including pulmonary inflammation, bacillary dysentery, gingival ulceration, and gangrenous stomatitis.

27.5.2 Acute Agranulocytosis

Its symptoms are high fever, extreme exhaustion, oropharyngeal ulceration, necrosis, local swollen lymph nodes, and substantial decrease or even absence of granulocyte in peripheral blood.

27.6 Diagnostic Examinations

27.6.1 Laboratory Tests

27.6.1.1 Serum Antibody Test

Serum antibody tests include enzyme-linked immunosorbent assay (ELISA), indirect hemagglutination assay (IHA), counter immunoelectrophoresis (CIE), indirect immunofluorescence test (IF), and direct agglutination test, all of which have high positivity and specificity. IFA and ELISA have a positive rate of 100 % but with possibility of false-positive findings.

27.6.1.2 Circulating Antigens Detection

Monoclonal antibody-antigen spot test (McAb-AST) can be used for the diagnosis of kala-azar, with favorable positive rate, sensitivity, specificity, and repeatability. The test only requires small quantity of serum and can be applied for therapeutic assessment.

27.6.1.3 Molecular Biological Examination

PCR and DNA probe technique can be used to detect kDNA and DNA fragments of *Leishmania donovani* in patients, with favorable sensitivity and specificity. In addition, their results are also applicable for early diagnosis and therapeutic assessment. However, due to its complex operational procedures, it has not been widely applied.

27.6.2 Examinations Following Puncture

27.6.2.1 Smear Test

Bone marrow smear is the most commonly used examination to detect *Leishmania donovani*, with a detection rate of 80–90 %. Smear test after lymph node puncture has a detection rate of 46–87 % for *Leishmania donovani*. Smear test after spleen or liver puncture also carries high detection rate.

27.6.2.2 Culture

Specimens harvested by abovementioned punctures can be inoculated into NNN culture medium, followed by placement in an incubator with a temperature of 22–25 °C for 1 week. Positive result can be then confirmed by visible active promastigotes in the cultured tissues.

27.6.2.3 Animal Inoculation Experiment

Specimens harvested from abovementioned punctures can be inoculated into susceptible animals, such as hamsters and

BALB/c mice. Tissue samples from the liver and spleen from these animals are collected in 1–2 months to prepare printing or smear, with following Wright-Giemsa staining and microscopic observation.

27.6.2.4 Skin Biopsy

Tissue fluid can be collected by puncture of skin nodules using a sterilized needle. Otherwise, a scalpel can be used to slightly scrape the skin nodules to collect tissues for smearing, staining, and microscopic observation.

27.6.3 Diagnostic Imaging

Ultrasonography, CT scanning, MR imaging, and other radiological examinations facilitate the detection of abdominal lesions and the related complications. However, radiological examinations cannot achieve qualitative diagnosis.

27.7 Imaging Demonstrations

27.7.1 Ultrasonography

Ultrasonography demonstrates enlarged liver and spleen. In some cases, megalosplenia can be demonstrated (Fig. 27.1).

Case Study 1
Visceral leishmaniasis

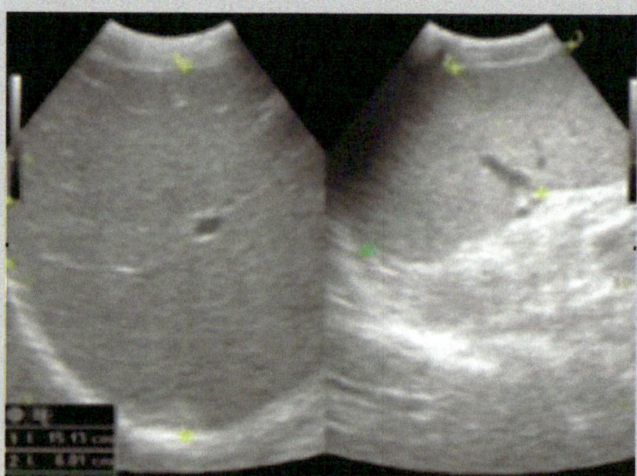

Fig. 27.1 Enlarged spleen in a patient with visceral leishmaniasis. Ultrasound demonstrates enlarged spleen

27.7.2 CT Scanning

CT scanning has no specific demonstration, with common findings of enlarged liver and spleen. In some cases, CT scanning can reveal conditions of splenic infarction and liver abscesses (Figs. 27.2, 27.3 and 27.4).

Case Study 2
Visceral leishmaniasis

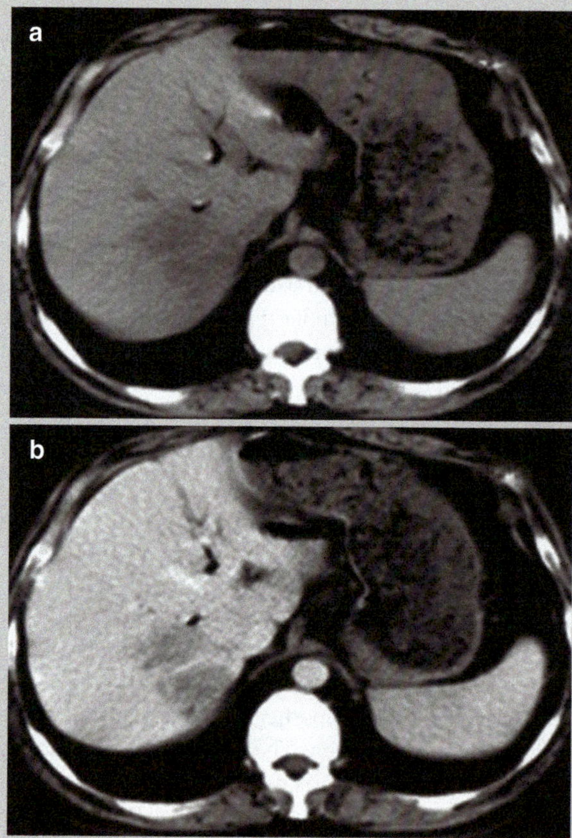

Fig. 27.2 Hepatic lesions of visceral leishmaniasis. (**a**, **b**) Plain CT scanning reveals multiple flakes of foci with low density in the right hepatic lobe, with unclearly defined boundaries. Contrast CT scanning demonstrates slightly enhanced foci still in low density

Case Study 3

A male patient aged 43 years was admitted to the hospital due to intermittent fever for 5 months. He had a history of living in an epidemic area of visceral leishmaniasis and a history of mosquito stings and bites. Serological test for visceral leishmaniasis is positive.

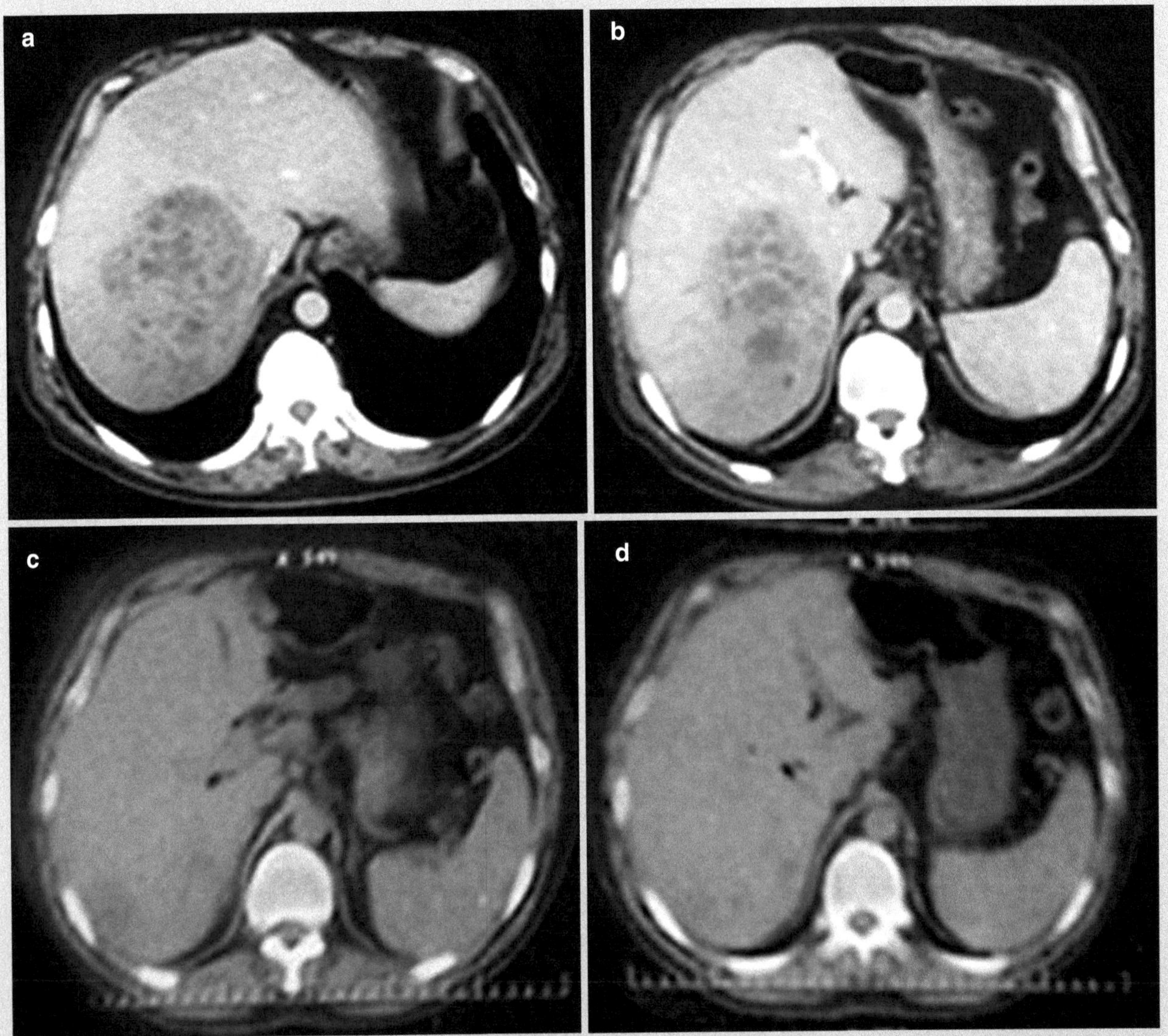

Fig. 27.3 Hepatic lesions of visceral leishmaniasis. (**a**, **b**) CT scanning demonstrates large flakes of honeycomb-liked low-density shadow in the right hepatic lobe, with quite clearly defined boundaries and uneven inner density. Contrast CT scanning demonstrates insignificantly enhanced foci. (**c**, **d**) CT scanning demonstrates absence of the hepatic lesions in the right hepatic lobe and decreased size of the spleen

Case Study 4

A male patient aged 38 years had persistent fever for 2 months, with a body temperature of 39 °C. He engaged in engineering construction in an area with epidemic of visceral leishmaniasis and had a history of mosquito stings and bites. Serological test for visceral leishmaniasis is positive.

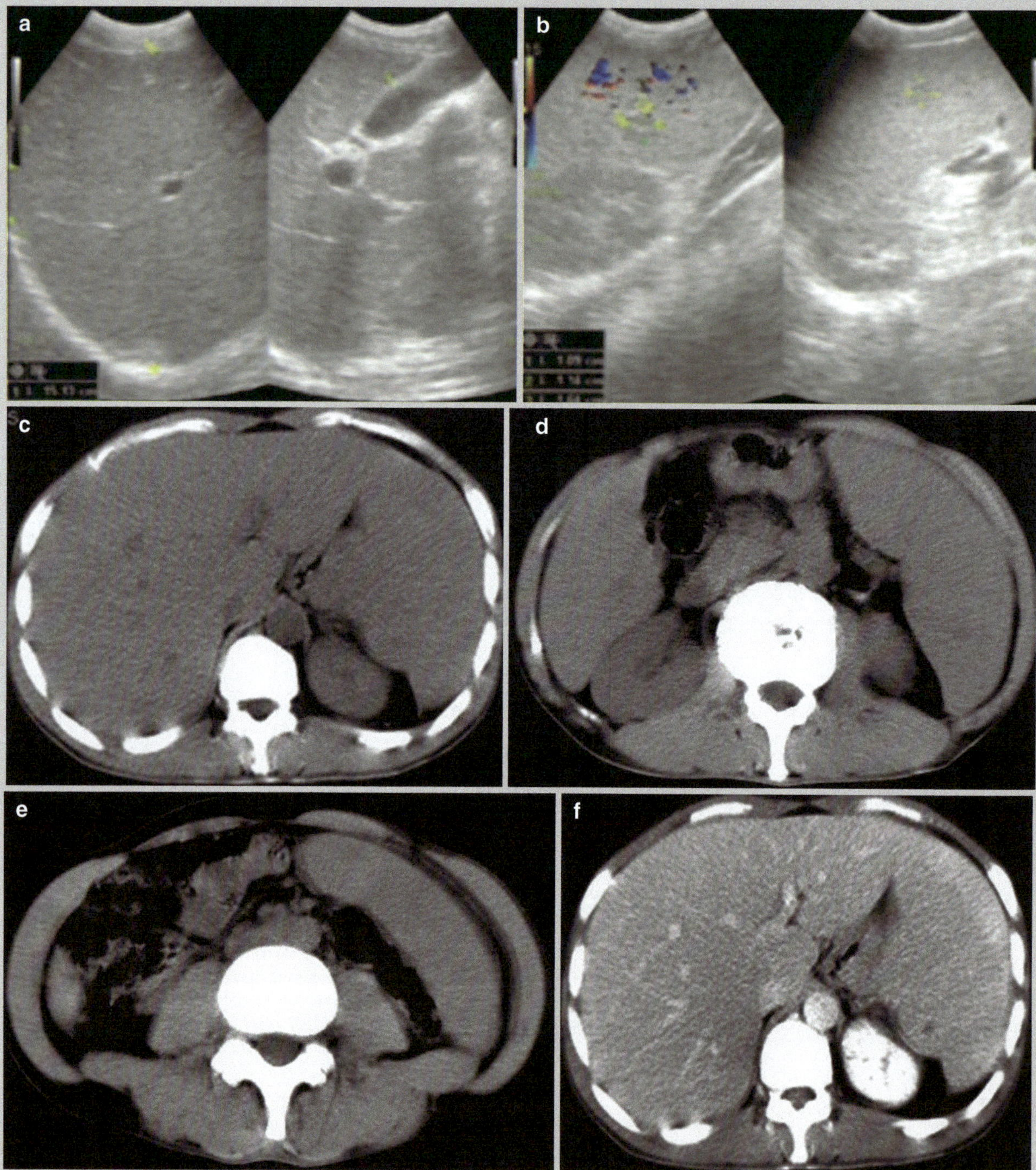

Fig. 27.4 Hepatic and splenic lesions of visceral leishmaniasis. (**a**, **b**) Ultrasonography reveals enlarged liver, with a maximum oblique diameter of 151 mm of the right hepatic lobe. The liver is morphologically well stacked, with two solid foci in different sizes in the upper segment of the right hepatic lobe. The foci have clearly defined borders and even inner echo, with no obvious blood flow signal around or in them. Ultrasonography also reveals enlarged spleen, with uneven echo of the splenic parenchyma and decreased echo from parts of the splenic parenchyma. In addition, there are multiple intermediate-weak echo areas in different sizes, with no blood flow signal in their peripheral and internal areas. (**c**–**h**) Plain CT scanning reveals enlarged spleen, with multiple low-density shadows in the spleen that have unclearly defined boundaries. Contrast CT scanning demonstrates no obviously enhanced foci

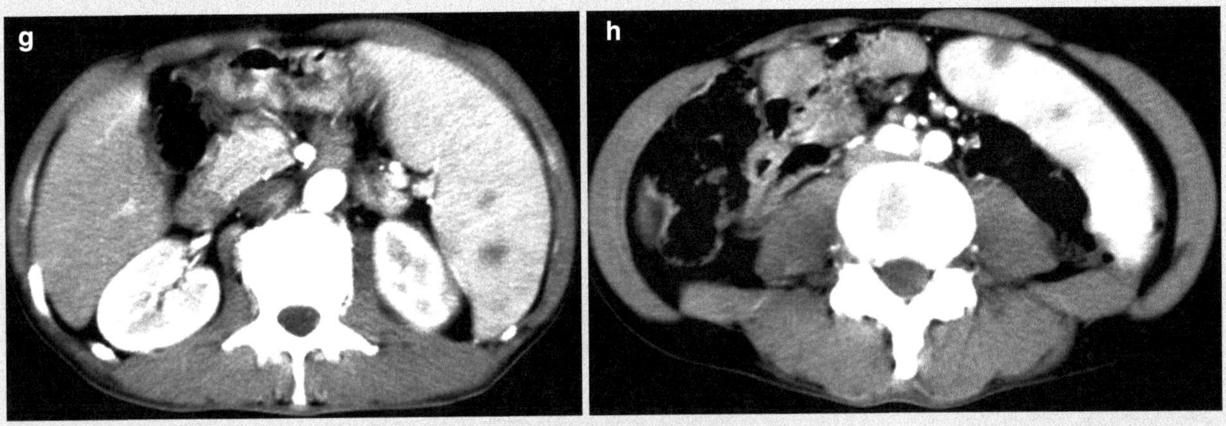

Fig. 27.4 (continued)

27.8 Diagnostic Basis

27.8.1 Epidemiological Data

For diagnosis, healthcare professionals should take into account a history of living or staying in epidemic area during the active seasons for sandflies.

27.8.2 Clinical Manifestations

The disease usually has a chronic onset, with persistent or repeated irregular fever, progressive splenomegaly, anemia, emaciation, and leukocytopenia. Systemic toxic symptoms are relatively mild.

27.8.3 Laboratory Tests

Patients with visceral leishmaniasis may have pancytopenia or even granulocytopenia, WBC count of $1.5–3.0 \times 10^9/L$, moderate anemia, and thrombocytopenia. In addition, there may be significantly increased plasma globulin, decreased albumin, and possibly reversed A/G. Detection of serum-specific antigen and antibody can facilitate the diagnosis. Punctures of bone marrow, lymph nodes, spleen, and liver can be performed for smear to detect Leishman-Donovan body or for culture to detect promastigote. Positive findings can define the diagnosis of visceral leishmaniasis.

27.8.4 Imaging Demonstrations

Imaging demonstrations include enlarged liver and spleen and intrahepatic large flake of honeycomb-liked low-density shadow with quite clearly defined boundary and uneven inner density. Contrast imaging demonstrates no obviously enforced foci. Intrasplenic demonstration resembling splenic infarction facilitates the diagnosis of visceral leishmaniasis.

27.9 Differential Diagnosis

During its acute stage, visceral leishmaniasis should be differentiated from tuberculosis, typhoid fever, malaria, typhus fever, acute schistosomiasis, and amebic liver abscess. During its subacute and chronic stages, visceral leishmaniasis should be differentiated from brucellosis, persisting *Salmonella* infections, leukemia, malignant histiocytosis, infectious mononucleosis, lymphoma, chronic schistosomiasis, and chronic malaria. Clinical manifestations and etiological findings of histoplasmosis capsulati have similarities to those of visceral leishmaniasis, which should be paid focused attention for differentiation. Post-kala-azar dermal leishmaniasis should be differentiated from leprosy, yaws, and syphilis.

Suggested Reading

Guan JJ, Chai LR. Leishmaniasis and sandfly in Xinjiang Wei Autonomous Region of China. Urumqi: Xinjiang People's Publishing House; 2006.

Mondal S, Bhattacharya P, Ali N. Current diagnosis and treatment of visceral leishmaniasis. Expert Rev Anti Infect Ther. 2010;8(8):919–44.

Palumbo E. Visceral leishmaniasis in children: a review. Minerva Pediatr. 2010;62(4):389–95.

Tan YF, Bi CY, Jiang LJ, et al. Clinical diagnosis and differential diagnosis of visceral leishmaniasis. Chin J Hosp Infect. 2012;22(4):756–7.

Zhan XM, Chen JP. Human parasitology. Beijing: People's Health Publishing House; 2003.

Zhang LP, Zhang FN. Epidemiological and clinical data of 166 cases of visceral leishmaniasis. Parasit Dis Infect Dis. 2010;8(4):181–6.

28 Schistosomiasis

Jiangfeng Pan

Schistosomiasis is a disease caused by parasitism of schistosoma in human body. There are mainly six types of schistosoma that are capable of parasitizing in humans. In China, schistosomiasis is commonly caused by *Schistosoma japonicum Katsurada*, which is known as *Schistosomiasis japonica*. In this chapter, we focus on *Schistosomiasis japonica*.

Schistosomiasis japonica is a disease caused by parasitism of *Schistosoma japonicum Katsurada* in the portal system of human body. Skin contact to contaminated water containing cercariae causes the infection, and the main pathological change is granuloma at the liver and colon caused by eggs of schistosome. In the acute stage, the symptoms and physical signs include fever, hepatomegaly, and liver tenderness, with accompanying diarrhea or bloody purulent stool and significant increase of eosinophilic granulocytes in the blood. In the chronic stage, the symptoms include hepatosplenomegaly. At the advanced stage, the lesions are mainly fibrosis around the portal vein, which may develop into portal hypertension, giant spleen, and ascites.

28.1 Etiology

Currently, it is recognized that schistosoma can be categorized into six types: *Schistosoma japonicum*, *S. mansoni*, S. *haematobium*, *S. intercalatum*, *S. mekongi*, and *S. malayensis*. In the life cycle of *S. japonicum*, human is its final host, and oncomelania is its necessary and unique intermediate host. *S. japonicum* has various animal reservoir hosts, which include livestock such as cow, pig, sheep, dog, and cat as well as various wild animals such as rats. A total of more than 40 kinds of animals can be its final hosts. *S. japonicum* is dioecious and parasitizes in the portal system, mainly in the inferior mesenteric vein of human body. Its survival period is averagely 4–5 years, and some can survive for 10–20 years or even longer. Female worms lay eggs in the terminal veins under the mucosa of intestinal wall, and each female worm can release about 1,000 eggs per day. After the eggs are discharged out of the human body along with feces into water, they are incubated in the water at an appropriate temperature of 25–30 °C into larvae (miracidia). Miracidia consequently invade into the intermediate host, oncomelania, and develop there. After two generations (mother sporocyst and daughter sporocyst) of development and multiplication, cercariae can be released after 7–8 weeks, whose quantity ranges from tens to hundreds per day. The cercariae float on water surface along with water flow. When human or animal touches the contaminated water, cercariae can penetrate human skin or mucosa within an extremely short period of time (usually 10 s). After invasion into human or animal body, cercariae finally reach the liver via lung along with blood flow, where they develop for 15–16 days. After that, male and female cercariae begin to pair with each other, with following maturation into adult worms in the liver within about 1 month. Subsequently, these adult worms flow against the blood flow to the terminal veins of the inferior mesenteric vein, where they lay eggs to begin another round of life cycle.

28.2 Epidemiology

Schistosomiasis is a parasitic disease that seriously threatens human health. It is widely distributed in 76 countries in Asia, Africa, South America, and the Middle East. In 2003, according to the estimation by WHO, about 200 million people were infected across the world and at least 779 million people were at high risk of infection. Therefore, WHO has listed it as one of the important diseases to be systematically prevented and treated.

J. Pan
Department of Radiology, City Central Hospital, Jinhua, Zhejiang, China
e-mail: panjiangfeng967@163.com

H. Li (ed.), *Radiology of Infectious Diseases: Volume 2*, DOI 10.1007/978-94-017-9876-1_28

28.2.1 Geographical Distribution

S. japonicum was first discovered in Kofu, Yamanashi-ken, Japan. Then, it has been prevailing in Japan, the Philippines, Indonesia, China, and other countries. In marshland regions, its prevalence is the most serious due to large flakes of distribution of oncomelania. In such regions, acute schistosomiasis is common. In the regions with river network, oncomelania are distributed in network along streams, and people living along the rivers are at high risk of infection due to life water use. In mountainous regions, oncomelania have a linear distribution along the water flow from the top downward. Since such regions are scarcely populated, patients are rarely found. The infection is commonly caused by field farm work.

28.2.2 Source of Infection

The sources of infection include the patients and the reservoir hosts, which vary in different epidemic areas. In the region with network of rivers, patients are the mainly source of infection; in marshland regions, in addition to the patients, infected cows and pigs are also important source of infection; in the mountainous regions, wild animals such as rats are also the source of infection.

28.2.3 Route of Transmission

The following three conditions are essential for transmission of the disease: (1) feces with schistosome eggs being discharged into water, (2) existence and growth of oncomelania, and (3) contact of human body to contaminated water.

28.2.4 Susceptible Populations

Populations are generally susceptible to schistosomiasis, whose occurrence is more common in farmers and fishmen because they are highly possible to contact contaminated water. For schistosomiasis, males are more commonly infected than females, and children aged under 5 years are less likely to be infected. Its infection rate increases along with the age, and the highest infection rate is demonstrated to be in adults aged 10–20 years.

28.3 Pathogenesis and Pathological Changes

28.3.1 Pathogenesis

At the different stages of development (egg, cercaria, larva, and adult schistosome), schistosoma can cause damaging effects to its host and trigger complex immunopathological responses. The early pathological changes of schistosomiasis japonica are mainly caused by the eggs. A large quantity of eggs deposit in the tissues to form granuloma. In egg-induced granuloma, soluble egg antigen can be detected at a high concentration. Around the eggs, rodlike substances can be found in radiating distribution that are acidophilic, which are actually immune complexes form by combination of antigens and antibodies. Such a finding is known as Hoeppli phenomenon. In the blood of patients with acute schistosomiasis, the positive rates of circulating immune complex and heterophilic antibody are quite high. Therefore, it is believed that acute schistosomiasis is the manifestation of mixed humoral and cellular immune responses. However, the immunopathogenesis of chronic and advanced schistosomiasis can be categorized into delayed allergic reaction. In the cases of schistosomiasis, hepatic fibrosis develops based on granuloma. All of the soluble egg factors, macrophagocytes and T lymphocytes, can produce fibroblast-stimulating factors to promote multiplication of fibroblasts and synthesis of collagen. Schistosomal fibrotic collagens mainly include two types: type I and type III. In the cases of advanced schistosomiasis, the intrahepatic collagens are mainly type I fibrotic collagen. Currently, two major theories have been proposed on the pathogenesis of central neuroschistosomiasis. The first theory is proposed based on egg embolism. It is believed that schistosome eggs go upstream along arteries or veins via the spinal Batson venous plexus that have no valves and deposit at any part that they have passed to cause spinal schistosomiasis. The other theory is mainly based on direct eggs laying, which refers to occurrence of schistosomiasis due to abnormal migration of adult schistosoma into the brain or spinal cord to lay eggs.

28.3.2 Pathological Changes

S. japonicum is mainly parasitic in the inferior mesenteric vein and the superior rectal vein. Its eggs deposit at the inferior layer of the mucosa of intestinal wall and reach the intrahepatic branches along with the blood flow in the portal vein. Therefore, the lesions are most obvious at the liver and colon.

28.3.2.1 Pathological Changes of Colon

The pathological changes are most serious at the colon, sigmoid colon and descending colon, with common involvements of the right colon and appendix. In the acute stage, the pathological changes include mucosa congestion and edema, nodules formed by deposited eggs at the inferior layer of mucosa that are surrounded by infiltration of a large quantity of eosinophilic granulocytes, and superficial ulceration after diabrosis of the nodules. In the chronic stage, proliferation of fibrous tissues and thickening of the intestinal wall can lead to polypoid hyperplasia and colon stenosis. The mesenteric membrane is subject to thickening and shortening, which is tangled with enlarged lymph nodes to form masses. These masses may cause intestinal obstruction. In the cases with deposit of schistosome eggs at the appendix, appendicitis is likely to occur.

28.3.2.2 Pathological Changes of Liver

In the acute stage, schistosome eggs arrive at the liver along with the blood flow in the portal vein to cause slightly enlarged liver. On the surface and section of liver, multiple grayish white or grayish yellow miliary nodules in different sizes can be observed. By microscopy, a large quantity of egg nodules can be observed adjacent to the portal area, and the hepatocytes might be subject to atrophy due to compression, degeneration, and small focal necrosis. In the chronic stage, chronic egg nodules and a large quantity of fibrous proliferation around the portal area can be observed in the liver. The liver may be subject to hardening and shrinkage due to serious fibrosis to cause schistosomal liver cirrhosis. The liver surface is rough that is divided into several slightly protruding areas in different sizes by shallow grooves. On the section, the hyperplastic connective tissues are distributed in tree-branch appearance along the portal vein branches, namely, trunk or pipe type of liver cirrhosis. Because the egg diameter is larger than that of terminal branch of the portal vein, the lesions caused by eggs are mainly found at the portal area, including fibrous proliferation and obvious fibrous septa. Consequently, preantral portal hypertension occurs, with no serious lesions at the hepatic lobules and no obvious regenerated nodules. These changes are different from those of portal liver cirrhosis, therefore, technically known as schistosomal liver fibrosis, which may develop into irreversible liver cirrhosis. The further outcomes of the disease include serious portal hypertension and even death.

28.3.2.3 Pathological Changes of Spleen

In the early stage, the spleen is subject to mild congestion, edema, and softness. In the advanced stage, liver cirrhosis causes portal hypertension, blood stasis at the spleen, tissue proliferation, fibrosis, and thrombosis. The spleen may be progressively enlarged, with occurrence of megalosplenia and secondary hypersplenism.

28.3.2.4 Ectopic Lesions

Ectopic lesions refer to lesions caused by eggs or/and adult worms parasitizing in organs other than the portal system. Such lesions are commonly found at the lungs and brain, but rarely found at the spinal cords.

Pulmonary Schistosomiasis

It mainly refers to delayed cell-mediated allergic reaction due to mechanical injuries and egg granuloma caused by penetration of schistosomulum into lung tissues. The pulmonary lesions include interstitial egg granuloma and accompanying inflammatory infiltration of peripheral alveoli.

Cerebral Schistosomiasis

In the cases of cerebral schistosomiasis, schistosome eggs can be found in the brain, cerebellum, brainstem, pia mater, and choroid plexus. By observation with naked eyes, acute egg nodules are grayish yellow nodules with their sizes ranging from miliary to soybean. By microscopy, one to several mature eggs can be observed at the center of nodule. Some radiating arranged acidophilic homogeneous rods adhere to the surface of nodule, which are actually antigen–antibody complex. Around the nodules, a flake of structureless coagulative necrosis can be observed, with accumulation of a large quantity of eosinophilic granulocytes and visible rhombic or polyhedral Charcot–Leyden crystal protein. The chronic egg nodules can be observed with granuloma formed by epithelioid cells and foreign-body multinuclear giant cells. Such changes may further develop into fibrosis and hyalinization, with formation of peripheral capillary network as well as occurrence of congestion and edema of adjacent brain tissues with accompanying gliosis. The lesions of cerebral egg granuloma are more commonly located in the parietal lobe and temporal lobe and are distributed at the interface of gray and white matters. However, no adult worms have been found in cerebral veins by autopsies or during surgical operations.

Spinal Schistosomiasis

Pathologically, spinal schistosomiasis shares commonalities with cerebral schistosomal granuloma, both with formation of pseudotubercles. By microscopy, necrotic, disintegrated, or calcified eggs can be observed. Around the eggs, there are mainly inflammatory cells in the acute stage and accumulation of epithelioid cells, foreign-body giant cells, and lymphocytes in the chronic stage.

28.4 Clinical Symptoms and Signs

The clinical symptoms of schistosomiasis are various and diversified, with variant severities. According to the stage, severity of infection, location of eggs deposition, and immune responses in human body, schistosomiasis is clinically divided into the following four types.

28.4.1 Acute Schistosomiasis

It is common in patients with primary infection, and its occurrence is more common in young male adults and children. The patients often have a definite history of contact to contaminated water, and about half of them experience flea-bite-like red skin lesion at the place where cercaria invades and cercarial dermatitis. These lesions are self-healed within 2–3 days. Fever is the major clinical symptom of acute schistosomiasis and is also a principal basis for assessing the conditions. It commonly occurs 1–2 months after contact to contaminated water, with intermittent fever as the most common. In the acute stage, gastrointestinal symptoms, such as anorexia, nausea, abdominal pain, diarrhea, and bloody purulent stool, are also found. Above 90 % of the cases experience hepatic pain and enlarged liver, and about 50 % of the cases experience slight enlargement of the spleen. There may be also allergic reactions such as urticaria, angioneurotic edema, and lymphadenectasis. The count of eosinophil granulocytes in the blood commonly increases remarkably, which has significant diagnostic value.

28.4.2 Chronic Schistosomiasis

In the epidemic area of schistosomiasis, chronic schistosomiasis accounts for the vast majority. It usually occurs in untreated patients with subsided acute symptoms or in patients with repeated slight infections in an epidemic area to acquire partial immunity. Such patients who experience schistosomiasis for above half a year can be diagnosed as chronic schistosomiasis.

28.4.2.1 Asymptomatic Patients

Most patients with chronic schistosomiasis are asymptomatic. The diagnosis is commonly defined by findings in the feces for general survey or when the patients seek medical care for other diseases.

28.4.2.2 Symptomatic Patients

The common symptoms include abdominal pain and diarrhea. The patients with chronic schistosomiasis often experience hepatosplenomegaly. At the early stage, hepatomegaly is the main manifestation, especially the left liver lobe. As the conditions progress, the spleen is gradually subject to enlargement.

28.4.3 Advanced Schistosomiasis

After repeated infection of cercaria or infection of a large quantity of cercariae, if treatment is delayed, the patients can develop serious lesions in the liver caused by eggs, which further progress into liver cirrhosis. The whole course often lasts for above 5–15 years. According to different organs that are involved and different severities, advanced schistosomiasis can be divided into four types. One patient may show manifestations of concurrent 2–3 types.

28.4.3.1 Megalosplenia Type

This type is the most common, with the inferior edge of spleen being lower than the umbilical level. Otherwise, the spleen is subject to medial swelling to exceed the midline of human body. The spleen has smooth surface, which is hardened possibly with tenderness and commonly with hypersplenism.

28.4.3.2 Ascites Type

Ascites is the manifestation of significant hepatic decompensation in the advanced stage of schistosomiasis. Along with progressive aggravation of ascites, the patients experience abdominal distention and protrusion, dyspnea, and commonly umbilical herniation and varicose vein of the abdominal wall.

28.4.3.3 Colon Granuloma Type

The patients often experience abdominal pain, diarrhea, constipation, or alternate episodes of diarrhea and constipation. At the left lower quadrant of the abdomen, lump or cord-like object can be palpated, with mild tenderness.

28.4.3.4 Dwarf Type

Currently, it rarely occurs. The patients experience delayed development, shortness, no secondary sex characteristics, and other clinical symptoms.

28.4.4 Ectopic Lesions

28.4.4.1 Pulmonary Schistosomiasis

It is more commonly in the cases of acute schistosomiasis, and it is an interstitial lung disease caused by deposition of eggs. Most of the respiratory symptoms are mild and are often misdiagnosed due to existence of systemic symptoms. The clinical manifestations include mild cough, dull chest pain, small quantity of sputum, and rarely found hemoptysis. The pulmonary physical signs are not obvious, sometimes with dry or moist rales.

28.4.4.2 Cerebral Schistosomiasis

Clinically, it can be divided into two types: acute cerebral schistosomiasis and chronic cerebral schistosomiasis, which are more common in young adult patients with schistosomiasis. The acute type is mainly manifested as meningitis, with symptoms and signs of consciousness disturbance, meningeal irritation sign, paralysis, convulsion, tendon hyperreflexia, and pyramid sign. Examination of cerebrospinal fluid demonstrates no abnormalities or slight increases of protein and WBC count. The main symptom of the chronic type is epileptic seizure, especially localized epilepsy.

28.4.4.3 Spinal Schistosomiasis

It is usually caused by deposit of schistosome eggs in spinal cord along with blood circulation. Most patients have a chronic onset, but there have been reports about its acute onset. The clinical manifestations include symptoms and signs of involved spinal segment, such as progressive weakness of lower limbs, pain, decreased sensations, and dysfunctions of urination and defecation. However, these symptoms and signs are nonspecific.

28.5 Schistosomiasis-Related Complications

28.5.1 Upper Gastrointestinal Hemorrhage

It is the main complication of advanced schistosomiasis, with an incidence rate of 10 %. The location of hemorrhage is commonly lower esophagus and gastric fundus veins, with manifestations of hematemesis and melena. The quantity of bleeding is commonly large.

28.5.2 Hepatic Encephalopathy

According to a report in China, the incidence rate of hepatic encephalopathy in the cases of advanced schistosomiasis is about 1.6–5.4 %, and its occurrence is commonly after splenectomy, portacaval shunt, and massive upper gastrointestinal bleeding.

28.5.3 Infection

The ascites type of advanced schistosomiasis can be complicated by primary peritonitis and septicemia caused by Gram-negative bacilli.

28.5.4 Intestinal Complications

28.5.4.1 Acute Appendicitis

Acute appendicitis is a common complication of schistosomiasis. In epidemic area of schistosomiasis, schistosome eggs can be found in 31 % of the surgically removed appendix specimens from patients with schistosomiasis. Acute appendicitis tends to cause perforation, which further induces peritonitis and localized abscess.

28.5.4.2 Incomplete Intestinal Obstruction

It is intestinal lumen stenosis caused by serious colon lesions in the cases of schistosomiasis. The stenosis is commonly found at the sigmoid colon and rectum, which can be further complicated by incomplete intestinal obstruction.

28.5.4.3 Colon Cancer

Colon granuloma in the cases of schistosomiasis can be complicated by colon cancer. The patients are commonly young adults, and the diagnosis is mostly adenocarcinoma with low malignancy and late metastasis.

28.6 Diagnostic Examinations

28.6.1 Laboratory Tests

28.6.1.1 Routine Blood Test

Acute schistosomiasis is characterized by a significant increase of eosinophilic granulocytes.

28.6.1.2 Liver Function Test

In the cases of acute schistosomiasis, seroglobulin level significantly increases, and serum ALT level slightly increases. In the cases of chronic schistosomiasis, especially asymptomatic patients, the liver function is mostly normal.

28.6.1.3 Parasite Examination

The direct evidence to define the diagnosis of schistosomiasis includes detection of eggs in feces or incubation of miracidia in feces. Generally, the detection rate is relatively high in the acute stage, and the positive rate is low in the cases of chronic and advanced schistosomiasis.

28.6.1.4 Rectum Mucosa Biopsy

It is one of the etiological examinations for the diagnosis of schistosomiasis.

28.6.1.5 Immunological Assays

The applicable assays are various, such as circumoval precipitin test, indirect fluorescence antibody test, enzyme-linked immunosorbent assay (ELISA), and cercaria membrane reaction test. Immunological assays have both high sensitivity and specificity, but fail to distinguish past infection from present infection. These assays may bear false-negative and false-positive results and have cross-reaction with other trematoda.

28.6.2 Diagnostic Imaging

28.6.2.1 Ultrasound

Ultrasound is an important examination for hepatic schistosomiasis. B-mode ultrasound demonstrates morphological changes of liver lesions and facilitates assessing the severity of hepatic fibrosis and locating for liver biopsy. Color Doppler ultrasound can also demonstrate the conditions of blood flow and portal hypertension.

28.6.2.2 X-Ray Radiology

X-ray is mainly applied for the diagnosis of pulmonary schistosomiasis.

28.6.2.3 CT Scanning

CT scanning facilitates in assessing severity of hepatic fibrosis and has a favorable demonstration for calcification of liver and intestinal wall. It also has favorable diagnostic value for pulmonary schistosomiasis and cerebral schistosomiasis.

28.6.2.4 MR Imaging

MR imaging is mainly applied for detecting lesions at the central nervous system and abdomen in the cases of schistosomiasis.

28.7 Imaging Demonstrations

28.7.1 Hepatic Schistosomiasis

28.7.1.1 Ultrasound

Acute Stage

The liver is demonstrated to be mildly enlarged or normal, with intensive echoes that are unevenly distributed. Sometimes, sporadic low echo areas are demonstrated. The lumen diameter of portal vein is demonstrated to be normal.

Chronic Stage

In most cases, the liver is demonstrated with shrinkage that is mainly the right liver lobe. The left liver lobe is demonstrated to be enlarged. The liver surface is unsmooth, and the intrahepatic echoes are demonstrated to be thickened and enhanced, with an uneven distribution or in small patches. The hepatic region is demonstrated with fibrous cord-like strong echoes, with maplike or broken cotton woollike areas in the effective sonolucent areas. The wall of portal vein is demonstrated to be thickened with thinner lumen. In some cases, enlarged diameter of the portal vein can be simultaneously demonstrated.

In the advanced stage of hepatic schistosomiasis, hepatic fibrosis commonly occurs. According to the guideline recommended by WHO/TDR, hepatic fibrosis is graded into the following 0–III levels. The respective manifestations are described as the following:

Level 0: normal light spots or slightly thick light spots type; normal morphology and size of the liver; normal demonstrations by liver ultrasonography or only coarse echo from the liver parenchyma

Level I: thickened light spots type; not obvious changes of morphology and size of the liver; coarse echo from the liver parenchyma with slightly uneven distribution

Level II: squamous and spider web type; hepatosplenomegaly; thickened Glisson's capsule line or wavy Glisson's capsule line; thickened and enhanced light spots at the liver parenchyma that diffusively distribute; concurrent fine light spots and flakes of echoes like spider web; enhanced echoes from the wall of portal vein

Level III: large network type; abnormal morphology of the liver; shrinkage of various diameters; unsmooth liver surface that is divided into countless irregular areas with a diameter of 3–5 cm by shallow grooves; irregular liver edge that is serration-like; thick reticular liver parenchyma with high-echo light strips and light patches that are demonstrated in maplike changes; simultaneous widened lumen of the splenic portal vein

28.7.1.2 X-Ray Radiology

Plain abdominal X-ray radiograph demonstrates splenomegaly, but poorly defined intrahepatic calcification. Barium meal examination can reveal esophageal and gastric varicose veins.

28.7.1.3 CT Scanning

For the cases of acute schistosomiasis, plain CT scanning demonstrates multiple low-density nodules. Contrast CT scanning demonstrates ring-shaped enhancement of the lesions at the arterial phase and slight central enhancement of the lesions at the venous phase. By delayed scanning, the lesions are demonstrated with low density (Fig. 28.1).

In the advanced stage, the patients with schistosomiasis experience liver cirrhosis of different degrees, namely, schistosomal liver cirrhosis.

Changes of Liver Volume

The liver is subject to enlargement or shrinkage of different degrees. The hepatic fissures are demonstrated to be widened and the liver lobes are demonstrated with percentage disproportion, that is, the most commonly enlarged left lobe with the second commonly enlarged caudate lobe (Fig. 28.2).

Liver Calcification

Liver calcification is caused by calcification of schistosome eggs and is the basic pathological change of schistosomal liver cirrhosis. It is also the main demonstration for CT diagnosis of schistosomal liver cirrhosis. The calcification has various morphologies, including linear, reticular, crab-like, maplike, mass-like, or subcapsular calcifications. Calcifications located at different positions have their own characteristic morphology. For instances, subcapsular calcification is mostly linear; calcification around the portal vein in portal area is mass-like; calcification extending along the surface or liver lobule is crab-like; connected interlobular calcification is curved; extensive linear calcifications intertwine into maplike or reticular appearance, which is the most serious pathologic change. Multiple morphologies of calcifications can be concurrently found (Figs. 28.3, 28.4, 28.5 and 28.6).

Changes of Portal Area

The portal area is broadened with decreased density, which is caused by fibrous tissue proliferation due to deposition of eggs at the portal area. At its center, vascular shadows can be observed, which are actually dilated and twisted branches of the portal vein. This is one of the characteristic pathological changes of advanced schistosomiasis.

Contrast CT Scanning of Liver

For the cases of hepatic schistosomiasis, contrast CT scanning demonstrates three types of intrahepatic enhancement: septal enhancement, capsular enhancement, and amorphous enhancement. The septal enhancement is linear and runs from deep liver to liver surface, which can be observed in the non-calcification area or calcification area. In some cases, septal enhancements interconnect to each other into a thick network. The capsular enhancement is demonstrated as curves in different lengths along the liver surface. The amorphous enhancements have irregular shapes, with no definite location and distribution.

Spleen Calcification

The schistosome eggs can flow contrarily the blood flow to the spleen and cause spleen calcification, which is commonly patchy clusters of calcification. However, capsular and amorphous enhancements are rarely found.

Calcification of Portal Venous System

It is calcification caused by deposition of the worm eggs at the vascular wall during their flow in the portal vein, which can be found at the portal vein, the splenic vein, and the superior mesenteric vein. The morphology of calcification is related to the running course of the blood vessels.

Portal Hypertension

Portal hypertension may result in splenomegaly and further develops into megalosplenia in the advanced stage. Most patients experience ascites, dilated portal vein, and its subordinating branches.

Complications

1. *Chronic cholecystitis or gallbladder stone*
   Sometimes, extensive fibrosis occurs in the portal area that causes unsmooth discharge of the bile. Otherwise, even gallbladder stone or cholecystitis occurs. By CT scanning, the gallbladder wall is demonstrated to be thickened to exceed 3 mm, with small volume of gallbladder and high-density stones in gallbladder and bile ducts.
2. *Liver cancer*
   Based on schistosomal liver cirrhosis, accompanying liver cancer is demonstrated, with similar radiological findings to those of ordinary liver cancer.

28.7.1.4 MR Imaging Demonstrations

In the liver, the wide fibrous septum is demonstrated to be linear, with low signal by T_1WI, high signal by T_2WI, and a morphology-like intrahepatic vascular shadow. Therefore, in the cases with the fibrous septum in deep liver parenchyma, SE sequence can hardly distinguish fibrous septum from regular blood vessel. Contrast MR imaging demonstrates the fibrous septum with significant enhancement, but with relatively low signal compared to the hepatic blood vessels. In demonstrating the septal calcification, MR imaging is less favorable than CT scanning. In addition, liver cirrhosis and portal hypertension can be demonstrated with enlarged or shrunk liver volume, disproportional liver lobes, and widened liver fissures. Other demonstrations include enlarged spleen, ascites, dilated and thickened portal vein, and opened collateral circulation. MRA can clearly demonstrate the location and running course of abnormal blood vessels.

Case Study 1

A male patient aged 45 years complained of abdominal distension and upset for more than 2 months. His circumoval precipitin test was positive.

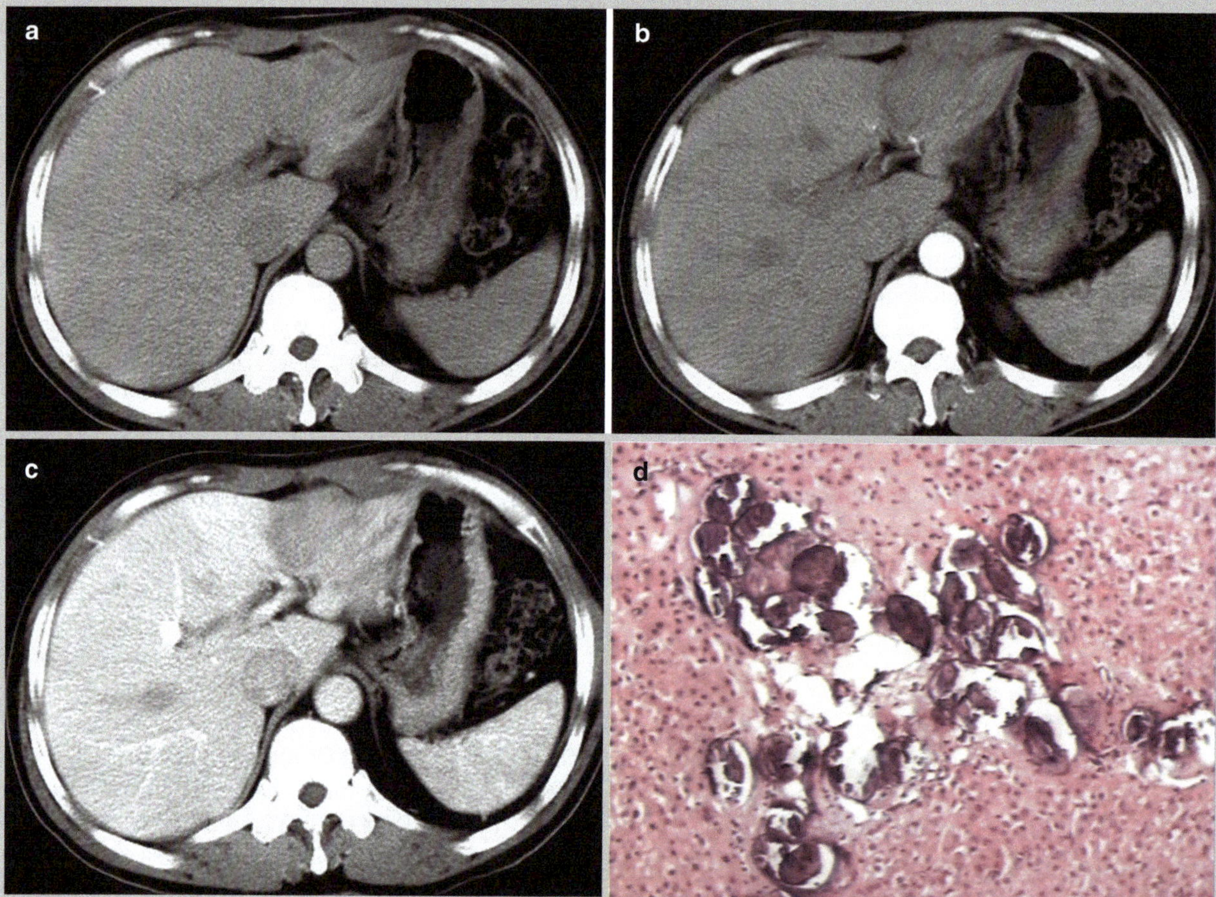

Fig. 28.1 Hepatic schistosomiasis. (**a**) Plain CT scanning demonstrates uneven low-density shadows in the left liver with poorly defined boundaries. (**b**, **c**) Contrast CT scanning demonstrates mildly uneven enhancement of the lesions in the arterial phase and portal vascular phase. (**d**) Postsurgical pathology demonstrates granuloma with accompanying deposition and calcification of schistosoma eggs

Case Study 2

A male patient aged 32 years complained of abdominal pain, aversion to cold, and fever for 2 weeks. He has a history of contact to contaminated water. His specific IgG antibody of schistosomiasis japonica was positive.

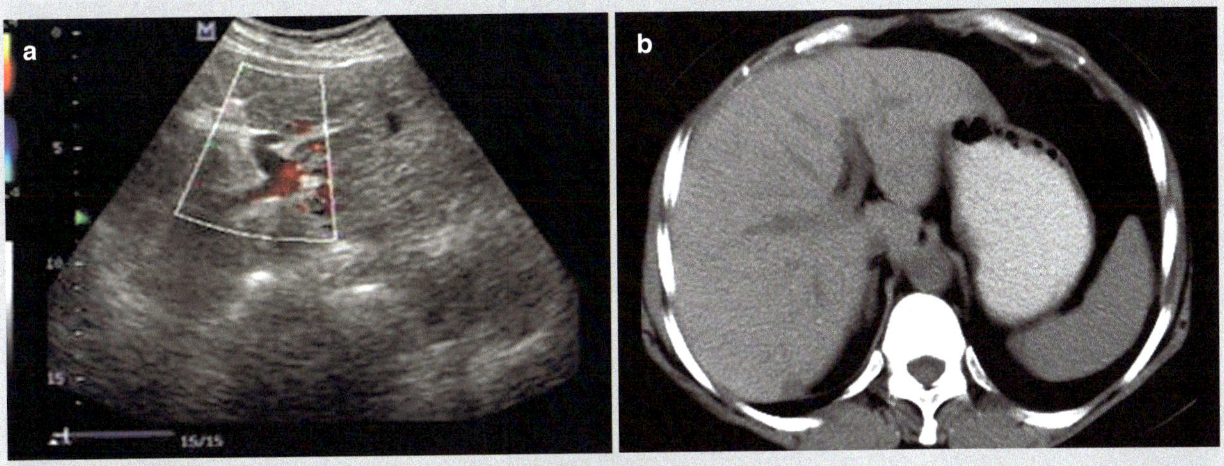

Fig. 28.2 Hepatic schistosomiasis. (**a**) Ultrasound demonstrates slightly increased echoes from the liver parenchyma, with thick and large light spots, and clear tubular network. (**b**) Plain CT scanning demonstrates slightly enlarged liver volume with even density

Case Study 3

A male patient aged 52 years had a medical history of schistosomiasis for more than 20 years.

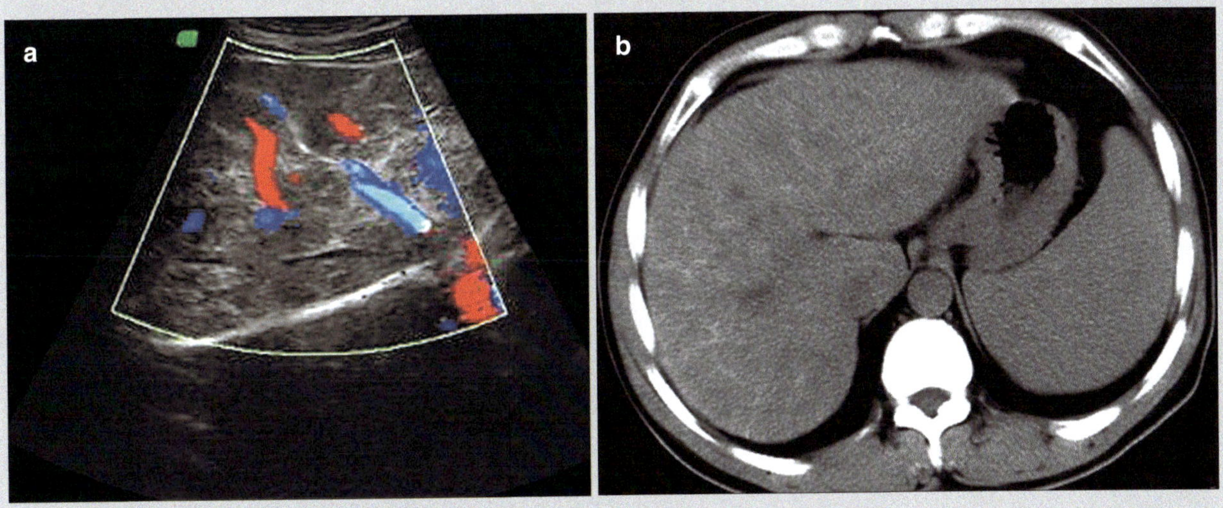

Fig. 28.3 Hepatic schistosomiasis. (**a**) Ultrasound demonstrates unsmooth Glisson's capsule, thickened but uneven echoes from the liver parenchyma with maplike appearance, and poorly defined tubular network. Plain CT scanning demonstrates enlarged liver. (**b**) The liver is demonstrated with uneven density, multiple linear calcifications in the liver parenchyma with grid-like appearance, and splenomegaly

Case Study 4

A male patient aged 64 years had a medical history of schistosomiasis for 30 years.

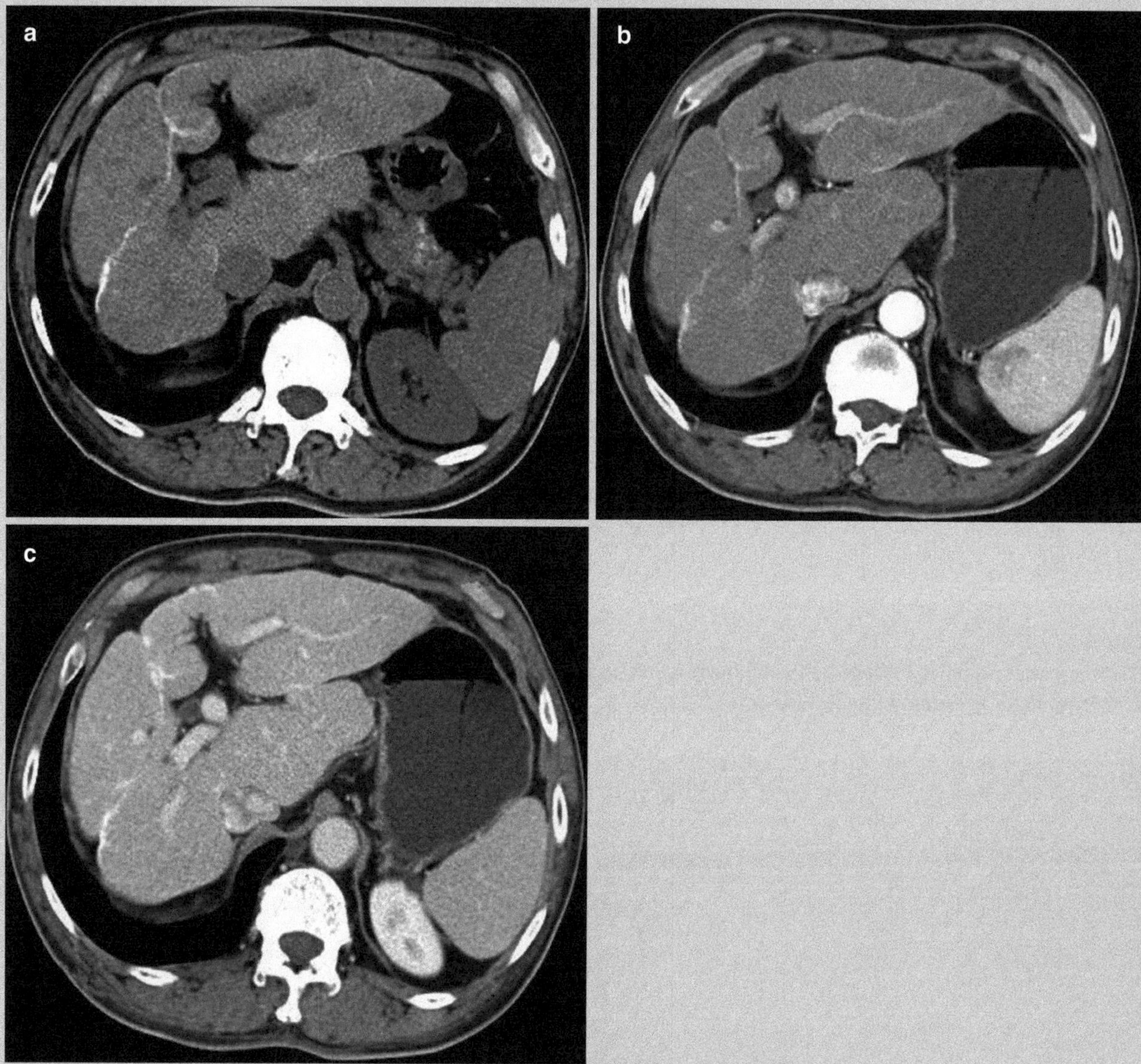

Fig. 28.4 Hepatic schistosomiasis. (**a**) Plain CT scanning demonstrates deformed liver with enlarged left and caudate lobes, increased density of the liver parenchyma, and strips of calcification at the liver and Glisson's capsule. (**b**, **c**) Contrast CT scanning demonstrates even enhancement of the liver parenchyma and linear enhancement of intrahepatic septum

Case Study 5

A male patient aged 67 years had a medical history of schistosomiasis for more than 30 years. He complained of dull pain at the middle upper abdomen for more than 10 years.

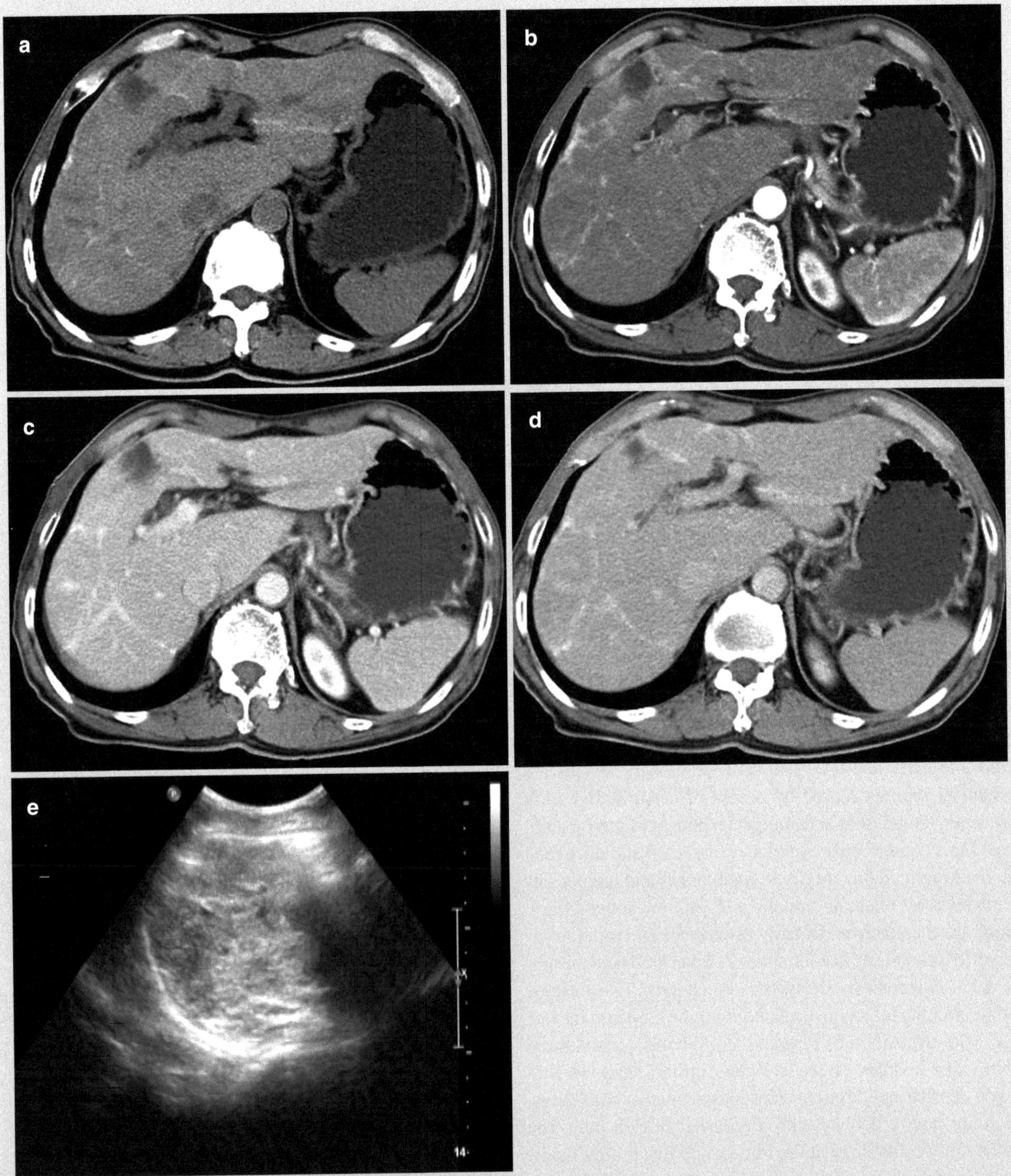

Fig. 28.5 Hepatic schistosomiasis. (**a**) Plain CT scanning demonstrates deformed liver and flakes of low-density lesions in the right liver lobe with maplike calcification. (**b**–**d**) Contrast CT scanning demonstrates no enhancement of the lesions in the right liver lobe and abnormal enhancement shadows of widened linear fibers in the liver parenchyma. (**e**) Ultrasound demonstrates thickened echoes from the liver parenchyma with maplike appearance

Case Study 6
A male patient aged 59 years had a medical history of schistosomiasis for more than 30 years.

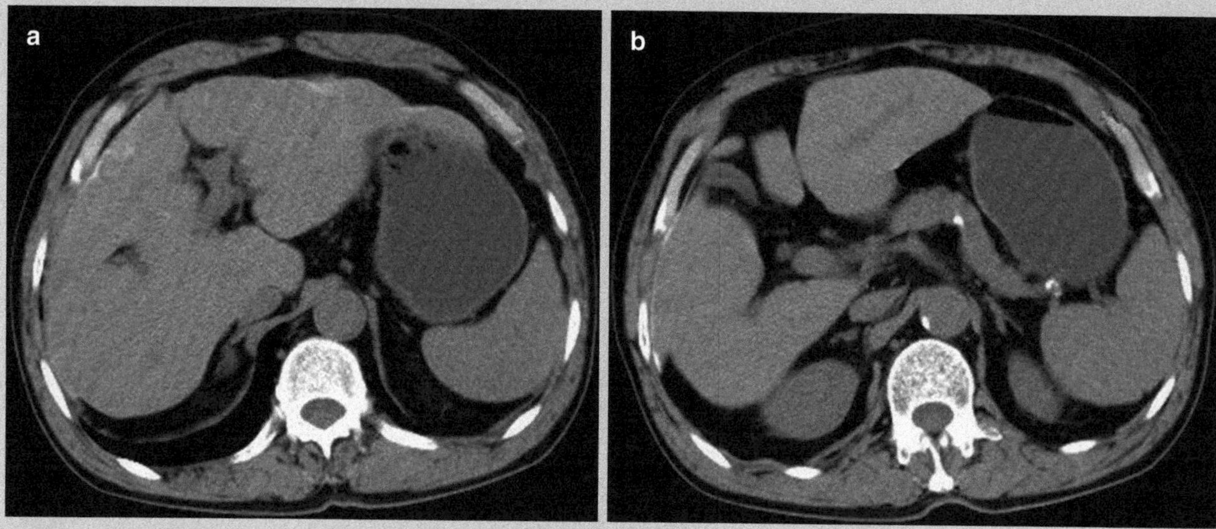

Fig. 28.6 Hepatic schistosomiasis. (**a**, **b**) Plain CT scanning demonstrates deformed liver, calcification of Glisson's capsule, and mild splenomegaly

28.7.2 Pulmonary Schistosomiasis

28.7.2.1 X-Ray Radiology

Acute Pulmonary Schistosomiasis

Pulmonary lesions caused by acute schistosomiasis can be staged into early and late. The early pulmonary lesions are mechanical injuries caused by access of cercaria and adult worms into lung tissues and allergic responses of their metabolites. Most patients only experience increased and thickened lung markings and, in rare cases, small flakes and large flakes of shadows at bilateral middle and inferior lungs. Early lesions are characterized by early occurrence and rapid residing, which commonly last for about 2–3 weeks. They are subject to misdiagnosis by delayed examinations. Two to three months after the infection, the conditions develop into the late stage, with deposition of eggs in the pulmonary interstitium to form false nodules. At the late stage, miliary shadows with uneven density and different sizes may scatter in both lungs, which are poorly defined with a diameter of 2–5 mm. The lesions mostly distribute in the middle and lower lung fields, with some fusing into flakes. The lesions have a higher central density and a light peripheral density, resembling to alveolar edema. Some lesions may also fuse into snowflake-like lesion, with a diameter of about 7–8 mm.

Chronic Pulmonary Schistosomiasis

X-ray demonstrations are nonspecific, with mainly changes of pulmonary interstitium.

Changes of Pulmonary Interstitium

The demonstrations include blurry lung markings in bilateral middle and lower lungs, with spots of shadows or network of nodular shadows.

Pulmonary Infection

The lungs are demonstrated with large flakes of dense shadows with internal fluid level and poorly defined boundaries. The shadows can also be demonstrated in patches or cloud-like, with poorly defined boundaries. Intrapulmonary flakes of shadows can also be demonstrated with well-defined boundaries, resembling to those of inflammatory pseudoneoplasm.

Pulmonary Atelectasis

The lesion is commonly found at the fundus of lungs adjacent to the diaphragmatic surface, with strip-like or plate-like dense shadow in length of 2–5 cm and width of 1–2 cm. The lesion moves along with breathing, mostly occurring in patients of ascites type.

Pleural Effusion

The demonstrations include dull costophrenic angle, infrapulmonary effusion, or confined encapsulated effusion. Sometimes, pleural effusion is the only chest X-ray demonstration of chronic pulmonary schistosomiasis.

28.7.2.2 CT Scanning

In patients with acute pulmonary schistosomiasis, micronodular shadows can be transiently demonstrated and alveolar parenchyma is rarely found. In this stage, thickened bronchial wall at the lesions can also be found.

Chronic pulmonary schistosomiasis can be demonstrated by CT scanning with fissure-shaped exudation shadows in the lung fields, multiple fibrous stripes of shadows in the lungs, and typical nodular or micronodular shadows. The nodules are commonly distributed in the middle and lower lung fields, subpleural area, or bronchial bifurcations. The nodules have central high density with poorly defined boundaries and surrounding hyaloid exudation, in halo sign (Fig. 28.7). As the course of the disease prolongs, CT scanning can also demonstrate pulmonary interstitial fibrosis and pulmonary hypertension.

Case Study 7

A male patient aged 30 years complained of cough and chest pain for 2 days. By tests and examinations, the count of eosinophilic granulocytes in the peripheral blood significantly increased, and schistosome eggs were detected in the feces.

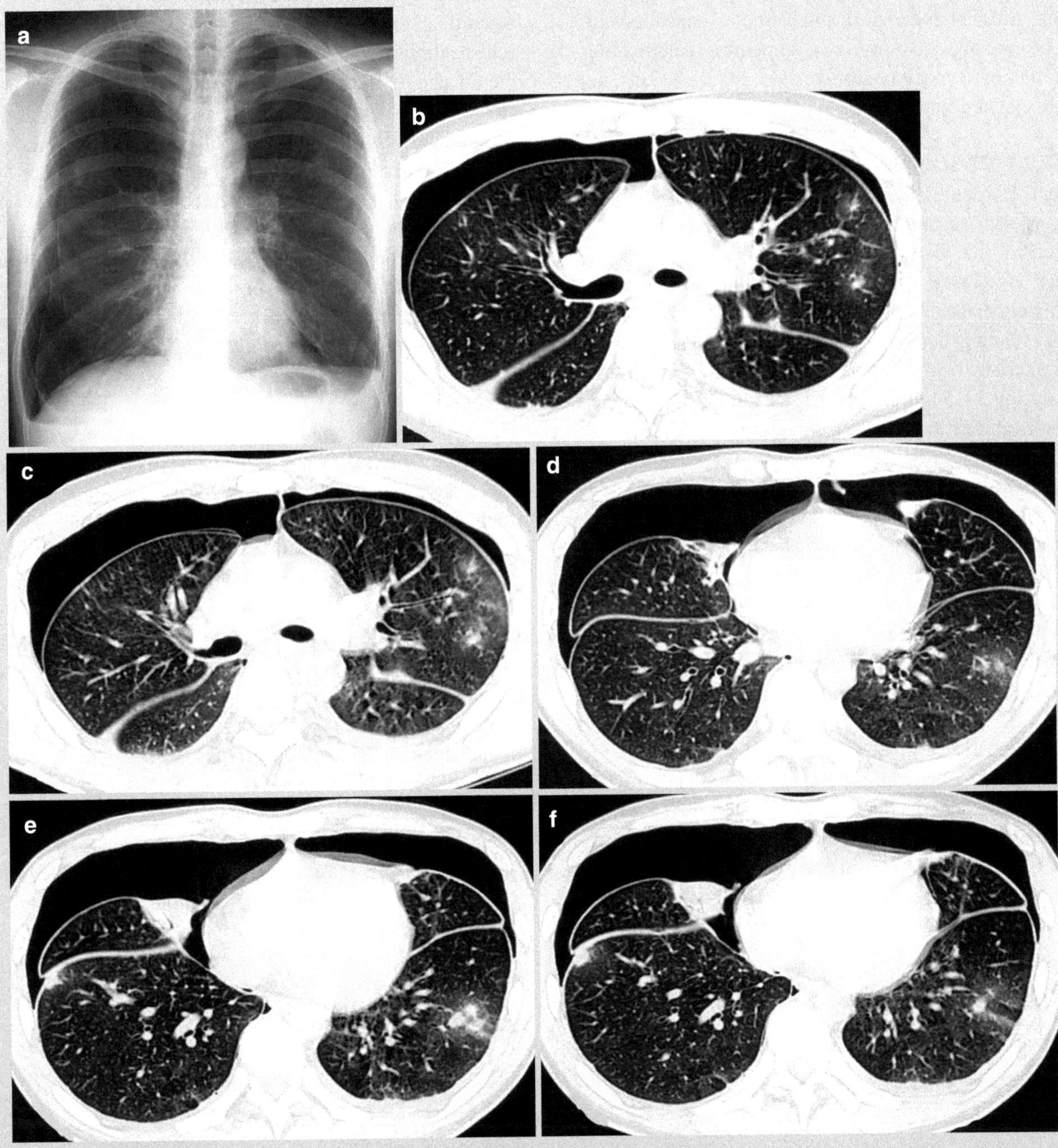

Fig. 28.7 Pulmonary schistosomiasis and pneumothorax. (**a**) X-ray demonstrates scattered patches of shadows in both lungs with poorly defined boundaries and bilateral pneumothorax. (**b–f**) Plain CT scanning demonstrates scattered nodular shadows in both lungs, with central high density and surrounding hyaloid changes, showing halo sign. There are also cord-like shadows that connect to the pleura and bilateral pneumothorax

28.7.3 Cerebral Schistosomiasis

Radiological demonstrations include multiple lesions in brain parenchyma, which are more common at the parenchyma of cerebral hemispheres, subcortex, and parietal lobe. The lesions are less commonly found at the brainstem, cerebellar hemispheres, cerebellopontine angle, and cerebral subdural space. In most cases, the main lesions are found at one certain area of the brain tissue. The lesions are multiple small nodules or nodules in different sizes that commonly fuse with each other. Contrast scanning demonstrates obvious even enhancement, with possible accompanying adjacent meningeal and vascular enhancements. In the lesions of schistosomiasis, sometimes calcification can be found in a typical target-like sign. In rare lesions, hemorrhage can be found.

28.7.3.1 CT Scanning

Plain CT scanning demonstrates low-density shadows of the lesions with surrounding low-density edema. Edema has a fingerstall-like distribution with significant space-occupying effect. By contrast scanning, the lesions are demonstrated with ring-shaped or mass-like enhancement. Dynamic contrast scanning demonstrates schistosomal granuloma with characteristic delayed enhancement, which is the most obvious during 5–15 min in delayed scanning. The characteristic demonstrations include slow enhancement and slow subsiding and fusion into masses. Perfusion CT scanning demonstrates significantly increased values of CBF, CBV, and PS of the schistosomal lesions, indicating significant vascular proliferation in the lesions, significant increased permeability, and severe damage of blood–cerebrospinal fluid barrier. In addition, MTT value is demonstrated with obvious decrease, indicating fast blood flow in the lesions, which is possibly related to the stimulation of inflammatory factors in the lesions as well as vascular dilations in the lesions.

28.7.3.2 MR Imaging

Plain MR imaging demonstrates equal or slightly low signal by T_1WI and high or slightly high signal by T_2WI, with obvious edema and space-occupying effect. Contrast imaging demonstrates various enhancements of the lesions, including nodular, sand-like, ring-like, or patchy enhancements, with multiple small nodules fusing into clusters. In the cases with enhancement at the cortex or subcortical interface between gray and white matters, there are surrounding large areas of edema, which extend toward the cortex-like fingerstall. DWI demonstrates the lesions with equal or slight high signals, which can be hardly distinguished from their surrounding edema and brain tissues. By ADC imaging, the lesions are demonstrated with increased ADC value, compared to the normal brain tissues. By eADC imaging, the lesions are demonstrated with decreased eADC value compared to the normal brain tissue.

28.7.3.3 Typing by CT and MRI

According to a series of pathological changes of cerebral schistosomiasis, some scholars have attempted to categorize the CT and MRI demonstrations of cerebral schistosomiasis. However, disagreement still exists. Peng RL et al. divided cerebral schistosomiasis into four types: encephalitis type, cerebral infarction type, granuloma type, and brain atrophy type. Sun JM et al. divided cerebral schistosomiasis into three types: encephalitis type, cerebral infarction type, and granuloma type, and they believed that localized brain atrophy is the common sequela of the above three types of cerebral schistosomiasis. We describe the detailed radiological demonstrations of each type as the following.

Encephalitis Type

This type is manifested as extensive edema of brain tissue induced by allergic responses and severe encephalitis due to toxins and metabolites secreted by schistosome eggs. No deposition of eggs can be found in the brain tissue. Plain CT plain demonstrates the lesions as low-density shadows with poorly defined boundaries. By MR imaging, the lesions are demonstrated as long T1 and long T2 signals. The lesions often involve multiple cerebral lobes and can be singular or multiple, which are more common at the parietal lobe. Contrast imaging demonstrates uneven patches of enhancement in the lesions. In the cases with pia mater involved, linear enhancement of meninges can be demonstrated (Figs. 28.8 and 28.9).

Granuloma Type

This type is the most common (Figs. 28.10 and 28.11). Based on the radiological demonstrations and the pathological findings of granuloma in the cases of cerebral schistosomiasis, Dong JN et al. further divided this type into four subtypes.

1. *Multiple small nodules type*
   The nodules have a diameter of 0.2–0.9 cm and have a scattering distribution or clusters of distribution, with no fusion of the nodules. By CT scanning and MR imaging, the cases of this type are demonstrated with stars-in-the-sky sign. The pathological basis of this type is acute nodules formed by worm eggs or small chronic nodules formed by worm eggs.
2. *Singular large nodule type*
   The singular nodule has a diameter of above 1.5 cm, with equal or slightly high density by plain CT scanning. The nodule clings to the gyrus, with a demonstration of gyrus hypertrophy. MR imaging demonstrates the nodule with equal or slightly low signal by T_1WI and slightly high signal by T_2WI. Contrast imaging demonstrates obvious uneven enhancement. Thin slice imaging demonstrates fusion of multiple small nodules with obvious enhancement into mass, which is the characteristic radiological demonstration of this type.
3. *Mixed nodule type*
   Both large nodules with a diameter of 1–3 cm and small nodules with a diameter of 0.2–0.9 cm are demonstrated with a scattering distribution. CT scanning and MR imaging demonstrate large nodules with enhancement with surrounding multiple small nodules.
4. *Nodule with ring-shaped enhancement type*
   Contrast scanning demonstrates the small lesions with a diameter of about 1 cm as ring-shaped enhancement. This type is commonly found in children, which is probably caused by deposition of schistosome eggs in the brain tissues of children that induces stronger local allergic responses than adults. And its pathological basis is probably acute egg nodules characterized by acidophilic necrosis.

Cerebral Infarction Type

This type is caused by ischemia and necrosis of brain tissues induced by worm eggs embolism or vasculitis. Plain CT scanning demonstrates fan-shaped low-density area in the brain, and MR imaging demonstrates long T_1 and long T_2 signals. The broad base is demonstrated to be attached to the inner plate of skull, with slight space-occupying effect. Contrast scanning or imaging demonstrates no enhancement or gyrus-like enhancement.

Brain Atrophy Type

Radiological demonstrations of this type are nonspecific, mainly with widened sulcus, localized dilation of ventricles. The separation of this type remains controversial. Some scholars believe brain atrophy is caused by formation of scars, some other scholars believe that the demonstrations are commonalities during prognosis of inflammatory lesions.

Case Study 8

A male patient aged 50 years complained of epileptic seizure for 2 weeks. His indirect hemagglutination test was positive and he was effectively treated by praziquantel therapy.

(Note: This case and the figures were provided by Wu WZ from Central Hospital, Jingzhou, Hubei, China.)

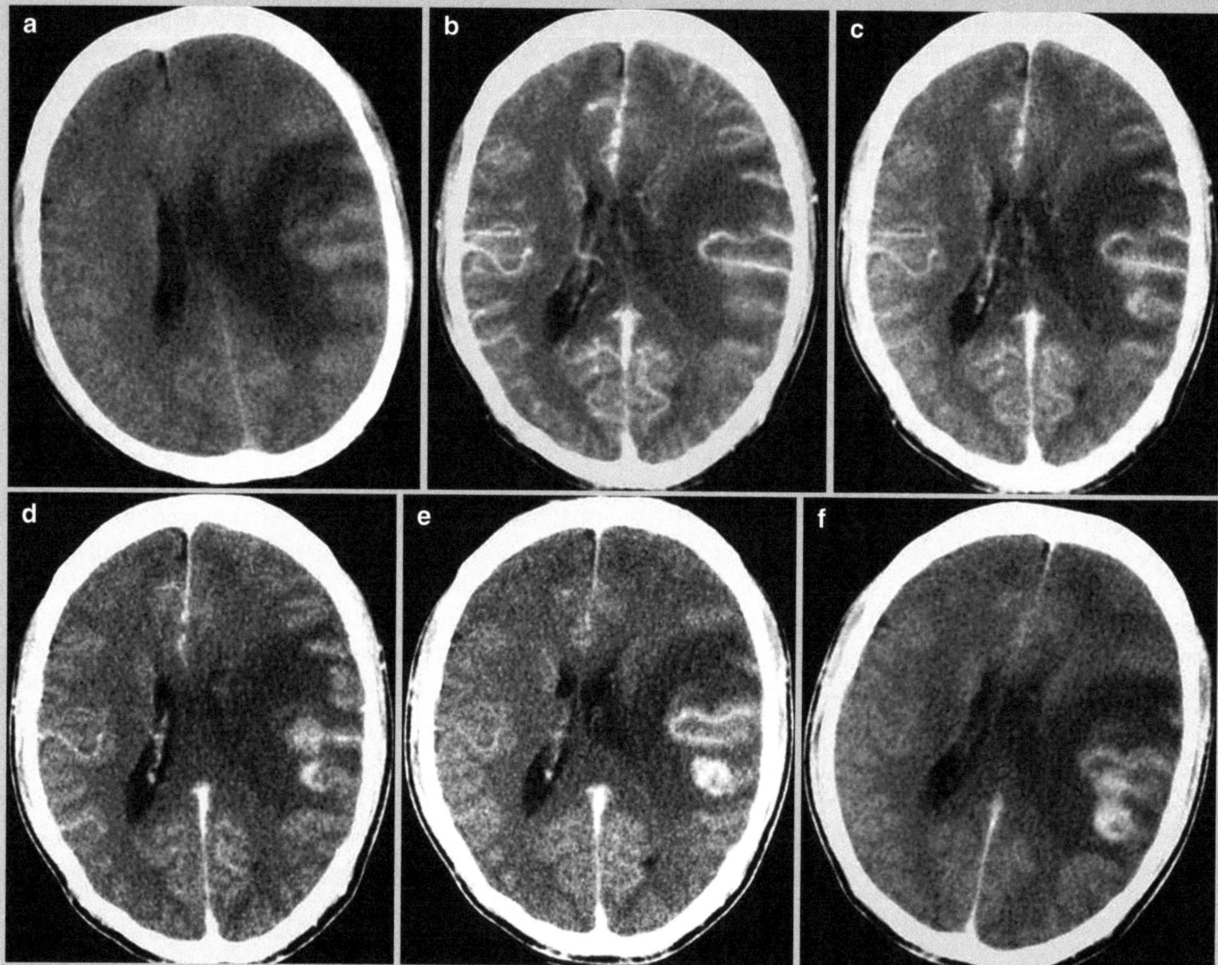

Fig. 28.8 Cerebral schistosomiasis. (**a**) Plain CT scanning demonstrates large flakes of mixed density shadows in the left temporal lobe with fingerstall-like edema. (**b**) Contrast CT scanning after 60–90 s demonstrates inflammatory congestion of the arteries, and scattering miliary spots of enhancement of the lesions. (**c**) Scanning during 2–5 min demonstrates multiple nodular enhancement of the foci in the lesions. (**d**) Scanning during 5–10 min demonstrates increased quantity of nodular lesions with enhancement and enlarged range. (**e**) Scanning during 10–15 min demonstrates significant enhancement of nodular lesions with enhancement and their fusion into mass. (**f**) Scanning during 15–20 min demonstrates gradual subsiding of the enhancement. The whole course of enhancement is characterized by slow enhancement and slow subsiding and fusion into mass

Case Study 9

A female patient aged 41 years complained of headache and nausea for 1 week. She had a history of contact to contaminated water. By ELISA for serum schistosome, the result was positive.

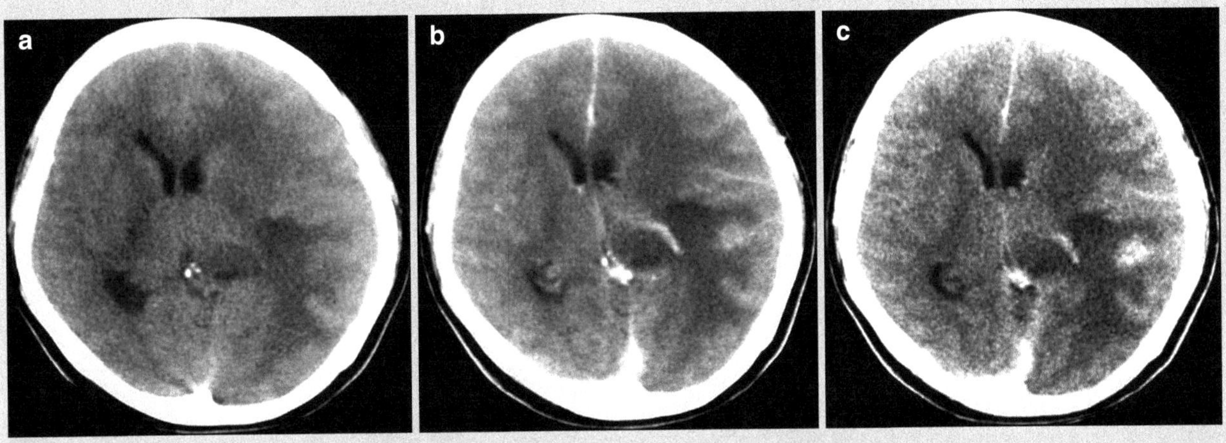

Fig. 28.9 Cerebral schistosomiasis. (**a**) Plain CT scanning demonstrates flakes of low-density areas in the left parietal lobe, deformed anterior horn of left lateral ventricle due to compression, and rightward shift of the midline structures. (**b**, **c**) Contrast CT scanning demonstrates gyrus-like enhancement

Case Study 10

A male patient aged 52 years experienced dizziness and accompanying convulsion and weakness of the left limbs. He had a history of contact to contaminated water. Circumoval precipitin test (CODT) for schistosome was positive with a titer of 1:20.

(Note: This case and the figures were provided by Liu HQ from Huashan Hospital, Shanghai, China.)

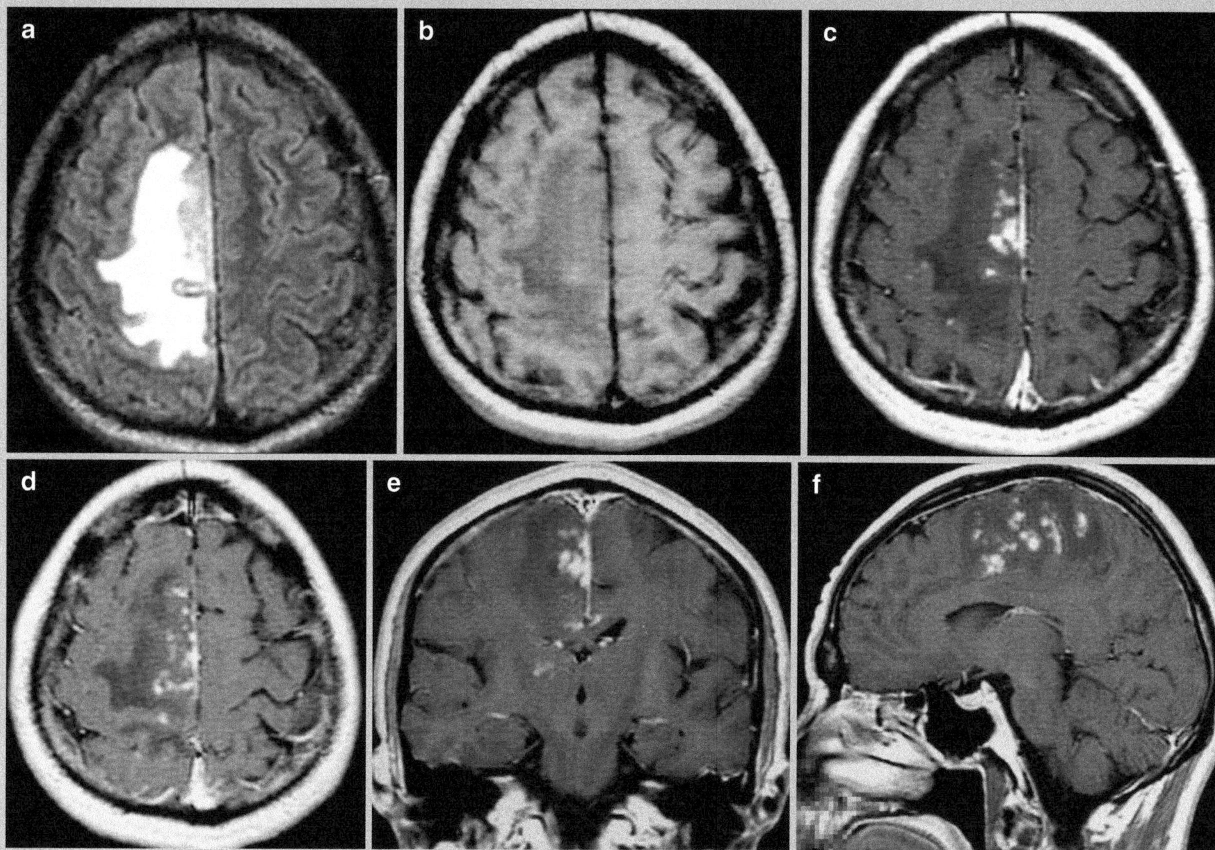

Fig. 28.10 Cerebral schistosomiasis. (**a**, **b**) By plain MR imaging, T_2WI demonstrates nodular high signal in the right parietal lobe, and T_1WI demonstrates slightly low signal, with surrounding large flakes of edema. (**c–f**) Contrast imaging demonstrates obvious spots, sand-like, and nodular enhancement of the lesions and enhancement of adjacent meninges

Case Study 11

A male patient aged 33 years complained of headache and vomiting for half a month.

Fig. 28.11 Cerebral schistosomiasis. (**a**, **b**) By MR imaging, T_2WI demonstrates multiple high-signal nodular shadows in the right parietal lobe, and T_1WI demonstrates slightly low signal. (**c**–**e**) Contrast imaging demonstrates obvious spots and nodular enhancement of the lesions. (**f**) Postsurgical pathology demonstrates granuloma of cerebral schistosomiasis

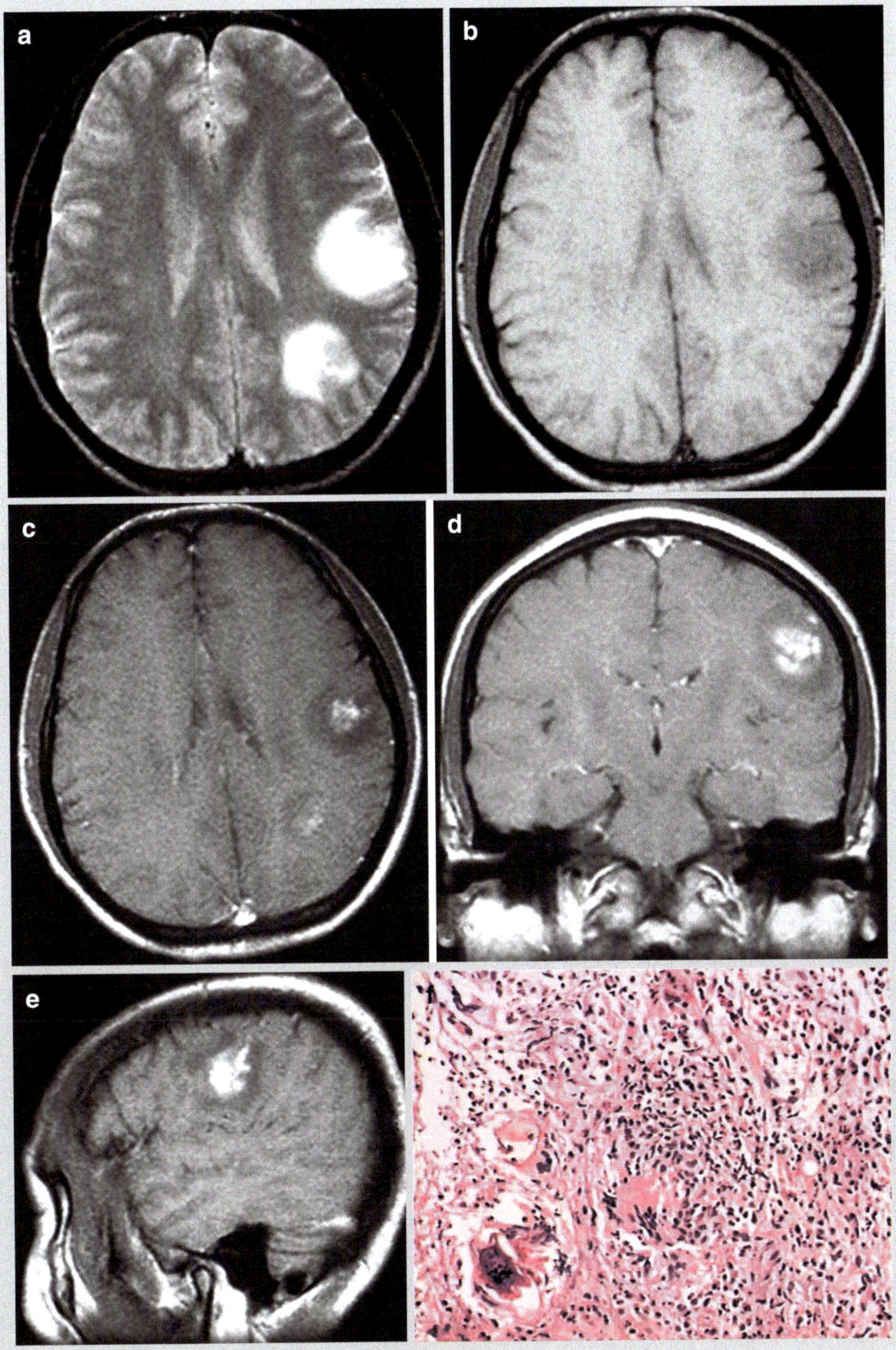

28.7.4 Spinal Schistosomiasis

Radiological examinations for spinal schistosomiasis include myelography, plain CT scanning, CT myelography, and MR imaging.

28.7.4.1 CT Scanning

CT myelography demonstrates cone enlargement or complete obstruction of CSF at the lower thoracic or lumbar segments. In some cases, transverse inflammation of the spinal cord is demonstrated with no abnormalities by routine myelography, plain CT scanning, or CT myelography. When the nerve roots of cauda equina are infected, irregular thickening or gathering adhesion can be found. In nonserious cases or cases with recent clinical symptoms, myelography and CT scanning may demonstrate no abnormalities.

28.7.4.2 MR Imaging

The lesions commonly involve medullary cone and the adjacent spinal segment. The spinal segment with lesions is demonstrated with slight swelling, with/without thickening of the cauda equina nerve roots. T_1WI demonstrates the lesions with equal or slightly low signal, while T_2WI demonstrates the lesions with slightly high signal, but the signal intensity is significantly lower than that of the spinal fluid. The medullary space is demonstrated to be narrowed and deformed due to compression. After injection of contrast agent, three types of enhancements are demonstrated: intramedullary nodule type, spinal cord periphery type, and spinal never root type. Linear and nodular enhancement of spinal cord often indicates spinal schistosomiasis. In the area with lesions, incomplete cystoid enhancement is sometimes demonstrated, which has pathologically confirmed to be necrotic tissue and incompletely disintegrated worm eggs in the cystoid enhancement area.

28.7.5 Intestinal Schistosomiasis

28.7.5.1 X-Ray Radiology

At the early stage, X-ray demonstrates no abnormalities, with manifestations of intestinal dysfunctions, and increased intestinal motility. Six to twelve hours after oral intake of barium meal, the whole colon is filled with barium, with increased tension of the intestinal canal, narrow intestinal lumen, as well as thick and deranged intestinal mucosa. Barium enema may demonstrate no abnormality. Otherwise, there are spasms of the descending colon and the sigmoid colon. At the late stage, X-ray demonstrations include:

Ulcer

The niche shadows are in different sizes in a small serration-like or grain-like shape. Serrated niches are often demonstrated at the barium-filling phase with manifestations of multiple needles protruding from enteric cavity. The scattering and shallow small ulcers are sometimes hardly demonstrated. Grain-shaped niches are the most favorably demonstrated by air-barium double-contrast examination, with spots of increased density shadows protruding out of the intestinal lumen, with a depth of 2–3 mm. The edge is commonly irregular, with scattering singular distribution or multiple dense distribution.

Mucosa Hyperplasia

Polypoid hyperplasia is very common, which is commonly found at the sigmoid colon and other intestinal parts. It is commonly scattered with a diameter of about 3–12 mm and is hardly distinguished at the filling phase. After barium evacuation, the mucosal phase has demonstrations of round-like or honeycomb-like filling defects. Air-barium double-contrast examination demonstrates fish scale-like lesions.

Enteric Lumen Stenosis

It is commonly found at the middle and lower segments of the descending colon. The stenotic part has variant lengths, generally ranging from 2 to 10 mm, and the stenotic degrees are various. The stenotic part migrates along with the normal segments, with no clearly defined borderline. In the cases with spasmodic stenosis of enteric lumen, the edge of enteric lumen is mostly smooth, and its morphology is variable. Stenosis caused by contraction of fibers is commonly demonstrated with coarse edge, and its morphology is hardly variable.

Rigid and Shortened Intestinal Canal

Rigid and shortened intestinal canal is commonly found at the inferior part of descending colon and the sigmoid colon. The involved intestinal segment disappears in bag pattern with rigid edge and confined expansion. In most cases, the mucosal striation disappears. And sometimes thick and deranged mucosa can be found. Even polypoid hyperplasia and ulceration concur. In the cases with large range of lesions, the colon is subject to shortening with round and blunt splenic flexure that migrates downward; the transverse colon is subject to straightening.

Granuloma

Granuloma of colonic schistosomiasis can develop into intraluminal and peri-intestinal lumps, with intraluminal lumps being more commonly found at the descending colon and the sigmoid colon. The demonstrations include large filling defects, possibly irregular edge and adjacent multiple small polypi. The local intestinal lumen is subject to stenosis, with its above segment dilated, which can be complicated by intestinal intussusception or intestinal obstruction. Peri-intestinal lumps are rarely found, which mostly occur at the lower abdomen or left iliac fossa. The lumps are usually large with a diameter of up to 20 cm. The lumps closely surround the intestinal canal, with rigidity of local intestinal canal.

Liver Cirrhosis

In the cases with ascites, the small intestines float, with widened space between intestinal canals. The enlarged spleen compresses the splenic flexure to migrate downward.

Cancerization

About 1–2 % cases of chronic schistosomal granuloma develops into colon adenocarcinoma. In the cases of cancerization, local mucosa is evidently destroyed with large filling defect. Large shallow niches might occur with surrounding fingerpressing sign. The lesions are abruptly defined from the adjacent intestinal segments.

28.7.5.2 CT Scanning

The worm eggs deposit at the colonic mucosa and inferior layer of mucosa. By CT scanning, linear or curved calcification can be demonstrated with a distribution along the intestinal wall. At the late stage, due to fibrosis of the intestinal wall, the intestinal wall is subject to thickening with narrowed intestinal lumen, which is the most obvious at the rectum and the sigmoid colon (Figs. 28.12, 28.13, 28.14, and 28.15).

Case Study 12

A male patient aged 53 years complained of right lower abdominal pain for 1 week.

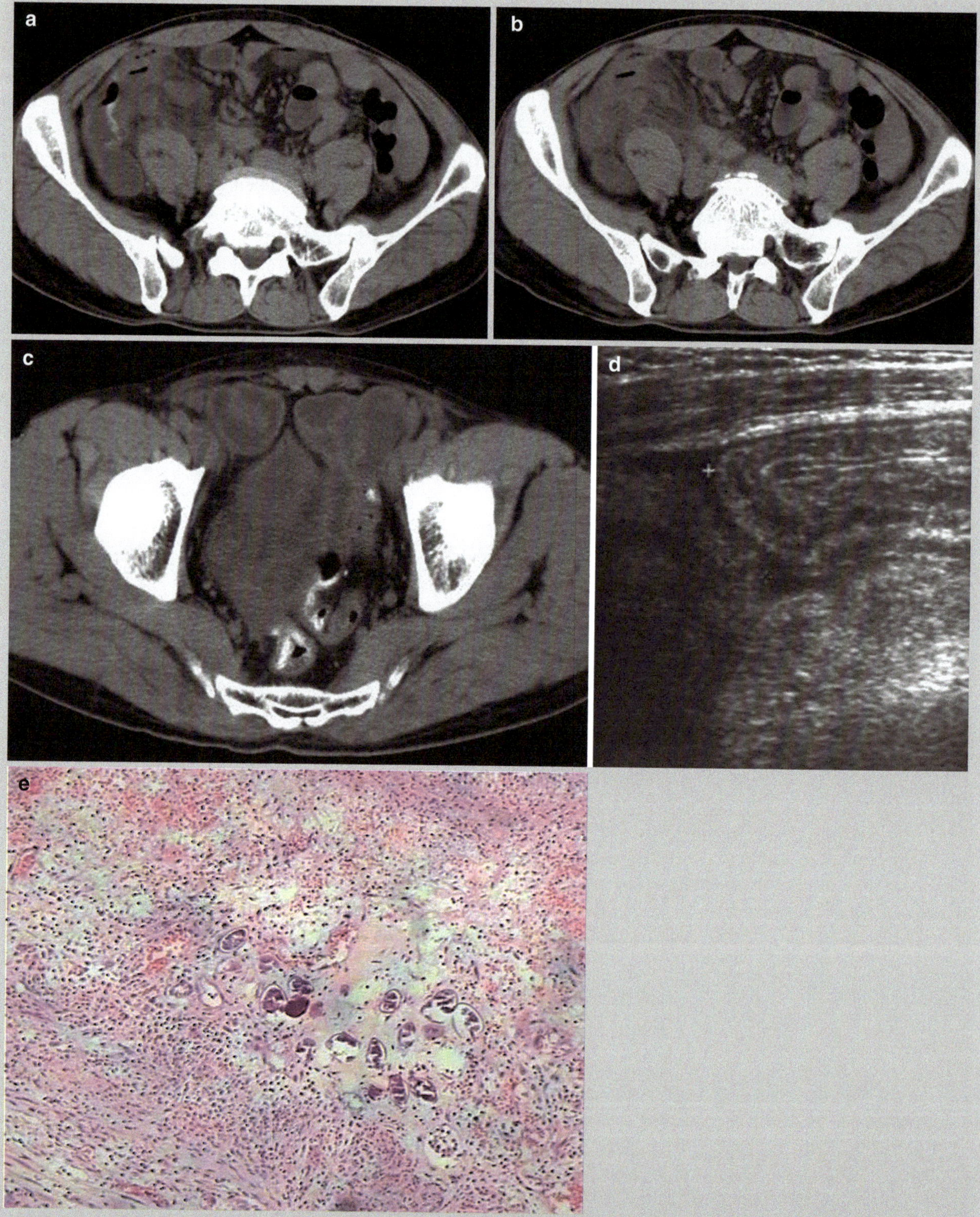

Fig. 28.12 Intestinal schistosomiasis. (**a**, **b**) Plain CT scanning demonstrates ileocecal swelling, blurry surrounding fat space, and fine strips of calcification at the intestinal wall. (**c**) Calcification is demonstrated at the intestinal wall of rectum and sigmoid colon. (**d**) Ultrasound demonstrates heterogeneous mass in the right lower abdomen with accompanying effusion. (**e**) Postsurgical pathology demonstrates acute suppurative appendicitis with accompanying deposition and calcification of schistosome eggs

Case Study 13

A male patient aged 62 years complained of abdominal distension for more than half a year.

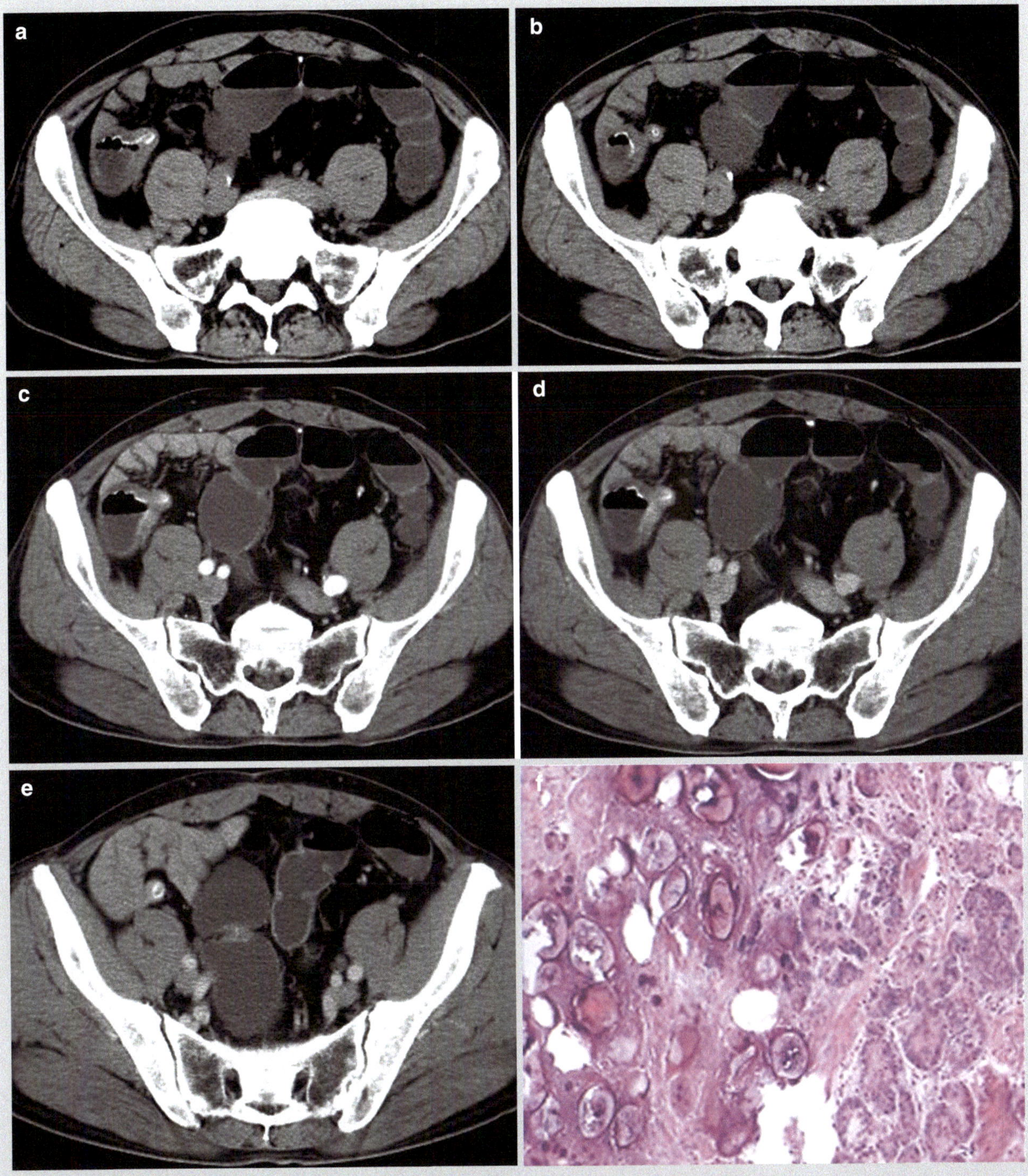

Fig. 28.13 Intestinal schistosomiasis. (**a**, **b**) Plain CT scanning demonstrates thickened intestinal wall at the ileocecal junction and appendix and accompanying calcification. (**c**–**e**) Contrast scanning demonstrates enhancement of the thickened intestinal wall and clearly defined surrounding fat space. (**f**) Postsurgical pathology demonstrates moderately to poorly differentiated adenocarcinoma at the ileocecal junction and appendix, infiltrative fibrous layer with accompanying deposition, and calcification of schistosome eggs

Case Study 14

A male patient aged 59 years had a medical history of schistosomiasis for more than 30 years.

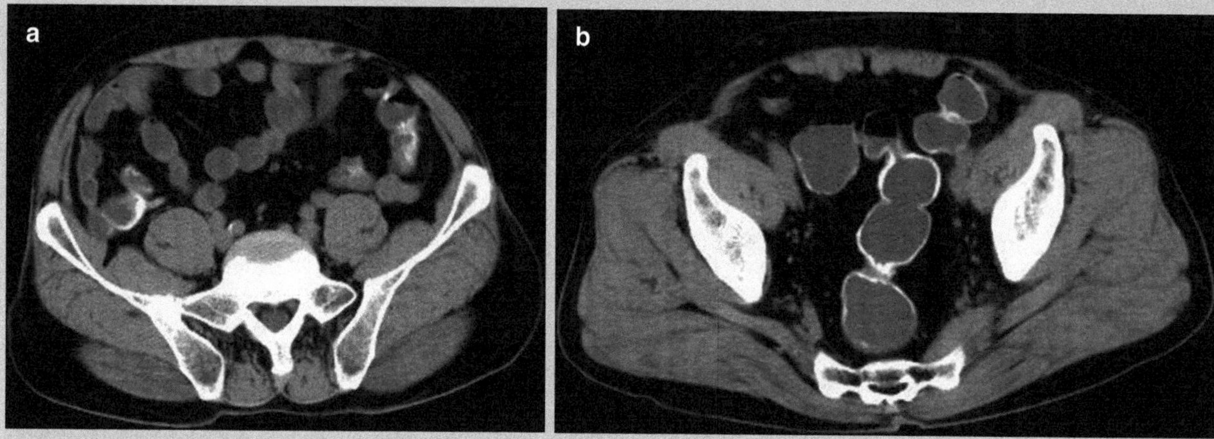

Fig. 28.14 Intestinal schistosomiasis. (**a**) Plain CT scanning demonstrates calcification at the intestinal wall of ileocecal junction, appendix, and descending colon. (**b**) Calcification is demonstrated at the intestinal wall of rectum and sigmoid colon

Case Study 15

A male patient aged 67 years complained of left lower abdominal pain for 1 month. He reported left lower abdominal pain 1 month ago with no known causes, which was persistent dull pain. At that time, he experienced no fever, jaundice, acid regurgitation, belching, diarrhea, hematemesis, and melena. In addition, he also experienced no discharges of feces or gas via the anus. However, he did not consider it serious. About 1 week ago, his abdominal pain aggravated, for which he paid clinic visit to a local hospital and received anti-infection and fluid replacement therapies. After treatment, his abdominal pain was relieved and abdominal CT scanning demonstrated lump at the posterior peritoneum which reminded him of a medical history of schistosomiasis 40 years ago with improved conditions after treatment. The patient was then hospitalized and received exploratory laparotomy. During the operation, a lump was found under the mesentery of terminal ileum, with a size of 4 cm×3 cm, which was hardened with poorly defined boundary and intact root. The lump was preliminarily diagnosed as appendiceal mass. The postsurgical pathology by frozen paraffin embedding defined the diagnosis of appendicular schistosomiasis.

(Note: The case and the figures were provided by Tang YH from Ruijin Hospital, Shanghai, China.)

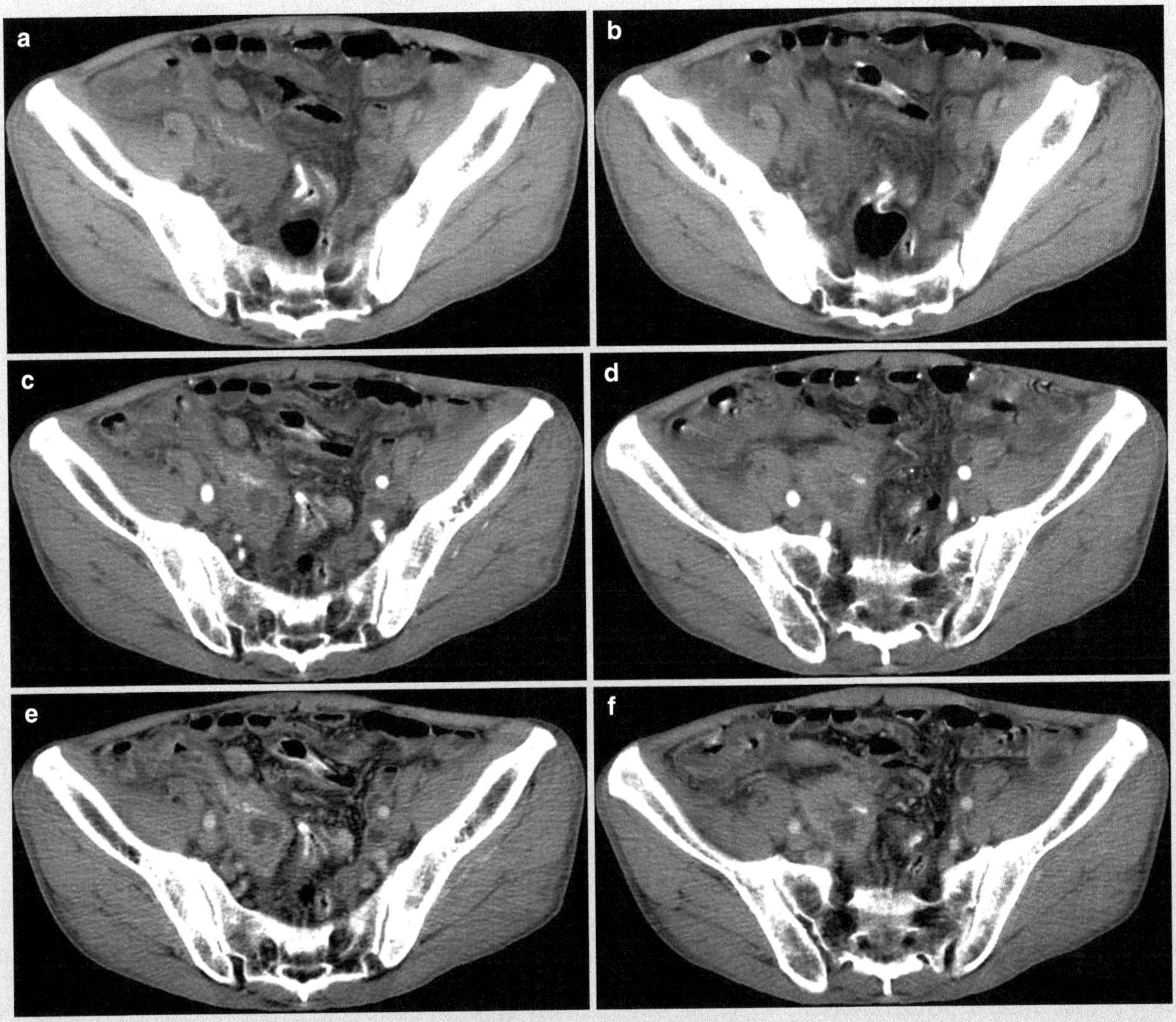

Fig. 28.15 Appendicular schistosomiasis. (**a**, **b**) Plain CT scanning demonstrates spindle-shaped lump in the pelvic cavity with soft tissue density, which has coarse boundary and uneven density. In the lump, strips of high-density shadows can be observed. (**c**–**f**) Contrast scanning demonstrates uneven enhancement of the lesions. In the lesions, irregular areas with no enhancement can be observed

28.8 Diagnostic Basis

28.8.1 Epidemiological History

A history of contact to schistosome contaminated water is an essential condition for the diagnosis.

28.8.2 Clinical Manifestations

The patients may experience symptoms and signs of acute, chronic, or advanced schistosomiasis, such as fever, dermatitis, urticaria, abdominal pain, diarrhea, and hepatosplenomegaly.

28.8.3 Laboratory Tests

In the cases with living eggs or hatched miracidia detected in feces, the diagnosis can be defined. The positive rate of detecting schistosome by rectum mucosa biopsy is very high. In the cases of acute schistosomiasis, the hemogram is characterized by significant increase of eosinophilic granulocytes.

28.8.4 Diagnostic Imaging

28.8.4.1 Hepatic Schistosomiasis

At the advanced stage of hepatic schistosomiasis, in addition to general symptoms of liver cirrhosis, there are also hepatic capsule calcification, maplike calcification at the liver parenchyma, low-density lesions at the intrahepatic portal area and central vascular shadows, septal enhancement at the parenchyma, and calcification of portal system and colon wall, which are highly characteristic. Such findings facilitate its diagnosis.

28.8.4.2 Pulmonary Schistosomiasis

At the early stage, X-ray radiology demonstrates flakes of shadows or military lesions that are mostly located at the middle and lower lung fields. At the advanced stage, old and new irregular flakes of shadows are demonstrated, with uneven densities or high densities and well-defined boundaries. Even pulmonary interstitial fibrosis can be observed.

28.8.4.3 Cerebral Schistosomiasis

Plain CT scanning or MR imaging demonstrates intracranial singular or multiple lesions, which are mainly located at the cortex or subcortex. The lesions are demonstrated with low density or with long T_1 and long T_2 signals. By contrast scanning or imaging, the lesions are demonstrated with diversified enhancements.

28.8.4.4 Spinal Schistosomiasis

The medullary cone expands, with the diseased spinal segment with equal or high signals. Contrast imaging demonstrates linear or nodular enhancement of the diseased spinal segment.

28.8.4.5 Intestinal Schistosomiasis

At the advanced stage, X-ray demonstrates ulceration of the intestinal wall, stenosis of intestinal lumen, rigidity and shortening of the intestinal canal, as well as granuloma.

28.9 Differential Diagnosis

Hepatic, pulmonary, cerebral, and spinal schistosomiasis should be differentiated from the following diseases.

28.9.1 Hepatic Schistosomiasis

28.9.1.1 Acute Hepatic Schistosomiasis

Typhoid Fever

In the cases of typhoid fever, the level of eosinophilic granulocytes significantly decreases or even be absent. The Widal's reaction is positive, and the cultures of blood and bone marrow demonstrate typhoid bacillus.

Amebic Liver Abscess

Amebic liver abscess is clinically characterized by fever and hepatalgia. In the feces collected from patients, amoeba trophozoite can be detected. Ultrasound or CT scanning demonstrates liquid space-occupying effect in the liver. By liver puncture, typical chocolate-like pus can be detected.

28.9.1.2 Chronic Schistosomiasis

Anicteric Viral Hepatitis

The patients experience loss of appetite, fatigue, hepatalgia, and obvious abnormalities by biochemical examination of the liver and no increase of eosinophilic granulocytes. Positive finding by etiological examination for hepatitis facilitates the differential diagnosis.

Amebic Dysentery and Chronic Bacillary Dysentery

In patients with schistosomiasis, those experience diarrhea and bloody stool are demonstrated with hatched miracidia, which are in a large quantity. In the patients with amebic dysentery, the feces can be detected with amoeba trophozoites. In patients with chronic bacillary dysentery, mucosa lesions can be observed directly by sigmoidoscopy, and specimens can be collected for culture, which facilitates the diagnosis.

28.9.1.3 Advanced Schistosomiasis

Schistosomal Liver Cirrhosis Should Be Differentiated from Cirrhosis Following Hepatitis

In the cases with cirrhosis after hepatitis, the liver is mostly subject to shrinkage, with more common occurrence of relatively enlarged caudate lobe. The liver edge is subject to homogeneously localized protrusion, with a diameter of less than 1 cm. No calcification can be found under the Glisson's capsule or in the liver parenchyma. However, in the cases of schistosomal liver cirrhosis, enlarged left liver lobe is more common. The liver edge is subject to heterogeneously localized protrusion, and multi-morphous calcifications are found under the Glisson's capsule or in the liver parenchyma. In combination to the clinical history, the differential diagnosis can be defined.

Primary Hepatic Carcinoma

Both the diseases are demonstrated with nodular low-density lesions. By contrast scanning or imaging, hepatic schistosomiasis is demonstrated with enhancement of the liver edge at the venous phase, and no obvious enhancement at the delayed phase. However, primary hepatic carcinoma is demonstrated with rapid increase and decrease with heterogeneous enhancement. In combination to other manifestations of hepatic schistosomiasis such as intrahepatic calcification, schistosomal liver cirrhosis, and low-density lesions in the portal area with central vascular shadows, the differential diagnosis can be defined. The diagnosis of schistosomal liver cirrhosis complicated liver carcinoma should be paid focused attention.

28.9.2 Pulmonary Schistosomiasis

The radiological demonstrations of pulmonary schistosomiasis are nonspecific. The demonstrations by X-ray and CT scanning are hardly distinguishable from acute military tuberculosis, pediatric lobar pneumonia, and bronchitis. In both epidemic area and nonepidemic area, the history of traveling as well as the clinical and laboratory data should be carefully collected and analyzed. In combination to radiological demonstrations, the conditions should be comprehensively assessed for the diagnosis.

28.9.3 Cerebral Schistosomiasis

Clinical and imaging manifestations of granuloma type of cerebral schistosomiasis resemble to those of intracranial space-occupying lesions. Therefore, cerebral schistosomiasis should be differentiated from the following diseases.

28.9.3.1 Glioma

After granulomas of schistosomiasis integrate with each other into a mass, the mass extremely resembles to malignant glioma. However, malignant glioma has more obvious space-occupying effect. By contrast scanning or imaging, irregular ring-shaped and lacelike enhancement of the lesions are demonstrated. Moreover, malignant glioma has rapid development of clinical conditions. All these findings facilitate the differential diagnosis.

28.9.3.2 Cerebral Cysticercus Granuloma

The locations commonly with lesions as well as the pathological changes of both diseases are similar. By MR imaging, nodular granuloma in the cases of cerebral cysticercus granuloma is demonstrated with obvious surrounding edema and enhancement. However, its lesion is commonly singular, involving a small range. In addition, in combination to serum antibody positive in the cases of cerebral cysticercus granuloma, the differential diagnosis can be defined.

28.9.3.3 Metastatic Tumor

The lesions are commonly singular or multiple nodules at the subcortex, possibly with central necrosis, cystic degeneration, hemorrhage, and no tendency to fusion. Clinically, the patients are commonly at an elderly age with a medical history of primary malignancies.

28.9.3.4 Cerebral Tuberculosis

The differentiation should be based on clinical symptoms and medical history. Cerebral tuberculosis is manifested clinically as small and singular tuberculous granuloma in the brain parenchyma, which is demonstrated with even or ring-shaped enhancement by contrast imaging. In the cases with multiple fused tuberculous granuloma, the lesions are demonstrated with beads-like or plum-shaped enhancement, with relatively regular boundary. Concurrently, there are accompanying hydrocephalus and abnormal meningeal enhancement at the basal cistern.

28.9.4 Spinal Schistosomiasis

28.9.4.1 Intramedullary Neoplasm

Intramedullary neoplasms such as ependymoma or astrocytoma have slow onset, and comparatively slight spinal dysfunction than those demonstrated by MR imaging. T_1WI commonly demonstrates abnormal signals of substantial space-occupying lesions or cystic degeneration with obvious space-occupying effect. By contrast imaging, enhancement of the spinal surface and arachnoiditis are rarely demonstrated.

28.9.4.2 Myelitis

Most cases of myelitis have acute onset and severe spinal dysfunction. MR imaging demonstrates multiple patches of long or equal T_1 and long T_2 signals at the thickened spinal cords. Contrast MR imaging demonstrates presence/absence of small flakes of enhancement, with rare occurrence of cystoid enhancement. The symptoms of arachnoiditis are rarely found.

Suggested Reading

Dong JN, Shi ZR, Wu HM, et al. CT scanning and MR imaging demonstrations of cerebral schistosomial granuloma and their categorization. Chin J Radiol. 2004;38(2):144–8.

Du CZ, Qiang YQ. Clinical manifestations and radiological demonstrations of pulmonary schistosomiasis. J Pract Radiol. 2006;22(11):1410–1.

Huang LX, Deng WC, Sun KY, et al. Ultrasonographic analysis of the liver in the cases of schistosomiasis japonica. Chin J Schistosomiasis Control. 2005;17(3):196–7.

Lei HW, Liu SY, Tao XF, et al. Advances in pathological and radiological studies on cerebral schistosomiasis. J Pract Radiol. 2007;23(8):1130–2.

Liu HQ, Chen YJ. Radiological diagnosis by MRI for cerebral schistosomiasis. Chin J Radiol. 2002;36(9):821–3.

Liu T, Song MF, Dong JS, et al. CT scanning and pathological demonstrations of the abdomen in the cases of chronic schistosomiasis. Chin J Radiol. 2005;39(11):1188–91.

Ma YL, Li LJ. Studies of infectious diseases. Shanghai: Shanghai Science and Technology Press; 2011.

Nascimento-Carvalho CM, Moreno-Carvalho OA. Neuroschistosomiasis due to Schistosoma mansoni: a review of pathogenesis, clinical syndromes and diagnostic approaches. Rev Inst Med Trop Sao Paulo. 2005;47(4):179–84.

Ren GH. Clinical studies of schistosomiasis. Beijing: People's Medical Publishing House; 2009.

Sliva LCS, Pereira ACF, Queiroz LC, et al. Disagreement between ultrasound and magnetic resonance imaging in the identification of schistosomal periportal fibrosis. Mem Inst Oswaldo Cruz. 2006;101 Suppl 1:279–82.

Waldman AD, Day JH, Shaw P, et al. Subacute pulmonary granulomatous schistosomiasis: high resolution CT appearances-another cause of the halo sign. Br J Radiol. 2001;74(887):1052–5.

Wu WZ, Du XH. Diagnostic value of delayed repeated spiral CT scanning for cerebral schistosomial granuloma: a report of 49 cases. J Pract Radiol. 2002;18(7):574–7.

Yeng SJ, Ren H. Studies of infectious diseases. Beijing: People's Medical Publishing House; 2011.

Zhang YY, Luo X, Feng J, et al. CT scanning demonstrations of hepatic lesions in the cases of chronic schistosomiasis: a report of 108 cases. J Pract Radiol. 2006;22(4):505–6.

29 Malaria

Li Li and Xiaochun Zhang

Malaria is an insect-borne infectious disease caused by infection of plasmodium via bites of anophelines. It is clinically characterized by repeated occurrence of periodic chills, high fever, headache, sweating, anemia, and splenomegaly. Tertian malaria and quartan malaria commonly recurs. Fever in the cases of malignant malaria is commonly irregular, with serious conditions, and may cause pernicious attacks such as cerebral malaria. Malaria ranks the first of fatal parasitic diseases in the world, with 300–500 million new cases per year, 3 million death cases per year. The pediatric cases are totally about 1 million. Malaria prevails in tropical and subtropical regions. In China, it prevails mainly in Yunnan, Hainan, and Guangdong provinces as well as in Guangxi Zhuang Autonomous Region. In the non-malaria-affected areas, the cases are mainly input malignant cases due to tourism, drug use, and blood transfusion.

29.1 Etiology

The pathogen of malaria is plasmodium, which parasitizes in the erythrocytes. There are four types of human pathogenic plasmodium, including *Plasmodium vivax*, *P. ovale*, *P. malariae*, and *P. falciparum*. *Plasmodium vivax* is the most commonly found pathogen, followed by *P. falciparum*. *P. ovale* and *P. malariae* are rarely found pathogens of malaria. The growth and development of plasmodium need two hosts, asexual reproduction in human and sexual reproduction in mosquito. Thus, human is its intermediate host, and mosquito is its terminal host.

L. Li (✉)
Department of Radiology, Beijing You'an Hospital,
Capital Medical University, Beijing, China
e-mail: sycrbyxx@126.com

X. Zhang
Department of Radiology,
The First Affiliated Hospital (Xinan Hospital),
The Third Military Medical University, Chongqing, China

29.1.1 Plasmodium in Human Body

The development and reproduction of plasmodium in human body can be divided into two stages: exoerythrocytic stage and erythrocytic stage.

29.1.1.1 Exoerythrocytic Stage

The infective sporozoites parasitizing in female anophelines are introduced into human body along with its salivary secretions at bites. Within 30–60 min, the sporozoites consecutively gain their access into the hepatic parenchymal cells along with the blood flow for schizogony to form tissue schizonts and stationary paulospores. The tissue schizonts continue their schizogony and develop into exoerythrocytic schizont (cryptozoite). This period, for *Plasmodium vivax*, lasts for about 8 days; for *P. falciparum*, 6 days; for *P. malariae*, 11–12 days; and for *P. ovale*, about 9 days. The mature merozoites overflow from the ruptured hepatocytes, and most of them are engulfed by macrophages after entering into the blood flow. And a small part of mature merozoites invade the erythrocytes after their binding with specific receptors on the erythrocytic membrane. Paulospores are only detected in recurrent infection of *P. vivax* and *P. ovale*. They are in stationary state for 6–10 months after the initial infection into the blood flow, and during this period, no clinical symptoms occur. After paulospores develop into tissue schizonts and release mature merozoites, the clinical symptoms reoccur. *P. malariae* and *P. falciparum* have no bradysporozoites and, therefore, no recurrence of their infection.

29.1.1.2 Erythrocytic Stage

After the merozoites escape from the ruptured hepatic cells to enter the erythrocytes, they develop into early trophozoites (malarial rosette), late trophozoites, immature trophozoites, and mature trophozoites. A schizont contains several to dozens of merozoites. The merozoites and their metabolites are released from the ruptured erythrocytes that they parasitize to cause the clinical onset of typical malaria. The released merozoites further invade the noninfected erythrocytes and

H. Li (ed.), *Radiology of Infectious Diseases: Volume 2*, DOI 10.1007/978-94-017-9876-1_29

begin another cycle of asexual reproduction. Correspondingly, periodic onsets are clinically found. A schizogony cycle in erythrocytic stage is about 48 h for both *P. vivax* and *P. ovale*, 24–48 h for *P. falciparum*, and about 72 h for *P. malariae*. The relatively fixed schizogony cycles of different plasmodia cause interval differences of clinical onsets, which facilitates to define the type of malaria.

29.1.2 Plasmodium in Mosquito

After the gametophytes are introduced into the body of female anopheline at their bites and stings, they begin their sexual reproduction to form infective sporozoites, which can actively move into the saliva gland of anopheline. When the anopheline bites again, the sporozoites gain their access into human body to continue their asexual reproduction cycle.

29.2 Epidemiology

29.2.1 Epidemiological Features

Malaria mainly prevails in tropical and subtropical zones, followed by the temperate zone, whose spread is closely related to the ecological environment factors. Infection of *P. vivax* has the most widely epidemic area, with infection of *P. falciparum* mainly prevailing in the tropical areas. Both infections of *P. malariae* and *P. ovale* are relatively rare. Apart from the mixed infections of *P. vivax* and *P. falciparum* prevailing in Yunnan and Hainan provinces in China, the infection of *P. vivax* mainly prevails in other epidemic areas. The occurrence is more common in summers and autumns. But in the tropical areas, its occurrence is rarely affected by seasonal factors. In addition, many imported malaria cases have been found in China.

Malaria ranks the first in fatal parasitic diseases in the world. About 300–500 million new cases of malaria are reported each year. About 3 million death cases from malaria are reported each year, with 1 million pediatric cases that are mostly young children under the age of 5 years. In some epidemic areas of malaria, about 10 % reported deaths are pediatric patients with malaria.

29.2.2 Source of Infection

The patients with malaria and asymptomatic plasmodium carriers are sources of infection. The infectious period of *P. vivax* is 1–3 years; that of *P. malariae*, 3–10 years; and that of *P. falciparum*, within 1 year.

29.2.3 Route of Transmission

The medium for spreading of malaria is female anophelines, which spread the disease via bites and stings. Some rare cases are transmitted via transfusion of contaminated blood with plasmodium or via the route vertically from mother to child.

29.2.4 Susceptible Population

Individuals living in the non-malaria-affected areas are susceptible to malaria. In the epidemic areas with high risk of infection, individuals above the age of 25 years have certain immunity against malaria. But those under the age of 25 years are still susceptible to the disease, with the highest incidence rate in infants aged under 2 years. After the infection, the patients can acquire certain temporary immunity. No cross immunity has been found between different types of malaria.

29.3 Pathogenesis and Pathological Changes

29.3.1 Pathogenesis

29.3.1.1 Pathogenesis of Typical Malaria

After invasion of plasmodium into the blood flow, it induces mononuclear macrophages to produce a large quantity of tumor necrosis factors (TNF), interleukin-1 (IL-1), interleukin-2 (IL-2), and γ-interferon (IFN-γ), which can play their role as factors stimulating the thermoregulatory center to cause clinical symptoms of malaria. In the cases with *P. falciparum-induced* malaria, the content of TNF in the body is significantly increased. TNF can kill the plasmodium. However, it can cause the release of oxygen free radicals to induce extensive damage to the vascular endothelium and pathological changes of various tissues and organs. Consequently, the production of erythrocytes in bone marrow is inhibited, and the phagocytes are more powerfully capable of destroying both the infected and normal erythrocytes. In combination to the destructive effects of the plasmodium itself on the erythrocytes, anemia and the following series of clinical symptoms occur.

29.3.1.2 Pathogenesis of Cerebral Malaria

The extensive filling of the infected erythrocytes in the cerebral vascular vessels and their adhesion to the endothelial cells of the cerebral capillaries result in vascular occlusion to interfere the gas exchange in brain tissues, with consequent occurrence of cerebral hypoxia and metabolic disturbance. Together with the virulence of plasmodium, serious cerebral lesions finally occur, which are known as cerebral malaria.

29.3.2 Pathological Changes

The pathological changes of malaria are mainly caused by hyperplasia of the mononuclear-phagocytic system. The proliferation of the plasmodium induces strong phagocytosis in the human body. Due to multiplication of schizonts of *P. vivax* and *P. malariae* in the peripheral blood in erythrocytic stage, mononuclear phagocyte system in the whole body is subject to systemic hyperplasia, with manifestations of hepatosplenomegaly, myelosis, increased mononuclear cells in the peripheral blood, and increased level of serum globulin. The multiplication of schizonts of *P. falciparum* in erythrocytic stage mostly occurs within microvascular vessels in the organs. The infected erythrocytes often adhere to capillary endothelial cells, leading to damages to organs. The brain has the most obvious lesions, followed by kidneys and other organs.

29.3.2.1 Spleen

In the acute stage, mild to moderate enlargement of the spleen can be found, with increased tension of the spleen capsule and dark red sections. By microscopy, large quantities of plasmodium and malarial pigment can be detected in the medullary cord. The patients sustaining long-term illness or with repeated infections show significant splenomegaly, with gradual fibrosis of the spleen medullary system, which is hardened with cinereous sections and deposition of a large quantity of malarial pigments. By microscopy, diffuse fibrosis can be detected in the splenic pulp, with thickened vascular walls and blood sinus walls as well as infiltration of large mononuclear cells.

29.3.2.2 Liver

The liver can be infected by all the 4 types of plasmodium. However, *P. falciparum* causes the most serious damage to the liver, with pathological changes of enlarged liver with edema in the color of blue brick or black. The hepatic sinus and the central vein are congested, and the hepatocytes are cloudy and swelling with degeneration. The Kupffer cells proliferate in a large quantity, containing malarial pigment, fragments of erythrocytes with or without plasmodium, and a small quantity of hemosiderin.

29.3.2.3 Brain

The pathological changes in the brain are commonly found in the cases with cerebral type of *P. falciparum* malaria, including congestion of pia mater, cerebral edema, dark grayish section due to deposition of malaria pigment in the cortex, and spots of bleeding in the white matter. By microscopy, lumen expansion of small vascular vessels in the brain tissue is observable, which is filled with erythrocytes containing plasmodia to block the vascular vessels. The vascular endothelial cells are swollen with phagocytosis as well as plasmodia and pigments. Free pigments are observable in the perivascular spaces. In the white matter, small focal necrosis is found, with ring-shaped hemorrhage and malaria granuloma. In small vascular vessels of necrotic lesion, transparent microthrombosis is found. And bleeding zone surrounds the lesion of necrosis. Many Durck nodules can be found in the brain, with central necrosis and surrounding hyperplasia of microglial cells to form malaria granuloma.

29.3.2.4 Lungs

By autopsy of death cases of malaria, pulmonary edema is definitely found. The pulmonary capillaries and venules are filled with inflammatory cells, mainly including neutrophils, plasma blood cells, macrophages with pigment deposition, and erythrocytes infected by plasmodia. Edema of vascular endothelial cells causes stenosis of capillaries, pulmonary interstitial edema, and formation of glassy membrane. Secondary bronchitis is also commonly found.

29.3.2.5 Kidneys

Nephropathies in patients with *P. falciparum* malaria are characterized by acute proliferative nephritis and nephrotic syndrome, which are reversible. Immune complex renal disease occurring in the cases of *P. malariae* malaria is a chronic progressive membranous glomerulonephritis. By kidney tissue biopsy of the patients, the antigen of *P. malariae* can be detected, as well as the specific antibody of *P. malariae*. It is an immune-responsive renal disease, which is irreversible after sufficient antimalarial treatment. In some serious cases, renal failure occurs.

29.3.2.6 Heart

The myocardial capillaries are filled with infected erythrocytes, macrophages containing malarial pigments, lymphocytes, and plasma cells. Hemorrhagic petechia is rarely found under the endocardium or in the pericardium.

29.3.2.7 Bone Marrow

Due to a large quantity of destroyed erythrocytes by invasion and reproduction of plasmodia, obvious hyperplasia of bone marrow cells can be found, with consequent proliferation of erythrocytic system in a large quantity. Plasmodia in different periods of development can be found parasitizing in the erythrocytes. Immature gametophytes can be occasionally found. And schizonts can be found in the cases of *P. falciparum* malaria.

29.4 Clinical Symptoms and Signs

The incubation periods of *P. vivax* malaria and *P. ovale* malaria last for 13–15 days; the incubation period of *P. malariae* malaria lasts for 24–30 days and that of *P. falciparum* malaria, 7–12 days.

The typical symptoms of malaria are sudden chills, high fever, and profuse sweating. The chills often last for 20–60 min, followed by rapid increase of the body temperature that is commonly above 40 °C, with accompanying headache, systemic soreness and pain, fatigue, and favorable consciousness. The fever usually persists for 2–6 h, with following profuse sweating and sudden decrease of the body temperatures, which lasts for 30–60 min. At this time, the patients commonly experience subjective improved conditions but complain of fatigue and thirst. Between two episodes of malaria, regardless of its type, there is an interval period, which can be irregular in patients of early stage. However, after several attacks, the interval is gradually regular. The interval periods of *P. vivax malaria* and *P. ovale* malaria are about 48 h; that of *P. malariae* malaria is around 72 h and that of *P. falciparum* malaria, 36–48 h. The repeated attacks cause destruction of erythrocytes in a large quantity, leading to anemia and splenomegaly of different degrees.

29.5 Malaria-Related Complications

29.5.1 Cerebral Malaria

Cerebral malaria is the most common complication. The initial symptoms include high fever and chills, with accompanying severe headache, nausea, vomiting, and lethargy, delirium, systemic convulsion, and gradual development into coma. Most patients have splenomegaly, and hepatomegaly is occasionally found. Anemia is also a common symptom of cerebral malaria but in different degrees. Cerebral malaria is dangerous, with a high mortality rate.

29.5.2 Pulmonary Malaria

Pulmonary malaria refers to lung lesions caused by various types of plasmodium. Clinically, in addition to typical or atypical systemic symptoms of malaria, pulmonary symptoms predominantly occur, including malarial bronchitis, malarial pneumonia, malarial asthma, malarial interstitial pneumonia, pulmonary edema, and acute respiratory distress syndrome.

29.5.3 Malarial Nephropathies

29.5.3.1 Acute Renal Failure

High fever, profuse sweating, and insufficient water intake caused by malaria can lead to a reduction of the effective blood volume, with following increased activities of compensatory sympathetic nerves. The increased secretion of catecholamine and strong contraction of renal vascular vessels cause significantly decreased renal blood flow and consequent acute renal failure. The mild cases have manifestations of edema, oliguria, increased blood pressure as well as proteins, red blood cells, and casts in the urine specimens.

29.5.3.2 Nephrotic Syndrome

Nephrotic syndrome commonly occurs after long-term repeated attacks of *P. malariae* malaria. And it also occurs in the cases of *P. falciparum* malaria. Nephritic syndrome is cause by deposition of malarial antigen and antibody complexes in the glomerular capillary basement membrane and vascular interstitium. Clinically, it is characterized by progressive proteinuria, anemia, edema, hypertension, and even renal failure.

29.5.4 Blackwater Fever

Blackwater fever, or hemolytic uremic syndrome (HUS), is a disease characterized by microangiopathic hemolytic anemia, acute renal failure, and thrombocytopenia. Its exact pathogenesis remains elusive. But the patients with congenital lack of glucose-6-phosphate dehydrogenase are susceptible to the disease. Antimalarial medications including quinine and primaquine contribute to the occurrence of the disease, which cause acute intravascular hemolysis. Its clinical manifestations include rapid onset of chills, high fever with accompanying lower back pain and abdominal pain, and suddenly decreased volume of urine. Within several hours, dark brown hemoglobinuria can be detected. The liver and spleen are subject to rapid enlargement with accompanying tenderness. There are also hemolytic jaundice, hemolytic anemia, and liver dysfunction. In some serious cases, renal tubular necrosis occurs.

29.6 Diagnostic Examinations

29.6.1 Laboratory Tests

29.6.1.1 Blood Smear

Successful detection of plasmodium by blood smear is the basis to define the diagnosis.

29.6.1.2 Immunological Diagnosis

Immunological diagnosis is based on the detection of antigen of plasmodium or its specific antibody.

29.6.1.3 Genetic Diagnosis

By PCR technique, the DNA of plasmodium can be directly detected, which is the diagnostic examination of malaria with the highest sensitivity and the highest specificity. It is especially appropriate for large-scale epidemiological studies.

29.6.2 Diagnostic Imaging

29.6.2.1 Ultrasound

Ultrasound is mainly applied to detect the abdominal lesions of malaria.

29.6.2.2 X-Ray

X-ray is a commonly applied diagnostic imaging examination for the diagnosis of malarial pneumonia.

29.6.2.3 CT

CT scanning is a commonly applied diagnostic imaging examination for the diagnosis of malarial pneumonia.

29.6.2.4 MRI

MR imaging is a commonly applied diagnostic imaging examination for the diagnosis of malarial encephalopathy.

29.7 Imaging Demonstrations

The lesion of plasmodial infection can be found in a single organ or in multiple organs, which is related to the types of plasmodium and the course of the disease. The relationship is nonspecific.

29.7.1 Cerebral Malaria

29.7.1.1 CT Scanning

By CT scanning, brain edema is commonly demonstrated, with multiple low-density lesions and spots of hemorrhagic lesions. Patankar et al. divided CT demonstrations of cerebral malaria into the following four types: (1) no abnormal demonstrations, (2) diffusive cerebral edema, (3) diffusive cerebral edema with accompanying low-density lesions in bilateral thalamus, and (4) diffusive cerebral edema with accompanying low-density lesions in bilateral thalamus and cerebellum. The low-density lesions in the cases of the latter two types are well defined, with no demonstration of hemorrhage. Patankar et al. reported that the cases with no abnormal demonstrations by CT scanning have favorable prognosis, and the cases with lesions involving the cerebellum usually have poor prognosis. All of the 5 cases they reported are death cases. Yang C reported 1 case with symmetrical low-density lesions in bilateral globus pallidus. The patient was reported to be cured.

Case Study 1

A male patient aged 17 years was diagnosed with infection of *P. falciparum* malaria, cerebral malaria. He experienced coma, convulsions, and slight paralysis of the right limbs. By Glasgow coma scale (GCS), he was scored 6 points.

(For case detail and figures, please refer to Patankar TF et al. *Radiology*, 2002, 224 (3): 811.)

Case Study 2

A male patient aged 20 years was diagnosed with infection of *P. falciparum* malaria, cerebral malaria. His GCS was scored lower than 6 points.

(For case detail and figures, please refer to Patankar TF et al. *Radiology*, 2002, 224 (3): 811.)

29.7.1.2 MR Imaging

The MR imaging demonstration of cerebral malaria is nonspecific, with common demonstration of diffusive brain edema. In the mild cases, MR imaging demonstrates no abnormalities or slight brain swelling. By T_2WI and FLAIR, the demonstrations may include multiple high-signal lesions in the white matter beside bilateral cerebral ventricles, parietal white matter, the genu and splenium of corpus callosum, thalamus, and semioval center (Fig. 29.1). The demonstrations may also include focal infarction in the basal ganglia, thalamus, pons, and cerebellum as well as demyelination of the pons and cerebellum. Nickerso et al. reported that the sensitivity to spots of hemorrhage by SWI is higher than that by T_2WI and FLAIR. SWI can show diffusive spots lesions of hemorrhage that are hardly demonstrated by T2WI and FLAIR. The lesions may be located at the interface between the gray and white matters, corpus callosum, and internal capsule. By DWI and ADC, the lesions are demonstrated with no limited diffusion. But they reported 1 pediatric case with demonstrations of limited diffusion of the lesions. Animal experiments have demonstrated the decreased NAA peaks of the striatum and thalamus in experimental mice.

Case Study 3

A female patient aged 22 years was diagnosed with infection of *P. falciparum* malaria. She experienced fever, chills and serious mental changes, and involuntary movements. By physical examination, deep reflex hyperfunctional and no meningeal irritation can be found.

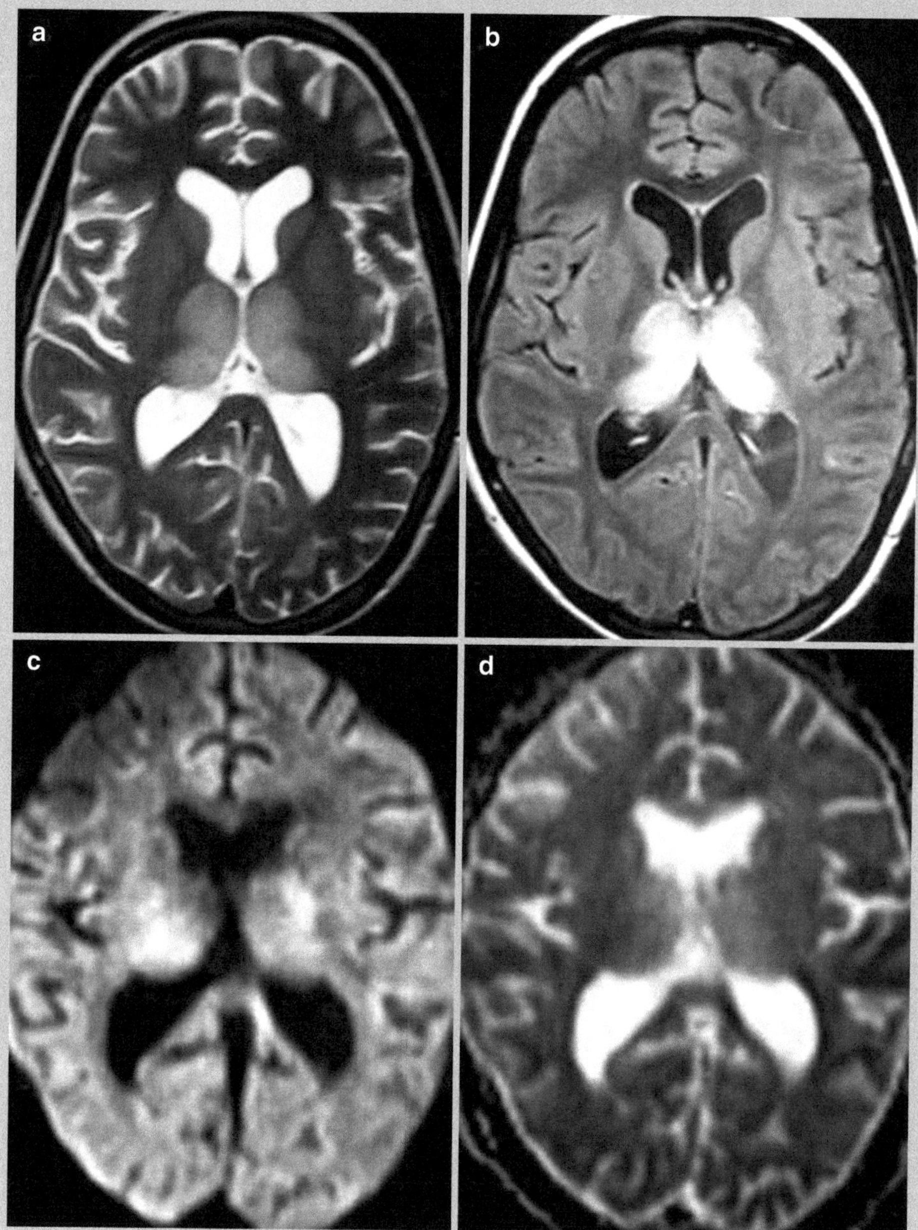

Fig. 29.1 Cerebral malaria. (**a**, **b**) Transverse T_2WI and FLAIR demonstrate symmetrical high signal in bilateral thalamus. (**c**, **d**) DWI and ADC demonstrate no limited diffusion of the lesions (Reprinted with permission from Yadav et al. 2008, 49(5):566)

Case Study 4

A male patient aged 30 years complained of headache, fatigue, and consequent coma. By GCS, he was scored 6 points. By laboratory tests, a large quantity of *P. falciparum* was detected by blood smear.

(For case detail and figures, please refer to Cordoliani YS et al. *AJNR*, 1998, 9 (5): 871.)

Case Study 5

A female patient aged 13 years was admitted to the hospital due to frequent convulsions. She suffered from malaria 1 month ago, with detected *P. falciparum* by blood smear. By neurological examination, she was normal. EEG demonstrated θ wave in the right temporal frontal lobe.

(For case detail and figures, please refer to Cordoliani YS et al. *AJNR*, 1998, 9 (5): 871.)

Case Study 6

A male patient aged 23 years was diagnosed with recurrent cerebral malaria. His GCS was scored 5.8 points. By blood smear, *P. falciparum* was detected.

(For case detail and figures, please refer to Cordoliani YS et al. *AJNR*, 1998, 9 (5): 871.)

Case Study 7

A female patient aged 31 years complained of periodic fever, chills, headache, nausea, and vomiting for 1 week. By blood smear, *P. falciparum* was detected.

(For case detail and figures, please refer to Nickerson JP et al. *AJNR*, 2009, 30 (6): e85.)

29.7.1.3 PET

The metabolic rate of glucose in the cerebral cortex diffusively decreases in experimental monkeys, but the changes in the basal ganglia are not obvious.

29.7.2 Pulmonary Malaria

29.7.2.1 X-Ray

According to different severities of the conditions, pulmonary X-ray demonstrations have great variance, which can be divided into the following five types.

Bronchitis Type

The demonstrations are commonly thickened and increased pulmonary markings in both lungs. These findings are mainly distributed in the middle and inner areas of both lower lung fields, and the findings in the outer area are usually along with interstitial changes. These demonstrations are nonspecific.

Interstitial Pneumonia Type

Concurrent with more, thickened and blurry pulmonary markings, X-ray demonstrates reticular shadow and small spots of changes in the interlobular septa. These findings are mainly distributed in the middle and outer areas. In some cases, these findings are distributed in the whole lungs (Fig. 29.2).

Bronchial Pneumonia Type

X-ray demonstrates the type with patches of blurry shadow in the thickened lung markings of both lower lung fields.

Lobar Pneumonia Type

X-ray demonstrates large flakes of cloudy high-density shadows that are distributed in pulmonary lobes or segments. The consolidation of pulmonary segments is characterized by lesions at the fundus (Fig. 29.3).

Pulmonary Edema Type

For the demonstrations, see Fig. 29.4. In addition, pleural thickening and pleural effusion can also be observable.

Case Study 8

A male patient aged 37 years complained of fever and cough for 10 days. By blood smear, plasmodia were detected positive.

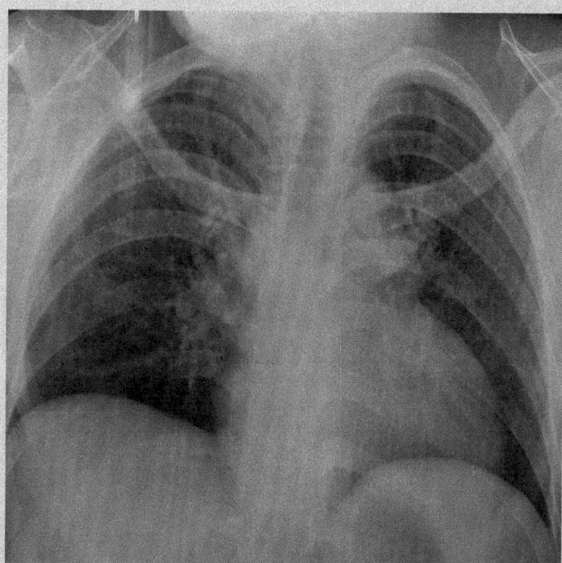

Fig. 29.2 Pulmonary malaria (interstitial pneumonia type). X-ray demonstrates more thickened and blurry lung markings in both lungs as well as reticular and small spots of shadows with increased density

Case Study 9

A boy aged 3.6 years complained of high fever and shortness of breath for 6 days. By blood smear, plasmodia were detected positive.

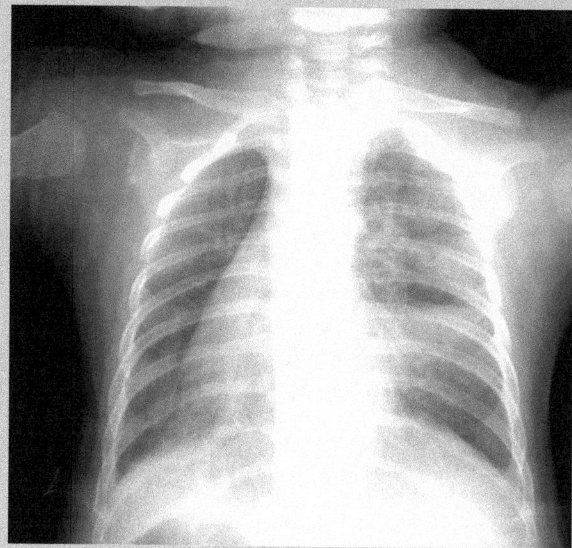

Fig. 29.3 Pulmonary malaria (lobar pneumonia type). X-ray demonstrates wedge-shaped dense shadow in the right middle lung lobe, with quite straight boundary

Case Study 10

A male patient aged 40 years complained of fever and paroxysmal dyspnea for 1 day. By blood smear, plasmodia were detected positive.

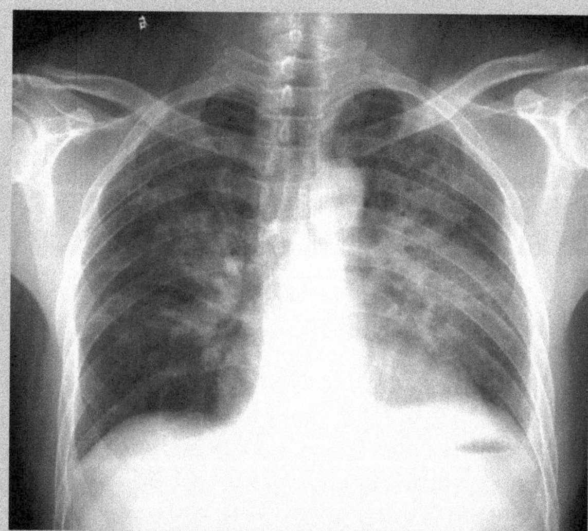

Fig. 29.4 Pulmonary malaria, with acute pulmonary edema and pleural effusion. X-ray demonstrates increased lung markings in both lungs, butterfly wing-shaped patches of shadows in the inner and middle areas of both lungs, and blunt bilateral costophrenic angles

29.7.2.2 CT Scanning

Pulmonary Edema

Symmetrical large flakes of effusive shadows in both lungs can be observed (Fig. 29.5).

Bronchitis

The bronchovascular bundles in both lungs are demonstrated to be thickened, increased, and deranged, which are especially obvious in the inferior lobes of both lungs (Fig. 29.6).

Pneumonia

The bronchovascular bundles are demonstrated to be thickened, increased, and deranged. There are patches, large flakes, and even segmental or lobar consolidation shadows with the pulmonary hilum as the center (Fig. 29.6).

Alveolar Blood Stasis

Patches or diffusive ground-glass opacities are demonstrated (Fig. 29.7).

Pleural Effusion

Case Study 11

A female patient aged 33 years complained of fever, cough, and chest pain for half a month. By blood smear, plasmodia were detected positive.

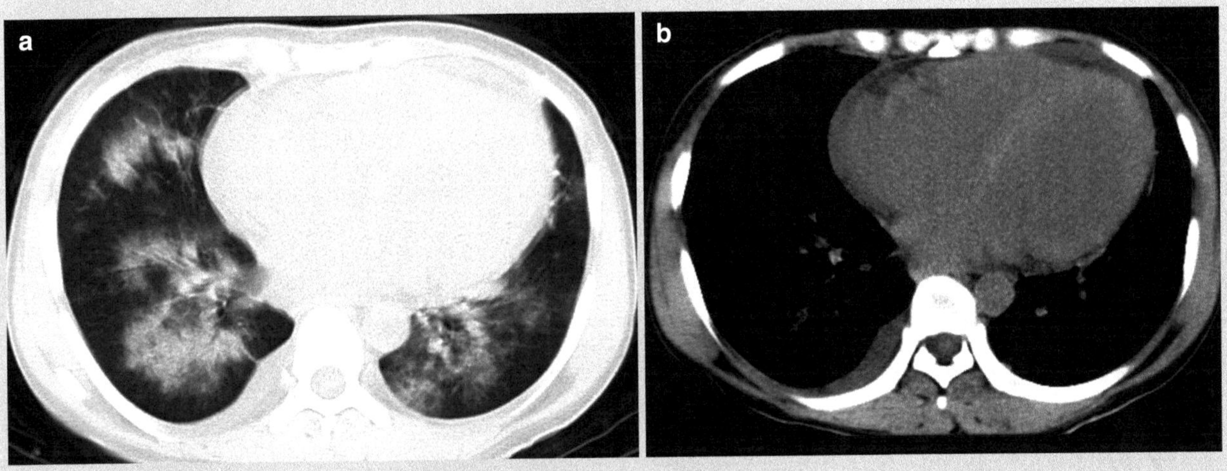

Fig. 29.5 Pulmonary malaria with pulmonary edema, pericardial effusion, and pleural effusion. (**a**, **b**) CT scanning demonstrates pulmonary edema in both lungs, enlarged heart, and a small quantity of liquid density shadows in the pericardial cavity, with right arch-shaped liquid density shadow

Case Study 12

A female patient aged 43 years complained of fever, cough, and chest pain for 7 days. By blood smear, plasmodia were detected positive.

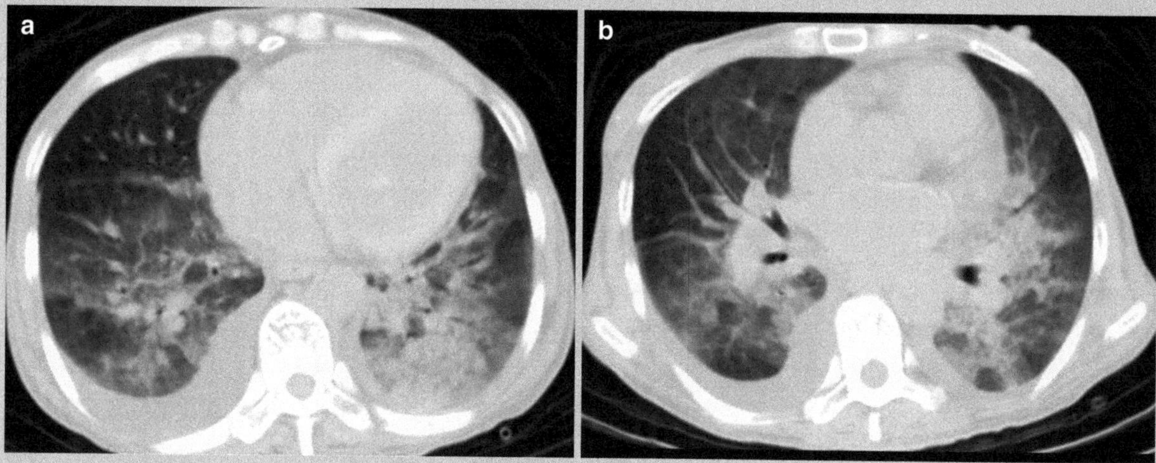

Fig. 29.6 Pulmonary malaria with pulmonary edema, pericardial effusion, and pleural effusion. (**a**, **b**) CT scanning demonstrates thickened, increased, and deranged bronchovascular bundles in both lungs, patches of consolidation shadows with the pulmonary hilum as the center, and small quantities of pleural effusion in both lungs

Case Study 13

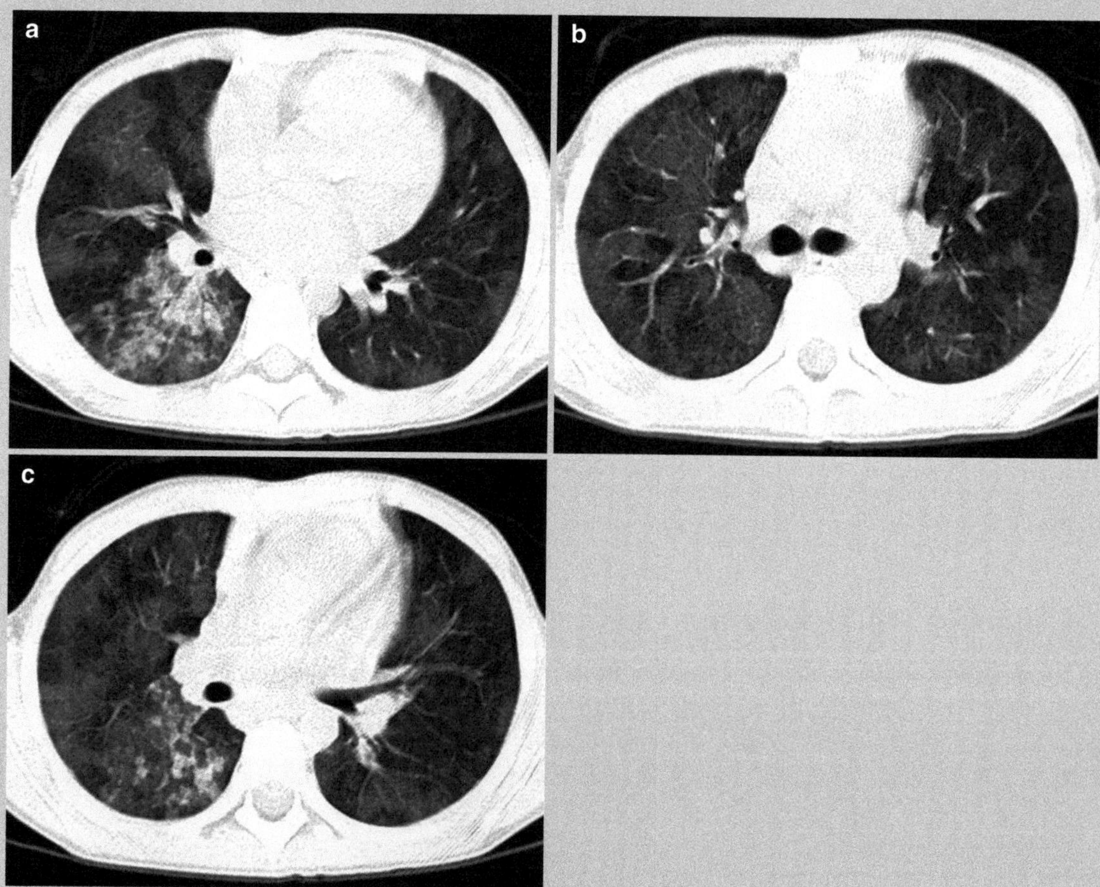

Fig. 29.7 Pulmonary malaria with alveolar edema. (**a**–**c**) CT scanning demonstrates diffusive ground-glass opacities in both lungs

29.7.2.3 PET

The metabolic rate of glucose in both lungs is demonstrated with diffusive decrease.

29.7.3 Abdominal Lesions

Abdominal malaria most commonly involves the liver and spleen, followed by the kidneys and gastrointestinal tract. The manifestations include hepatomegaly, liver dysfunction, gallbladder wall edema, splenomegaly or megalosplenia, spleen infarction, spleen rupture and hemorrhage, portal hypertension, gastrointestinal wall swelling, ascites, and mild edema of both kidneys.

29.7.3.1 Ultrasound

Hepatosplenomegaly is commonly demonstrated. There are also thickened echoes from the liver parenchyma, dilated hepatic portal vein and splenic vein as well as ascites. In the cases with spontaneous spleen rupture, the area under the splenic capsule on the diaphragmatic surface is demonstrated with crescent-shaped low echo. Ultrasonography and color Doppler ultrasound can provide valuable information for the diagnosis of spleen infarction, which is demonstrated with enlarged spleen and singular or multiple wedge-shaped or irregular low echo area in the spleen parenchyma. In the cases with complicating hemorrhage, the hemorrhage lesions are demonstrated with high echo. Ultrasonography demonstrates irregular or wedge-shaped filling defects in the spleen. Gallbladder wall edema is demonstrated with thickened gallbladder wall and decreased echo. Kidney edema is demonstrated with poorly defined corticomedullary interface and decreased echo.

29.7.3.2 CT Scanning

Hepatosplenomegaly is commonly demonstrated, and in some cases even megalosplenia, with enlarged volume. By plain scanning, the density of the enlarged spleen and the enlarged liver is demonstrated to be decreased, while by contrast scanning, the density is progressively enhanced, with stronger enhancement of the liver than that of the spleen (Fig. 29.8). Occasionally, the liver is enlarged with increased density, which is speculated to be the result of hemosiderosis in the liver due to extensive rupture of erythrocytes (Fig. 29.9). By plain scanning, spleen infarction is demonstrated as multiple wedge-shaped, bar-shaped, or map-like low-density lesions at the margin of the spleen, whose pathogenesis may be related to hyperplasia of reticuloendothelial system due to hyperfunctional removal of the spleen. By contrast scanning, infarction of the spleen is demonstrated with no enhancement of the lesions. And the wedge-shaped lesions are typical demonstration of splenic infarction. Radiological studies of animal models have demonstrated that bar-shaped low-density lesions are organized thrombi formed by infected erythrocytes in the dilated splenic vein. Kim et al. reported that the lesions in the spleen are reversible. By follow-up reexaminations, the bar-shaped low-density lesions in the spleen can disappear, with simultaneous normal size of the spleen. The liver dysfunction is demonstrated with intrahepatic lymphatic stasis (Fig. 29.10). Megalosplenia and multiple splenic infarctions are common in the cases of severe *P. falciparum* malaria (Fig. 29.11). In addition, there are also edema surrounding the gallbladder wall and the portal vein, ascites, spontaneous rupture of the spleen, and subcapsular hemorrhage, which are common in the patients with *P. vivax* malaria.

The involvement of kidney has manifestations of acute renal insufficiency or failure. Plain scanning demonstrates decreased density of both kidneys and poorly defined corticomedullary interface. Otherwise, the enhanced lesions with patchy attenuation are demonstrated (Fig. 29.12). Gastrointestinal malaria is commonly demonstrated as extensive gastrointestinal wall edema and ascites (Fig. 29.13).

Case Study 14

A male patient aged 30 years, an enthusiastic traveler, complained of fever, chills, and poor appetite for 1 month. By blood smear, plasmodia were detected positive.

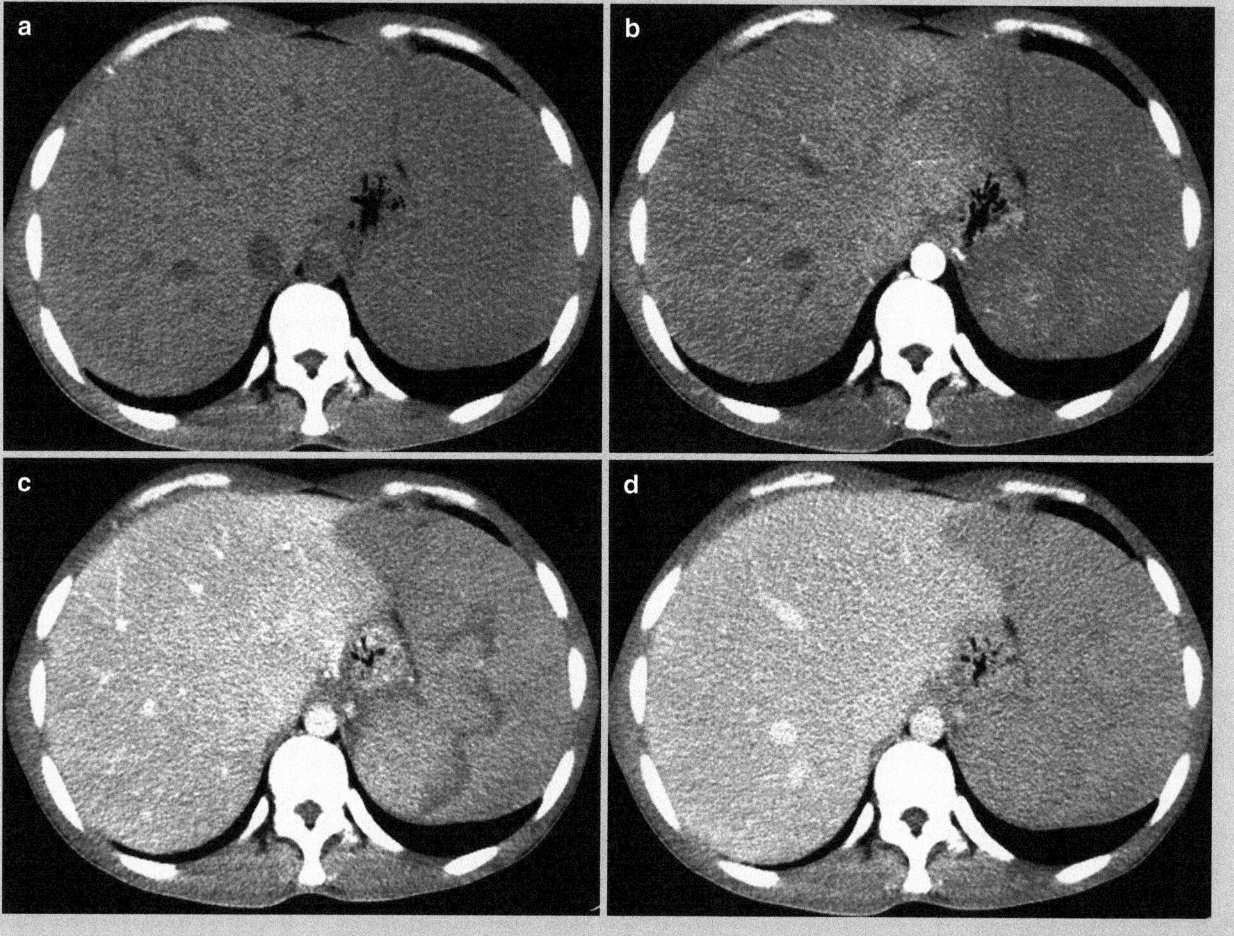

Fig. 29.8 Abdominal malaria with hepatosplenomegaly and splenic infarction. (**a**) Plain CT scanning demonstrates increased volumes of the liver and the spleen. (**b**) Contrast CT scanning demonstrates irregular-shaped low-density area at the arterial phase in the spleen, with internal spots and flakes of slightly high-density shadows. (**c**) By contrast scanning, the spleen is demonstrated with wedge-shaped and strips of low-density shadows in the spleen at the venous phase, with stronger enhancement of the liver than that of the spleen. (**d**) By contrast scanning, the spleen is demonstrated still with wedge-shaped slightly low-density areas in the spleen at the equilibrium phase

Case Study 15

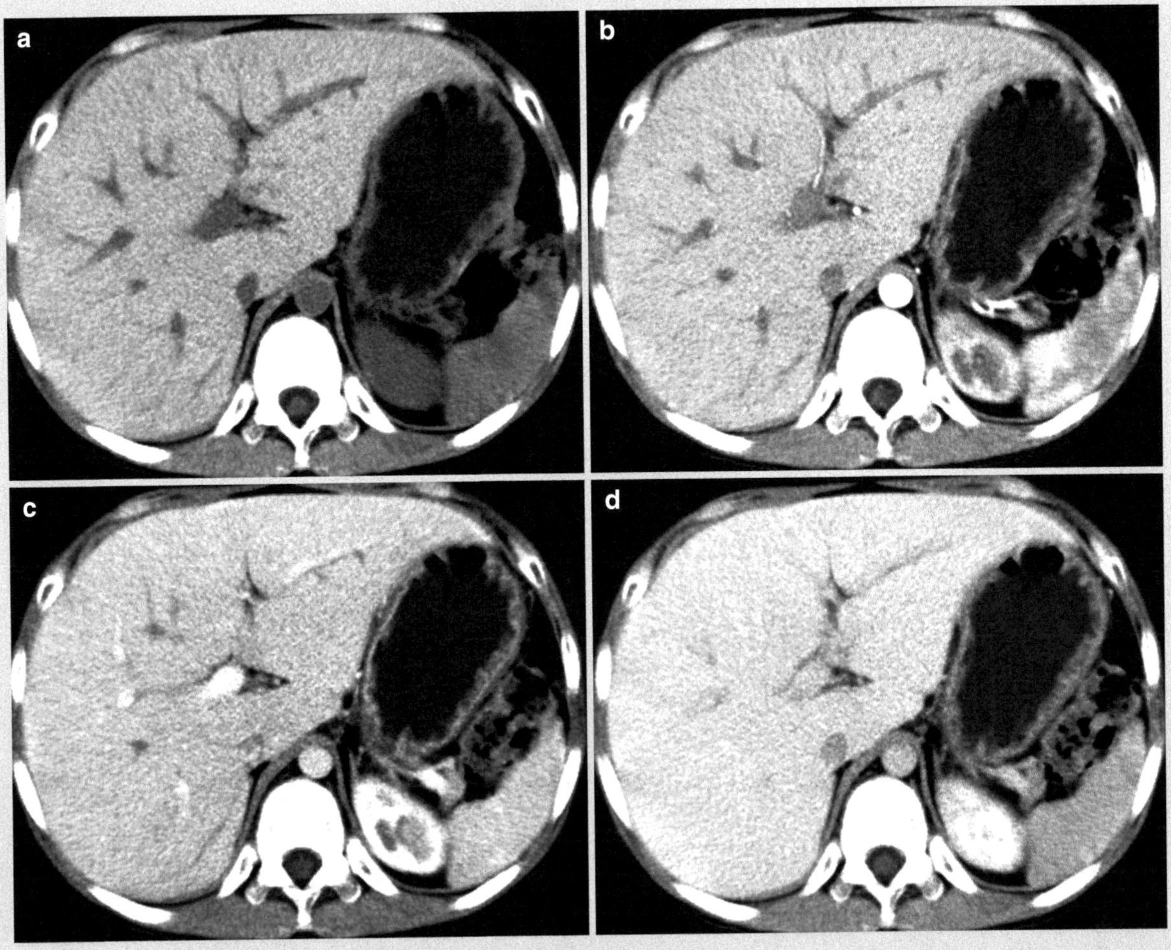

Fig. 29.9 Abdominal malaria with hepatomegaly. (**a**) Plain CT scanning demonstrates increased volume of the liver as well as obviously higher density of the liver parenchyma than that of the spleen parenchyma. (**b–d**) Contrast scanning demonstrates stronger enhancement of the liver than that of the spleen

Case Study 16

A male patient aged 52 years complained of fever and chills.

(For case detail and figures, please refer to Kim EM et al. *Am J Trop Med Hyg*, 2010, 83 (6): 1202.)

Case Study 17

A male patient aged 17 years, with a history of traveling in the epidemic area of malaria, complained of high fever and poor appetite for 7 days. By blood smear, plasmodia were detected positive.

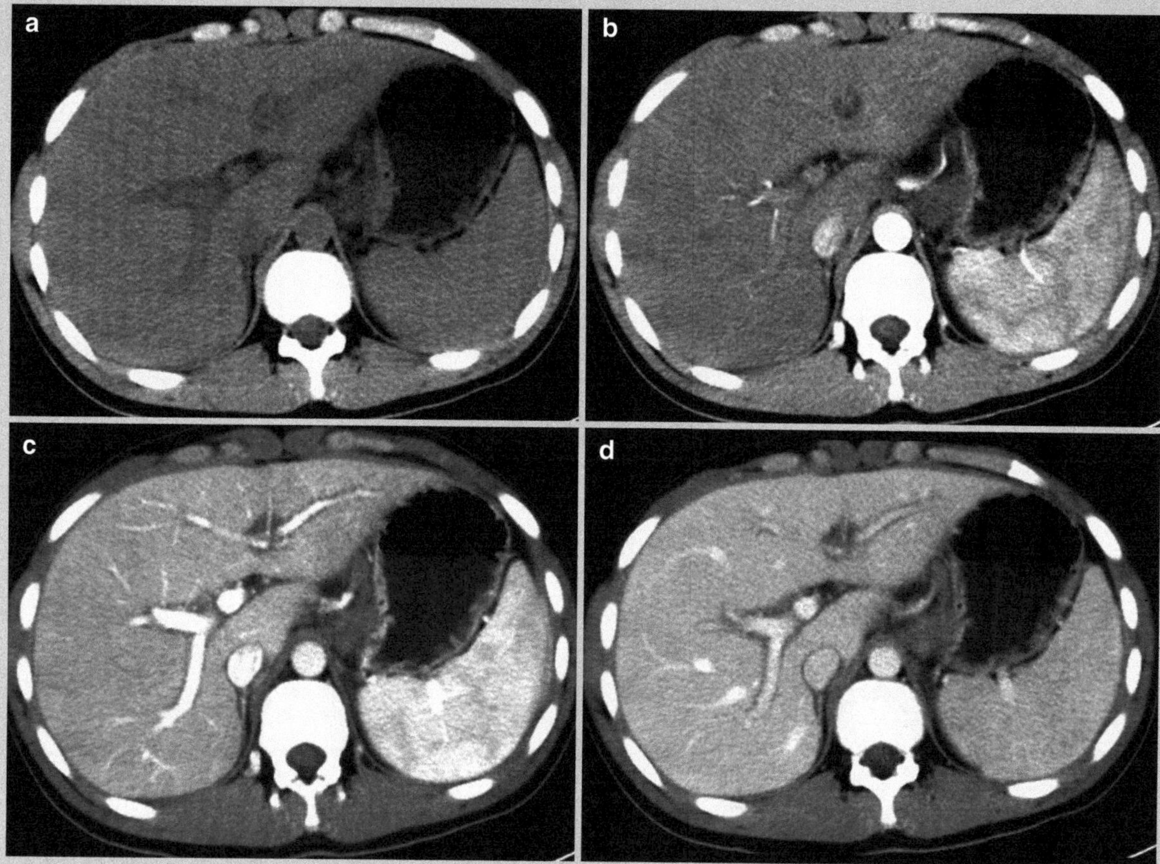

Fig. 29.10 Abdominal malaria with hepatosplenomegaly and intrahepatic lymphatic stasis. (**a**) Plain CT scanning demonstrates slightly enlarged volume of the liver, strips, and ring-shaped slightly low-density shadows at both sides of the right and left branches of the intrahepatic portal vein and slightly enlarged volume of the spleen. (**b–d**) Contrast scanning demonstrates no enhancement around the intrahepatic portal vein and inferior vena cava, with strips of low-density track sign and circular low-density halo sign

Case Study 18

A female patient aged 65 years, a woman living in a rural area, complained of intermittent fever, nausea, and anorexia for half a month. By blood smear, plasmodia were detected positive.

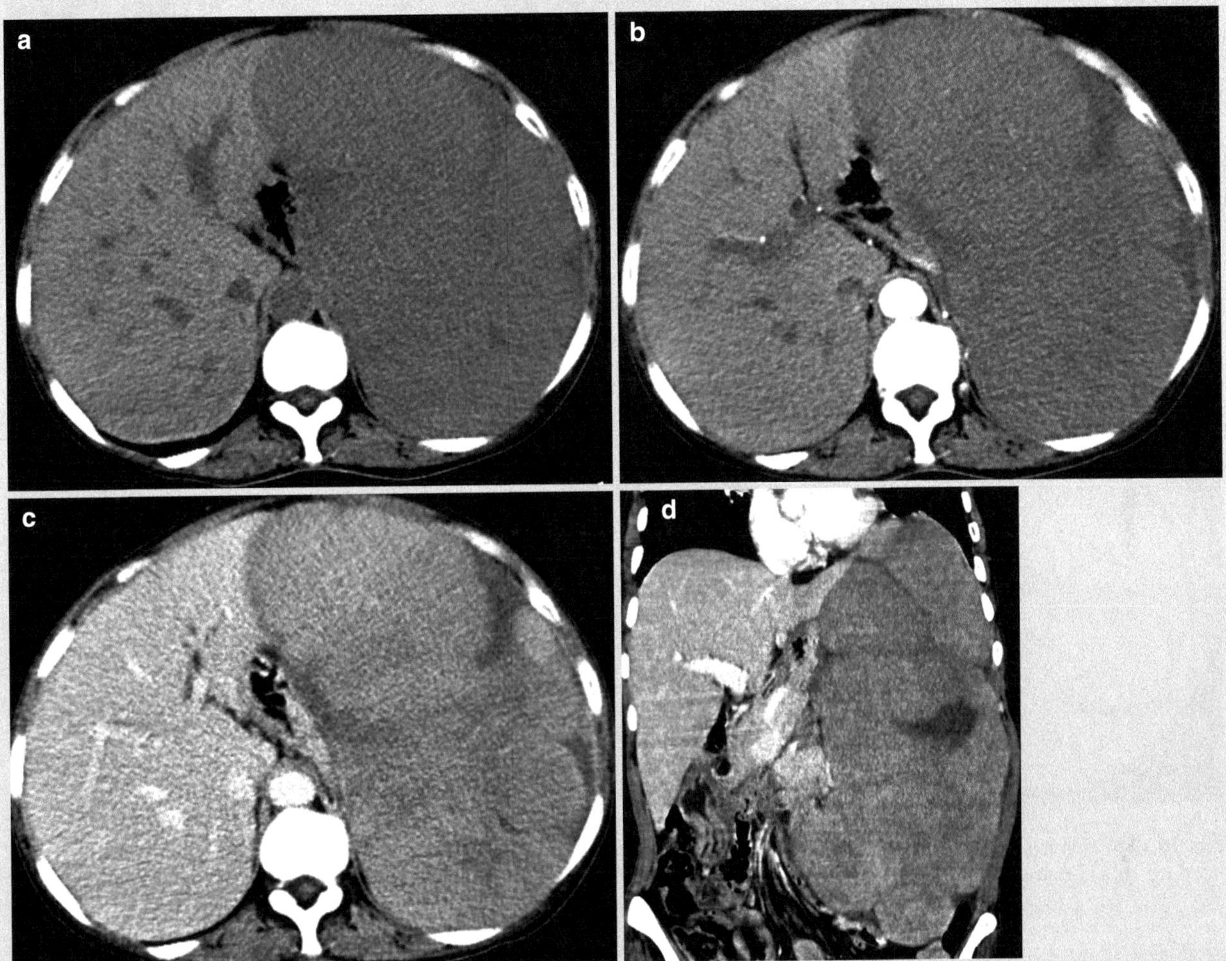

Fig. 29.11 Abdominal malaria with megalosplenia and splenic infarction. (**a**) Plain CT scanning demonstrates obviously increased volume of the spleen, which exceeds the abdominal midline, as well as rightward shifts of the stomach and abdominal aorta due to compression. Multiple strips of low-density lesions are demonstrated in the spleen with blurry boundaries. (**b**, **c**) Contrast scanning demonstrates no enhancement of the low-density lesions in the spleen with well-defined boundaries. (**d**) Demonstrations by sagittal scanning

Case Study 19

A female patient aged 52 years complained of fever and left abdominal pain. She reported no history of trauma. By laboratory test, she was definitively diagnosed with *P. vivax* infection.

(For case detail and figures, please refer to Kim EM et al. *Am J Trop Med Hyg*, 2010, 83 (6): 1202.)

Case Study 20

A male patient aged 17 years complained of fever and low back pain for 7 days and oliguria for 1 day.

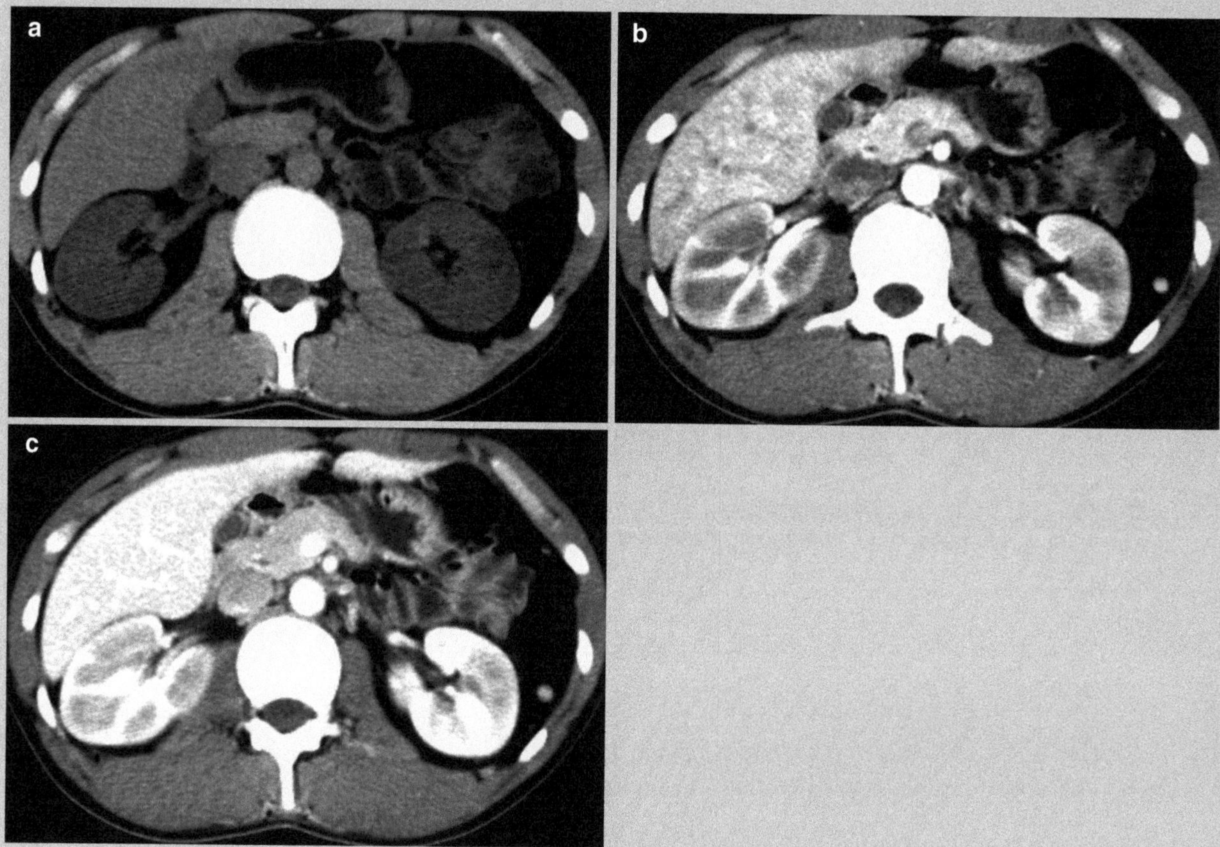

Fig. 29.12 Renal malaria. (**a**) Plain CT scanning demonstrates decreased density of both kidneys and poorly defined corticomedullary interface. (**b**, **c**) Contrast scanning demonstrates enhancement of the lesions with patchy attenuation

Case Study 21

A male patient aged 47 years complained of fever, nausea, abdominal pain, and diarrhea for 4 days. By blood smear, plasmodia were detected positive.

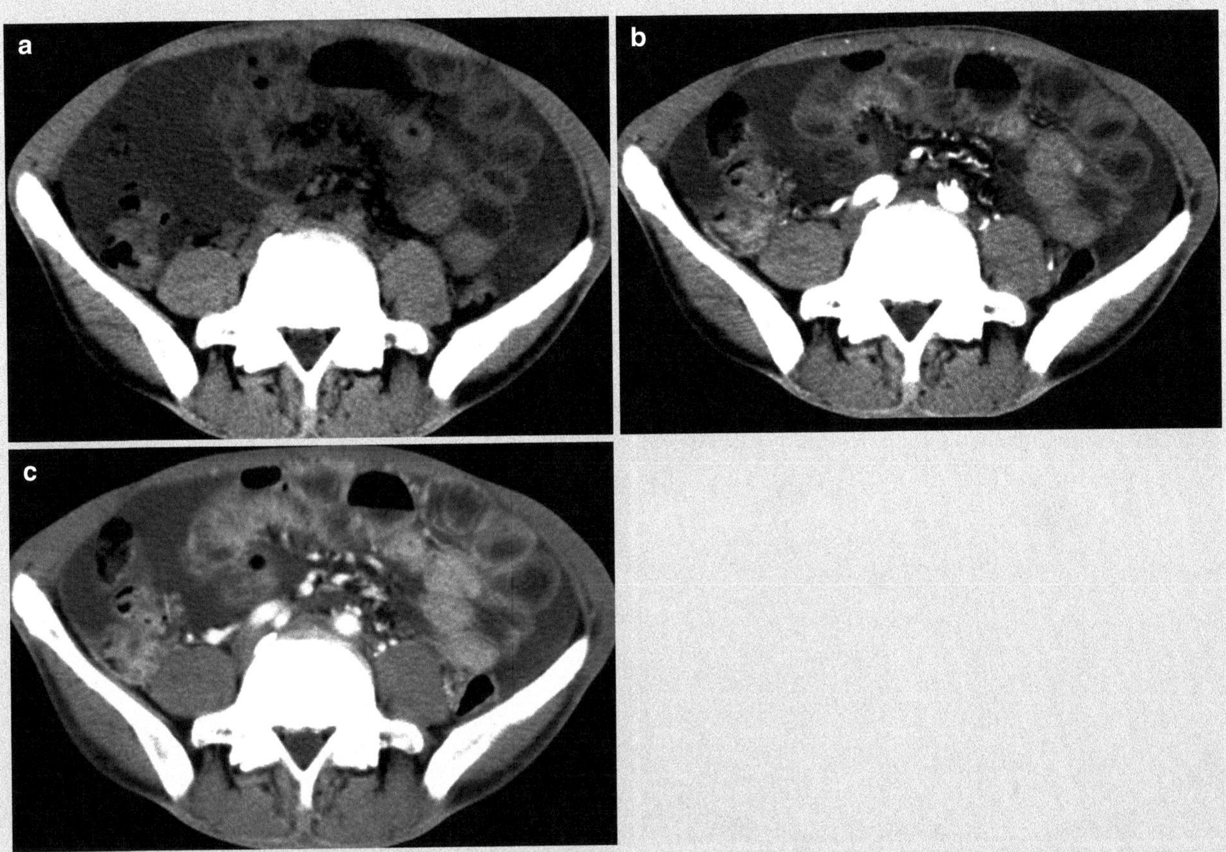

Fig. 29.13 Intestinal malaria and ascites. (**a**–**c**) CT scanning demonstrates swelling of the intestinal wall and the colon wall. Contrast CT scanning demonstrates no abnormal enhancement. There are also liquid density shadows surrounding the intestinal canal

29.7.3.3 MR Imaging

The liver is demonstrated with enlarged volume in slightly long or equal T_1 and slightly long T_2 signals. The gallbladder is demonstrated with thickened wall in slightly long or equal T_1 and slightly long T_2 signals. The portal vein and the splenic vein are demonstrated to be widened. The spleen is demonstrated with increased volume or megalosplenia in slightly long or equal T_1 and slightly long T_2 signals. Splenic infarction is demonstrated with irregular, wedge-shaped, or map-like long T_1 and long T_2 signals in the spleen; otherwise, strips of filling are detected in the dilated splenic vein by Gd-DTPA contrast imaging. Spleen rupture is demonstrated as short T_1 signal lesions under the spleen capsule or in the spleen parenchyma. By routine imaging, there are thickened wall of the gastrointestinal tract and absence of the 3-layered structure of the intestinal wall with slightly long T1 long T2 signals that are poorly defined. In the abdominal cavity, multiple long T_1 and long T_2 signal shadows are demonstrated, which are high signals by T_2WI fat-suppression imaging. The parenchyma in both kidneys is poorly defined in long T1 long T2 blurry signals.

29.7.3.4 PET

A group of animal experiments have demonstrated diffusively increased ^{18}F-FDG uptake in the whole spleen of the experimental monkeys infected by plasmodia, with an average SUV of 5.1 ± 0.6 that is significantly higher than that before the infection (the average SUV is 1.6 ± 0.7).

Case Study 22

Animal experiments

(For case detail and figures, please refer to Kawai S et al. *Am J Trop Med Hyg*, 2006, 74 (3): 353.)

29.7.4 Subcutaneous Soft Tissue Changes

In the cases of malaria, extensive swelling of the subcutaneous soft tissues can be observed.

29.7.4.1 Ultrasound

Ultrasound demonstrates decreased echo of subcutaneous soft tissues.

29.7.4.2 CT Scanning

CT scanning demonstrates thickened subcutaneous soft tissues and increased density of the subcutaneous fat (Fig. 29.14).

Case Study 23

A female patient aged 49 years complained of fever, diarrhea, and systemic soreness and pain for 11 days. By blood smear, plasmodia were detected positive.

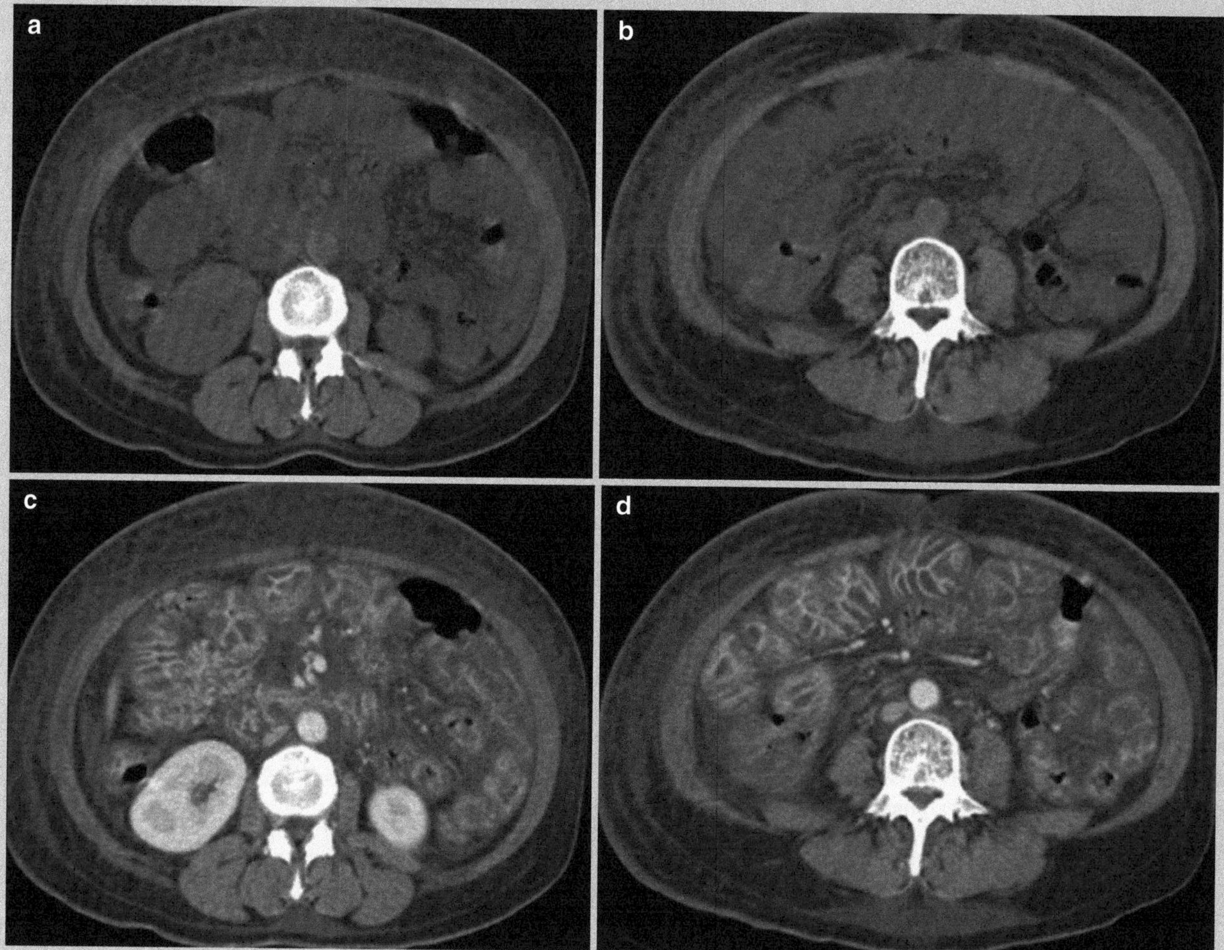

Fig. 29.14 Abdominal wall edema and the intestinal wall of malaria and ascites. (**a–d**) CT scanning demonstrates extensive swelling of the abdominal wall and the intestinal wall as well as liquid density shadows surrounding the intestinal canal

29.7.4.3 MR Imaging

MR imaging demonstrates thickened subcutaneous soft tissues. The high signals of the subcutaneous fats are partly or wholly replaced by slightly long T_1 and slightly long T_2 signals. T_2WI fat suppression demonstrates no obvious decrease of the signals.

29.7.5 Multiple Organ Involvement

Simultaneous involvement of the liver, spleen, and lungs is the most common (Fig. 29.15), followed by simultaneous involvement of the liver, spleen, and brain (Fig. 29.16) and simultaneous involvement of the liver and lungs (Fig. 29.17). And simultaneous involvement of the liver, spleen, lung, brain, gastrointestinal tract, and soft tissues is rare.

Case Study 24

A female patient aged 18 years complained of high fever, cough, and hepatic pain for 3 days. By blood smear, plasmodia were detected positive.

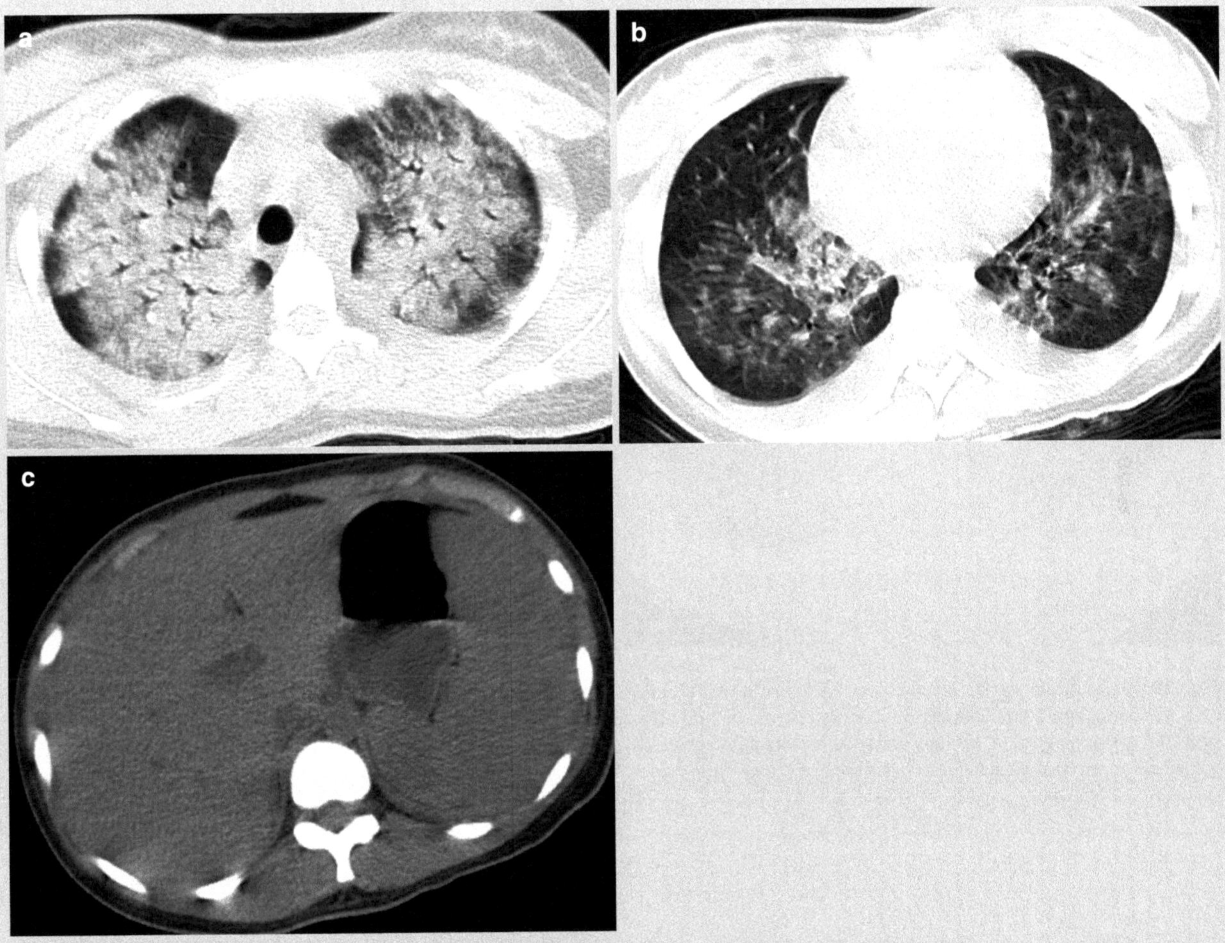

Fig. 29.15 Multiple organ involvement of malaria with pulmonary edema, pleural effusion, and hepatosplenomegaly. (**a**, **b**) CT scanning demonstrates diffusive distribution of ground-glass opacities in both lungs and bilateral pleural effusion in small quantities. (**c**) The liver and the spleen are demonstrated with enlarged volumes

Case Study 25

A female patient aged 39 years complained of fever, cough, and headache for 3 days. By blood smear, plasmodia were detected positive.

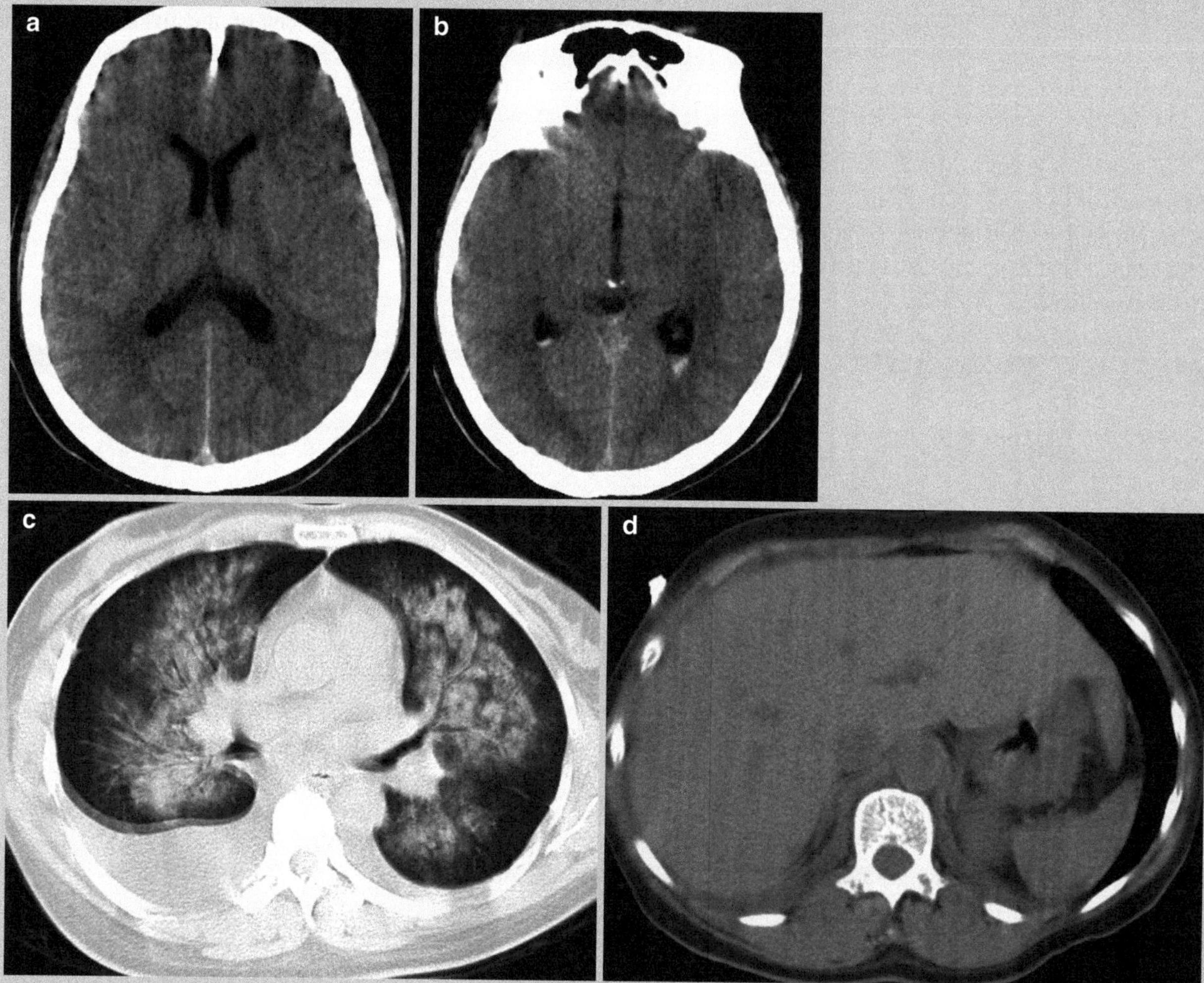

Fig. 29.16 Multiple organ involvement of malaria with brain edema, subarachnoid hemorrhage, pulmonary edema, pleural effusion, and hepatomegaly. (**a**, **b**) Sulci and fissures in bilateral cerebral hemispheres are demonstrated to be narrowed or blurry. Some sulci are demonstrated with slightly increased density. Small strips of high-density shadows are observable at the posterior horn of bilateral cerebral ventricles. (**d**) Diffusive distribution of ground-glass opacity in both lungs is demonstrated, with bilateral pleural effusion. (**c**, **d**) The liver is demonstrated with an enlarged volume

Case Study 26

A female patient aged 43 years complained of fever, hepatic pain, and poor appetite for 5 days. By blood smear, plasmodia were detected positive.

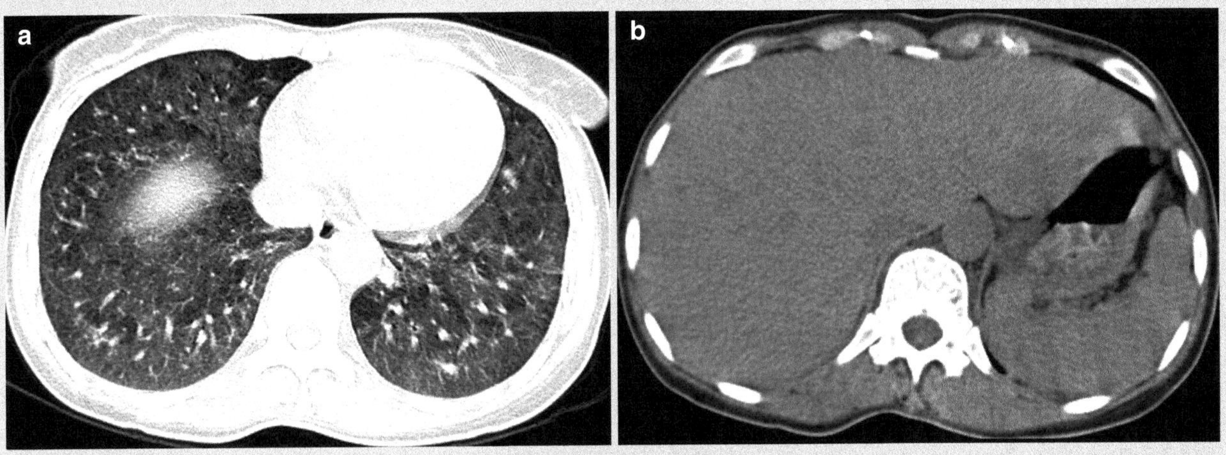

Fig. 29.17 Multiple organ involvement of malaria with pulmonary infection and hepatomegaly. (**a**) CT demonstrates diffusive distribution of ground-glass opacities in both lungs. (**b**) The liver is demonstrated with an enlarged volume

29.8 Diagnostic Basis

29.8.1 Diagnosis of Malaria

Patients with a history of visiting the epidemic area during the prevailing season of malaria or patients with a history of blood transfusion within past 2 weeks, who complain of periodic chills, fever, and sweating but no obvious symptoms during the intervals or with accompanying progressive anemia and splenomegaly, should be suspected with malaria. The following blood smear with positive finding of plasmodia can define the diagnosis. Some patients have clinical manifestations resembling to those of malaria but with negative finding by blood smears. For these cases, if the possibility of other diseases can be excluded, chloroquine medication to treat malaria can be administered as a trial for 3 days. Those with alleviated symptoms after treatment can be diagnosed with malaria.

29.8.2 Diagnosis of Malaria-Related Complications

29.8.2.1 Cerebral Malaria

1. In the epidemic area of malaria during summers and autumns, patients with fever, chills, sleepiness, or convulsion and coma, with accompanying severe headache, vomiting, and anemia, should be suspected with malaria.
2. Blood smear with positive finding of plasmodia provides important basis to define the diagnosis.
3. Brain CT scanning and MR imaging of patients with malaria demonstrate different degrees of brain edema and hemorrhage as symmetrical low-density areas or long T1 long T2 signals in the basal ganglia. The lesions can also be found in the frontal lobe, the occipital lobe, the semioval centrum, and the corpus callosum, which are radiologically demonstrated as inflammatory edema or hemorrhage.
4. Patients with malaria may also experience increased pressure, cell counts, and protein level in their cerebrospinal fluid but normal glucose level.

29.8.2.2 Pulmonary Malaria

1. Patients with malaria are clinically characterized by respiratory symptoms, such as cough and expectoration. By auscultation, scattering dry and moist rales can be heard in both lungs.
2. X-rays and CT scanning demonstrate thickened lung markings, butterfly sign, patchy shadow, and consolidation shadow.

29.8.2.3 Malarial Nephropathy

Blackwater Fever
Microangiopathic hemolytic anemia and thrombocytopenia are necessary for the diagnosis of HUS. Radiological examinations can demonstrate hepatosplenomegaly and edema surrounding the portal vein.

Malarial Nephropathy
Malarial nephropathy can be diagnosed based on clinical symptoms, such as hematuria, proteinuria, oliguria, or urodialysis, and laboratory findings of CREA and BUN levels.

29.9 Differential Diagnosis

29.9.1 Pneumonia

Most cases of pulmonary malaria are radiologically demonstrated with thickened pulmonary markings or interstitial changes, which are nonspecific. In some severe cases, the radiological demonstrations include lobular pneumonia, segmental pneumonia, and lobar pneumonia, which are similar to pulmonary changes caused by other pathogenic bacteria. However, pulmonary malaria has short course of illness and rapid absorption of the lesions. Most of the pulmonary lesions are absorbed within 1 week. Antimalarial medication is especially effective to alleviate and cure malaria.

29.9.2 Encephalitis

By blood smear, plasmodia may not be detected positive in the cases of cerebral malaria. Therefore, it should be differentiated from encephalitis B and viral meningoencephalitis. Cerebral malaria is common in children and adults visitors, with common manifestations of anemia and hepatosplenomegaly. They usually have no obvious meningeal irritation sign and basically normal findings by the cerebrospinal fluid examination. If necessary, blood smear can be repeatedly performed for the diagnosis and differential diagnosis. Viral encephalitis has a chronic onset and commonly occurs in teenagers, with symptoms of fever and accompanying fatigue, dizziness, temperament changes, and mental abnormalities. By the cerebrospinal fluid examination, the findings indicate virus infection of the central nervous system, with increased cells counts and protein and normal levels of glucose and chlorides. T2WI of MRI demonstrates scattered or infused high-signal area, while T1WI demonstrates equal or low signal with different degrees of space-occupying effect.

29.9.3 Brain Tumors

Brain tumors have chronic onset with the conditions progressively aggravate. The patients commonly experience symptoms of headache, vomiting, visual impairments, epilepsy, limb paralysis, and no fever or low-grade fever. Brain radiology demonstrates substantial space-occupying lesion in brain tissue, which enlarges along with the illness course.

29.9.4 Amebic Liver Abscess

The disease is clinically characterized by remittent fever with profuse sweating. Chloroquine has certain curative effect for it, especially for swelling and pain of the liver. In such cases, the WBC count and the neutrophil percentage obviously increase. X-ray demonstrates elevated right diaphragm and limited movement. Ultrasound can demonstrate liquid level segment in the hepatic region. Chocolate pus can be drawn by liver puncture.

References

Cordoliani YS, Sarrazin JL, Felten D, et al. MR of cerebral malaria. AJNR Am J Neuroradiol. 1998;9(5):871–4.

Kawai S, Ikeda E, Sugiyama M, et al. Enhancement of splenic glucose metabolism during acute malarial infection: correlation of findings of FDG-PET imaging with pathological changes in a primate model of severe human malaria. Am J Trop Med Hyg. 2006;74(3):353–60.

Kim EM, Cho HJ, Cho CR, et al. Abdominal computed tomography findings of malaria infection with Plasmodium vivax. Am J Trop Med Hyg. 2010;83(6):1202–5.

Nickerson JP, Tong KA, Raghavan R. Imaging cerebral malaria with a susceptibility-weighted MR sequence. AJNR Am J Neuroradiol. 2009;30(6):e85–6.

Patankar TF, Karnad DR, Shetty PG, et al. Adult cerebral malaria: prognostic importance of imaging findings and correlation with postmortem findings. Radiology. 2002;224(3):811–6.

Yadav P, Sharma R, Kumar S, et al. Magnetic resonance features of cerebral malaria. Acta Radiol. 2008;49(5):566–9.

Suggested Reading

Bae K, Jeon KN. CT findings of malarial spleen. Br J Radiol. 2006;79(946):e145–7.

Das CJ, Sharma R. Central pontine myelinolysis in a case of cerebral malaria. Br J Radiol. 2007;80(960):e293–5.

Gamanagatti S, Kandpal H. MR imaging of cerebral malaria in a child. Eur J Radiol. 2006;60(1):46–7.

Xu RG, Pei XP, Zhang MC, et al. X-ray demonstrations of pulmonary lesions in the cases of malaria: a report of 27 cases. Northwest J Natl Def Med. 2009;30(4):268–70.

Index

H. Li (ed.), *Radiology of Infectious Diseases: Volume 2*, DOI 10.1007/978-94-017-9876-1

9789401798754